NATURE AND TREATMENT OF STUTTERING

NEW DIRECTIONS

SECOND EDITION

Edited by

RICHARD F. CURLEE
University of Arizona

GERALD M. SIEGEL
University of Minnesota

Allyn and Bacon
Boston   London   Toronto   Sydney   Tokyo   Singapore

Executive Editor: Stephen D. Dragin
Editorial Assistant: Christine Svitila
Editorial-Production Administrator: Joe Sweeney
Editorial-Production Service: Walsh Associates
Composition Buyer: Linda Cox
Manufacturing Buyer: Suzanne Lareau
Cover Aministrator: Suzanne Harbison

Library of Congress Cataloging-in-Publication Data

Nature and treatment of stuttering : new directions / edited by
    Richard F. Curlee, Gerald M. Siegel. — 2nd ed.
        p.   c m.
    Includes bibliographical references and index.
    ISBN 0-205-16336-X
    1. Stuttering.   I. Curlee, Richard F. (Richard Frederick), 1935–   .
II. Siegel, Gerald M., 1932–   .
    [DNLM: 1. Stuttering.   2. Stuttering—therapy.   WM 475 N285 1996]
RC424.N38   1996
616.85'54—dc20
DNLM/DLC
for Library of Congress   96-22777
                                                                    CIP

Printed in the United States of America

10 9 8 7 6 5 4 3 2   00 99 98 97

Contents

PART TWO
STUTTERER-NONSTUTTERER DIFFERENCES   97

CHAPTER 5   **STUTTERING: A PSYCHOLINGUISTIC PERSPECTIVE**   **99**

Nan Bernstein Ratner

CHAPTER 6   **RESPIRATORY AND LARYNGEAL CONTROL IN STUTTERING**   **128**

Margaret Denny & Anne Smith

CHAPTER 7   **BRAIN IMAGING CONTRIBUTIONS**   **143**

Ben C. Watson & Francis J. Freeman

PART THREE
ETIOLOGICAL VIEWS OF STUTTERING   167

PART FOUR
CLINICAL MANAGEMENT OF CHILDREN   237

PART FIVE
CLINICAL MANAGEMENT OF ADULTS   333

PREFACE

The goals of science are to describe, explain, predict, and control events in nature. And as a science matures, more time and effort are devoted to the prediction and control of events than to their description or explanation. Most areas of speech-language pathology are still largely involved in the description of the signs and symptoms of communication disabilities and in efforts to understand the conditions or impairments that cause them. Such is the case for stuttering.

Stuttering is a disability of spoken language that emerges most often at a time when young children's cognitive, linguistic, and motor abilities are undergoing rapid maturation and development. It is generally accepted that stuttering affects about 5 percent of the population, that its incidence is highest during preschool years, and that remission rates are high, especially during the first twelve to eighteen months after onset. It is also widely believed that one's ancestors and gender influence a child's odds of beginning to stutter and, perhaps, of recovery. How these and other observations about stuttering may contribute to an understanding of its nature and treatment are the focus of this text.

More than a decade has passed since the first edition of this volume was published. During that period a substantial amount of new information has been published about stuttering and added to an ever-growing accumulation of data, clinical observations, hypotheses, beliefs, and speculations. Indeed, it is doubtful that any other communication disorder has received as much attention from historians, philosophers, theoreticians, clinicians, researchers, even next-door neighbors, as has stuttering. Clearly, it is time for a progress report on the state of knowledge about stuttering and the art of its clinical management.

This revision, as did the first edition, relies on colleagues whose research, clinical experience, and scholarship permit them to sift through all of this information, critically examine it, and write about it in a clear, responsible manner. But instead of a compendium of updated findings and restated views from the initial edition of this text, this volume provides a new take on stuttering by a largely new team of researchers, clinicians, and thinkers who were assembled to share their understanding of what we know about stuttering. With the help of this new team and the invaluable assistance of a new co-editor, Gerald Siegel, I believe you'll find that this revision of *Nature and Treatment of Stuttering: New Directions*, lives up to all that its title promises.

We would also like to acknowledge the following reviewers: E. Charles Healey, University of Nebraska–Lincoln; Samuel K. Haroldson, University of Minnesota; and Barry Guitar, University of Vermont.

LIST OF CONTRIBUTORS

Klaas Bakker, PhD
Department of Communication Disorders
Southwest Missouri State University

Ellen Bennett, PhD
Department of Communication Disorders and
    Speech Science
University of Colorado at Boulder

Oliver Bloodstein, PhD
Department of Speech
Brooklyn College

Edward Conture, PhD
Communication Sciences and Disorders
Syracuse University

Anne K. Cordes, PhD
Department of Speech Pathology and Audiology
University of Georgia

Margaret Denny, PhD
Boston University
Sargent College of Allied Health Professionals

Susan Felsenfeld, PhD
Department of Communication
Division of Communication Sciences and
    Disorders
University of Pittsburgh

Francis Freeman, PhD
University of Texas at Dallas
Callier Center for Communicative Disorders

Barry Guitar, PhD
Department of Communication Sciences
University of Vermont

Roger Ingham, PhD
Department of Speech and Hearing Sciences
University of California at Santa Barbara

Ellen Kelly, PhD
Department of Audiology and Speech Sciences
Purdue University

Herman Kolk, PhD
Nijmegen Institute of Cognition and
    Information (NICI)
University of Nijmegen
The Netherlands

Dale Metz, PhD
Department of Communication Sciences and
    Disorders
State University of New York–Geneseo

Florence Myers, PhD
Department of Speech Arts and Communicative
    Disorders
Adelphi University

Mark Onslow, PhD
Australian Stuttering Research Center
The University of Sydney
Lidcombe NSW 2141
Australia

Ann Packman, PhD
Australian Stuttering Research Center
The University of Sydney
Lidcombe NSW 2141
Australia

William Perkins, PhD
Professor Emeritus
University of Southern California

Albert Postma, PhD
Department of Experimental Psychology
University of Utrecht
The Netherlands

David Prins, PhD
Department of Speech and Hearing Sciences
University of Washington

Peter Ramig, PhD
Department of Communication Disorders
    and Speech Science
University of Colorado at Boulder

Nan Bernstein Ratner, PhD
Department of Hearing and Speech Sciences
The University of Maryland at College Park

Kenneth O. St. Louis, PhD
Department of Speech Pathology and Audiology
University of West Virginia

Nicholas Schiavetti, PhD
Department of Communication Sciences and
    Disorders
State University of New York-Geneseo

Anne Smith, PhD
Department of Audiology and Speech Sciences
Purdue University

C. Woodruff Starkweather, PhD
Speech, Language, and Hearing Sciences
Temple University

Ben Watson, PhD
Department of Otolaryngology
New York Medical College

Ehud Yairi, PhD
Department of Speech and Hearing Science
University of Illinois at Urbana-Champaign
and
Department of Communication Disorders
Sachler School of Medicine
Tel Aviv University

PART ONE

CHILDHOOD STUTTERING

Although a substantial amount of information has been accumulated about childhood stuttering and a number of promising leads have been uncovered, conclusive evidence is not yet available to implicate any of these leads as contributing factors to either the onset or the remission of stuttering. We know more about childhood stuttering than we understand. That is, we have more facts than we can integrate into a coherent theory of the origins and the course of this puzzling disorder, and we have long since lost the simple assurance that motivated Johnson and his colleagues in pursuit of the diagnosogenic theory of stuttering.

In this initial section, Felsenfeld and Yairi examine current knowledge concerning endogenous and exogenous factors associated with childhood stuttering. Their chapters touch on issues that have long intrigued students of stuttering. Felsenfeld reviews the tantalizing evidence that stuttering may be the expression of a genetic disorder, a view that has never been far from the consciousness of stuttering researchers, even when cloaked in the form of an interaction hypothesis involving genes and environment. Yairi has done the unthinkable and has confronted Johnson on his own ground by replicating Johnson's earlier, extensive studies of the conditions that surround stuttering, bringing to that investigation the advantages of modern methods for identifying and collecting data from children who stutter and their families, and a mindset that may be more neutral, or at least differently disposed, than was Johnson's when the original research was done. The result is a rare example of classic research being revisited in terms of contemporary approaches. Perhaps not surprisingly, Yairi's results differ in critical ways from Johnson's interpretations of evidence favoring an environmental explanation for stuttering onset, and find a place in Felsenfeld's review of genetic variables associated with stuttering.

Despite the importance of recent findings, a major area of information is still lacking. Only retrospective data are available concerning the conditions under which childhood stuttering emerges, though Yairi has significantly reduced the interval between its diagnosis and data collection. Prospective studies are still needed to answer many of the most crucial questions about which children are at risk to develop stuttering and how the environment can be modified to eliminate or ameliorate the problem of even those children who may be disposed to stutter. Both Felsenfeld and Yairi suggest directions that further research might take to fill in some of the missing information.

We conclude this section with Starkweather's discussions of the role that learning may play in the development or remission of stuttering. The issue is not one of nature or nurture but how endogenous capacities and exogenous events interact to shape the kind of people we become. In many ways, this chapter is a bridge between the information on childhood stuttering covered in this section and that covered in subsequent sections. It describes the kinds of interactions between a child's behaviors and the environment that result in behavioral changes that are attributed to learning. Such changes may also account for many of the differences found between groups of stuttering and nonstuttering speakers, the correlates between stuttering and psycholinguistic, physiological, and neurological events, and the signs and symptoms of stuttering that require clinical management.

CHAPTER 1

EPIDEMIOLOGY AND GENETICS
OF STUTTERING

SUSAN FELSENFELD

*If 20,000 genes are unique to the brain, perhaps 19,000 will be effective-
ly the same in almost all people, whereas only 1,000 will give rise to
individual differences. From a genetic perspective, what people have in
common vastly exceeds what makes us different . . .*
—Wahlsten, 1994

*An individual inherits a developmental pattern for his body as a whole—
his body must have a skin, which then develops a certain color; it must
have a brain to appreciate music before musical ability can be manifested. Abilities and disabilities are not inherited as separate entities; they
are merely aspects of the developmental pattern of the organism.*
—Dobzhansky, 1956

INTRODUCTION

Genetic breakthroughs are occurring with such
regularity that they seem almost commonplace.
In 1995 alone, for example, genes that increase
some individuals' susceptibility for breast, blad-
der, and cervical cancer; dyslexia; obesity;
autism; and schizophrenia may have been located.
Researchers in centers across the globe are engaged in the painstaking process of cataloguing
the details of the entire human genome. This bur-
geoning knowledge base is both provocative and
a little intimidating, since most of us have been
ill-prepared to place such laboratory breakthroughs into perspective.

Is it, in fact, the case that many pathological
conditions, including stuttering, may soon be
identifiable in early or even asymptomatic stages
through a simple genetic blood screen? Once
pathological genes are identified in an individual's
genome, can they simply be supplanted using
"gene replacement therapy"? Can medications be
developed to counteract the pernicious effects of a
renegade gene? Will there be differences in prognosis or in treatment of individuals with and without family histories of stuttering? Should parents
be alerted that their offspring are at an increased
risk for a disorder in families having multiple affected members? Is it ethical not to? For those interested in the assessment and treatment of

ACKNOWLEDGMENTS: This chapter was developed concurrently with a review paper on genetics that has been accepted for publication in the *Journal of Fluency Disorders*. The
author wishes to thank Richard Curlee and Michael Pogue-
Guile for their careful editorial review and insightful suggestions.

disorders, these questions are highly relevant, because knowledge of a condition's "heritability" does not by itself enhance outcomes for individual patients.

The present chapter has three main objectives. First, a brief discussion of some central principles and methods in the field of behavior genetics will be presented to provide a common theoretical foundation for interpreting later results. Secondly, a critical review and discussion of the methods and results from the field's most influential family and twin studies of stuttering will be presented. Finally, the implications of the findings from genetic studies will be explored and future research needs in this area will be highlighted.

Much of what we know about the genetics of stuttering has come from a small number of twin and family studies conducted between 1960 and 1985. Unfortunately, since that time, empirical work in this area has decreased considerably, probably due in large part to the methodological complexity of this research. While not rare, neither is stuttering a particularly commonplace condition. The incidence of stuttering (the percentage of the population who has stuttered at any time during their lives, sometimes referred to as lifetime risk) is estimated to approximate 5 percent for stuttering that persists for at least six months (Peters & Guitar, 1991). In contrast, the point prevalence of stuttering (the percentage of the population who stutter at a given time) is considerably less: about 1 percent for children and somewhat less than 1 percent for adults (Andrews, Craig, Feyer, Hoddinot, Howie, & Neilson, 1983; Peters & Guitar, 1991). The difference between the incidence and prevalence rates for stuttering probably reflects recovery, which occurs for 50 to 80 percent of prepubescent stutterers for reasons that are still unclear (Peters & Guitar, 1991).

The prevalence rate suggests that at any given sampling time, about 1 in 100 individuals of all ages in the population will be diagnosed as active stutterers. Of these, an unknown number will be available for study participation, or will meet basic inclusion criteria. Subjects are also likely to differ in age, stuttering severity, and symptomology, all of which may be unwanted sources of variability. Moreover, because of the characteristic nature of this disorder, there are dangers of both including false positive cases in the database (e.g., young children with transient fluency problems, or high levels of normal nonfluency) and of missing true cases of disorder (e.g., failing to identify very mild stutterers or those who have recovered). Because genetic modeling procedures are highly sensitive to misclassifications or misdiagnoses, these types of errors pose serious threats to internal validity. Finally, these studies require large sample sizes (i.e., data from hundreds of twin pairs and/or relatives), making it difficult for individual investigators to gather sufficient data, particularly within special populations such as twins. Such obstacles highlight the need for developing collaborative projects across institutions that can engage in the uniform collection of twin and family (and ultimately molecular) data.

WHAT IS BEHAVIOR GENETICS?

Behavior genetics is a branch of psychology whose primary focus is to identify factors responsible for individual differences within a population. It has two principal divisions: the study of animal behavior and human behavior genetics. These divisions interact with and inform one another and also maintain close scholarly ties with molecular and medical genetics. However, because animal models are of limited value for modeling a phenotype such as stuttering and our knowledge about the loci of "stuttering genes" is nonexistent, neither animal geneticists nor molecular geneticists have become involved in the analysis of fluency disordered subjects.

The study of humans from a behavior genetics perspective is really a study of variances, of what makes people in a population different from one another. Rather than asking, "What is the mean or average for trait X in such and such a population?" a behavior geneticist might ask, "What factors create the variance around the mean for trait X?" For many traits, these factors are likely to include both genetic differences and differences that result from nongenetic factors (in a broad sense, the "environment"). Behavior geneticists assume that such interactions occur. What interests them is whether the *relative* importance of variables can be identified and help us understand the pathogenesis of a particular condition or behavior. Any trait or behavior that varies within a population can be studied. Musicalness, athleticism, verbal ability, height, and extroversion have all been studied, for example, and "speech fluency" might very appropriately be added to this list. Although fluency is seldom conceptualized as a continuously distributed trait, it is likely that there are substantial individual differences for this ability within the population. If so, then the relative contribution of genetic and environmental factors to fluency can be investigated using behavior genetic methodologies. We might ask, for example, whether highly fluent adults also have highly fluent parents, offspring, and siblings. If one member of a monozygotic twin pair is highly fluent, is his or her co-twin likely to be so identified? Through twin or family studies, we might begin to isolate intrinsic variables (e.g., oral-motor sequencing performance or laryngeal reaction time) and extrinsic variables (e.g., pre- or perinatal, medical, or educational factors) that correlate with fluency in a sampled population.

Classic behavior genetic methodologies (i.e., family, twin, and adoption paradigms) are founded upon mathematical principles and predictions derived from knowledge of how genes are transmitted in different family constellations. For example, full biological siblings and dizygotic (fraternal) twins, on average, share one-half of their polymorphic genes (i.e., genes with two or more alleles, or alternate forms), while half-siblings and first cousins, on average, share only one-quarter of their polymorphic genes. Similarly, a parent shares half of his or her genes at each polymorphic locus with each child. With the exception of monozygotic twins, who are genetically identical, the particular genes that are shared by family members cannot be predicted. This is what makes family members, on average, resemble one another more than unrelated individuals, but also show substantial individual differences. Within my family, for example, there is a characteristic "Felsenfeld phenotype" of which I am a prime exemplar. This phenotype—petite stature, wavy dark hair, small and very dark brown eyes, and fair skin—reflects our shared genetic background and can be identified quite easily in photographs of the extended Felsenfeld family. Of course, this phenotypic similarity for some features belies the many ways in which members of my family differ. Indeed, our varied rearing backgrounds, our unique experiences, and our genotypic differences all conspire to ensure that the Felsenfelds are and will continue to be a very diverse group.

Behavior Genetic Methodologies

Family Studies.   There are two principal family study methodologies: pedigree or high-density designs and case-control designs. In a high-density paradigm, which is also called a consanguinity study, families with multiple affected members are studied intensively. Usually, data are collected across several generations and include assessments of both first-degree relatives (parents, siblings, and offspring) and second-degree relatives (aunts, uncles, cousins, grandparents, and grandchildren).

After multiple pedigrees of highly affected families have been obtained, a statistical technique called segregation analysis can be performed to identify possible modes of transmission for the condition under study. A segregation analysis examines the way in which a condition is actually distributed in affected families and compares these observations with predicted patterns of transmission. By comparing observed with expected results under several potential transmission models, segregation analyses can indicate which models provide the best statistical fit to the observed data. Rarely can one model be conclusively proven; rather, these computations serve primarily to eliminate models whose modes of transmission are incompatible with empirical observations.

In addition to providing evidence that is consistent with a hypothesized mode of transmission, the data gathered from high-density families can be used in molecular linkage analyses. In the ideal case, linkage studies are performed only after segregation analyses have provided statistical evidence that a major gene is involved in the transmission of a condition (Suarez & Cox, 1985). By analyzing the chromosomal structure of affected and unaffected individuals within families with high a incidence of a condition, linkage analysis attempts to identify the "susceptibility locus" that is transmitted within affected families and that co-occurs with the disorder phenotype. Even if a susceptibility locus is identified in some families, this site may be implicated in the etiology of only a fraction of affected individuals in the population. Cox (1988) has argued that this limitation should not diminish the importance of this procedure, since the identification of a major gene in even a subsample of affected individuals increases our general understanding of the pathogenesis of a condition.

The second family study methodology, and the one that has been used most often for assessing the familial aggregation of stuttering, is the case-control design. In this design, an affected individual is identified by the investigators, which serves to "flag" immediate or extended family members for further study. This individual, typically called the proband, may be any subject for whom an accurate diagnosis is made. After a proband is selected as a subject for a family study, information about family members is obtained by using the proband (or parents) as the primary informant (the "family history method") or by assessing the status of relatives directly (the "family study method"). It is important in a case-control family study that probands be selected without regard for the disorder status of their family members. Thus, investigators should not seek out probands with a known family history of a condition or disorder, since the purpose of this methodology is to establish the extent to which a condition occurs in the families of a representative sample of affected cases.

Twin Studies. Twin studies provide another methodology for examining the role of genetic factors in the etiology of specific traits or conditions. Unlike family studies, whose primary role is to establish familial aggregation of a condition and to explicate its modes of transmission, twin studies are particularly useful for deriving heritability estimates (i.e., the proportion of phenotypic variance that can be attributed to genetic factors in a given population at a given time). Briefly, this is accomplished by examining differences in the resemblance of a trait or condition between pairs of identical, or monozygotic (MZ), twins and pairs of fraternal, or dizygotic (DZ), twins. For continuously distributed traits (such as height and intelligence), this is usually done by calculating intra-class correlation coefficients for the MZ and DZ pairs. For categorical conditions, such as the presence or absence of stuttering, resemblance is more often reported as concordance rates that are analyzed using a chi-square statistic.

Twinning is a relatively common event, occurring in approximately 1 of 83 live births in the United States (Plomin, DeFries, & McClearn, 1980). Approximately one-third of all twin births produce monozygotic (MZ) twins who are genetically identical. The remaining two-thirds of twin births produce dizygotic (DZ) pairs; of these, approximately half are same-sex and half are opposite-sex twins (Plomin et al., 1980). Genetically, fraternal twins share, on average, half of their polymorphic genes, the same as full siblings. Because accurate zygosity classification is of critical importance in twin studies, strict criteria for determining zygosity (preferably, using blood group analysis) should be used.

The theory underlying twin studies is straightforward. If a condition is heritable, genetically identical MZ twins will display greater resemblance for that condition than will the less genetically similar DZ twins (i.e., MZs will be more highly correlated or concordant). For MZ twins reared together, the only factors contributing to intra-pair variance are (theoretically) nonfamily environmental influences; that is, unique experiences that are not shared by the twins. For DZ twins reared together, within-pair variance can result from both nonfamily environmental factors and genetic factors, since fraternal twins differ in both. What interests behavior geneticists, then, is the difference in intra-class correlations or concordance rates between pairs of MZ and DZ twins, in addition to the magnitude of the associations.

Adoption Studies.   Adoption studies provide the most powerful of all behavior genetic methodologies for establishing the relative importance of genetic factors in the expression of traits or conditions. In this design, information is typically collected from both the biological and adoptive relatives of individuals who were adopted near the time of birth. Because adopted subjects in these studies are known to have had little if any contact with biological relatives during their formative years, any resemblance between adopted individuals and their biological relatives must reflect their shared genetic background. In like manner, the degree of resemblance between adopted subjects and their adoptive families (parents and siblings) reflects their shared environmental background, given there is no biological association between them. With the exception of a small anecdotal report by Bloodstein (1993), adoption studies of stuttering have not been performed. The time and cost associated with these designs, as well as the increasingly difficult access to adoption records, make it unlikely that a carefully controlled adoption study of stuttering will ever be feasible to pursue. Felsenfeld (1995) obtained some preliminary information on the occurrence of speech disorders (primarily stuttering) in three groups of adopted and nonadopted children who were participating in the longitudinal Colorado Adoption Project. The children in these groups were considered to be at varying risk for a developmental speech or language disorder, based upon their biological and/or adoptive parents' speech history. The results of this study suggested that having a biological parent with a reported history of speech disorder appeared to be more important for the development of these conditions than being reared by a parent with a positive history. However, because of modest sample sizes and other methodological complications, this finding should be viewed with caution.

Case-Control Studies of Stuttering

References to the familiality of stuttering and to "stuttering families" have appeared in the literature for more than fifty years (Andrews & Harris, 1964; Gray, 1940; Johnson, 1959; Wepman, 1939; West, Nelson, & Berry, 1939). Sheehan and Costley (1977) and Bloodstein (1981) reviewed many of these early studies and concluded that, on average, about one-third to one-half of all stutterers will report the presence of other current or former stutterers in their immediate families, a conclusion that has been supported by more recent investigations (Ambrose, Yairi, & Cox, 1993; Kidd, Heimbuch, & Records, 1981). Although these early reports are of historical interest, they are of limited usefulness as sources of data for quantitative genetic analyses that are being performed today.

Much of our recent knowledge about the transmission of stuttering comes from three relatively large case-control family history studies that have obtained information about the fluency status of family members of proband subjects with widely varying ages (Ambrose et al., 1993; Kay, 1964; Kidd, 1984). Table 1.1 summarizes methodological details such as proband sample size and characteristics, recruitment sites, and classification criteria for each of these investigations.

As can be seen, these studies were similar methodologically. In each case, relatives were classified as stutterers or nonstutterers using the family history method, with little or no direct assessment of speech status. Although this type of dichotomous classification is appropriate for the performance of segregation analysis, it does not allow researchers to examine qualitative or quantitative aspects of the phenotype or related behaviors (e.g., frequency of stuttering, duration of longest moments, stuttering type, number of associated behaviors, articulatory competency, etc.).

TABLE 1.1   Summary of Methods in Three Case-Control Family Studies of Stuttering

INVESTIGATORS	NUMBER OF PROBANDS	AGE OF PROBANDS	RECRUITING SITES	DIAGNOSIS OF PROBANDS	DIAGNOSIS OF FAMILY MEMBERS
Kay (1964) [Newcastle Study]	213	161 children; 52 adolescents and adults	clinics, schools, and hospitals	diagnosis as current or recovered stutterer by self or SLP	informant report
Kidd (1984) [Yale Family Study]	approx. 600	older adolescents and adults	private and university clinics	diagnosis as current or recovered stutterer by self or SLP	informant report
Ambrose, Yairi, & Cox (1993)	69	preschool children	university clinic	diagnosis as current stutterer by SLP	informant (parent) report

Relatives were classified as "affected" in these studies if they currently stuttered or were reported ever to have stuttered. Although these subgroups of relatives were found to be of approximately equal size in the Yale sample (Seider, Gladstein, & Kidd, 1983), they were grouped for analysis in all three investigations. This is unfortunate, because collapsing active and recovered stutterers may have obscured important information about the relationship between recovery and family history variables. The affected proband subjects who participated in these studies were recruited primarily from private or university clinics and hospitals. Accordingly, they may not represent a random sample of all stutterers in the population, since those who seek treatment are often more severely affected and more economically advantaged than those who do not.

In addition to these concerns, each of these studies suffers from the absence of control families and the potential for diagnostic imprecision. These particular issues are of sufficient concern to warrant a more elaborated discussion.

Absence of Control Families.   Control families were not included in any of these investigations, and none can be considered a well-designed family history study. Instead, rates of stuttering found within the proband families were compared with incidence rates expected within the general population. The inclusion of matched control families in a case-control design is more desirable than comparing the disorder rates observed in proband families with pre-established population rates reported in the literature for several reasons. Because both incidence and prevalence rates reported in the literature are typically pooled estimates derived from a number of sources, it is difficult to assess the degree of uniformity in diagnostic criteria across studies and to determine if these criteria are comparable to those used in a particular family study. The probability that an individual will "ever stutter" (i.e., the lifetime incidence) is typically reported to be about 5 percent (Bloodstein, 1981; Peters & Guitar, 1991); however, this is a consensus figure based upon a rough average of several epidemiological studies of varying size and quality, and may therefore only approximate the true disorder rate. Moreover, unless control families are included, there is no opportunity for examiners to evaluate subjects blindly, thereby increasing the likelihood that inadvertent biases will contaminate the classification process.

Potential for Diagnostic Imprecision.   The precision and reliability of classification of both probands and family members are important for case-control family studies. For disorders such as schizophrenia and alcoholism, standard interview scales are used for diagnostic classification. For these conditions, phenotype measurement is, at the very least, fairly uniform across investigations, and, presumably, the sensitivity and specificity of diagnoses based upon these instruments are adequate. Even within these areas of research, however, there is some disagreement on the degree of involvement that is sufficient to warrant a positive diagnosis. In family studies of alcoholism, for example, some investigators have found that rates of disorder among the relatives of alcoholic probands will vary depending upon the strictness of the definition used to classify individuals as alcoholic (Kendler, Neale, Heath, Kessler, & Eaves, 1994).

For a disorder such as stuttering, which lacks a universally recognized or standardized diagnostic protocol, the classification problem is even more complex. Because different investigators use different standards for identifying a fluency disorder, the criteria that have been communicated to informants and used to classify affected individuals almost certainly have varied in significant but unknown ways from one study to the next. Because validations of subjects' classifications were not done in these studies (e.g., comparing informant reports with other diagnostic data), the degree of measurement error introduced by lack of precision is unknown, but potentially significant (Roy, Walsh, Prescott, & Kendler, 1994). Moreover, a number of variables that are known to influence the reliability of informants' reports were not controlled in these studies. A partial list includes the extent of the informant's knowledge about immediate and extended relatives, his or her own disorder status, and gender (Hedges, Umar, Mellon, Herrick, Hanson, & Wahl, 1995; Kendler, Silberg, Neale, Kessler, Heath, Phil, & Eaves, 1991; Roy et al., 1994). For stuttering, little attention has been paid to the impact of these variables on the accuracy of informants' reports, although a recent study suggested that underreporting of stuttering (i.e., poor sensitivity) is a concern, particularly when nonstuttering relatives are providing family history information (Hedges et al., 1995).

Summary of Results.   Table 1.2 presents the rates of stuttering among first-degree relatives that have been reported in these three studies. In light

TABLE 1.2   Percentage of Relatives Affected in Three Family Studies

RELATIVES	KAY (1964) SAMPLES POOLED (N=213)[a]	KIDD (1980) SEXES POOLED (N=396)	AMBROSE ET AL. (1993) SEXES POOLED (N=69)
Mothers	6.8%	6.6%	4.3%
Fathers	19.1%	18.4%	23.2%
Sisters	8.4%	6.8%	18.4%
Brothers	20.3%	20.4%	26.1%
Sons	NA	26.3%	NA
Daughters	NA	11.5%	NA

[a]indicates number of proband subjects in sample

NA indicates that data are not available

of the caveats just noted, it would be prudent to view these percentages as rough estimates of the "true" disorder rates in affected families.

If the percentages for all affected relatives are averaged, these results indicate that approximately 15 percent of the first-degree relatives of proband subjects are current or recovered stutterers. In comparison to a reported incidence rate of 5 percent for the general population, a 15 percent rate of stuttering (i.e., a threefold increase) is considered significant (Andrews et al., 1983; Kidd, 1984). It is worth noting that proband subjects in the Yale sample who were considered severe stutterers were no more likely than mild stutterers to report stuttering relatives, suggesting that although the presence of stuttering may be familial, its severity is not (Kidd, Heimbuch, Records, Oehlert, & Webster, 1980).

Table 1.2 makes clear that the probability, or risk, of stuttering is not uniform for all family members. Rather, male relatives of a stutterer (fathers, brothers, and sons) are at greater risk than are female relatives of a stutterer (mothers, sisters, and daughters). For instance, these findings suggest that 20 to 26 percent of all brothers of proband subjects will be current or recovered stutterers, but only 4 to 7 percent of all mothers. The studies by both Kay (1964) and Kidd (1980) are consistent in reporting male:female ratios that range from 2.3:1 to 3.0:1 for all relevant comparisons: affected fathers versus mothers, brothers versus sisters, and sons versus daughters. These results also agree with the well-accepted epidemiological finding that approximately three times as

many males in the population stutter (Andrews et al., 1983; Van Riper, 1982).

The gender data from the Ambrose and colleagues (1993) investigation did not conform to these expected values. In their study, the ratio of affected fathers to affected mothers was higher than in previous reports (approximately 5.4:1), while, somewhat paradoxically, the ratio of affected brothers to affected sisters was lower (1.4:1). These discrepancies may simply reflect an instability due to small cell sizes. Alternatively, these findings may provide additional information about the natural course of the disorder. In particular, it may be that both brothers and sisters of very young proband subjects have similar risks for stuttering in their early and middle childhood years. However, because there is some evidence that female relatives of stutterers are more likely to recover from stuttering than are male relatives, and to do so at earlier ages (Seider et al., 1983), the gender ratio should become more pronounced with increasing subject age. If Ambrose and her colleagues continue to obtain longitudinal speech data from proband subjects and their affected siblings, then recovery profiles by gender can be examined more carefully and may permit more definitive conclusions.

Table 1.3 presents the percentage of affected first-degree relatives by sex of the proband in these three case-control studies.

Once again, the findings of the Newcastle and Yale family studies were similar to one another and different from those of Ambrose and her colleagues. In the two former studies, significantly

TABLE 1.3 Percentage of Affected First-Degree Relatives by Sex of Proband in Three Family Studies.

	KAY (1964) (N=213)[a]	KIDD (1980) (N=512)	AMBROSE ET AL. (1993) (N=69)
Male proband	12.2%	13.8.%	18.0%
Female proband	20.2%*	18.0%*	14.8%

[a]indicates number of proband subjects in sample

* p<.05 for gender differences

more immediate family members were reported to stutter when the proband was a female. Additional analyses demonstrated that this risk was particularly high for sons of stuttering mothers, with rates as high as 39 percent reported in the literature (Kidd, Kidd, & Records, 1978). These findings have been used to support the hypothesis that the liability for stuttering is different for the two sexes, with females having a higher liability threshold, and, by implication, requiring greater "genetic loading" for stuttering to be expressed (Kidd et al., 1981). The negative findings of Ambrose and colleagues (1993) suggest that this increased risk to family members might operate only for female probands who are still stuttering as adults, presumably the most severe cases in the population.

Although the sex-specific genetic threshold interpretation may be correct, there are alternative, nongenetic explanations for the reports of increased stuttering among family members of female probands. In particular, gender-based and/or projection biases among informants may influence reporting rates in family history studies and can pose problems for studies that rely on this method. To use alcoholism as an example again, it has been observed that males and females differ in their tendency to over-report family members as alcoholic, with female informants significantly more likely to identify unaffected relatives as problem drinkers than are males (Roy et al., 1994). In addition, there is a well-documented tendency for affected informants of both genders to project falsely their own disorder onto unaffected family members, which is termed projection bias (Chapman, Mannuzza, Klein, & Fyer, 1994; Roy et al., 1994). In the present context, it is possible that the increased incidence of stuttering among family members of female probands reported in some studies may be explained by a complex interaction between these two sources of bias—a tendency for affected subjects to project their disorder to family members coupled with a lower tolerance for dysfluency among women. The best way to determine if these sources of bias are relevant for family history studies of stuttering is to verify informant diagnoses by direct evaluations of relatives. Until this is done, the often-reported finding of increased stuttering among family members of female stutterers should be considered a preliminary finding.

Results of Pedigree and Segregation Analyses

Probably the most famous pedigree study of stuttering was an early investigation by Gray (1940) of the "X" family. This was a large family with two independent branches (the Iowa and Kansas branches), both of which descended from a stuttering female. The incidence of stuttering in these two branches diverged over time, with the Iowa branch containing multiple stuttering members and the Kansas branch containing only a few. Because both branches descended from the same stuttering proband, it was concluded that the large difference in stuttering frequency was related to a familial culture of anxiety about stuttering that was typical of Iowa but not Kansas family members. At the time this study was published, it was used as evidence to support environmental but not hereditary transmission of stuttering. Subsequently, this pedigree has been examined by others, and genetic transmission has been judged to provide an equally viable explanation for the data (Wingate, 1986).

More recently, MacFarlane, Hanson, Walton, and Mellon (1991) reported data from 269 family members of a multigeneration pedigree that had a stuttering rate that was five to fifteen times higher than that of the general population. Although a formal segregation analysis was not performed, the data were interpreted as theoretically consistent with transmission at a single major autosomal locus (a major gene on a nonsex chromosome), with different thresholds for males and females. Unfortunately, environmental analyses that may have identified relevant coexisting cultural transmission variables in this family were not performed.

Formal segregation analyses of family data have appeared in two studies (Ambrose et al., 1993; Cox, Kramer, & Kidd, 1984). Both of these studies evaluated transmission patterns within nuclear families using a segregation program called POINTER (Lalouel & Morton, 1981). This program evaluates several alternative transmission models (e.g., single major locus, polygenic, mixed) and either accepts or rejects each model based upon distributional properties of the available family data. For POINTER to operate, investigators must specify two parameters: the estimated lifetime incidence of the condition, by gender if applicable (referred to as the population affection rate), and a parameter termed ascertainment probability (the probability that any proband who meets selection criteria is actually identified for study, which is typically set low at .01 or .001 percent). These analyses also require that the phenotype is coded as a binary trait, with all cases classified as either affected or unaffected. Table 1.4 presents the results of the POINTER analysis for both of these investigations.

As can be seen, these segregation studies found evidence for a genetic component in the transmission of stuttering. There was not, however, complete agreement about which transmission model provided the best fit for the data. Although both studies found evidence for polygenic inheritance, only the Ambrose study found evidence for transmission at a single major locus. If a major locus is involved, the pattern of transmission does not conform to classic Mendelian probabilities (i.e., it is not a fully penetrant dominant, recessive, or sex-linked gene), because incidence figures in relatives are too low (Vandenberg, Singer, & Pauls, 1986). Interestingly, although the analysis by Cox and colleagues (1984) rejected a major locus transmission of stuttering, Kidd himself argued for a major locus model with sex-specific thresholds in at least two separate publications (Kidd, 1980; Kidd, 1984).

Table 1.5 presents the single major locus parameter estimates provided by POINTER for these two studies. For this analysis, a fully penetrant major gene influence is assumed. The reported parameters, then, reflect the probability that an individual of a given genotype will be affected with a disorder, based upon the estimated frequency of a "pathological" major gene in the population. For stuttering, three genotypes are theoretically possible: NN (two normal alleles at a given locus), NS (one normal and one stuttering allele), and SS (two stuttering alleles). The frequency of this hypothetical "stuttering gene" has been estimated to be fairly low by these methods, occurring in only about 4 percent of individuals (Kidd, 1984). Within the general population, then, about 91 percent of all individuals would be expected to have the [NN] genotype, 8 percent would be heterozygotes [NS], and only .16 percent would be homozygotic for the stuttering allele [SS] (Kidd, 1980).

The parameter estimates derived from both of these segregation analyses indicate that almost no individuals with the [NN] genotype in the population would be expected to stutter. Among heterozygotes, 23 to 30 percent of males but only 8 to 12 percent of females would be predicted to stutter. This suggests that most individuals who

TABLE 1.4   Results of Genetic Model-Fitting Procedures in Two Segregation Studies

MODEL TESTED	AMBROSE ET AL. (1993)	COX ET AL. (1984)
Is there evidence for genetic transmission?	YES	YES
Is there evidence for transmission at a major locus?	YES	NO
Is there evidence for polygenic transmission?	YES	YES

TABLE 1.5   Single Major Locus Parameter Estimates in Two Segregation Studies.

INVESTIGATORS	NUMBER OF FAMILIES	POPULATION AFFECTION RATES (MALES, FEMALES)	MALES			FEMALES		
			NN	NS	SS	NN	NS	SS
Ambrose et al. (1994)	69	.05, .01	.00	.23	.90	.00	.08	.58
Cox et al. (1984)	383	.035, .01	.02	.30	1.0	.00	.12	1.0

Note: NN = 2 nonstuttering alleles (homozygotic noncarrier)

NS = 1 nonstuttering allele and one stuttering allele (heterozygote)

SS = 2 stuttering alleles (homozygotic carrier)

carry only one copy of the "stuttering" gene (i.e., one [S] allele) will not manifest the stuttering phenotype, although more heterozygote males than females will be affected. Both models predict that virtually 100 percent of males who are homozygotic for the stuttering gene [genotype SS] will stutter. The principal difference between these analyses is reflected in the findings for homozygotic carrier females. The analysis by Cox and her colleagues predicts that most females with the [SS] genotype will stutter (i.e., there is very high penetrance for both males and females), while that by Ambrose and colleagues indicates that only about half of all [SS] females (58%) will display the stuttering phenotype. The latter investigators do not provide an explanation for the reduced penetrance among homozygotic carrier females, although, presumably, some intrinsic or extrinsic protective factors would need to be invoked to explain how females, but not males, are able to compensate for such a powerful genetic liability. It is also worth noting that a single gene model of inheritance does not eliminate the role of the environment. Environmental factors are acknowledged to be important in determining the degree to which a phenotype will be expressed (including no overt expression), particularly among heterozygotes (Kidd, 1980). In other words, the predisposing conditions that result from the effects of a major gene are not considered impervious to outside influences and can be over-ridden by circumstances that are either extremely damaging or extremely facilitating.

Although it has received less elaboration, the polygenic-multifactorial model should still be considered an equally viable if not frankly preferable transmission model for stuttering (Vandenberg et al., 1986). In multifactorial-polygenic inheritance, genetic susceptibility is believed to be transmitted through the cumulative contribution of multiple unspecified genes and multiple environmental factors. Implicit in this model is the existence of an underlying liability distribution in the population whose shape resembles a bell-shaped curve. Most individuals in the population will possess "normal" or "average" fluency control skills, with a small percentage of very fluent and a small percentage of very dysfluent (stuttering) speakers. (We do not have a name for nor do we study hyperfluent speakers, although, theoretically, they do exist and should be of interest.) At some point in this hypothetical distribution lies a threshold that, if exceeded, will result in stuttering. Such thresholds can be gender-specific, with one gender (in the case of stuttering, males) requiring fewer disruptive factors for expression of the disorder. Because both genetic and environmental factors are shared by first-degree relatives, this model predicts that the mean performance of the relatives of stuttering probands should be poorer on fluency-related tasks than that of control individuals. That is, although they may not all stutter, the family members of proband subjects should be, on average, less "fluency competent" than are randomly selected control speakers, due to a combination of multiple shared genetic liabilities and environmental exposures.

Although a multifactorial-polygenic explanation may be considered less satisfying and more "messy" than a single-gene hypothesis, it may be the most viable transmission model for most cases. Alternatively, a mixed model, which allows for a multifactorial background (familial and nonfamilial environmental effects and/or polygenic influences) in addition to a single major locus, might ultimately account best for the observed pattern of familial resemblance (c.f. Vogler, Gottesman, McGue, & Rao, 1990). Obviously, we do not yet have enough pedigree information or sufficient statistical power to obtain a reasonable discrimination between competing transmission hypotheses, although it does appear safe to conclude that the null hypothesis of no familial transmission of stuttering can be rejected. The next step in this investigative sequence requires molecular analyses using blood samples collected from high-density pedigrees so that the location of a candidate major gene, if one exists, can begin to be isolated. Once such a gene is found, its functions and products can be identified, thereby increasing the probability that appropriate remediative measures (e.g., pharmacological treatments) may be developed. Although clearly desirable, our present state of knowledge makes it impossible to predict the likelihood that this outcome will occur.

Twin Studies of Stuttering

Very little information is available about the concordance of stuttering in twin pairs whose zygosity has been rigorously established. In her now classic study, Howie (1981a) evaluated thirty same-sex twin pairs (ages 6 to 27 years) in which at least one member was reported to be a current or recovered stutterer. Care was taken to ensure accuracy in determining zygosity, and stuttering diagnoses were made independently and blindly by trained judges. Howie found that the age-corrected pairwise concordance rates differed signif-

icantly between twin types, with 10/16 of the monozygotic pairs (63%) and 3/13 (19%) of the dizygotic pairs concordant for stuttering. Although this is the most robust twin study completed to date, the small sample size limits its usefulness for further quantitative genetic analyses, such as estimates of heritability.

In addition to classifying co-twins as either affected or unaffected, Howie (1981b) examined the degree of resemblance within twin pairs for specific dysfluency topographies, using intra-class correlations. Perhaps due to the large number of discordant DZ twin pairs, the DZ correlations were not significantly different from zero for any type of dysfluency except interjections ($r = .52$). For monozygotic twins, all of the intra-class correlations were positive, ranging from a low of .27 for phrase repetitions to a high of .83 for interjections. For the characteristics typically considered as "core" stuttering behaviors (blocks, prolongations, and syllable repetitions), MZ correlations were .55, .25, and .38, respectively, which suggests a moderate degree of resemblance for stuttering type within MZ twin pairs. However, because of the small number of core behaviors, these correlations may be inflated.

Of greater interest is the significant difference between the MZ and DZ correlations. If these results are reliable, they argue that genetic factors may play a significant role in determining the form that dysfluencies take, particularly core stuttering behaviors. However, since both MZ and DZ twins showed a moderate to high degree of resemblance for interjections, nongenetic familial factors appear to be more important than genetic factors alone in influencing the rate of production of this particular dysfluency topography.

In a recent study by Andrews, Morris-Yates, Howie, and Martin (1991), information about the incidence of stuttering was obtained from several thousand Australian adult twins who were participating in a large, population-based, twin study. In a population study such as this, twins are not selected through an affected proband. Instead, a representative sample is selected (in this case, all twins born between 1981 and 1982 in a particular location), and broad-based assessment data are obtained. These studies can be quite useful in confirming incidence data for a variety of conditions but are usually less useful for capturing large numbers of subjects who have the specific disorder under study.

In this particular twin investigation, a question about past or present stuttering was included in a lengthy questionnaire that was mailed to twin pairs participating in the study. This item was answered by 64 percent of the pairs, resulting in a sample size of 3810 pairs. Among these respondents, 1.9 percent indicated that they had "ever stuttered"—3.2 percent of males and 1.2 percent of females. These rates are lower than the reported lifetime incidence rate of 5 percent for stuttering (Bloodstein, 1981; Peters & Guitar, 1991), and suggest that either underreporting of stuttering occurred in this sample, or that the "true" incidence of stuttering in the population is less than five percent. Parenthetically, these findings suggest that the incidence of stuttering in twins is probably not higher than that of singletons, as had been reported in early investigations (Berry, 1938; Nelson, Hunter, & Walter, 1945).

The pairwise concordance rates found in this unselected twin sample were, in fact, lower than those reported in Howie's (1981a) study. Of the fifty monozygotic twin pairs containing at least one self-reported stutterer, only ten pairs were concordant for stuttering (20%). Among same-sex dizygotic twin pairs with at least one self-reported stutterer, only 3 percent (3/85) were concordant, less than that expected for non-twin same-sex siblings. Although these pairwise agreements are lower than expected, the substantial difference between the MZ and DZ twin types yields a pairwise concordance ratio of 5.7:1. Somewhat paradoxically, despite the small number of concordant pairs, this ratio indicates a substantial genetic effect for stuttering. In fact, genetic model fitting procedures estimated that 71 percent of the variance in these data could be attributed to genetic factors, with the remaining 29 percent attributable to the nonfamilial environment.

Although this heritability estimate is impressively large, the low concordance rates that were obtained for both the MZ and DZ twin pairs is puzzling. It seems unlikely that subject identification procedures alone would cause such large discrepancies between these and Howie's earlier findings, although they almost certainly had some effect. It would be interesting to know if comparably low concordance rates would have been obtained if twin pairs having a self-reported stutterer had been assessed by trained examiners, as was done in the Howie study. Although it seems that adults should be able to recall their own speech history accurately, the reliability of such self-reports has never been well established. Moreover, it is conceivable that this type of self-disclosure might be particularly questionable for twins, who sometimes assess their own performance relative to that of their co-twin, a phenomenon referred to as the twin contrast effect (Loehlin, 1992). Since the severity of stuttering does not appear to be inherited (Kidd et al., 1980), it follows that a twin with mild stuttering or one who has recovered may not consider his or her speech disordered when compared to a more severely affected co-twin. Since diagnoses were based upon a single self-report item, measurement sensitivity may not have been adequate. Whatever the explanation, future studies should try to clarify this inconsistency by analyzing the speech of twins directly, obtaining more sensitive interview measures, and by validating self-reports through external records. At the very least, the results of this Australian twin study serve to highlight the importance that such factors as subject recruitment, sampling, and measurement sensitivity may have on the outcome of behavior genetic investigations.

FUTURE RESEARCH NEEDS

The family and twin studies reviewed here provide a solid foundation for future behavior genetic investigations of stuttering. It is probably safe to conclude that stuttering runs in families and is influenced by genetic factors. Lest we conclude, however, that we already know all that we need to know in this area, it should be emphasized that the methodology of these studies resembles that done twenty to thirty years ago to investigate other behavior disorders, such as alcoholism or schizophrenia. Consequently, they provide only the necessary first steps in the process of analyzing a complex disorder from a genetic perspective. It is to be hoped that future behavior genetic studies will bring us closer to identifying the actual genes and gene products that are involved in stuttering, using a combination of behavior, biochemical, and anatomical technologies. If so, multidimensional behavior and physiological measures will have to be obtained from both co-twins and family members of stuttering probands, as well as from control individuals and their families. The following suggestions for future research could be refined, reordered, and extended in a number of ways. Their chief purpose here is to stimulate the thinking of both new and veteran fluency investigators in the hope that some may be enticed into pursuing questions that contribute to this important knowledge base.

1. *Develop a standard assessment battery for the diagnosis of stuttering across the lifespan.*

The development of an accepted protocol for the diagnosis of stuttering is a priority for those interested in behavior genetic studies of stuttering. Ideally, such a protocol would elicit a representative sample of the range of behaviors that are integral to identifying this disorder at various points in its progression (e.g., stuttering type and frequency, avoidance behaviors, self-concept, etc.). While a small percentage of classification errors is unavoidable, the objective of this protocol should be to maximize sensitivity and specificity for identifying respondents of all ages who stutter, who used to stutter, and who have never stuttered. To do this effectively, it would be helpful to know more about the relationship between stuttering and other disfluencies in the general population so that appropriate boundaries that demarcate these behaviors may be identified either perceptually, physiologically, or by report (Borden, 1990; Alfonso, 1990). Long standing professional debates

about the optimal definition of stuttering and its relationship to normal nonfluency will undoubtedly complicate efforts to develop a classification protocol. However, these debates should not preclude serious attempts to draft a viable classification system for widespread use.

Recently, for example, Shriberg (1993) developed a classification system for genetic research to assess the articulation performance of individuals across the lifespan. This system was developed so that both normal and disordered speakers could be placed into one of ten polychotomous speech categories, based upon specific age-sensitive articulation and phonological production characteristics in a sample of continuous conversational speech. There are two categories for coding speech that is perceptually normal ("normal" and "normalized" speech), and eight for coding speech that is considered perceptually abnormal or disordered. Shriberg maintains that a wide range of potentially important phenotypic variability in speech production, including normalization of previously disordered speech, can be identified through the use of this system.

Although Shriberg's taxonomy is of tremendous interest, it is likely that a more multidimensional assessment protocol will be required for classifying fluency disordered subjects at all levels of severity, including cases that are controlled, relatively covert, or have normalized (Ludlow, 1990). To increase diagnostic precision, a protocol might combine interviews with direct assessments of spontaneous speech and reading, perceptual rating scales, physiological measures, and tasks designed to tax a speaker's fluency (Alfonso, 1990). An optimal protocol would be one that maximizes classification accuracy in a relatively short period of time, preferably without requiring specialized equipment or elaborate experimental procedures. Since genetic studies require very large sample sizes, it would be ideal if a structured interview, perhaps in conjunction with a specialized perceptual rating scale of connected speech (c.f., Franken, Boves, Peters, & Webster, 1995), would serve this purpose. One logical step to advance this process would be to cross-correlate several types of diagnostic measures with fluency status in a manageable number of affected and control cases. Once this is done, a preliminary classification protocol could be developed and made available for pilot testing at several research and clinical centers.

2. *Identify the relationship between family history status and epidemiological variables.*

Understanding the relationship between family history status and epidemiological variables such as stuttering severity, probability of spontaneous recovery, and potential for relapse is of importance for both theoretical and clinical reasons. In the clinic, family history status is being used already as an indicator to predict which children are more likely to recover spontaneously (Cooper, 1972; Cooper & Cooper, 1985; Pindzola & White, 1986), and several writers have suggested that relapse among adults may be partly determined by biological (i.e., genetic) vulnerability (Boberg, Howie, & Woods, 1979; Kamhi, 1982). Clinically, it is often presumed that a positive family history decreases the likelihood of spontaneous recovery and increases the probability of relapse, but these presumptions are still just intuitive (albeit plausible) hypotheses that may or may not mirror true epidemiological outcomes (see Chapter 2 by Yairi). For this reason, it is important that future longitudinal and case-control family studies obtain and analyze separately the developmental histories, speech and non-speech behaviors, and fluency outcomes of incipient and adult stutterers who are grouped according to family history status. Although the absence of familial aggregation does not necessarily imply the absence of genetic influence (individuals may carry deleterious genes that are not expressed for a number of complex reasons), these subgroup analyses are of value in estimating the influence of family history on outcome.

On a more theoretical level, it would be useful for family study researchers to formulate testable models a priori that would lead to specific predictions for family history negative [FHN] versus family history positive [FHP] stutterers. By way of example, one might start with the hypoth-

esis that adult stutterers with a positive family history are more likely than FHN stutterers to evidence deficits that reflect an inherited and fairly isolated impairment in systems that coordinate precisely timed sequential motor movements, including speech (Janssen, Kraaimaat, & Brutten, 1990; Webster, 1993). If this were true, we might predict that FHP stutterers' speech would include a high proportion of dysfluency types that reflect problems in the timing of speech-motor onsets and offsets, such as prolongations and blocks (Janssen et al., 1990) and would also have more difficulty with sequential behaviors that are unrelated to speech (such as sequential finger tapping). Finally, and perhaps most important, *family members* of FHP stutterers should evidence less efficient or atypical sequential motor performance when taxed than that found among FHN family members or controls (Felsenfeld, 1994). Because FHN stutterers might be dysfluent for a variety of idiopathic reasons that are unlikely to aggregate within families, they would be predicted to display a more diffuse behavior profile and, perhaps, a higher frequency of adverse prenatal, postnatal, or early childhood events that might have precipitated the stuttering disorder (Poulos & Webster, 1991). The point of this discussion is not, of course, to present or defend this particular causal model, but to illustrate how a "top-down" experimental program can be of value in integrating seemingly isolated subgroup findings into a coherent and internally consistent theoretical framework.

3. *Examine extrinsic factors that may precipitate or maintain the disorder.*

Plomin (cited in Wachs, 1992) recently observed that "we know more than we think about genes and . . . less than we think about environment." Although it is clear that nongenetic factors are important in the etiology of stuttering, identifying these environmental influences is not straightforward. The environment is a complex system of interactions whose influences operate simultaneously on a number of levels, including those originating from culture and society, from unique nonfamilial experiences (e.g., effects due to prenatal or perinatal events, school or peer experiences, etc.), and from the family directly (Rowe, 1994; Wachs, 1992). Although we often assume that within-family (i.e., shared) environmental factors are the most influential in determining developmental outcomes, nonfamilial (nonshared) environmental forces may actually be of greater importance for many developmental phenotypes (Rowe, 1994). In light of this counterintuitive observation, perhaps research efforts should focus attention on the role of *nonshared* environmental factors in stuttering etiology, in addition to assessing traditional within-family environmental influences.

In socialization science, the environment is frequently conceptualized as a static, monolithic entity that provides uniformly "good" or "bad" input. In reality, however, the impact that any one environmental variable has on a condition is almost always mediated by other influences and may operate only during particular age-sensitive periods (Wachs, 1992). Using rapid parental speaking rate (a shared environmental variable) as an example, it might be the case that fast parental speech has deleterious consequences for fluency only for those children having a highly reactive temperament during a specific developmental period (e.g., 2 to 4 years). For younger or older children, or those with different constitutional dispositions, rapid parental speech may have a neutral or even a facilitating effect. Thus, rather than considering speaking rate as a static entity (wherein "fast is bad and slow is good"), it might be more appropriate to frame future questions about this variable in interactional terms. Are children with neonatal problems more intolerant of fast parental speaking rate than are children without neonatal problems? Do children with a positive family history of stuttering respond to parental speaking rates differently than do children without such a history? Does a rapid parental speaking rate differentially affect boys and girls? If so, during what developmental periods? At the risk of belaboring the point, it should be understood that extrinsic factors interact with one another and with the intrinsic capabilities and

susceptibilities of each individual to precipitate a disorder as complex as stuttering (Adams, 1990; Smith, 1990; Wachs, 1992).

Although the number of extrinsic factors that might bear upon the emergence of stuttering seems theoretically limitless, in practice there are a few sets of variables that have received primary attention. These include developmental influences, particularly those relating to the emergence of speech and language competency (Bloodstein, 1981; Starkweather & Gottwald, 1990), and aspects of within-family environment such as parental verbal behavior and standards for maturity and achievement (Johnson, 1959; Starkweather & Gottwald, 1990). Although rarely discussed, extrinsic factors that may have initially helped to precipitate a fluency disorder are likely to be different from those that serve to maintain it. Among chronic adult stutterers, for example, unique experiences, perhaps even cultural and societal factors, may play a larger role than direct family influences in shaping and perpetuating their disorder. To identify sets of precipitating and maintaining variables that are common across cases, it would be optimal for a standard environmental assessment protocol to be developed that could be applied to probands and proband families at various stages in the disorder process, from onset through remission or relapse.

Several behavior genetic methodologies have the potential to clarify nongenetic factors that may be important in the etiology of stuttering. For example, using a case-control family study design, the home environment of families having several affected members (high-density families), those with an isolated affected member, and matched control families with no affected members could be evaluated systematically, with particular attention directed to the types of verbal and psychosocial variables cited above. If specific within-family transmission factors are important in precipitating or maintaining stuttering, then these factors should be most evident in families containing multiple members who stutter and least apparent in control families. However, when assessing within-family factors such as these, the direction of effects is not always clear. Even if parents of stuttering children are rated as less verbally responsive, on average, than control parents during a structured interaction, can we conclude that this lack of responsiveness caused the affected children to stutter? Alternatively, might these differences reflect a learned parental reaction to their child's escalating stuttering behavior, perhaps a misguided attempt to minimize the amount of talking the child must do? Within biologically intact families, these directional ambiguities complicate the identification of within-family environmental factors. However, if appropriate experimental controls are included in study designs, the confounding influence of direction of effects can be addressed.

The existence of discordant MZ pairs indicates that nongenetic factors must be relevant for stuttering to emerge and to persist. These discordant monozygotic pairs provide an interesting sample for study. By examining the histories of young monozygotic twin pairs containing at least one stutterer, nonshared variables that might have precipitated different fluency outcomes may be identified. For example, within a discordant pair, a twin who developed a fluency problem might have experienced a serious medical trauma at age two that was not shared by his unaffected co-twin. This kind of post hoc design cannot establish the role that such constituents play in etiology; however, if similar types of discriminating events characterize several discordant monozygotic twin pairs, inferences about the importance of such nonshared environmental factors may be made with more confidence. Although more methodologically complex, it might also be of value to examine adult monozygotic twins having discordant treatment outcomes or maintenance profiles. The results of a study such as this in which one twin has maintained treatment gains while his or her monozygotic co-twin has relapsed might be useful in identifying factors that facilitate the maintenance process.

4. *Increase the pool of high-density pedigrees for genetic modeling and linkage analyses.* Because evidence to support a major gene effect for stuttering has been identified in at least

one segregation study, there is justification for the aggressive pursuit of families for molecular linkage analyses. Recently, there has been a trend in psychiatry to improve the generalizability of linkage findings by examining family members from multiple, "typical" pedigrees, rather than selectively recruiting one or two unusually dense families. This strategy has several advantages, not the least of which is simplified family identification, and should be considered for future molecular studies of stuttering.

Investigators should be alert to the possibility that stuttering may co-occur with other phenotypic markers in some families when assessments are done. Hays and Field (1989), for example, reported on three families in which stuttering and manic-depressive disorder coexisted at rates that were much greater than chance. Although the significance of this observation is unknown, the possibility that bipolar disorder may provide a useful marker for some families should encourage stuttering researchers to include a psychiatric screening in pedigree assessment batteries.

SUMMARY

Some clinicians and graduate students may view genetics research as a remote enterprise that has limited relevance to real-world clinical problems. After all, there is no reason to believe that findings from behavior genetics studies will lead to an imminent cure for stuttering or will be useful in determining the most suitable therapy program for a given client. In fact, some clinicians may feel uncomfortable with this line of investigation, fearing that some clients will use cries of genetic predisposition to abdicate responsibility for their own recovery. Similarly, some may perceive that the probability for long-term maintenance of treatment gains among adult clients will be further compromised if stuttering is found to have a genetic basis. Trepidations such as these must be accepted as reasonable and countered with empirical evidence. There is no reason to expect that behavioral treatment will change dramatically if stuttering is found to be a highly heritable condition. We will still need well-trained speech-language pathologists to work individually with dysfluent clients, even if supplementary forms of intervention, such as palliative drugs, are developed as an outgrowth of genetics research. Perhaps most importantly, both researchers and clinicians must be cognizant of the emotionality that discussions of genetic predisposition can incite in the public, particularly within families with stuttering members. Accordingly, when communicating the results of genetic studies of stuttering to others, it is important that both the promise and the limitations of the work be clearly represented. At the beginning of this chapter, a number of provocative questions about gene therapy, pharmacological treatments, and genetic counseling were posed. By now, it should be apparent that we are still a substantial distance away from having definitive answers to these questions. While it is clear that genetic factors will play a role in our ultimate understanding of this complex and puzzling disorder, the prominence, nature, and implications of these factors remain over the horizon.

REFERENCES

Adams, M.R. (1990). The demands and capacities model I: Theoretical elaborations. *Journal of Fluency Disorders, 15*, 135–141.

Alfonso, P.J. (1990). Subject definition and selection criteria for stuttering research in adult subjects. In J.A. Cooper (Ed.), *Research needs in stuttering: Roadblocks and future directions* (ASHA Reports 18, pp. 15–24). Rockville: American Speech-Language Hearing Association.

Ambrose, N.G., Yairi, E., & Cox, N. (1993). Genetic aspects of early childhood stuttering. *Journal of Speech and Hearing Research, 36*, 701–706.

Andrews, G., Craig, A., Feyer, A., Hoddinot, S., Howie, P., & Neilson, M. (1983). Stuttering: A review of research findings and theories circa 1982. *Journal of Speech and Hearing Disorders, 48*, 226–246.

Andrews, G., & Harris, M. (1964). *The syndrome of stuttering*. London: Spastics Society Medical Education and Information Unit.

Andrews, G., Morris-Yates, A., Howie, P., & Martin, N. (1991). Genetic factors in stuttering confirmed (letter). *Archives General Psychiatry, 48*, 1034–1035.

Berry, M.F. (1938). A common denominator in twinning and stuttering. *Journal of Speech Disorders, 3*, 51–57.

Bloodstein, O. (1981). *A handbook on stuttering*. (3rd ed.). Chicago: National Easter Seal Society.

Bloodstein, O. (1993). *Stuttering: The search for a cause and cure*. Boston: Allyn and Bacon.

Boberg, E., Howie, P., & Woods, L. (1986). Mainte- nance of fluency: A review. In G.H. Shames & H. Rubin (Eds.), *Stuttering: Then and now* (pp. 489–500). Columbus: Charles E. Merrill Publishing Co.

Borden, G.J. (1990). Subtyping adult stutterers for research purposes. In J.A. Cooper (Ed.), *Research needs in stuttering: Roadblocks and future directions* (ASHA Reports 18, pp. 58–62). Rockville: American Speech-Language Hearing Association.

Chapman, T.F., Mannuzza, S., Klein, D.F., & Fyer, A.J. (1994). Effects of informant mental disorder on psychiatric family history data. *American Journal of Psychiatry, 151*, 574–579.

Cooper, E.B. (1972). Recovery from stuttering in a junior and senior high school population. *Journal of Speech and Hearing Research, 15*, 632–638.

Cooper, E.B., & Cooper, C.S. (1985). *Cooper personalized fluency control therapy handbook*. Allen: DLM Teaching Resources.

Cox, N. (1988). Molecular genetics: The key to the puzzle of stuttering? *Asha, 30*, 36–40.

Cox, N., Kramer, P., & Kidd, K. (1984). Segregation analyses of stuttering. *Genetic Epidemiology, 1*, 245–253.

Dobzhansky, T.G. (1956). *The biological basis of human freedom*. New York: Columbia University Press.

Felsenfeld, S. (1994). Developmental speech and language disorders. In J.C. DeFries, R. Plomin, & D.W. Fulker (Eds.), *Nature and nurture during middle childhood* (pp. 102–119). Oxford: Blackwell.

Felsenfeld, S. (1995). Speech outcomes in adopted children with a positive and negative parental history of speech disorder. Paper presented at the annual meeting of the Behavior Genetics Association. Richmond, Virginia.

Franken, M., Boves, L., Peters, H.F.M., & Webster, R.L. (1995). Perceptual rating instrument for speech evaluation of stuttering treatment. *Journal of Speech and Hearing Research, 38,* 280–288.

Gray, M. (1940). The X family: A clinical and laboratory study of a "stuttering" family. *Journal of Speech and Hearing Disorders, 5,* 343–348.

Hays, P., & Field, L.L. (1989). Postulated genetic linkage between manic-depression and stuttering. *Journal of Affective Disorders, 16,* 37–40.

Hedges, D.W., Umar, F., Mellon, C.D., Herrick, L.C., Hanson, M.L., & Wahl, M.J. (1995). Direct comparison of the family history method and the family study method using a large stuttering pedigree. *Journal of Fluency Disorders, 20,* 25–33.

Howie, P. (1981a). Concordance for stuttering in monozygotic and dizygotic twin pairs. *Journal of Speech and Hearing Disorders, 24,* 317–321.

Howie, P. (1981b). Intrapair similarity in frequency of disfluency in monozygotic and dizygotic twin pairs containing stutterers. *Behavior Genetics, 11,* 227–238.

Janssen, P., Kraaimaat, F., & Brutten, G. (1990). Relationship between stutterers' genetic history and speech-associated variables. *Journal of Fluency Disorders, 15,* 39–48.

Johnson, W. (1959). *The onset of stuttering.* Minneapolis: University of Minnesota Press.

Kamhi, A.G. (1982). The problems of relapse in stuttering: Some thoughts on what might cause it and how to deal with it. *Journal of Fluency Disorders, 7,* 459–467.

Kay, D.W. (1964). The genetics of stuttering. In G. Andrews & M. Harris (Eds.), *The syndrome of stuttering* (pp. 132–143). London: The Spastics Society Medical Education and Information Unit.

Kendler, K.S., Neale, M.C., Heath, A.C., Kessler, R.C., & Eaves, L. (1994). A twin-family study of alcoholism in women. *American Journal of Psychiatry, 151,* 707–715.

Kendler, K.S., Silberg, J.L., Neale, M.C., Kessler, R.C., Heath, A.C., Phil, D., & Eaves, L. (1991). The family history method: Whose psychiatric history is measured? *American Journal of Psychiatry, 148,* 1501–1504.

Kidd, K. (1980). Genetic models of stuttering. *Journal of Fluency Disorders, 5,* 187–201.

Kidd, K. (1984). Stuttering as a genetic disorder. In R.F. Curlee & W.H. Perkins (Eds.), *Nature and treatment of stuttering: New directions* (pp. 149–169). Boston: Allyn and Bacon.

Kidd, K., Kidd, J., & Records, M.A. (1978). The possible causes of the sex ratio in stuttering and its implications. *Journal of Fluency Disorders, 3,* 13–23.

Kidd, K., Heimbuch, R., & Records, M.A. (1981). Vertical transmission of susceptibility to stuttering with sex-modified expression. *Proceedings of the National Academy of Sciences, 78,* 606–610.

Kidd, K., Heimbuch, R., Records, M.A., Oehlert, G., & Webster, R. (1980). Familial stuttering patterns are not related to one measure of severity. *Journal of Speech and Hearing Research, 23,* 539–545.

Lalouel, J.M., & Morton, N.E. (1981). Complex segregation analysis with pointers. *Human Heredity, 31,* 312–321.

Loehlin, J.C. (1992). *Genes and environment in personality development.* Newbury Park: Sage Publications.

Ludlow, C.L. (1990). Research procedures for measuring stuttering severity. In J.A. Cooper (Ed.), *Research needs in stuttering: Roadblocks and future directions* (ASHA Reports 18, pp. 26–31). Rockville: American Speech-Language Hearing Association.

MacFarlane, W.B., Hanson, M., Walton, W., & Mellon, C.D. (1991). Stuttering in five generations of a single family. *Journal of Fluency Disorders, 16,* 117–123.

Nelson, S.F., Hunter, N., & Walter, M. (1945). Stuttering in twin types. *Journal of Speech Disorders, 10,* 335–343.

Peters, T.J., & Guitar, B. (1991). *Stuttering: An integrated approach to its nature and treatment.* Baltimore: Williams and Wilkins.

Pindzola, R.H., & White, D.T. (1986). A protocol for differentiating the incipient stutterer. *Language, Speech, and Hearing Services in Schools, 17,* 2–15.

Plomin, R., DeFries, J.C., & McClearn, G.E. (1980). *Behavioral genetics: A primer.* San Francisco: W.H. Freeman and Company.

Poulos, M., & Webster, W. (1991). Family history as a basis for subgrouping people who stutter. *Journal of Speech and Hearing Research, 34,* 5–10.

Rowe, D.C. (1994). *The limits of family influence: Genes, experience, and behavior.* New York: The Guilford Press.

Roy, M., Walsh, D., Prescott, C.A., & Kendler, K.S. (1994). Biases in the diagnosis of alcoholism by the family history method. *Alcoholism: Clinical and Experimental Research, 18*, 845–851.

Seider, R., Gladstein, K., & Kidd, K. (1983). Recovery and persistence of stuttering among relatives of stutterers. *Journal of Speech and Hearing Disorders, 48*, 394–402.

Sheehan, J., & Costley, M.S. (1977). A reexamination of the role of heredity in stuttering. *Journal of Speech and Hearing Disorders, 42*, 47–59.

Shriberg, L. (1993). Four new speech and prosody-voice measures for genetics research and other studies in developmental phonological disorders. *Journal of Speech and Hearing Research, 36*, 105–140.

Smith, A. (1990). Factors in the etiology of stuttering. In J.A. Cooper (Ed.), *Research needs in stuttering: Roadblocks and future directions* (ASHA Reports 18, pp. 39–47). Rockville: American Speech-Language Hearing Association.

Starkweather, C.W., & Gottwald, S.R. (1990). The demands and capacities model II: Clinical applications. *Journal of Fluency Disorders, 15*, 143–157.

Suarez, B.K., & Cox, N.J. (1985). Linkage analysis for psychiatric disorders I: Basic concepts. *Psychiatric Developments, 3*, 219–243.

Van Riper, C. (1982). *The nature of stuttering* (2nd ed.). Englewood Cliffs: Prentice-Hall.

Vandenberg, S.G., Singer, S.M., & Pauls, D.L. (1986). *The heredity of behavior disorders in adults and children* (pp. 231–235). New York: Plenum Medical Book Company.

Vogler, G.P., Gottesman, I.I., McGue, M.K., & Rao, D.C. (1990). Mixed-model segregation analysis of schizophrenia in the Lindelius Swedish pedigrees. *Behavior Genetics, 20*, 461–472.

Wachs, T.D. (1992). *The nature of nurture*. Newbury Park, CA: Sage Publications.

Wahlsten, D. (1994). The intelligence of heritability. *Canadian Psychology, 35*, 244–260.

Webster, W.G. (1993). Hurried hands and tangled tongues: Implications of current research for the management of stuttering. In E. Boberg (Ed.), *Neuropsychology of stuttering* (pp. 73–127). Edmonton: The University of Alberta Press.

Wepman, J. (1939). Familial incidence of stammering. *Journal of Heredity, 30*, 199–204.

West, R., Nelson, S., & Berry, M. (1939). The heredity of stuttering. *Quarterly Journal of Speech, 25*, 23–30.

Wingate, M. (1986). Physiological and genetic factors. In G.H. Shames & H. Rubin (Eds.), *Stuttering: Then and now* (pp. 49–69). Columbus: Charles E. Merrill Publishing Co.

SUGGESTED READINGS

Cooper, J. (Ed.) (1990). *Research needs in stuttering: Roadblocks and future directions* (ASHA Reports 18). Rockville, MD: American Speech-Language-Hearing Association. This edited volume highlights several prominent research areas in stuttering, with an emphasis on directions for future research. Several of the chapters are of particular relevance for those interested in behavioral genetics topics; notably, chapters by Alfonso on subject selection criteria, Ludlow on measuring stuttering severity, Pauls on genetic factors, Smith on intrinsic and extrinsic etiological factors, Borden on subtyping adult stutterers for research, and McClean on neuromotor aspects of stuttering.

Gould, S.J. (1981). *The mismeasure of man*. New York: W.W. Norton & Company. This is a lively and very engaging nonacademic text written by an evolutionary biologist. The author's principal thesis is that our current and historical proclivity to measure individual differences, particularly intelligence, from a hereditarian perspective has been misguided. While not without its faults, this text makes several important points and provides a well-reasoned critical perspective that should be understood and valued by those interested in the "nature-nurture" debate.

Loehlin, J.C. (1992). *Genes and environment in personality development*. (Individual Differences and Development Series). Newbury Park, CA: Sage Publications. This is a brief and readable text that provides an excellent introduction to the theoretical underpinnings and principal methodologies of the field of behavior genetics. Although the text focuses on behavioral genetic studies of personality development (itself an interesting area), the principles can be translated easily to fit content areas of more direct interest to stuttering researchers.

Wachs, T.D. (1992). *The nature of nurture*. (Individual Differences and Development Series). Newbury Park, CA: Sage Publications. This text provides a discussion of concepts and evidence pertaining to the effect of the environment on human development, with particular emphasis on "organism-environment covariance." Issues such as how individuals respond differently to stress, medical treatment, parenting styles, teaching approaches, and day-care centers are explored, often from a cross-cultural perspective. Perhaps more importantly, the author provides valuable guidance about ways in which the environment can be conceptualized and measured for research purposes, a topic that has received too little attention in the speech and language development literature.

CHAPTER 2

HOME ENVIRONMENT AND PARENT-CHILD INTERACTION IN CHILDHOOD STUTTERING

EHUD YAIRI

INTRODUCTION

The home environment of people who stutter, especially during early childhood, has played a central role in theory, research, and clinical intervention with early childhood stuttering. Some theoretical views blame stuttering on parental behavior, and parents are the targets of intervention in several clinical programs. Indeed, the importance placed on the home environments of stuttering children is clearly reflected in the large number of references in the literature on this topic. Schuell (1949) underlined this point with her statement that "it is impossible to escape the need for working with the parents of the young child who stutters" (p. 251). Because of the unusual crossing of theoretical-clinical interests and the inclusion of parents and sometimes the entire nuclear family in stuttering treatment, ongoing reassessment of the accumulating data in light of this view about stuttering and its pathognomy is necessary. In my opinion, advancement of knowledge about stuttering has greatly outpaced knowledge about the stutterer's home environment.

ACKNOWLEDGMENT: This chapter was prepared with the support of grant #2 R01-DC00459 from the National Institute on Deafness and Other Communication Disorders, National Institutes of Health.

Thus, as the level of sophistication in advising parents about the nature of the disorder has increased, the database needed to enhance counseling them has lagged behind. For example, although it has been demonstrated that slow speech ameliorates stuttering, the effect of advising parents to use slow speech has not been adequately tested.

This chapter explores the sources that have contributed to the information on stuttering children's home environments and reviews, organizes, and critiques the pertinent research literature as I understand it. Each area of information is briefly summarized with specific conclusions. Because this review is research oriented, references that do not report quantified or otherwise organized data have not been included. On the other hand, you will also find several sources that were not included in previous reviews of the literature. Additionally, due to space limitations and my effort to minimize overlap with chapters on clinical intervention, I have focused on the home environment in its unaltered state. Thus, studies reporting descriptive data on parental speaking rate are included, but those that have manipulated parents' speech are not. Lastly, I assess the overall impact of these findings, derive specific clinical implications, evaluate the quality of available research, and suggest future directions for study.

SIGNIFICANCE OF THE HOME ENVIRONMENT

The impact of home environments can best be appreciated by recognizing the multiple, widely different sources that have contributed to highlighting the importance of this aspect to childhood stuttering. There are eight such contributors.

Psychoanalytic Perspectives

Psychogenic perspectives of stuttering were the earliest major influence. Brill (1923), Coriat (1943), Fenichel (1945), Glauber (1958) and others expressed the psychoanalytic view that stuttering represents a symptom of psychosexual fixation that originated from a child's unconscious conflicts over unsatisfied needs. It was suggested that these conflicts could be traced to neurotic parental personalities and their conflict-motivated behaviors. Such views led to research on parents' personalities and emotional adjustment (e.g., LaFollette, 1956), as well as to parent-oriented psychotherapies (Glauber, 1958; Glasner, 1962; Wakaba, 1992).

Child's Conscious Awareness of Stuttering

The writings of Froeschels (1921) on the mild nature of incipient stuttering and especially Bluemel's (1932) view of "primary" stuttering as simple, effortless repetitions of which the child is not aware, set the stage for the widely accepted belief that becoming aware of disfluencies is a necessary element in the transition to "secondary" stuttering, which is characterized by negative emotions and physical tension. Minimizing a child's awareness of speaking difficulties as a means of preventing an advanced, more severe form of the disorder became a significant theoretical issue that soon had clinical consequences. Indeed, several years later, Van Riper (1939) amplified Bluemel's concept of "primary" and "secondary" stuttering and drew attention to the home environments of children who stutter. He emphasized that prevention of awareness was es-

sential in treating primary stuttering and advocated that parents become the focus of treatment while "letting the child alone."

Diagnosogenic Theory and Its Implications

The subsequent emergence of Johnson's diagnosogenic theory (Johnson, 1942; Johnson et al., 1959) hypothesized a multifaceted, pressure-creating home environment that was destined to foster stuttering in young children. A scenario was drawn that depicted parents as being overly sensitized to their child's speech by virtue of their familial history of stuttering. These worrisome parents were also seen as being driven by inner perfectionistic attitudes and high standards for both their children and themselves. With this hypothesized home atmosphere in the background, Johnson's belief that calling attention to the child's speech is the immediate cause of stuttering was crystallized and resulted in the often repeated epigram that stuttering begins in the parent's ear, not in the child's mouth (Johnson, 1955). Because much of the blame was placed on parents of young stutterers, they were the prime targets of therapy, namely counseling, with the dual objectives of preventing the child from becoming aware of disfluencies while modifying the pressure-inclined parental attitudes.

Research into Parental Role

Research of stutterers' home environment prompted by the diagnosogenic and psychogenic theories of stuttering had an influence of its own. During the 1950s and 1960s, scientific work in this area peaked and findings were generally interpreted to indicate that stutterers, as a group, were subject to more adverse parental pressures and negative attitudes than were control group children. Domination, overprotection, high expectations, and perfectionism in child rearing (e.g., cleanliness, eating, toilet habits, manners, speech) as well as feelings of rejection and undesirable evaluations of the child's personality, were among the characteristic parental behavior patterns identified

(Abbott, 1957; Darley, 1955; Despert, 1946; Glasner, 1949, Goldman & Shames, 1964a; Johnson et al., 1959; Kinstler, 1961; Moncur, 1951, 1952). Such findings reinforced stereotypic concepts about stutterers' parents that were originally formed under the influence of the diagnosogenic and psychogenic theories. They also reinforced the inclination to focus treatment on reducing parental pressure and improving parent-child interactions.

Sociocultural Factors

Reported differences in the incidence of stuttering in different cultures (e.g., Lemert, 1953; Snidecor, 1947) and socioeconomic groups (Morgenstern, 1956) also drew attention to child-rearing practices as a causative agent in stuttering onset. The typical interpretation of the inconsistent findings supporting such differences emphasized pressure from either high cultural values for speech skills or familial aspirations for social and economic advancement.

Parental Role in Spontaneous Recovery

A relatively late influence that highlighted the role of home environments in stuttering emerged from interpretations of data on spontaneous recovery. Acceptance of the frequent remissions observed among young stutterers as "spontaneous" was challenged by Wingate (1976), Ingham (1981), and Martin and Lindamood (1986) in critical reappraisals of the literature. They concluded that, far from being "spontaneous," such recoveries were likely to have been effected, at least partially, by parental corrections of their children's stuttering. This view, then, shifted the focus from the home environment as an etiologic factor to its presumed therapeutic benefits. The implications of this view, which were incompatible with those of counseling, encouraged active parental reaction to a child's overt stuttering. Curiously, both Wingate and Ingham advocated a belief in parents' power to change stuttering into normal speech through correction and negative reactions to the child's disfluencies but expressed doubt about the diagnosogenic theo-

ry's supposition that similar parental behaviors could change normal speech into stuttering.

Parental Role in Clinical Intervention

Beliefs that parents' speech can greatly affect the onset, maintenance, and complexity of stuttering have found expression in both parent counseling and speech therapy strategies. Advice that parents should employ "good speech," "smooth speech," "slow speech," and "simple language" can be found in the professional literature dating back several decades (e.g., Bender, 1943; Bluemel, 1959; Murphy & Fitzsimmons, 1960; Van Riper, 1939; Wyatt & Herzen, 1962) and has become standard advice in parent counseling. Recently, efforts to facilitate slow or paced speaking patterns in stuttering children in direct treatment programs (Coppola & Yairi, 1982; Shine, 1980) have become popular, as has the inclusion of parents in therapeutic programs. Empirical support of the belief that parents' speech patterns influence their child's fluency is minimal, and the data are not easily interpreted (Bernstein Ratner, 1993). Nevertheless, having parents slow their speaking rates has been advocated as an efficient way to slow a child's speech rate (Ramig, 1993; Starkweather, Gottwald, & Halfond, 1990). Other aspects of communication, such as eliminating or decreasing interruptions and slowing turn-taking, are also used (Botterill, Kelman, & Rustin, 1994; Rustin, 1987). Thus, parents' presence in therapy sessions as observers or active participants and their implementation of home programs to facilitate generalization and maintenance increased significantly in recent years. The growing role of parents' verbal and nonverbal communication behavior in the therapeutic process has also instigated experimental scrutiny of the assumed relation between parents' and children's speech.

Genetic Perspectives

The fact that stuttering runs in families has been documented over a long period (Bryngelson & Rutherford, 1937; Yairi & Ambrose, 1992). Genetic interpretations were offered relatively early in the history of modern research (Nelson, 1939), but psychosocial explanations that stuttering runs in families by virtue of the adoption of anxious attitudes by successive generations of the family prevailed for several decades (Johnson, 1942; Johnson et al., 1959). Although the etiologic weakness of Johnson's psychosocial interpretations of familial incidence is now recognized, it is reasonable to assume that the presence of family members who stutter, or the memory of deceased ones, would likely promote comments, comparisons, and a general atmosphere of interest in, or concern about, the disorder. More recently, the evidence for a major genetic factor in stuttering, including specific models of transmission (Ambrose, Yairi, & Cox, 1993; Kidd, 1984), has become so strong that genetics appears to be the most solidly established source of influence in the home environments of children who stutter.

RESEARCH OF THE HOME ENVIRONMENT

In what kind of family is a child who stutters raised? This is the basic question posed by investigators of the home environment of people who stutter. As we will see, a broad spectrum of research methods has been employed to study the many facets of these environments. Incidence surveys were used to examine the relation of stuttering to the socioeconomic status of families, while familial pedigree analyses have been used to test genetic models. Formal psychological tests, personal interviews, and questionnaires appear to have been the most commonly used techniques for studying parents' personality and attitudes. Direct observations of parent-child interactions as well as analyses of the speech characteristics of parents have increased recently. Most investigators have focused on parents, although a few have studied the child's perception of the parents. In addition, most of this research has been descriptive in nature, with only a few studies relying on controlled, experimental manipulation.

The following review is organized around issues that are related to the major sources of influ-

ence just discussed. The number of areas covered is expanded, however, and their order is not directly parallel. To facilitate a better appreciation of the strengths and weaknesses of research findings, information about the subjects, children and/or parents, is included when available so that the characteristics of the population samples employed can be considered. Careful analysis reveals several important limitations or weaknesses. For example, one critical problem is that much of this information has been gathered at a time that was far removed from the onset or early stages of the disorder. In many studies in which groups of parents were compared, the children were matched but not the parents. Finally, little if any attention has been given to subgrouping families on familial history of stuttering.

Genetic Considerations

According to Andrews and Harris (1964), the chances that children who stutter will have other family members who stutter are three to four times higher than that of nonstutterers. Support for this conclusion began with an early study by Bryngelson and Rutherford (1937) which reported a positive familial history of stuttering in 46 percent of 74 stuttering children, but only 18 percent among nonstuttering comparison subjects. This pattern occurs in many later studies that gathered data on the percentage of subjects having positive family histories of stuttering, although the percentages found have varied greatly. Accordi and colleagues (Accordi, Bianchi, Consolaro, Tronchin, DeFilippi, et al., 1983) reported familial history of stuttering in 50 percent of 2802 stutterers, but only 6.6 percent in 1602 nonstuttering control subjects. In 1977, Sheehan and Costley reviewed nineteen such studies and reported that the percentages of stutterers having a family history of stuttering ranged from 12 percent to 74 percent. The mean of the means of these studies, which I calculated, approximates 42 percent. The percentages among the nonstuttering comparison subjects ranged from 1.3 percent to 42 percent, with a mean of means approximating 14 percent. These differences likely reflect sampling biases related to age, sex, type of relatives included, or knowledge of family history, among other factors. (See review of the literature on genetics of stuttering by Yairi, Ambrose & Cox, in press) Subjects' ages in the large Accordi and colleagues (1983) investigation were not specified; therefore, two investigations of preschool children near the onset of stuttering in which information on familial incidence was obtained are of particular interest. As a consequence of the subjects' young age and the investigators' long-term contact with subjects' families, information about family history could be verified because most relatives of interest were still alive. Additionally, because of the subjects' proximity to onset, samples were not biased by an overrepresentation of older, chronic stutterers, or by an alteration in sex-ratio that typically occurs with age. In the first study, Yairi (1983) reported stuttering in the immediate family of 45 percent of twenty-three young stutterers, ages 2 to 3, which increased to 64 percent when extended families (grandparents, aunts, uncles, and cousins) were included. In the second study, which included sixty-nine stuttering children and their families (Ambrose, Yairi, & Cox, 1993), a preschool child who begins to stutter had a 43 percent chance of having a stutterer in the immediate family and a 71 percent chance in the extended family.

Reporting percentages of families with histories of stuttering is common, but such data do not provide adequate genetic information, because they fail to account for differences in family size. A single occurrence of stuttering in a large family carries the same weight as a single occurrence in a small family in such studies. For accurate analyses, complete pedigrees and total counts of family members are required (Kidd, 1984). Using this method, Ambrose, Yairi, and Cox (1993) calculated the chances of preschool children who stutter (mean age = 40 months) and are at early stages of the disorder having stuttering relatives in various categories. Their results are presented, with minor modifications, in Table 2.1. As can be seen, as many as 27 percent of these children had one parent who stuttered, and 43 percent had members of their immediate family with a stuttering history. In addition, the percentage of boys having parents with a positive stuttering history was about three times higher than that of girls, whereas the percentages of girls having siblings who stuttered were nearly twice as high as those of boys.

Such basic epidemiologic information about stuttering has been largely overlooked in research

TABLE 2.1 Proportion of Stuttering Family Members in Each Class of Relatives of Male and Female Children Who Stutter

RELATIVES	MALE PROBANDS	FEMALE PROBANDS	TOTAL
Fathers	15/48=.313	1/21=.048	.232
Mothers	2/48=.042	1/21=.048	.043
Brothers	9/37=.243	3/9=.333	.261
Sisters	3/28=.107	4/10=.400	.184
Grandfathers	6/96=.063	1/42=.024	.051
Grandmothers	3/96=.031	4/42=.095	.051
Uncles	10/146=.068	3/50=.060	.066
Aunts	1/114=.009	0/71=.000	.005
Male cousins	14/192=.073	6/85=.071	.072
Female cousins	5/183=.027	0/71=.000	.020

Adapted from Ambrose, N., Yairi, E., & Cox, N. (1993). Genetic aspects of early childhood stuttering. *Journal of Speech and Hearing Research, 36,* 701–706.

of home environments of children who stutter. In view of the evidence from family relations and child development disciplines that parents' childhood histories serve as a working model for parenting style (Puttalaz, Constanzo, & Smith, 1991), it is plausible that the home environments of 27 percent of stuttering children whose parents had stuttered would differ from those of children not having such backgrounds. As will be discussed later, several aspects of home environments—such as parents' education and social status—might be better understood if genetic factors were accounted for. Unfortunately, except for a single study (Cox, Seider, & Kidd, 1984), differences in this important factor have not been considered by investigators who have looked at the psychosocial or speech characteristics of parents of stutterers.

Nevertheless, genetic influences on the home environment of children who stutter may be gaining in practical significance. One potential contribution is the early prediction of the course of stuttering. In a preliminary report of a three-year, longitudinal investigation, Yairi, Ambrose, Paden, and Throneburg (1996) presented findings from twenty preschool age children who recovered from stuttering without receiving therapy and from twelve who persisted in stuttering. They found that chronicity and recovery were significantly related to the outcomes reported among relatives. Thus, children from families with chronic stutterers among immediate or extended family members had a higher risk of continuing to stutter than did children from families with recovered stutterers.

Family Structure and Style

Other researchers have explored a variety of other familial characteristics. For example, Johnson and colleagues (1959) compared parents of 150 children who stuttered, ages 2 to 8, with a like number of parents of matched nonstuttering children using extensive interviews guided by a standard questionnaire. Parents of stutterers had significantly less formal education than did parents of nonstutterers, and they also tended to be older than the

control parents were at the time of the interview, their marriage, and the birth of the stuttering child. The two groups also differed significantly on several items believed to reflect social attitudes. Mothers and fathers of stuttering children reported having fewer social interests, such as belonging to organizations, assigned lower ratings to the value of friendship, evaluated neighbors as less friendly, and said they spent less time in family activities (e.g., games and picnics) than did control parents. Parents of children who stutter were less satisfied with their spouses' behaviors, reporting more that were likely to create a tense, undesirable, emotional, and unfavorable home environment. The latter findings were supported by Rustin and Purser (1991) whose study of the families of 209 stuttering children, but no control group, reported that a high proportion of couples in their sample did not enjoy fulfilling relationships.

Perhaps the most in-depth research on familial characteristics was conducted by Andrews and Harris (1964) in a study of eighty English school-age children who stuttered and a matched control group. Unfortunately, information on families was obtained only from mothers. Findings from structured interviews indicated that there were no statistically significant between-group differences in mothers' ages at marriage or at birth of the stuttering child, fathers' ages relative to the mothers', or the number of children in the family. Andrews and Harris also coded interview responses as they related to intactness of the family, quality of joint family life, housing, and relationships with extended family. Although the families of stutterers did more poorly on each of these indices, only the difference in housing (number of rooms) was statistically significant. One of the more important findings of this study, however, was that mothers of stutterers were significantly poorer in school achievement and work history, and more were below average intelligence.

These two investigations, which are among the largest and most cited studies on familial characteristics of stutterers, agree on three tendencies. Compared with nonstuttering children, stuttering children are more likely to be raised (1) in less harmonious families, (2) in less sociable and less close families, and (3) by parents having less formal education and/or lower intelligence. Although these are characteristics of many families whose children do not stutter, such home environments may exacerbate conditions that lead to speech difficulties and withdrawal tendencies. Whether such tendencies are forged primarily by parents who stutter, especially fathers, whose personal inhibitions led them to marry later, maintain more isolated social lives, and obtain lower levels of education, is not known. It is also plausible that the lower parental education levels reported by Johnson and colleagues (1959), and the poorer education achievements and lower intelligence of mothers reported by Andrews and Harris (1964), may contribute to the increased incidence of difficulties in speech, language, and academic development that has been found among stuttering children.

Minimal attention has been given to family size and structure. Morgenstern (1956) and Andrews and Harris (1964) reported no difference in the number of children in families of children who stutter and that of control families. Several investigators, however, have examined the family positions of children who stutter. An early study by Rotter (1939) surveyed 522 stutterers, 425 males and 97 females, who ranged in age from 2.5 to 44 years (median = 14 years). Only 18 were below age 5. The percentages of only, oldest, youngest, and middle children were compared to census norms for junior high students, and significantly more only children (20% vs. 12%) and fewer middle children (27% vs. 36%) were found among the stuttering group than in the census data. Ten years later, Boland (1949) reported that the number of older and only children was significantly higher in a sample of 262 white persons who stuttered and ranged from 4 to 56 years of age (M = 17 years) than that among a large sample of the general population. Similarly, Johnson and colleagues (1959) found more stuttering than control children were the first or only child and that the combined category of "oldest" and "only" children accounted for 54 percent of the stuttering group but only 37 per-

cent of the control group, a difference that was statistically significant. Morgenstern (1956) and Andrews and Harris (1964), on the other hand, concluded that being an older or a younger child was not related to stuttering. The previously cited study of Rustin and Purser (1991), whose sample comprised 209 stuttering children of mostly school and high school age, reported that the birth order of their subjects "clearly shows a bias toward youngest and eldest children . . ." There was, however, no control group.

Some research has also been directed toward age differences between siblings. Rotter (1939) reported that the age gaps between stutterers and their nearest sibling was significantly greater, by an average of one year, than the gaps between siblings in nonstuttering families. Assuming that only children and more widely spread children receive more attention, Rotter concluded that such gaps are likely to encourage parents to pamper or overprotect these children in ways that promote stuttering. Findings of larger spacings between children in families of children who stutter than in families with nonstuttering children were also reported by Morgenstern (1956). He, too, hypothesized that children who are further apart in age from siblings are likely to draw more parental attention, including comments on their speech, which may lead to heightened self-consciousness and stuttering. Andrews and Harris (1964), however, appear to be the main source of contradictory findings in this area. They reported no group differences in the number of children or age gaps between siblings.

In summary, the connections, if any, between sibling constellation and stuttering are unclear because of contradictory data. Three studies concluded that stutterers tend to be only or oldest children more frequently than are control speakers, two found no differences, and one study reported a double bias toward either the oldest or youngest position. Likewise, two studies reported wider age gaps between siblings in families of stuttering children than in control families, but one study found no such differences.

Socioeconomic Status

The socioeconomic distribution of a disorder cannot be assessed with an acceptable level of precision if reliable data on national norms are not available, if samples are not carefully selected to represent the population at large, or if referral trends in various segments of the population are not known. Four investigations, three American and one British, all published during the middle 1950s, examined this factor.

In a study whose main focus was the educational adjustment of stutterers, Schindler (1955) surveyed 20,000 school-age children, grades K through 12, in five Iowa counties. Information on parent occupation revealed no statistically significant differences across the seven occupational categories studied between the parents of seventy-nine children who stuttered and those of nonstuttering children in the survey. It was noted, however, that about one-third of the parents of stutterers were in the upper three occupation categories, whereas only one-sixth of control parents were in these levels. A stronger trend in this direction was indicated in two studies that were primarily concerned about the onset of stuttering. Darley (1955) found that 80 percent of his fifty stuttering children, ages 2 to 14, came from middle and upper socioeconomic class homes. Johnson and colleagues (1959) reported that approximately 70 percent of the 150 stuttering children in their sample came from middle and upper class families, although middle class subjects represented the lower end of this class. Only a single investigation, which was conducted in Scotland (Morgenstern, 1956), was designed specifically to analyze the incidence of stuttering in relation to the distribution of socioeconomic characteristics of families in the population. Morgenstern's main advantage was a national survey on socioeconomic characteristics, which had been completed in Scotland several years earlier. In his survey of 355 11-year old Scottish children who stuttered, 289 boys and 66 girls, Morgenstern found significant differences between the social class distribution of

this sample and that of the national survey. The number of stutterers in families of semiskilled laborers exceeded the number expected in nine classes of fathers' occupations. At the same time, the percentage of stuttering children living in less crowded quarters was higher than expected.

Thus, American studies have reported that stuttering occurs more often in families in the upper half of the population's socioeconomic groups, whereas Morgenstern's Scottish investigation found more in those families just above the low end of the socioeconomic distribution. Considering its superior norms, the latter is probably more accurate, but further verification is needed. It is interesting to note that in spite of the disparity in their results, all investigators speculated that higher incidences of stuttering, whether in semiskilled or middle class workers, may have resulted from upward social mobility pressures. If there are socioeconomic influences, they appear to be quite diffuse.

Parents' Personality and Affect

A logical consequence of theoretical notions that the etiology of stuttering rests within parental psychopathologies and disturbed parent-child relations was research that examined parents' personalities. A total of eleven investigations, many of which were conducted in the early-to-mid 1950s, explored this possibility using formal tests of personality or emotional adjustment that were administered to parents of stuttering children. Five yielded positive, and six, negative findings.

Projective techniques were used by two investigators. Wilson (1951) administered the Travis-Johnson Projection Test, the Thematic Apperception Test, and the Rorschach test to both parents of thirty stuttering children, ages 4 to 12. No control groups were included. Wilson interpreted mothers' responses as significantly high on the aggression-hostility factor of the Travis-Johnson Test, and as showing strong anxiety tendencies on the Rorschach. Fathers were reported to be high in their projection of hostile feelings. A year later,

Christensen (1952) administered the Rorschach to the same group of parents. His interpretation of their responses was that none of the fathers or mothers could be rated as adequate.

Three paper-and-pencil personality tests were employed in a third study conducted by LaFollette in 1956. This investigation was larger in scope than the previous two and included eighty-five sets of parents whose stuttering offspring ranged from 3 to 30 years of age. A control group of fifty parents of nonstutterers was also employed. Fathers of stuttering subjects were found to be less well adjusted on the McFarland and Seitz Psycho-Somatic Inventory than were fathers of nonstutterers. They were also more submissive on the Allport Ascendance-Submission Reaction Study than were mothers of stutterers or fathers of non-stutterers. Most of the differences between the two groups of fathers were contributed by fathers of older stutterers, those between 19 and 30 years of age. No differences were found on the California Test of Personality, and none of the tests differentiated the two groups of mothers.

Two later investigations also reported positive findings. Zenner, Ritterman, Bowen, and Gronhovd (1978) compared the anxiety levels of three groups of seven parents, each, of stuttering, articulatory defective, and normal-speaking children who were 4 to 10 years of age. Parents' general anxiety was measured first using the A-Trait portion of the Self-Evaluation Questionnaire. Then, following observation of videotapes of their own child and a child from each of the other two groups, parents were administered the situational anxiety portion (A-State) of the scale. Both parents of stutterers exhibited significantly higher levels of general anxiety than did parents of non-stutterers, with mothers having significantly higher levels than fathers. Parents of stutterers also evidenced significantly higher levels of situational anxiety after observing videotapes than did parents of the other two groups. A year later, Fluegel (1979) administered the Maudsley Personality Inventory to 124 mothers of stuttering children and 97 mothers of normally speaking control children. He reported significantly higher levels of Neuroti-cism and Extraversion compared to parents of nonstuttering children.

In a second group of investigations, all six studies used paper-and-pencil techniques, included both parents, and employed control groups. All yielded negative results. Three studies employed the well-known Minnesota Multiphasic Personality Inventory (MMPI). It was administered by Grossman (1951) to both parents of twenty-one stuttering children, ages 5 to 12,[1] by Goodstein and Dahlstrom (1956) to parents 100 young stutterers (mean age = 5:0 years), and by Goodstein (1956) to parents of fifty older children who stuttered (mean age = 10:10). Although all three investigations concluded that there were no major group differences, the parents of children who stuttered scored significantly higher than did parents of nonstuttering children on the anxiety scale. The latter parents scored significantly higher on dominance and defensiveness scales. Additionally, Grossman reported that parents of stutterers scored significantly higher on the F-Scale of MMPI. Higher scores on this scale are believed to indicate an inability to comprehend items or a tendency to interpret them in an atypical fashion. Also during the middle 1950s, Darley (1955) used the Inventory of Factors STDCR (Guilford, 1940) to assess two emotionality and three introversion-extroversion factors of personality. Again, no statistically significant differences were found between fifty pairs of parents of stuttering children (mean age = 9 years) and a like number of control parents.

An unusual research target in this area was described in the 1976 study by Feldman that examined parents' openness tendencies. He used a Self-Disclosure Questionnaire to compare thirty-two pairs of parents of stuttering children, ages 4 to 16 years (mean = 8.6), with a closely matched control group of parents. Although results indicated that the two groups did not differ significantly, Feldman noted that mothers of stutterers declined to disclose information more often than did con-

---

[1]Parents ranged from 26 to 52 years of age (M = 39).

trol mothers when requested by their spouses or children. Such behavior was interpreted as stifling spontaneity.

A more in-depth investigation of parent personality was conducted in Scotland by Andrews and Harris (1964). In this previously mentioned study, mothers of eighty school-age stuttering children and a control group of mothers underwent psychiatric interviews that revealed the two groups to be "remarkably similar" in the adequacy of the mothers' previous family life, childhood emotional adjustment, adolescence period, sexual maturation, sociability, and neuroticism. Two personality tests, the Maudsley Personality Inventory and the Cattel 16 Personality Factor Inventory, also indicated no significant differences. On the latter test, however, intelligence differences approached the level of statistical significance. The investigators realized from other parts of the study that there was a tendency for mothers of stutterers to fail in their school and work history and in providing an adequate home environment for their children, and they related such tendencies to these mothers' lower mental abilities.

In summary, of the five studies reporting positive findings, two (Christensen, 1952; Wilson, 1951) had no control subjects. In a third study (LaFolette, 1956), positive findings were limited to fathers, primarily those with adult stuttering offspring. Considering the number and scope of these investigations, the strength of the test instruments, and the use of control groups, the balance of research outcomes concerning the personality and emotional adjustment of parents of stuttering children clearly tips in favor of negative findings, that is, no major differences. Nevertheless, the heightened anxiety levels reported in three investigations (Fluegel, 1979; Goodstein, 1956; Zenner et al., 1978) should not be dismissed.

Parents' Attitudes and Behavior Management

A number of studies have focused on parents' day-to-day behavior and interactions with their children rather than on personality type or psychopathologic characteristics. Personal inter-

views and questionnaires have been the most commonly used procedures. Three investigators, Despert (1946), Glasner (1949), and Ritzman (1941), used informal, nonquantitative clinical assessment techniques without control groups. The earliest work, by Ritzman (1941)[2] as reported by Wingate (1962), described the attitudes of parents of stutterers as nonaccepting and coercive, which repressed the child's self-assertion. The more widely known report by Despert (1946) was based on clinical interviews of mothers of fifty stuttering children, ages 6 to 15 years. He concluded that most were domineering and anxious about food and the child's physical health. Early toilet training and daily use of coercive, punitive methods were also reported. Generally, these mothers were characterized as being overprotective and encouraging emotional dependency in their children. Fathers played only secondary roles. Similar observations of parental high standards plus overanxiousness, were reported by Glasner (1949) based on the case studies of seventy young stutterers, who were under age 5 years (M= 3:6), and their parents. Glasner concluded, however, that these parents' indecision and inconsistent behavior were the major adverse influences.

Several investigators obtained quantitative data from parents of stutterers and nonstutterers, primarily through structured interviews. A 330-item questionnaire was administered by Moncur (1951) to mothers of forty-eight children who stuttered, ages 5 to 8 years (Median = 6.6) and mostly boys, and to mothers of nonstuttering control children. He concluded that mothers of stutterers introduced adverse influences into their child-training practices of eating, sleeping, and toilet training by being overprotective and hypercritical and using oversupervision and harsh disciplinary measures. A further analysis of these data using parental domination criteria (Moncur, 1952) indicated that mothers of stutterers were more dominant than were mothers of nonstutterers and also

---

[2]I was unable to locate this reference or its discussion in other sources.

demanding and limiting in ways that subordinated their stuttering children. Grossman (1951) administered the Minnesota Scale of Parents' Opinion (MSPO), an 80-item questionnaire, to parents of twenty-one child stutterers. No significant difference was found on the first part of the instrument, which measures the degree of unfavorable control that parents exert over a child. The second part of the instrument measures parental ability to evaluate the desirability or undesirability of selected child behavior traits in terms of their contribution to the child's social and personality adjustment. Parents of stuttering children scored significantly lower than did control parents.

Considerably longer interviews, which were guided by questionnaires of nearly 850 items, were administered by Darley (1955) and Johnson and colleagues (1959) to both parents of stuttering and nonstuttering children.[3] The first study included the parents of two groups of fifty children each, ages 2 to 14 years. The second study interviewed the parents of two groups of 150 children each, all of whom were between 2 and 8 years of age. Questions covered a wide range of child-rearing practices and parent-child interactions. Both investigations concluded that parents of stuttering and nonstuttering children are more similar in attitudes than different. Powell (1966) arrived at a similar conclusion and presented the only racial perspective on this topic. He employed a 233-item questionnaire for his interviews with mothers of fifty Black stuttering children, ages 6 to 10 years (M = 8:9), and the mothers of fifty matched control subjects. His study was also unusual in its attempt to differentiate mothers' attitudes relative to stuttering severity. Results, however, indicated there were no differences between the two groups of mothers or among the mothers of children having different stuttering severities.

In spite of the general lack of significant findings across a wide range of parental attitudes in the Darley (1955) and Johnson and colleagues (1959) studies, there were several important exceptions. Both investigations agreed that parents of stutterers, especially mothers, had higher child development standards and were more demanding and less satisfied with their children. According to Darley's (1955) data, parents of stutterers more often reported that their children failed to meet their expectations in intelligence, school achievements, and speech development. Johnson and colleagues (1959) commented that they seemed to behave in ways "calculated to make tension in the home" (p. 227). Quarrington (1974), however, in a reanalysis of data from the Johnson study concluded that both parents of young, beginning stuttering children can be characterized as showing submissiveness, passivity, and low social domination. The emergence of punitive attitudes, he claimed, occurs in parents of older, chronic stutterers.

A potentially powerful test of the impact of familial attitudes and other home environment factors on stuttering was used in a unique investigation by Cox, Seider, and Kidd (1984) that yielded negative results. Reasoning that important home environment factors should be particularly apparent in families having high incidences of stuttering, the experimenters compared fourteen high-density, extended families having at least five members who stutter, with ten extended families free of stuttering as controls. Results of case interview questionnaires revealed no differences in the two groups' familial histories, and when one extreme case was eliminated from the data, no differences were found in the ways that parents of control subjects, parents of stutterers, recovered stutterers, and nonstutterers in the high-density families rated their children on the Child Trait Checklist (CTC). One problem with this study was that the age of the participants, the number of those who stuttered or were children or parents of stutterers, were not reported. Because most of the families had participated in previous studies of these investigators, it is likely that most were adults.

A crucial conclusion of Johnson and col-

---

[3]The first study in this series of "Iowa Studies" was published by Johnson in 1942 and also relied on extensive interviews with parents of forty-six young stuttering children and a group of matched control parents. These interviews, however, focused on health and developmental histories, and the circumstances surrounding the onset of stuttering with only minimal attention to parents' attitudes.

leagues (1959) was that parents of children who stutter view, as well as react to, normal disfluencies in their children's speech more negatively than do parents of nonstuttering children. This belief, which served as the main basis of the diagnosogenic theory, has not been supported by a number of studies. Some of Darley's (1955) less widely published data indicated there were no significant differences between the parents of stuttering and nonstuttering children on the Iowa Scale of Attitudes Toward Stuttering. Glasner and Rosenthal's (1957) study of parents of 153 first graders who stuttered concluded that parents' evaluations of disfluency as "stuttering" were not a matter of attitude but had an objective basis, because they correlated with the amount and type of disfluency exhibited by the child.

Three of four experimental studies that had parents judge tape-recorded speech samples have also provided evidence contrary to the Johnson (1959) conclusion. A classic study by Bloodstein, Jaeger, and Tureen (1952) asked parents of twelve stuttering children, ages 3 to 8 years, and parents of twelve age-matched nonstuttering children to identify stutterers from a series of speech samples recorded by these children but which excluded their own child's sample. Parents ranged in age from 25 to 43 years. Those whose children stuttered made "stutterer" judgments more frequently than did parents of nonstuttering children. Using a more elaborate design, Berlin (1960) compared the reactions of parents of children who stutter, of articulatory disordered children, and of normally speaking children as they listened to speech samples containing various amounts of simulated disfluencies. There were no group differences in concern expressed about disfluencies. Similarly, no differences were found by Curran and Hood (1977) between parents (sex unspecified) of ten stuttering and ten normally fluent children in grades 1 through 6 in evaluating tape-recorded samples of simulated disfluencies as "stuttering." More recently, Zebrowski and Conture (1989) instructed the mothers of ten children who were 3 to 5 years of age (M = 4:1) and within 12 months of stuttering onset, and ten mothers of nonstuttering

children to judge recordings of various types of simulated disfluencies as either "stuttered" or "not stuttered." Results indicated that the two groups of mothers did not differ significantly in overall judgments of disfluency, although they did differ on some specific disfluency types.

The information on parental attitudes described thus far was obtained from parents' reports. Some investigators, however, have directly observed interactions between stuttering and nonstuttering children and their parents. Presumably, this approach would provide more objective assessments. Abbott (1957) observed thirty mothers of stuttering children, ages 4:9 to 11:11, and thirty mothers of nonstuttering children matched for sex and age, as they interacted with their child during free play. Ten behavioral qualities were rated by an unseen observer. Mothers of stutterers were rated as displaying more affection, empathy, and overprotection toward their child than were mothers of nonstutterers. The tendency for overprotection was supported by results of a paper-and-pencil questionnaire, Parental Attitude Research Instrument (PARI), which was also administered to these mothers.

Using a different approach, Goldman and Shames (1964a) studied fifteen pairs of parents of stutterers and fifteen pairs whose children did not stutter. The groups were matched for socioeconomic status, education, age, and children's age. Parents estimated their performances on a simple motor task using the Rotter Board, which is sometimes called the Level of Aspiration Board (Rotter, 1942). The two groups of parents did not differ significantly in goal setting behavior for themselves. In a follow-up study, Goldman and Shames (1964b) matched twenty-four pairs of parents of stuttering children (M = 10:9) with those of normally speaking children and asked them to predict their child's performance on the Rotter Board task and on a storytelling task. The authors indicated that parents of stutterers, particularly fathers, expressed slightly higher expectations and set somewhat higher goals for their children on both tasks than did those of nonstutterers. They also implied that these parents should be counseled in order to realize the possible consequences of their unrealistic expectations, even though these tendencies were not statistically significant.

A few years later, Quarrington, Seligman, and Kosower (1969) replicated the Goldman and Shames (1964b) investigation, doubling sample size to twenty-eight parents of 2- to 6-year old stuttering children (M = 3:10 years) and twenty-eight control parents. Another strength of this study was that all of the stuttering children were within 4 to 32 weeks of stuttering onset (M = 21 weeks). Their results, in contrast to previous studies, indicated that mothers of stuttering children set lower goals for their children than did control group mothers. No differences were found for fathers.

Meyers and Freeman (1985c) compared twelve mothers of stuttering children, ages 4:0 to 5:11, with twelve mothers of nonstuttering children during social-communicative interactions. Parents were videotaped for ten minutes in free play with their own child, an unfamiliar stuttering child, and an unfamiliar nonstuttering child. Videotapes and transcripts were analyzed for language measures, interactional measures, such as time spent talking, how verbal interactions were initiated, and the types of utterances spoken. The two groups of mothers interacted with children similarly. Only one of thirteen variables yielded a significant group difference; mothers of nonstutterers used more routine statements, such as "thank you," "bye," "hi," and "let's see."

Overall, the investigations just summarized, whether based on parental reports or direct observations, have revealed few attitudinal, interaction, child-rearing, or goal-setting characteristics that distinguish the fathers and mothers of children who stutter from those of normally fluent children. The failure to find differences in parental goal-setting and/or expectations, does not support important assumptions of the diagnosogenic theory about the onset of stuttering. As we shall see later, the assumption about parents' negative evaluations of disfluencies has also been challenged. Although inconsistent findings characterize this area of study, there is one common, positive finding: Parents of children who stutter are overprotective and overanxious about their children more frequently than are parents of normally fluent children. Both clinically oriented reports of Despert (1946) and Moncur (1951) as well as more structured studies, several of which were large in scale, by Abbott (1957), Darley (1955), Glasner and Rosenthal (1957), and Johnson and colleagues (1959), all point to the same conclusion. In this context, it is interesting to recall Rotter's (1939) interpretations of findings that children who stutter are more likely to be a first child and/or more separated in years from siblings than are other children. Assuming that only children and/or more isolated children receive extra attention while middle children receive less attention than other siblings, Rotter stated that "this order can best be looked on as that in which we would expect the child to be pampered . . ." (p. 145). Such "pampering" as overprotection, oversolicitous and overanxious parental attitudes was assumed by Rotter to promote the development of stuttering.

Parents' Underlying Feelings and Perceptions of a Stuttering Child

Parents' underlying feelings toward a child, which may be reflected in subtle behavior, could be as critical to the child's mental health as their observable behavior—perhaps even more so. The assumption that how a parent feels is more important than what the parent does led to Kinstler's (1961) study. It utilized a projective-type questionnaire, the Maternal Attitude Scale, to study overt and covert rejection in thirty mothers of children who stuttered, ages 3:6 to 14 (M = 7.46), and a matched group of mothers of nonstuttering children. Mothers of stutterers responded to more items that expressed rejection of their children than to those expressing acceptance. The opposite was true for mothers of nonstutterers. Kinstler interpreted these results as showing that mothers of stutterers reject their children covertly far more, but overtly far less than do mothers of nonstutterers.

Another facet of parents' feelings may be found in how they describe their children's personalities. Such information has been reported in portions of several of the studies mentioned earlier. Christensen (1952) had both parents of thirty stuttering children, ages 4 to 12 years, rate their stuttering child and a sibling, who was not always of the same sex, on a 69-item questionnaire. A more negative perception of the stuttering child was reflected in the finding that he or she was seen by both parents as more nervous and more easily upset than the sibling. Darley (1955) reported that the nonstuttering children in his study were rated more favorably by parents on twelve of fifteen personality traits than were stuttering children. Mothers of young stutterers interviewed by Glasner (1949) described their children as sensitive, nervous, unsocial, and stubborn, and high percentages of parents of stuttering children in both the Darley (1955) and Johnson and colleagues (1959) investigations expressed the belief that stuttering is due to such personality characteristics as nervousness, inferiority complex, and immaturity.

Except for the Kinstler (1961) study, the findings summarized in this section have received only limited attention in the literature and are probably among the least familiar. Yet, together, they present some of the more cohesive, consistent research findings about stutterers' home environments, which depict a rather strong tendency on the part of parents to hold images of a stuttering child that are unfavorable in personal and social terms. This may be construed as reflecting their discomfort with, or less than full acceptance of, such children.

Children's Perceptions of Parents

A different approach to the study of home environment has been taken by investigators who attempted to assess it through the eyes of stuttering children, how they perceive and react to their parents. This group of nine investigations involves diverse methodologies, a wide age range of subjects, including adults, and presents a confusing mix of findings.

In 1958 Wyatt tested the hypothesis that stuttering results from a crisis in the mother-child relationship. She administered a battery of projective tests to twenty stuttering children, ages 5:6 to 8:11 (M = 7 years), and a nonstuttering control group matched for age, sex, and intelligence scores. The stuttering children showed more "Distance Anxiety" (distance from mother) and fear of "Devaluation of Mother." Projective techniques were also used by Broida (1962) to study the parental preferences of forty-five Caucasian, middle-class, stuttering boys, ages 5 to 10 years, who had been stuttering from one to eight years. She used the Structured Story Completion Test to evaluate the boys' perceptions of parents as a source of nurturance and/or punishment, and the Structured Puppet Play Test to estimate parental preferences. Broida concluded that boys who stutter are more ambivalent in their sex role identification and parent preferences than are nonstuttering boys. She said they perceived their fathers as more punishing than nurturing, a perception that differs from the balance assumed to characterize well-adjusted children. Such disturbances in identification in early childhood were said to result in neurotic conflicts that may lead to stuttering.

Clinically based data derived from systematic analyses of counseling and psychotherapy materials were reported by two investigators. Schultz (1947) analyzed tape-recorded sessions of twenty adult stutterers, eighteen males and two females (mean age = 29 years), during nondirective counseling. Approximately 75 percent of the group expressed the feeling that they lacked affection at home and that their parents were dominant, irritating, and had high standards. There was no comparison group. Whitman (1942) relied on data from intensive psychotherapy with fifteen stuttering boys in concluding that there is an age-related, changing pattern in parent-child relations. During early childhood, boys perceive their mothers as hostile, while the father becomes much more prominent around age seven. According to Whitman, there is a feeling of dissatisfaction with an inadequate father who, in spite of his "inadequacy," is portrayed in a severely punishing role, allowing the mother to become a relatively easy person to identify with. The ever-present threat of punishment for supplanting the father is hypothesized to prevent complete identification, and the boy wavers passively, caught in a conflict, without developing strong masculine or feminine characteristics.

Other investigators have employed standardized, quantifiable measuring instruments. Duncan (1949) compared the perception of home environment by sixty-two college-age stutterers (median age 18) with that of students having other speech problems. She administered a Home Adjustment subtest from Bell's Adjustment Inventory which included many questions requiring subjects to evaluate their parents' personalities, behavior, and attitudes toward them. Duncan reported that there were large group differences on at least five items indicating that college-age stutterers perceive parental disappointment, lack of real affection, and underestimates of their maturity. Gildstone (1967) compared fifty-five junior high school stuttering students, fifty-one males and four females, who ranged in age from 11:10 to 16:2 years (M = 14:1), with a control group using the Hilden Q-Sort, which uses fifty self-referents to assess parental acceptance. The correlation between how subjects sorted items as they thought mothers or fathers see them and how they thought parents would like to see them, was taken as a measure of perceived parental acceptance. Stutterers were found to perceive parents as less accepting than were nonstutterers, but there were no differences in perceived acceptance of mothers and fathers.

Different results were obtained in two investigations, both of which focused on school-age children. The Children Reports of Parent Behavior Inventory (CRPBI), which consists of eighteen scales that assess the bipolar dimensions of Love-Hostility and Autonomous-Control, was administered by Bourdon and Silver (1970) to twenty-four school-age stutterers of unspecified age and sex, and by Yairi and Williams (1971) to thirty-four sixth- and seventh-grade male stutterers. Both studies employed matched control groups. Yairi and Williams (1971) also included scales to assess students' attitudes toward speech. Contrary to expectation, Bourdon and Silver found no differences on any of the scales between the two groups,

or between mild and severe stutterers. In contrast, Yairi and Williams found that stuttering children perceived their parents as more accepting, less controlling, instilling less anxiety, and having less negative attitudes toward speech. Cox, Seider and Kidd (1984) used a similar instrument, the Parent Behavior Instrument (PBI), in their study of high-density families. No differences were found between control subjects' ratings of parents' attitudes and those of stutterers, recovered stutterers, and nonstutterers in the high-density group.

To summarize, six of the nine investigations reviewed in this section reported data that suggest several problem areas in the relations of parents and stuttering children. These include ambivalence in sex-role identification (Broida, 1962; Whitman, 1942), distance anxiety (Wyatt, 1958), inadequate and/or punishing fathers (Whitman, 1942), lack of affection and disappointment (Duncan, 1949; Schultz, 1947); lack of acceptance (Gildstone, 1967), and underestimation of the child's maturity (Duncan, 1949). Two studies, Bourdon and Silver (1970) and Cox, Seider, and Kidd (1984), reported no differences in stuttering children's perceptions of parents, whereas Yairi and Williams (1971) reported more positive perceptions of home relations by stuttering than by normally fluent children. It is not clear if such findings are applicable only to families with one or more stuttering children, or may also apply to families having children with other speech-language disorders and families with children having other disorders.

Parent-Child Interactions and Parental Reaction to Stuttering

Much of the preceding discussion traces the history of research oriented by theoretical interests to various personality factors and psychosocial attitudes of parents toward their stuttering children. In spite of the central theoretical notions of the importance of parental attitudes in the onset and development of stuttering and the importance assigned to them in counseling and in direct intervention programs, data on parent-child verbal interactions and parental overt reactions to their child's speech, especially disfluencies, has received relatively little experimental attention.

Much of the available information concerning parental reactions to disfluency has been obtained as byproducts of studies based on parental self-reports. A study by Glasner and Rosenthal (1957) focused on the relation between the occurrence of disfluencies in young children, parents' diagnoses of stuttering, and their attitudes and reactions to it, in a sample of 153 first graders, ages 5 to 7, having histories of stuttering. Using a standard brief questionnaire in personal interviews with parents, the authors reported that 65 percent of the parents took active corrective measures, such as asking the child to slow down, stop and start again, stop stuttering, and other similar comments. Parents were more apt to respond actively if a child was exhibiting several disfluency patterns or when parents presumed the cause of stuttering was emotional in nature. Thirty percent of the parents tried to minimize the problem by just waiting or ignoring stuttering. Fewer than 3 percent sought professional help. Because 47 percent of the children who were actively corrected stopped stuttering, the authors concluded that direct parental correction may have contributed to the recovery of many of them. They made no reference to the 53 percent who continued stuttering in spite of parental correction.

Evidence of active parental reactions to a child's stuttering has been provided by a number of other investigators. In the Johnson (1959) study of 150 children, ages 2 to 8 years, two-thirds of the fathers and three-fourths of the mothers indicated they had said something to the child about stuttering. Most commonly, suggestions had been made to slow down, take it easy, or stop and start over. In a follow-up study with ninety of these children, 75 percent showed either improvement or complete recovery. About one-third of this group of parents related the child's improvement to their corrective measures. Parental reactions were noted also in an investigation by Dickson (1971) concerning the remission of stuttering among 369 elementary and junior high school children. Responses to questionnaires indicated that suggestions or admonishments were offered by 65 percent of the parents whose children recovered and by 84 percent of the parents of persistent stutterers. Parents had typically reacted to their child's stuttering with such admonishments as "start over again," "slow down," "think before you talk," and "take a deep breath." Recovery was reported in over 53 percent of the children who received such parental corrections.

More recent investigations of parent reactions to speech during verbal interactions have relied on direct observations. Mordechai (1979) rated eighteen parent-interactive behaviors during 30-minute conversations. He reported that both parents of ten preschool-age stuttering children, ages 37 to 60 months (M = 47 months), did not allow adequate opportunities for their children to respond to questions before asking another question more frequently than did parents of matched controls. Meyers and Freeman (1985a) observed the frequency of interruptions of mothers of twelve 4- and 5-year-old boys who stuttered and twelve matched nonstuttering children. The crucial finding of this study was that all mothers interrupted disfluencies much more frequently (16.3%) than fluent speech (2.2%). The fact that no statistically significant differences were found between the two groups of mothers in the proportion of disfluencies they interrupted blurs the real (nonrelative) significance of these results. It is apparent from the data that, in absolute terms, mothers of stuttering children exhibit considerably larger numbers of interruptions, on any type of disfluency, than do mothers of nonstuttering children. The proportional similarity between the two groups of mothers does not provide much relief to the child who is experiencing a larger number of interruptions. Because the number of interruptions increases as the number of disfluencies increases, interruptions are magnified for more severe stutterers. The findings from this study, however, were not corroborated by Kelly and Conture (1992). These investigators found no differences in parents' interruptive behavior.

A study of the content of parents' verbal messages using direct observations was reported by Kasprisin-Burrelli, Egolf, and Shames (1972).

They compared the verbal interactions of fourteen parents and their school-age stuttering children, ages 6 to 13 (M= 10:4), to those of parents talking with age- and gender-matched nonstuttering control children. Fifteen minutes of conversational speech were analyzed for negative and positive statements. Parents of stuttering children produced a mean of 78 negative statements compared to 34 of the control parents. In a subsequent study, Egolf, Shames, Johnson, and Kasprisin-Burrelli (1972) reported observations, but not quantified data, of parents' negative responses to school-age stuttering children during unstructured conversations. Negative reactions included interruptions, silent periods, even holding hands over their ears when the child stuttered. Direct observations of verbal interactions were also employed by Langlois, Hanrahan, and Inouye (1986). Their analyses of recorded conversations in home settings between eight 5- to 9-year-old school-age stuttering children, a control group of nonstuttering children, and their respective mothers indicated that mothers of stutterers asked significantly more questions and made more demands of their children than did mothers of control children. Although not negating the possibility that excessive questioning by parents may contribute to an atmosphere of pressure at home, Weiss and Zebrowski (1992) reported that responses to questions by eight stuttering children, ages 4 to 10, during a 10-minute conversation with a parent were significantly less likely to contain disfluencies than were assertions.

Meyers (1990) was more interested in comparing the verbal interactions of children who stutter with their mothers and fathers. She recorded twelve 2- to 6-year-old stuttering children (M = 4:5) during thirty minutes of play, ten minutes each, with their mother, father, and a familiar peer. Although fathers used more utterances and words than did mothers, there were no significant differences in the number of positive, negative, or general statements they made to the child or in the number of questions asked. Stuttering children used more positive statements when talking to fathers than to mothers. In general, the fluency failures of stuttering children were not affected by their conversational partner. Finally, LaSalle and Conture (1991) examined mother-child eye contact during conversations. Their sample included ten stuttering boys, between ages 3:6 and 5:11 (M = 57 months), their mothers, and a matched control group. Their investigation took place about 24 months, on average, after stuttering onset. The authors reported that most eye contact was initiated by the mother's gaze and that mothers of stuttering children established eye contact with their children during fluent and disfluent speech more frequently than mothers of nonstuttering children did. Mothers of stutterers gazed at their children during 49 percent of their stuttering events, and the authors suggested that these mothers' extra eye contact could have been the result of previous advice, or an effort to both monitor the child and assure him that she was attentive. Interestingly, the possibility that mothers were anxiously concerned was not mentioned.

For the most part, research findings on parents' responses to a stuttering child's speech portray a rather unfavorable speaking environment. There is strong evidence that most parents of children who stutter react with admonitions, and, at times, outright negative criticisms of a child's stuttering. There are also indications that such direct, aversive responses to stuttering are complemented by a disproportionately high number of generally negative-in-content statements during verbal interactions with a stuttering child compared to parents of nonstuttering children. Data concerning parent's interruptive behaviors, however, are inconsistent.

Parental Speech Characteristics

Both genetic and learning accounts of stuttering would be expected to generate considerable research directed at parents' speech as a possible influence on their children's speech. Research in this area has been minimal, however, and totals three studies that were motivated by theoretical interests about the possible influences of parental disfluences in the etiology of stuttering.

In 1965, Knepflar reported that fathers and mothers of twenty-one stuttering subjects had significantly more disfluencies in conversational speech than did a matched group of parents of nonstuttering controls. Additional information about the children and parents was not made available. A few years later, in a master's thesis I directed, Roman (1972) compared the disfluencies in conversational speech samples of mothers and fathers of thirteen children who stutter (mean age = 8:10) to those of thirteen control parents. To minimize effects of aging, all parents were under age 40. No significant differences were found between the two parent groups.[4] Meyers (1989) recorded speech samples of fathers and mothers of twelve 2- to 6-year-old children who stutter (M = 4:5) as each conversed with the child. No significant differences were found between the fathers and mothers in total disfluency or in any disfluency type. No control group was employed.

Recent years have also seen an increased interest in parents' speaking rate, although such studies have been limited in scope. The potential implications of findings to treatment programs that modify speaking rate have served as important catalysts. Four studies have compared the speaking rates of parents of stuttering children with those of parents of nonstuttering controls. Meyers and Freeman (1985b) measured the speaking rates of mothers of twelve 4- and 5-year-old boys who stuttered and those of mothers of a matched nonstuttering control group. Mothers of stuttering children exhibited rates that were significantly faster, a half syllable per second on average, than were the rates of control mothers. No differences, however, were found by Schultze (1991) who compared the speaking rates of parents of ten preschool stuttering children (mean age = 5:0 years) with those of ten parents, each, of

children having articulatory disorders or normal speech. Negative results were also found by Kelly and Conture (1992) for mothers of thirteen 3- and 4-year-old stuttering boys (M = 4:0) compared to mothers of nonstuttering controls, and by Kelly (1994) for fathers of eleven stuttering children, ages 2 to 10 years (M = 5:1), compared to fathers of eleven matched nonstuttering children. Other investigations, as well as portions of the studies just mentioned, have studied the manipulation of parents' speech rates or the relative differences in speech rates of parents and children (e.g., Bernstein Ratner, 1992; Stephenson-Opsal & Bernstein Ratner, 1988). Current findings on differences in the speaking rates of parents of stuttering and nonstuttering children are mostly negative, and it would appear that any differences in relative speaking rates are more likely to reflect the child's rather than the parent's behavior. More detailed discussions of these studies can be found in Kelly (1993).

Overall, the current body of data on parents' speech is small in terms of the number and scope of studies completed. Available information does not provide sufficient support for any hypothesis that the parents of children who stutter, in contrast to parents of nonstuttering children, talk in ways that present either more disfluent or faster speech models or that could be viewed as stressful or having other negative influences. Nor are there indications that parents of stuttering children, on their own, have altered (e.g., slowed) their speech patterns in order to make them easier to imitate.

SUMMARY

The research literature pertaining to the home environments of children who stutter is extensive but spread over many areas. As a result, some areas have been barely examined. For example, parent personalities and parent-child psychosocial interactions have been extensively researched, but only three studies have examined the disfluency characteristics of parents. A similar imbalance has also characterized research methodology. A substantial majority of studies have employed subjective re-

---

[4]Similarly, a study of the relation between various types of disfluency in normally speaking preschool-age children and their parents' speech was undertaken by Yairi and Jennings (1974). All but one correlation between the disfluencies of parents and children were not significant. Only that between boys and fathers for disrhythmic phonation was significant.

sponses to tests, questionnaires, and personal interviews of parents or children, and only a few have used direct, objective observations of behavior. Because the home environments of stutterers have not been investigated with consistent rigor, various areas of investigation cannot be discussed at similarly informed levels.

More than fifty years of home environment research has yielded a body of data characterized by differing interpretations, conflicting results, and few definitive answers. Keeping in mind the reservations about the quality of current data, my conclusion is that children who stutter have higher chances of encountering unfavorable home conditions than do normally speaking children, a conclusion similar to that of Wingate's (1962). I also concur with Adams' (1993) view that children who stutter do not grow up in a home environment that is clearly pathologic. Organizing the accumulated information into several related components allows a more analytic assessment. Taken at face value, the findings reviewed support the following sets of conclusions:

Similarities between Parents of Stuttering and Nonstuttering Children

1. Familial characteristics, such as socioeconomic background, family size, and sibling order, await further clarification but seem unlikely to have strong relations to stuttering.
2. The weight of the evidence does *not* support the hypothesis that parents of stutterers typically have abnormal personalities or significant emotional or adjustment problems. There are, however, repeated indications that they tend to have heightened anxiety levels.
3. There appear to be no significant differences in most aspects of the two groups of parents' day-to-day attitudes or child-rearing practices.
4. There are no differences in speech disfluencies or speaking rates of parents of stuttering children and those whose children do not stutter.

Differences between Parents of Stuttering and Nonstuttering Children

1. The most solidly established, predictable difference between the families of stuttering and nonstuttering children is a familial history of stuttering. Up to 43 percent of children who stutter have parents, mainly fathers, or siblings who stutter. Up to 71 percent are raised in families having a history of stuttering in the extended circle of relatives. These percentages are three to four times higher than those in other families. The full implication of this factor to home environments is not yet understood, but recent evidence suggests that familial history of stuttering may be an important factor in determining a stuttering child's chance of having a persistent problem.
2. Findings from two major investigations (Andrews & Harris, 1964; Johnson et al., 1959) suggest that parents of stuttering children have lower intelligence scores and fewer years of formal education than do parents of normally fluent children. If the reliability of these findings is confirmed, they may have implications for the pathogenesis of stuttering as well as other spheres of the home environment.
3. There are consistent reports that children who stutter are raised more frequently than are nonstuttering children in less harmonious, more socially withdrawn families that take less time to enjoy each other's companionship.
4. There are consistent reports that parents are more frequently or to a greater degree overprotective or anxious about their children who stutter than they are about their normally speaking children.
5. There are indications that parents of a child who stutters have negative evaluations of the child's personality and that the child perceives these negative attitudes as well.
6. There is consistent evidence of overt, sometimes negative, parental reactions to a child's stuttering. No credible evidence has been reported, however, to support the contention

that such reactions have either positive or negative influences on recovery from stuttering.

Many of these conclusions should be tempered in light of my overall concerns that much of the research in this area suffers major weaknesses. This review has revealed that many investigations have studied parents of stuttering children several to many years after the onset of stuttering. Hence, considerable portions of these data are not directly related to the early stage of stuttering, etiologically or otherwise. Moreover, these data have not been collected in ways that clearly tie them to either the development or the maintenance of the disorder.

Two possibilities should be considered in light of the fact that much of the data have been obtained from parents of chronic stutterers. First, the home environments of a large proportion, perhaps a majority, of the preschool stuttering children who have recovered from stuttering have not been investigated. Recent data by Yairi and Ambrose (1992), Yairi, Ambrose, and Niermann (1993), and Yairi, Ambrose, Paden, and Throneburg (1996) have confirmed previous reports by Andrews and Harris (1964) of both high rates, 65 percent to 80 percent, and early, spontaneous recoveries among preschool-age stutterers. The parents of this group of children may prove to be even less distinguishable from parents of normally speaking children. Second, many findings in the literature, such as parents' overprotectiveness, negative evaluations of the child, and negative reactions to his or her stuttering, may reflect changing parental attitudes over the years and their efforts to cope with a chronically speech-handicapped child. Certainly, such reactions are not "causal" in isolation, but they may contribute to a constellation of factors that exacerbates speech breakdowns and their emotional consequences. As such, they may reflect factors that lead to, or result from, the emergence of chronic stuttering.

No less detrimental to the quality of this area of research is the failure of nearly all investigators to control for genetic factors in selecting subject samples. As was suggested earlier, families with current or past histories of stuttering may be more inclined to harbor or exercise attitudes and behaviors toward a stuttering child that differ from those of families without such backgrounds. Furthermore, in light of the apparent relationship of genetic factors to stuttering, parents having a stuttering history or a high risk for stuttering may also score differently on personality or intelligence tests or on other tasks that are related to the pathogenesis of stuttering. If their responses or performances are indeed different from normal, such differences may have been obscured in studies that did not distinguish such parents from those not having this background. Parents' intellectual capacity and level of education provide particularly interesting possibilities. Because it has been reported that stutterers, as a group, have lower mean intelligence scores than do nonstutterers (e.g., Andrews & Harris, 1964; Schindler, 1955), it is reasonable to suspect that findings of lower formal education among parents of stutterers (Johnson et al., 1959) may reflect their intellectual capacity. Unfortunately, this variable has not been controlled. Intellectual functioning may, in turn, be related to findings concerning both socioeconomic status and familial styles.

Another obvious neglect is the failure to control for familial history in studies of parents' disfluency and speaking rates. Parents with a history of stuttering would be more likely to perform differently than would parents of stutterers without such history. The absence of these subgroups in research may have obscured important differences between them and parents of normally speaking children. Finally, although many more fathers than mothers of stutterers have a history of stuttering, several investigations, including the well-known Andrews and Harris (1964) study, were limited to mothers. Overlooking such epidemiologic-genetic features of stuttering has clearly compromised the validity of these data. In my opinion, considerably more attention should be directed to fathers, especially those with a history of stuttering.

There is a great need to revisit the area of the home environment armed with research designs that consider epidemiological factors. Just as subgrouping should be an important principle of research with stuttering children (Yairi, 1990), so should research with their parents. Future research should also focus on changes in a stuttering child's home environment as a function of the developmental course of the disorder and should consider such influences as the impact of a handicapped child on family dynamics (Margalit, 1990). Finally, future research should be pursued beyond the narrow theoretical notions of stuttering and explore some of the recent theoretical models in such fields as family relations and special education (e.g., Turnbull, Patterson, Beh, Murphy, Marquis, & Blue-Banning, 1993).

The research data that I have reviewed and interpreted have several clinical implications for early childhood stuttering:

1. It is clearly time to declare that the belief that parents' personalities or attitudes are causally related to stuttering is null and void for purposes of counseling and treatment. For many years, too many parents have been, either directly or indirectly, wrongly faulted for their child's stuttering.
2. Clinicians should become familiar with the home environment of a stuttering child as a potential problem area that may complicate the child's stuttering, interfere with progress, or cause additional personal-social difficulties that affect the quality of the family's life and the child's healthy development. The conclusions about conditions likely to characterize the homes of these children that were summarized earlier (p. 42) may be helpful guides.
3. Although there is no credible evidence to support the contention that parents' overt reactions to their child's stuttering contributes to recovery, the data do not negate the potential usefulness of their participation in therapeutic programs. Research pertinent to this issue was not critically examined in this chapter.
4. Recent data have provided evidence that recovery and chronicity in young stuttering children are related to familial history of stuttering. As knowledge concerning genetic contributions to stuttering increases in coming years, the clinical significance of a child's family will increase, especially as it may relate to differential diagnosis and prognosis, and an understanding of genetics and pedigree analyses will likely become an important clinical skill.

REFERENCES

Abbott, T. (1957). A study of observable mother-child relationships in stuttering and non-stuttering families. Unpublished Ph.D. dissertation, University of Florida.

Accordi, M., Bianchi, R., Consolaro, C., Tronchin, F., DeFilippi, R., Pasqualon, L., Ugo, E., & Croatto, L. (1983). L'Eziopatogenesi della balbuzie: Studio statistico su 802 casi. *Acta Phoniatrica Latina, 5,* 171–180.

Adams, M. (1993). The home environment of children who stutter. *Seminars in Speech and Language, 14,* 185–192.

Ambrose, N., Yairi, E., & Cox, N. (1993). Genetic aspects of early childhood stuttering. *Journal of Speech and Hearing Research, 36,* 701–706.

Andrews, G., and Harris, M. (1964). *The syndrome of stuttering.* Clinics in Developmental Medicine, No. 17. London: Spastic Society Medical Education and Information Unit in association with Wm. Heineman Medical Books.

Bender, J. (1943). The prophylaxis of stuttering. *Nervous Child, 2,* 181–198.

Berlin, C. (1960). Parents' diagnosis of stuttering. *Journal of Speech and Hearing Research, 3,* 372–379.

Bernstein Ratner, N. (1992). Measurable outcome of instructions to modify normal parent-child verbal interaction: Implications for direct stuttering therapy. *Journal of Speech and Hearing Research, 35,* 14–20.

Bernstein Ratner, N. (1993). Parents, children, and stuttering. *Seminars in Speech and Language, 14,* 238–250.

Bloodstein, O., Jaeger, W., & Tureen, J. (1952). A study of the diagnosis of stuttering by parents of stutterers and nonstutterers. *Journal of Speech and Hearing Disorders, 17,* 308–315.

Bluemel, C. (1932). Primary and secondary stammering. *Quarterly Journal of Speech, 18,* 187–200.

Bluemel, C. (1959). If a child stammers. *Mental Hygiene, 43,* 390–393.

Boland, J. (1949). An investigation of certain birth factors as they relate to stuttering. Unpublished M.A. thesis, University of Michigan.

Botterill, E., Kelman, E., & Rustin, L. (1994). Parents and their pre-school stuttering child. In L. Rustin (Ed.), *Parents, families, and the stuttering child.* San Diego: Singular Publishing Company.

Bourdon, K., & Silver, D. (1970). Perceived parental behavior among stutterers and nonstutterers. *Journal of Abnormal Psychology, 75,* 93–97.

Brill, A. (1923). Speech disturbances in nervous and mental diseases. *Quarterly Journal of Speech Education, 9,* 129–135.

Broida, H. (1962). An empirical study of sex role identification and sex-role preference in a selected group of stuttering male children. Unpublished Ph.D. Dissertation, University of Southern California.

Bryngelson, B., & Rutherford, B. (1937). A study of laterality of stutterers and non-stutterers. *Journal of Speech Disorders, 2,* 15–16.

Christensen, A. (1952). A quantitative study of personality dynamics in stuttering and nonstuttering siblings. *Speech Monographs, 19,* 187–188.

Coppola, V., & Yairi, E. (1982). Rhythmic speech training with preschool stuttering children. *Journal of Fluency Disorders, 8,* 447–457.

Coriat, I. (1943). The psychoanalytic conception of stammering. *Nervous Child, 2,* 167–171.

Cox, N., Seider, R., & Kidd, K. (1984). Some environmental factors and hypotheses for stuttering in families with several stutterers. *Journal of Speech and Hearing Research, 27,* 543–548.

Curran, M., & Hood, S. (1977). Listeners' ratings of severity for specific disfluency types in children. *Journal of Fluency Disorders, 2,* 87–97.

Darley, F. (1955). The relationship of parental attitudes and adjustments to the development of stuttering. In W. Johnson (Ed.), *Stuttering in children and adults.* Minneapolis: University of Minnesota Press.

Despert, J. (1946). Psychosomatic study of fifty stuttering children: I. Social, physical and psychiatric findings. *American Journal of Orthopsychiatry, 16,* 100–113.

Dickson, S. (1971). Incipient stuttering and spontaneous remission of stuttered speech. *Journal of Communication Disorders, 4,* 99–110.

Duncan, M. (1949). Home adjustment of stutterers versus nonstutterers. *Journal of Speech and Hearing Disorders, 14,* 255–259.

Egolf, D., Shames, G., Johnson, P., & Kasprisin-Burrelli, A. (1972). The use of parent-child interaction patterns in therapy for young stutterers. *Journal of Speech and Hearing Disorders, 37,* 22–232.

Feldman, R. (1976). Self-disclosure in parents of stuttering children. *Journal of Communication Disorders, 9,* 227–234.

Fenichel, O. (1945). *The psychoanalytic theory of neurosis.* New York: Norton.

Froeschels, E. (1921). Beitrage zur symptomatoligie des stotterns. *Monatsschrift fur Phrenheilkinde, 55,* 1109–1112.

Fluegel, F. (1979). Erhenbungen von personalichkeitsmerkmalen an muttern stotternderkinder und jugendlicher. *Disorders of Speech and Hearing Abstracts, 19,* 226.

Gildstone, P. (1967). Stutterers' self acceptance and perceived parental acceptance. *Journal of Abnormal Psychology, 72,* 59–64.

Glasner, P. (1949). Personality characteristics and emotional problems in stutterers under the age of five. *Journal of Speech and Hearing Disorders, 14,* 135–138.

Glasner, P. (1962). Psychotherapy for the young stutterer. In D. Barbara (Ed.). *The psychotherapy of stuttering.* Springfield, IL: Charles Thomas.

Glasner, P., & Rosenthal, D. (1957). Parental diagnosis of stuttering in young children. *Journal of Speech and Hearing Disorders, 22,* 288–295.

Glauber, P. (1958). Stuttering and personality dynamics. In J. Eisenson (Ed.), *Stuttering: A symposium.* New York: Harper and Row.

Goldman, R., & Shames, G. (1964a). A study of the goal-setting behavior of parents of stutterer and parents of nonstutterers. *Journal of Speech and Hearing Disorders, 29,* 192–194.

Goldman, R., & Shames, G. (1964b). Comparisons of the goals that parents of stutterers and nonstutterers set for their children. *Journal of Speech and Hearing Disorders, 29,* 381–389.

Goodstein, L. (1956). MMPI profiles of stutterers' parents: A follow-up study. *Journal of Speech and Hearing Disorders, 21,* 430–435.

Goodstein, L., & Dahlstrom, W. (1956). MMPI differences between parents of stuttering and nonstuttering children. *Journal of Consulting Psychology, 20,* 365–370.

Grossman, D. (1951). A study of the parents of stuttering and nonstuttering children using the Minnesota Multiphasic Personality Inventory and the Minnesota Scale of Parents' Opinions. Unpublished M.A. thesis, University of Wisconsin.

Guilford, J. (1940). *Manual of directions and norms: An inventory of factors STDCR* (Revised edition). Beverly Hills, CA: Sheridan Supply Company.

Ingham, R. (1981). Spontaneous remission of stuttering: When will the emperor realize he has no clothes on? In D. Prins and R. Ingham (Eds.), *Treatment of stuttering in early childhood: Methods and issues.* San Diego: College Hill.

Johnson, W. (1942). A study of the onset and development of stuttering. *Journal of Speech Disorders, 7,* 251–257.

Johnson, W. (1955). A study of the onset and development of stuttering. In W. Johnson (Ed.), *Stuttering in children and adults.* Minneapolis: University of Minnesota Press.

Johnson, W., Boehmler, R., Dahlstrom, G., Darley, F., Goodstein, L., Kools, J., Neeley, J., Prather, W., Sherman, D., Thurman, C., Trotter, W., Williams, D., & Young, M. (1959). *The onset of stuttering.* Minneapolis: University of Minnesota Press.

Kasprisin-Burrelli, A., Egolf, D., & Shames, G. (1972). A comparison of parental verbal behavior with stuttering and nonstuttering children. *Journal of Communication Disorders, 5,* 335–346.

Kelly, E. (1993). Speech rates and turn-taking behaviors of children who stutter and their parents. *Seminars in Speech and Language, 14,* 203–214.

Kelly, E. (1994). Speaking rates and turn-taking behaviors of children who stutter and their fathers. *Journal of Speech and Hearing Research, 36,* 1284–1294.

Kelly, E., & Conture, E. (1992). Speaking rates, response time latencies, and interrupting behavior of young stutterers, nonstutterers, and their mothers. *Journal of Speech and Hearing Research, 35,* 1256–1267.

Kidd, K. (1984). Stuttering as a genetic disorder. In R. Curlee & W. Perkins (Eds.) *Nature and treatment of stuttering: New directions.* San Diego: College Hill.

Kinstler, D. (1961). Covert and overt maternal rejection in stuttering. *Journal of Speech Disorders, 26,* 145–155.

Knepflar, K. (1965). Speaking fluency in the parents of stutterers and nonstutterers. *Asha, 7,* 391.

LaFollette, A. (1956). Parental environment of stuttering children. *Journal of Speech and Hearing Disorders, 21,* 202–207.

Langlois, A., Hanrahan, L., & Inouye, L. (1986). A comparison of interactions between stuttering children, nonstuttering children, and their mothers. *Journal of Fluency Disorders, 11,* 263–273.

LaSalle, L., & and Conture, E. (1991). Eye contact between young stutterers and their mothers. *Journal of Fluency Disorders, 16,* 173–200.

Lemert, E. (1953). Some Indians who stutter. *Journal of Speech and Hearing Disorders, 18,* 168–174.

Margalit, M. (1990). *Effective technology integration for disabled children: The family perspective.* New York: Springer-Verlag.

Martin, R., & Lindamood, L. (1986). Stuttering and spontaneous recovery: Implications for speech-language pathologists. *Language, Speech, and Hearing Services in Schools, 17,* 207–218.

Meyers, S. (1989). Nonfluencies of preschool stutterers and conversational partners: Observing reciprocal relationships. *Journal of Speech and Hearing Disorders, 54,* 106–112.

Meyers, S. (1990). Verbal behaviors of preschool stutterers and conversational partners: Observing reciprocal relationships. *Journal of Speech and Hearing Disorders, 55,* 706–712.

Meyers, S., and Freeman, F. (1985a). Interruptions as a variable in stuttering and disfluency. *Journal of Speech and Hearing Research, 28,* 428–435.

Meyers, S., & Freeman, F. (1985b). Mother and child speech rate as a variable in stuttering and disfluency. *Journal of Speech and Hearing Research, 28,* 436–444.

Meyers, S., & Freeman, F. (1985c). Are mothers of stutterers different? An investigation of social communicative interaction. *Journal of Fluency Disorders, 10,* 193–209.

Moncur, J. (1951). Environmental factors differentiating stuttering children from non-stuttering children. *Speech Monographs, 18,* 312–325.

Moncur, J. (1952). Parental domination in stuttering.

Journal of Speech and Hearing Disorders, 17, 155–165.

Mordechai, D. (1979). *An investigation of the communicative styles of mothers and fathers of stuttering versus nonstuttering preschool children during a triadic interaction.* Unpublished doctoral dissertation, Northwestern University.

Morgenstern, J. (1956). Socio-economic factors in stuttering. *Journal of Speech and Hearing Disorders, 21,* 25–33.

Murphy, A., & Fitzsimmons, R. (1960). *Stuttering and personality dynamics.* New York: Ronald.

Nelson, S. (1939). The role of heredity in stuttering. *Journal of Pediatrics, 14,* 642–654.

Powell, H. (1966). Childrearing practices reported for young male Negro stutterers and nonstutterers in two South Carolina school districts. Unpublished Ph.D. dissertation, Pennsylvania State University.

Puttalaz, M., Constanzo, P., & Smith, R. (1991). Maternal recollections of childhood peer relations: Implications for their children's social competence. *Journal of Social and Personal Relationships, 8,* 403–422.

Quarrington, B. (1974). The parents of stuttering children: The literature re-examined. *Canadian Psychiatric Association Journal, 19,* 103–110.

Quarrington, B., Seligman, E., & Kosower, E. (1969). Goal setting behavior of parents of beginning stutterers and parents of nonstuttering children. *Journal of Speech and Hearing Research, 12,* 435–442.

Ramig, P. (1993). Parent-clinician-child partnership in the therapeutic process of preschool- and elementary-aged children who stutter. *Seminars in Speech and Language, 14,* 226–237.

Ritzman, C. (1941). Notes on psychodynamic interpretation of stuttering. Unpublished Ph.D. dissertation, University of Iowa.

Roman, G. (1972). An investigation of the disfluent speech behavior of parents of stuttering and nonstuttering children. Unpublished M.A. thesis, Texas Tech University.

Rotter, J. (1939). Studies in the psychology of stuttering: XI. Stuttering in relation to position in the family. *Journal of Speech Disorders, 4,* 143–148.

Rotter, J. (1942). Development and evaluation of a controlled method. *Journal of Experimental Psychology, 312,* 410–422.

Rustin, L. (1987). The treatment of childhood disfluency through active parental involvement. In L.

Rustin, H. Purser, & H. Rowley (Eds.), *Progress in the treatment of fluency disorders.* London: Whurr Publishers.

Rustin, L., & Purser, H. (1991). Child development, families, and the problem of stuttering. In L. Rustin (Ed.), *Parents, families, and the stuttering child.* San Diego: Singular Publishing Company.

Schindler, M. (1955). A study of the educational adjustment of stuttering and nonstuttering children. In W. Johnson & R. Leutenegger (Eds.), *Stuttering in children and adults.* Minneapolis: University of Minnesota Press.

Schuell, H. (1949). Working with parents of stuttering children. *Journal of Speech and Hearing Disorders, 14,* 251–254.

Schultz, D. (1947). A study of nondirective counseling as applied to adult stutterers. *Journal of Speech Disorders, 12,* 421–427.

Schultze, H. (1991). Time pressure variables in the verbal parent-child interaction patterns of fathers and mothers of stuttering, phonologically disordered and normal preschool children. In H.F.M. Peters & W.H. Hulstijn (Eds.), *Speech motor control and stuttering* (pp. 441–452), New York: Exerpta Medica.

Sheehan, J., & Costley, M. (1977). A reexamination of the role of heredity in stuttering. *Journal of Speech and Hearing Disorders, 42,* 47–59.

Shine, R. (1980). Direct management of the beginning stutterer. In W. Perkins (Ed.), *Strategies in stuttering therapy.* New York: Thieme-Stratton.

Snidecor, J. (1947). Why the Indian does not stutter. *Quarterly Journal of Speech, 33,* 493–495.

Starkweather, W., Gottwald, S., & Halfond, M. (1990). *Stuttering prevention: A clinical method.* Englewood Cliffs, NJ: Prentice Hall.

Stephenson-Opsal, D., & Bernstein Ratner, N. (1988). Maternal speech rate modification and childhood stuttering. *Journal of Fluency Disorders, 13,* 49–56.

Turnbull, A., Patterson, J., Beh, S., Murphy, D., Marquis, J., & Blue-Banning, M. (1993). *Cognitive coping, families and disabilities.* Baltimore: Brooks Publishing.

Van Riper, C. (1939). *Speech correction: Principles and methods.* New York: Prentice-Hall.

Wakaba, Y. (1992). Process of recovery from stuttering of a three year old stuttering child. *Tokyo Gakugei University Research Institute for The Education of Exceptional Children, 41,* 35–46.

Weiss, A., & Zebrowski, P. (1992). Disfluencies in the

conversations of young children who stutter: Some answers about questions. *Journal of Speech and Hearing Research, 35,* 1230–1238.

Whitman, D. (1942). The role of the father in the development of the personality of the stutterer. *Psychological Bulletin, 39,* 476.

Wilson, D. (1951). A study of the personalities of stuttering children and their parents as revealed through projection tests. *Speech Monographs, 18,* 133.

Wingate, M. (1962). Evaluation of stuttering: II. Environmental stress and critical appraisal of speech. *Journal of Speech and Hearing Disorders, 27,* 244–257.

Wingate, M. (1976). *Stuttering theory and treatment.* New York: Irvington.

Wyatt, G. (1958). Mother-child relationships and stuttering in children. Unpublished Ph.D. dissertation, Boston University.

Wyatt, G., & Herzen, J. (1962). Therapy with stuttering children and their mothers. *American Journal of Orthopsychiatry, 23,* 645–659.

Yairi, E. (1983). The onset of stuttering in two- and three-year-old children. *Journal of Speech and Hearing Disorders, 48,* 171–177.

Yairi, E. (1990). Subtyping child stutterers for research purposes. *ASHA Reports, 18,* 50–57.

Yairi, E., & Ambrose, N. (1992). Onset of stuttering in preschool children. Journal of Speech and Hearing Research, 35, 782–788.

Yairi, E., Ambrose, N., & Cox, N. (In press). Genetics of stuttering: A critical review. *Journal of Speech and Hearing Research.*

Yairi, E., Ambrose, N., & Niermann, R. (1993). The early months of stuttering: A developmental study. *Journal of Speech and Hearing Research, 36,* 521–528.

Yairi, E., Ambrose, N., Paden, N., & Throneburg, R. (1996). Predictive factors of persistence and recovery: Pathways of childhood stuttering. *Journal of Communication Disorders, 29,* 51–77.

Yairi, E., & Jennings, S. (1974). Relationship between the disfluent speech behavior of normal speaking preschool boys and their parents. *Journal of Speech and Hearing Research, 15,* 714–719.

Yairi, E., & Williams, D. (1971). Reports of parental attitudes by stuttering and by nonstuttering children. *Journal of Speech and Hearing Research, 14,* 596–604.

Zebrowski, P., & Conture, E. (1989). Judgments of disfluency by mothers of stuttering and normally fluent children. *Journal of Speech and Hearing Research, 32,* 625–634.

Zenner, A., Ritterman, S., Bowen, S., & Gronhovd, D. (1978). Measurement and comparison of anxiety levels of parents of stuttering, articulatory defective, and normal-speaking children. *Journal of Fluency Disorders, 3,* 273–284.

SUGGESTED READINGS

This list comprises the major literature reviews published during the past thirty-five years on the home environments of people who stutter. Together, they provide not only comprehensive coverage of this topic but also different points of view that should enlighten the interested reader.

Bernstein Ratner, N. (1993). Stuttering and parent-child interaction. *Seminars in Speech and Language. 14,* (3).

Bloodstein, O. (1995). *A Handbook on stuttering* (Fifth edition). San Diego, CA: Singular Publishing Group.

Quarrington, B. (1974). The parents of stuttering children: The literature re-examined. *Canadian Psychiatric Association Journal, 19,* 103–110.

Wingate, M. (1962). Evaluation of stuttering: II. Environmental stress and critical appraisal of speech. *Journal of Speech and Hearing Disorders, 27,* 244–257.

CHAPTER 3

DISFLUENCY CHARACTERISTICS OF CHILDHOOD STUTTERING

EHUD YAIRI

INTRODUCTION

Interruptions in the speech flow of people who stutter, commonly referred to as "disfluencies," are the most obvious feature of their disorder. Stuttering and disfluency, however, are not to be equated. Stuttering is a complex, multidimensional disorder in which disfluency is but one component. Indeed, some disfluencies occur in the speech of normally speaking persons and not all those produced by people who stutter are necessarily stuttering; some are perceived as normal. Furthermore, the same disfluencies may be perceived as either stuttering or normal by the same listeners under different conditions (Williams & Kent, 1958). Nevertheless, disfluent events are obligatory signs of "stuttering" and have become the single most frequently used parameter to describe and define stuttering or stutterers. Reflecting a deep-rooted view that stuttering comprises discrete events, disfluency counts have been the classic metric of the disorder as well as the dependent variable of interest in both clinical and experimental studies.

For seven decades, disfluency has had a prominent role in theories of stuttering, especially those pertaining to its inception during early childhood. For example, failure to differentiate normal from abnormal disfluency (Johnson & Associates, 1959) and selective reinforcement of initially normal disfluency (Shames & Sherrick, 1963) have been regarded as essential components in learning processes presumed to result in stuttering. It is also worth noting that when Bluemel (1932) coined the term "primary stammering" to designate an incipient stage of the disorder, his concept that it was a pure speech disturbance relied heavily on the nature of the observed disfluency. He proposed that this early stage of stuttering consists exclusively of easy repetitions devoid of physical or emotional tension, and that physical tension and other reactions ". . . have nothing to do with primary stammering" (p. 188). Many similar ideas, centered around disfluency, continue to this day.

In the clinical realm, disfluent speech has special importance with respect to early identification of childhood stuttering and is often the only obvious characteristic observed by laypersons and clinicians alike. Because other components of stuttering, such as awareness or emotionality, are not always apparent during early stages of the disorder and because of difficulties encountered in their measurement, analyses of disfluency have been weighted heavily in instruments and methods of diagnosis and evaluation of early childhood stuttering (Adams, 1977; Curlee, 1980; Gordon & Luper, 1992; Pindzola & White, 1986).

Thus, what constitutes normal and abnormal disfluency is a significant question. Johnson's (1959) "axiom" was that the distinction between "normal" disfluency and "stuttering" is, in the

ACKNOWLEDGMENT: This chapter was prepared with the support of grant #2R01-DC00459 from the National Institute on Deafness and Other Communication Disorders, National Institutes of Health.

final analysis, a matter of the listener's evaluative judgment in which "right" or "wrong" criteria do not apply. Following similar reasoning, Bloodstein (1970) stated that, "There is no test for determining the precise point at which speech repetitions stop being 'normal' and become stuttering . . . it is not a scientific question" (p. 31). Given the prospect that an absolute distinction is impossible, there remain two avenues of inquiry. As Bloodstein (1970) elegantly pointed out, we may seek an answer in terms of statistical probability and identify disfluency features or elements that carry a high probability of being perceived as stuttering under certain conditions. A second, complementary approach would be to attempt to isolate disfluent features that are usually produced differently by people who stutter than by normal speakers.

This chapter utilizes evidence from listeners' perceptions and from speech data but relies most heavily on speech characteristics. It does *not*, however, cover information pertaining to linguistic or environmental factors that influence disfluency. While recognizing that it is not yet possible to identify a distinct demarcation between normal and abnormal disfluency, it is apparent to me that, by combining measures of various aspects of disfluent speech in young children, differentiation is possible at an acceptable and increasing level of confidence.

METHODOLOGY AND MEASUREMENT ISSUES

Information on the speech characteristics of early childhood stuttering comes in two major forms: subjective descriptions and analyses of speech data. Both should be reviewed with regard to the research methodologies that have been employed.

Subjective Descriptions

A common weakness of descriptive studies of early stuttering has been their reliance on indirect or unquantified data. Early studies of speech characteristics at the onset of stuttering (Johnson &

Associates, 1959) used retrospective parental reports that are subject to the respondent's bias and selective memory. Bloodstein's (1960a; 1960b) landmark study on the development of stuttering utilized descriptions retrieved from old diagnostic reports, which included both parents' and children's reports. The fact that two of the most influential studies in the field are based on either second-hand or unquantified data often seems to be underappreciated.

Although retrospective data in research of the onset of stuttering are useful, their inherent weakness is exacerbated if there is inadequate control of the interval between the date of stuttering onset and the interview. Obviously, the shorter the post-onset interval, the greater the accuracy. Long intervals increase the chance of memory failures and the influence of recent features of the disorder. Unfortunately, most of the information on early stuttering (Darley, 1955; Johnson & Associates, 1959) includes data from interviews conducted as late as eleven years after onset. The validity of parental descriptions of subtle speech characteristics, such as the number of times a child repeated syllables several years earlier, is highly questionable.

Another critical methodological issue is the age of stuttering subjects. The importance of this factor has been overlooked even though it threatens the meaningfulness of appreciable portions of often cited information. Bloodstein's (1960b) descriptions of Phase I stuttering, for example, were based on the speech characteristics described in the diagnostic reports of children who ranged from 2 to 6 years of age and who must have had stuttering histories of very different lengths. Considering Bloodstein's own conclusions on age-related variations in stuttering, and recent studies reporting rapid changes in stuttering during the first few months after onset (Yairi, Ambrose, & Niermann, 1993), "composite profiles" across wide age ranges, particularly ages 2 to 6, disregard basic facts about the pathognomonic course of stuttering. Froeschels' (1964) classic description of early stuttering suffers similar deficiencies because of unspecified ages and post-onset intervals.

Direct Speech Analyses

Much of the information about speech characteristics in young, beginning stutterers has focused on the frequency of specified types of disfluency, such as "syllable repetition" and "sound prolongation." In spite of abundant research during the past fifty-five years, comparisons and generalizations of data are difficult because inconsistent methodologies and measures have been used. Other aspects of disfluent events, including their duration, extent (number of repetition units), clustering, associated physical movement, or acoustic features, have received relatively little attention until recently.

One problem is the selection of *target phenomena*: What disfluencies should be included, and how should they be grouped? Early studies (Branscom, Hughes, & Oxtoby, 1955) counted only three types of repetition. Later, Johnson and Associates (1959) introduced an eight-type disfluency scheme that has been employed, with modifications, in many studies. Yairi (1981), for example, introduced separate counts for monosyllabic and multisyllabic words, and Campbell and Hill (1987) included no fewer than ten disfluency types. Other investigators combined several disfluency categories to create other measures. Conture (1982) defined "stuttering" as *within-word* disfluency types, particularly sound repetition, syllable repetition, and prolongation. Unfortunately, the status of monosyllabic word repetitions, a common element in the disfluent speech of young stutterers, was left unclear, and later studies (Conture & Caruso, 1987; Schwartz & Conture, 1988) did not mention this disfluency type.[1] This definition also excludes *between-word* phenomena, such as tense pauses, which often occur in the speech of stutterers. It is also confusing if disfluencies that are called "stuttering" are counted in the speech of nonstuttering children, which, in this context, seems to contradict common sense. Recently, Yairi and Ambrose (1992b) introduced two global disfluency measures for children, Stuttering-Like Disfluencies (SLD) and Other Disfluencies (OD), which will be discussed later.

Problems also arise in how best to treat multiple disfluencies occurring on the same word. Although many studies, including those of Branscom, Hughes, and Oxtoby (1955), Johnson and Associates (1959), and myself (e.g., Yairi, 1981), counted multiple disfluency types separately, some investigators either count only one type per word or per syllable or report data that reflect this position (Meyers, 1986). The confusion on this issue was recently discussed by Onslow and colleagues (Onslow, Gardner, Bryant, Stuckings, & Knight, 1992), and in my opinion, counting only one disfluency-type per word if two or three actually occurred results in a misrepresentation of data. For example, important information is lost when bu-bu-bu——>t-but is counted only as a word repetition when, in fact, a part-word repetition and sound prolongation were produced.

Another source of problems is the *metric* used to express data. The more common metrics—percent of disfluent words, number of disfluencies per 100 words, and number of disfluencies per 100 syllables—yield different results. To illustrate, in a sample of 300 words containing 400 syllables, if a child has 25 disfluencies on 15 different words, Meyers (1986) and Zebrowski (1991) would report the child as being "5 percent disfluent," Johnson and Associates (1959) would report 8.33 disfluencies per 100 words, and Yairi and Lewis (1984) would report 6.25 disfluencies per 100 syllables. These are substantial differences. Furthermore, as the number of syllables in the same number of words increases, so does the discrepancy. As can be seen, the "percent disfluent" metric discards appreciable portions of the data by counting only the words affected regardless of how many disfluencies occurred. The "number of disfluencies per 100 words," on the other hand, tends to be inflated, because shorter words receive the same weight as longer ones. Furthermore, both metrics obscure other disfluency phenomena. For

---

[1]Recently, however, Conture (1994) stated that monosyllabic should be included.

example, limiting analyses to percent of disfluent words discards information about the clusters resulting from multiple occurrences of disfluencies on the same word.[2]

Thus, a syllable-based metric more accurately reflects the amount of speech affected by disfluency. Although word length may vary little among school-age children and adults, such is not the case in early childhood. During this critical period, a six-month age difference is often associated with a substantial increase in the length of words as well as in the percentage of longer words spoken. In my experience, approximately 85 percent of the words produced by 2- to 3-year-olds are monosyllabic, whereas for 5-year-old children, the figure is 65 to 70 percent. Unfortunately, the significance of this fact to early childhood stuttering is not always appreciated and has resulted in biased data. For example, Davis' (1939) study of the changes in disfluencies between ages 2 and 5 used the disfluencies per 100 words metric. This overlooked the fact that 100 words of 5-year-old children undoubtedly consist of more syllables than 100 words of 2-year-olds and that eight repetitions for a given number of words in the speech of a 5-year-old likely constitutes less disfluency than eight repetitions in the speech of a 2-year-old. Thus, the age-related downward slope in disfluency that Davis reported may have been considerably steeper. Other studies of early childhood disfluencies that combined data from children across a wide age range are also likely to contain serious errors. So are clinical reports or efficacy studies of young stutterers that describe disfluency changes over long periods of time. The incompatibility of these metrics was demonstrated in data reported by Hubbard and Yairi (1988) from speech samples of children obtained near the onset of stuttering. Their frequency of disfluency per 100 words was 25.10 but fell to 22.57 per 100 syllables for the same samples. Based on this evidence and the above discussion, I cannot agree with Conture and Caruso's (1987) opinion that this

is an insignificant issue, especially in evaluating young children.

A third factor is *speech sample size*. Disfluencies do not occur regularly; they are separated by periods of fluent speech that vary in length within and between subjects. As a result, the size of a speech sample influences the representativeness of data describing subjects' disfluency. Yet, speech-sample size has varied widely across different studies and different subjects in the same study. Meyers (1986) obtained approximately 350-word samples, whereas Yairi, Ambrose, and Niermann (1993) had approximately 1000 words per sample. In other studies of disfluency, investigators have used speech samples that ranged from 31 to 2044 words (Johnson & Associates, 1959), 342 to 2529 words (Silverman, 1971), and 85 to 650 words (Schwartz & Conture, 1988). Such inconsistency gives rise to multiple sources of errors. Short samples may contain only the peaks or valleys of a child's fluctuating disfluent output. Also, if different sample sizes are used and subjects' ages differ by more than just a few months, disfluency measures may be distorted by the less representative shorter samples of younger subjects close to stuttering onset or by the longer samples of older subjects with more chronic stuttering. This problem extends beyond the number of subjects studied. For example, in research on the duration of disfluencies, there is no standard for the number of disfluent events to be used in deriving means for each subject. Yairi and Hall (1993) averaged 2 to 5 disfluent events per subject, Throneburg and Yairi (1994) averaged all measurable events in a subject's sample, while Zebrowski (1991) collapsed the data from her entire group without deriving individual subjects' scores. In studies that quantified associated facial and head movements (e.g., Conture & Kelly, 1991; Yairi, Ambrose, & Niermann, 1993), only 10 disfluent events per subject were analyzed.

A fourth methodological issue is the *frequency and timing of sampling*. Early studies of disfluency (see Branscom, Hughes, & Oxtoby, 1955) obtained speech samples during several sessions conducted over at least two days. In contrast, most

---

[2]The within-word definition discussed earlier also interferes in the analyses of clusters that include between-word phenomena.

TABLE 3.1   Interjudge Reliability Data for Studies on Speech Disfluencies in Preschool Children

STUDY	TYPE OF RELIABILITY	RELIABILITY VALUE
Hughes (1955)*	Total numbers of instances: For individual type of instances For total repetitions	0.62–0.92 0.90
Johnson & Associates (1959)	Counts of each of 8 disfluency types	0.90–0.97
Yairi (1981)	Point-by-point	0.92
Wexler (1982)	Identify specific type	0.86–1.00
Colburn and Mysak (1982)	Identify and classify disfluencies	0.88
Yairi and Lewis (1984)	Point-by-point	0.93
Zebrowski (1991)	Identify instances Identify types Repetition units	0.92 0.92 0.89
Yairi, Ambrose, & Niermann (1993)	Point-by-point for SLD Point-by-point for other disfluencies	0.84 0.90

*From Branscom, Hughes, and Oxtoby (1955).

later studies have relied on a single recording session, although Yairi, Ambrose, and Niermann (1993) and Yairi and Ambrose (1996) obtained speech samples over two different days. In addition, little if any attention has been paid to the time of day when recordings are made, and with 2- to 4-year-old children, this could be a critical factor. Children who have missed their nap or have just awakened are less likely to produce adequate speech samples. Because early stuttering tends to fluctuate throughout the day and from day to day, lack of a standard protocol for recording speech samples increases the variability in disfluency data.

The lack of a standard protocol has also affected *reliability estimates* in disfluency research. Studies have varied from reporting only intrajudge agreement for overall number of disfluencies and for type of disfluency (e.g., Silverman, 1971) to calculating agreement based on the presence and/or absence of disfluency (e.g., Wexler, 1982), to reporting point-by-point (type and location) agreement only for the presence of disfluency (Hubbard & Yairi, 1988).[3] Large variations are also found in the size of speech samples that were remeasured, ranging from 10 percent (Zebrowski, 1991) to 100 percent (Yairi, Ambrose, & Niermann, 1993). It appears, however, that children's disfluency data, when analyzed by trained investigators, has yielded remarkably satisfying reliability levels. Table 3.1 lists the reliability types and coefficients reported in several studies. The point-by-point interjudge agreement reported during the 1980s and 1990s generally falls between .82 and .93. Based on these data, the position advocated by some investigators (Cordes & Ingham, 1994; Ingham, Cordes, & Gow, 1993; Kully & Boberg, 1988) that low agreement among observers threat-

---

[3]Calculations that include agreement on both the absence of disfluency (i.e., the utterance or word is fluent) and presence of disfluency typically yield higher estimates of reliability than do calculations limited to agreement on its presence.

ens the validity of results from several decades of research on stuttering may be questionable.[4] It is apparent that the disfluency data obtained on early childhood stuttering, as well as those derived from routine clinical recordings and analyses, can be significantly affected by methodological variations. Awareness of the impact of such variations should emphasize the urgent need for more uniform standards in recording, counting, and calculating disfluency measures.

DESCRIPTIONS OF INCIPIENT STUTTERING

The last 100 years have seen a significant evolution in the conceptualization of early childhood stuttering that has resulted from changes in the nature, quantity, and quality of information about this stage of the disorder. Much of this information stems from three types of sources: summaries of clinical impressions, record analyses, and parent interviews.

There are obvious obstacles in documenting authentic "first stuttering." First, the chances for trained investigators to be present when stuttering onset occurs are slim; and second, parents of beginning stutterers frequently assume a wait-and-see strategy, often on advice of pediatricians (Yairi & Carrico, 1992). Consequently, researchers who focused specifically on the onset of stuttering have had to rely almost exclusively on retrospective parental recollections, whereas those directing more broadly based inquiries have used direct clinical observations or record analyses. Much of their work, however, was based on children who were first observed several months to several years after they began stuttering.

Summaries of clinical impressions characterized the writings of early authors. For example, Gutzmann (1894) suggested that a stuttering child's thoughts run ahead of an awkward motor

speech system that repeats initial sounds or syllables. Hoepfner (1911) described the earliest form of stuttering as excessive syllable repetitions resulting from neurological deficits, whereas Bluemel (1913) emphasized the effortless nature of those repetitions. Similar emphases on repetitions can be found in Froeschels' writings (1921; 1943; 1952). His personal observations and case histories of 800 patients led him to state emphatically that the first signs of stuttering were ". . . exclusively word or syllable repetitions" (1952, p. 221). Froeschels also considered repetition rate and physical tension as signs of stuttering. He stated that in the primary clonus stage, a child's repetitions were of normal tempo and without tension and that faster repetitions appeared a bit later.

The singling out of repetitions as the main, if not only, speech characteristic of the incipient stage of stuttering prevailed throughout the first half of the current century and was supported by a host of case studies (see Van Riper, 1971). A departure from this view began in the second half of the century with two influential investigations that used the second source of information, analyses of clinical records. In Bloodstein's (1960a; 1960b) cross-sectional study of the development of stuttering, information from initial evaluation reports of various age groups of children who stuttered was coded according to symptoms. Although Bloodstein concluded that the predominant speech feature of the earliest phase of stuttering is repetition of syllables and words, he reported that 40 percent of the thirty 2- to 3-year-old children had exhibited hard contacts and that 33 percent had associated physical symptoms. Bloodstein (1987) flatly stated, "Practically any of the integral or associated symptoms of stuttering may be seen in some of the youngest stutterers and in some cases there seems to be little or no repetition" (p. 41).

A few years later, the realization that stuttering symptomatology at onset is diverse, and perhaps, not categorically different from advanced forms of the disorder, was reinforced by Van Riper's (1971) description of developmental heterogeneity, a report that was also based on his analyses of clinical records. Although unhurried

[4]Although Kully and Boberg (1988) emphasized the disagreement among clinics in identifying stuttering and disfluencies, inspection of their Table 2 reveals that agreement between the two clinics that counted "percent disfluency" averaged 81.7% considerably better than those counting "percent stuttering.

multiple- and single-syllable word repetitions maintained their top ranking for children in the largest group, Track I, other characteristics were listed as prominent also, such as fast-rate repetitions and silent gaps, for Track II; prolongations, complete blocks, vocal fry, breathing abnormalities, and struggle for Track III; and stereotyped repetitions of whole words and sentences, pauses associated with grunting, tongue protrusions, wide-open jaw, and lip tremors for Track IV. In a later separate study, Van Riper (1982) analyzed the clinical records of sixty-one children whom he personally examined within three weeks of stuttering onset. In this relatively large sample, 80 percent of the children repeated syllables or words at least three times per instance, 28 percent had prolongations longer than two seconds, and 15 percent indicated awareness of stuttering. Similar observations were also reported in several case studies. For example, Wyatt (1969) emphasized the compulsive nature of repetitions by a young, stuttering child, and Yairi (1974) described the severe, complex symptomatology of his son's stuttering and provided rare, quantified data on disfluencies at the time of onset. He reported up to fifteen consecutive repetition units of words or syllables within days of onset and noted their compulsive, tense nature.

Parent interview studies, the third major information source about early stuttering, also began to describe more complex/severe stuttering symptomatology during this period. The first such investigation was a little-known study conducted at the University of Iowa by Taylor (1937) with parents of forty-seven stuttering children, ages 3 to 7 years. Eighty-five percent of these parents reported repetitions as the only initial symptom, with repetition of whole words the most frequently reported (25%). Still, 12 percent of the children were reported to have sound stoppages and 11 percent such secondary characteristics as head movements and gasping. A few years later, Johnson's (1942) first investigation of stuttering onset revealed that forty-two of forty-six parents reported that their children's "stuttering" consisted initially of effortless, brief

repetitions of parts of words, whole words, or phrases, usually at the beginning of speech attempts. Significantly, "brief" was casually described by Johnson as two to four iterations of a repeated segment. As we shall see later, this detail received minimal attention but may be an important feature of early stuttering. In Darley's (1955) study, which included the parents of fifty stuttering children (mean post-onset interval = 50 months) and an equal number of control parents, the main characteristic of initial stuttering was recalled as repetitions of syllables and words "averaging about three repetitions per stutter" (p. 138). Nevertheless, 16 percent of the stuttering children were reported to have blocks, 8 percent prolongations, and 4 percent severe articulatory fixations and respiratory abnormalities.

The largest parent interview study, by Johnson and his colleagues (1959), published data for 150 children who stuttered (mean post-onset interval = 18 months) and their nonstuttering controls. The most frequently reported characteristics of early stuttering were syllable (60%) and word (50%) repetitions; however, 12 to 15 percent of these parents reported sound prolongations, and 3 percent noted complete blocks. Although the authors inferred that the disfluencies described by these parents were normal, McDearmon's (1968) reanalyses of the same data led him to conclude that parental descriptions of at least 63 percent of these children resembled "primary stuttering" (e.g., repetitions and prolongations of syllables with as many as 36% having light tension), and that "secondary stuttering" characteristics, such as interruptions accompanied by struggle, tension, and emotional reactions, were reported for 4.1 percent. He concluded, therefore, that the descriptions of only 28 percent of the children could be considered as "normal disfluencies."

Two recent parent interview studies of stuttering onset were carried out for twenty-two and eighty-seven beginning stuttering children, respectively (Yairi, 1983; Yairi & Ambrose, 1992b). These investigations were conducted, on average, less than six months from the time of onset, a significant procedural improvement. In a departure from previous findings,[5] these investigators reported that stuttering onset was a distinct sudden event for 31 to 36 percent of the children, respectively, and that initial stuttering was rated as moderate to severe for 28 to 36 percent. Among the children in the first study, 95 percent were reported to exhibit syllable repetitions at onset; 40 percent also exhibited word repetitions. Significantly, 85 percent of parents reported that syllables or words were repeated three to five times per instance, 36 percent reported sound prolongations, 23 percent conspicuous silent periods, 14 percent blocks, 18 percent facial contortions, and 18 percent respiratory irregularities. Only 32 percent of these parents described the onset of stuttering as consisting of easy, simple repetitions, devoid of any sign of tension or force. Most parents perceived early stuttering to be associated with some degree of force, and 36 percent reported moderate to severe tension. More than 20 percent thought their child was aware of the problem. Observing the positive relationship between sudden onset and severity of stuttering, Yairi and Ambrose (1992b) pointed out the potential of such information in differentiating stuttering subgroups and developmental patterns that might permit early prognoses of chronicity and recovery. Such advances would place clinical intervention decisions on sound empirical information, a position urged by Curlee (1992a).

Keeping in mind the limitations of this information, speech-language clinicians should be aware of the increasing indications that early childhood stuttering is a heterogeneous disorder from its inception. It may begin gradually or suddenly and be either mild or severe. The most common speech characteristics are repetitions of syllables or words, many of which may be associated with some degree of tension and repeated *twice or more* per instance. Sound prolongations, articulatory fixations (blockages), and associated physical movements, though less frequent, are not uncommon, and are not necessarily signs of advanced stuttering. Researchers and clinicians should be alert to the possibility that initial variations in type of onset and in speech characteristics may provide diagnostic and prognostic differentiation of young stutterers (Yairi & Ambrose, 1992b).

FREQUENCY OF DISFLUENCIES: NONSTUTTERING CHILDREN

Historically, scientific interest in the disfluent speech of children began independently of interest in stuttering. For example, in the late nineteenth century, Kirkpatrick (1891) suggested that babies babble (repeat sounds and syllables) because they are not aware that they have been understood, whereas Conardi (1904) described it as playful exploration of speech. Systematic research of disfluent speech began with the study of language development. Early investigators (Brandenburg, 1915; Nice, 1920) studied a single child and noted the occurrence of repetitions; later studies (Adams, 1932; Fisher, 1932; McCarthy, 1930; Smith, 1926) involved groups of preschool children. Although investigators commented on the presence of repetitions and reported some quantitative data (e.g., Adams, 1932), repetitions were neither defined nor differentiated. A later study that described age-related variations in repetitions of preschool children but did not provide quantified data was published by Metraux (1950). Quantitative research of disfluency began at the University of Iowa in the late 1930s and early 1940s with the emergence of Johnson's diagnosogenic theory that linked stuttering onset to erroneous parental reactions to normal disfluencies. If it could be demonstrated that disfluencies were commonplace, the theory would receive important support. Thus, the disfluent speech of nonstuttering young children became a significant research objective.

Between 1939 and 1946, five investigations of preschool children's speech disfluency were completed at the University of Iowa. These included a doctoral dissertation by Dorothy Davis published in 1939, master's theses by Margaret

---

[5]Sudden onset was reported by Preus (1981) in 17 percent of 100 cases and by Van Riper (1971) in 10 percent of 114 cases.

Branscom (1942), Jeannette Hughes (1943), and Eloise Tupper Oxtoby (1943), and an unpublished study by Wendell Johnson. Altogether, these five studies (summarized in Branscom, Hughes, & Oxtoby, 1955) included 193 nonstuttering preschool-age children, comprising 104 boys and 89 girls. Because tape-recorders were not available, a child's verbal output was handwritten, and disfluencies were simultaneously marked on the transcripts. Such technological disadvantages reduced precision in recording a child's utterances and disfluencies and limited the disfluency types studied to only three: syllable, word, and phrase repetitions. Nevertheless, it was one of the first times that disfluencies were defined and differentiated, with careful attention given to discrete ages of children between ages 2 and 5 years. Another early study by Egland (1938) with kindergarten children, who were mainly 5-year-olds (M = 5:5), used electronic recordings and a different disfluency system. As it turned out, the results of these studies led to two widespread, long-lasting beliefs: (1) Repetitions and other disfluencies are common and frequent in nonstuttering children (e.g., Bloodstein, Jaeger, & Tureen, 1952) and (2) these same kinds of "normal disfluencies" also characterize the speech of young beginning stutterers (Johnson & Associates, 1959).

A careful scrutiny of the data should provide an objective evaluation of these beliefs. The upper portion of Table 3.2 presents a summary of the results of the six studies for two measures: Total Disfluency, as reported by the investigators, and Short-Element Repetitions (SER), which I calculated by combining the counts of syllable and word repetitions.[6] Because the latter types of repetitions are typical of early stuttering, this count provides the data most pertinent to the beliefs stated above. As can be seen, data sets for mean Total Disfluency vary narrowly between 1.83 and 5.41 per 100 words, and of greater interest, between 1.20 and 3.73 per 100 words for mean SER. These means are considerably closer to the lower end (0.0) than to the upper end (11.00) or even midpoint of the individual data distributions. In Davis' study, the SER for 2-year-olds, her most disfluent age group, was 2.27. Even if two extrapolated standard deviations of .65 were added to this mean, the upper limit for SER would only be 3.75.

More than twenty-five years later, a second wave of studies reporting the frequency/type distribution of disfluencies in nonstuttering preschool children began to appear. These studies used electronic recordings that permitted repeated listening for additional disfluency types; they were undoubtedly more accurate. The expanded disfluency system developed by Johnson and Associates (1959) was later modified by Williams, Silverman, and Kools (1968) and included the following categories: Part-Word Repetition, Word Repetition, Disrhythmic Phonation (sound prolongation and broken words), Tense Pause (audible tension between words), Phrase Repetition, Interjection, and Revisions-Incomplete Phrases. This modified system was employed in a series of three studies reported by Yairi and his students (Yairi & Clifton, 1972; Yairi & Jennings, 1974; Yairi, 1981) for discrete, single-year age groups of preschool children, and their data are summarized in the middle section of Table 3.2. The studies by Silverman (1972) and Wexler (1982) included only boys. The data in the lower part of Table 3.2 were obtained from normally fluent children who were controls for stuttering subjects in the studies listed.

With additional disfluency types now available, I recently proposed another data index, Stuttering-Like Disfluency (SLD), which encompasses part-word and monosyllabic word repetition, disrhythmic phonation, and tense pause. Although these disfluency types occur much more often in the speech of stutterers,[7] all of them occur in the speech of normal speakers. Thus, "stutter-

---

[6]Egland used a more elaborate system and reported more total disfluencies than are shown here. Table 3.2 calculations include only data that are equivalent across all of the studies that are listed.

[7]See Wingate (1962) and Young (1984). As will be discussed later, data on disfluent speech near the onset of stuttering (Yairi & Lewis, 1984; Yairi & Ambrose, 1996) also justify the inclusion of monosyllabic word repetitions.

TABLE 3.2   Group Means per 100 Words, or per 100 Syllables (X), or as Percent of Disfluent Words (XX) of Total Disfluency, Short-Element Repetition (SER), Stuttering-Like Disfluency (SLD) and the Percent of SLD in Total Disfluency for Various Age Groups of Nonstuttering Children in Three Groups of Studies***

INVESTIGATOR	AGE	N	TOTAL	SER	SLD	% SLD
BHJ (1955)*	2	18	5.17	3.73		
Davis (1939)	2	15	5.41	2.27		
BHJ (1955)*	3	26	3.90	2.73		
Davis (1939)	3	20	4.48	1.79		
Oxtoby (1955)**	3	25	4.76	2.51		
BHJ (1955)*	4	42	2.93	1.20		
Davis (1939)	4	27	3.97	1.62		
BHJ (1955)*	5	20	3.42	2.26		
Egland (1955)	5	26	1.83	1.48		
Yairi (1981)	2	33	6.49	2.54	3.44	52%
Yairi & Jennings (1974)	4	24	7.86	1.49	2.17	28%
Yairi & Clifton (1971)	5	15	7.65	1.84	2.67	35%
Silverman (1972)	4	10	8.86	2.95	4.30	48%
Wexler (1982)	2	12	14.56	2.84	5.86	40%
Wexler (1982)	4	12	9.10	1.28	3.36	37%
Wexler (1982)	6	12	9.08	1.43	2.77	25%
Johnson et al. (1959)	2–8	68	7.28	1.62	1.88	26%
Yairi & Lewis (1984) X	2–3	10	6.18	2.24	3.02	49%
Hubbard & Yairi (1988) X	2–4	15	5.90	1.90	2.59	43%
Yairi & Ambrose (1996) X	2–5	50	5.73	1.33	1.39	24%
Zebrowski (1991) XX	2–5	10	5.00			36%
Meyers (1986) XX	4–6	10	5.12	2.2	3.50	34%

*Includes the combined means of the studies by Branscom, Hughes, and Johnson. From Branscom, Hughes, and Oxtoby (1955).

**From Branscom, Hughes, and Oxtoby (1955).

***Upper part: early studies; middle part: later studies; lower part: studies in which subjects were used as controls for stutterers.

ing-like" indicates that they are not exclusively "stuttering." SLD data were calculated by me for studies listed in Table 3.2. As can be seen in the middle and lower portions of the table, the total disfluencies reported by studies that used the expanded disfluency system are larger than those in the upper part of the table, whereas SER means remain close to those of the early Iowa studies.

Overall, with the exception of the Wexler (1982) study, the table reveals impressively similar findings from sixteen studies conducted by different investigators over a period of fifty-five years.

For those studies employing the full range of disfluency types, most Total Disfluency means for nonstuttering preschool children fall between 6 and 8 disfluencies per 100 words. In contrast, SLD means approximate 3, and SER means cluster around 2 per 100 words. With the exception of one study, the percentages of SLD suggest an important guideline: The percentage of SLDs in the Total Disfluency of nonstuttering children is always under 50 percent and is mostly near 35 percent. Among recent sources, the study with the largest sample size (Yairi & Ambrose, 1996) places it at a low of 24 percent. The importance of this guideline will be apparent when the disfluency of children who stutter is discussed in a later section.

Two additional studies used either unclear or unusual definitions of disfluencies that prevented their listing in Table 3.2. Floyd and Perkins (1974) found that twenty normally speaking children, between 2 and 5 years old, had mean percent disfluent syllables of 1.22. Bjerkan (1980) reported a mean percentage of 6.2 percent repeated words in the speech of 108 Norwegian children who were 2 to 6 years old. The frequency of "fragmentation" was virtually zero.[8] Generally, these data agree with those of the studies summarized.

If these data, especially SER and SLD, question the traditional view that disfluencies are common and frequent in the speech of young, nonstuttering children, examination of individual subject data further reinforces such doubts. Typically, when individual disfluency data were reported in the studies listed in Table 3.2, they were extremely heterogeneous. In the Yairi (1981) investigation of thirty-three 2-year-old children, the largest recent study of disfluency in this age group, total disfluency ranged from 0 to 25.6 per 100 words. Moreover, a substantial number of children were disfluent rather infrequently; nine had 2 or fewer total disfluencies, and over half had 1 or fewer syllable- or word-repetitions per 100 words. This point is supported by the fact that the disfluencies of the upper quartile subjects equaled the sum of the lower three quartiles combined. This finding is consistent with Davis' (1939) report that sixteen of her sixty-two subjects, ages 2 through 5 years, produced no syllable repetitions, and twenty-eight had fewer than 0.5 per 100 words, a finding that is often overlooked in the literature.

Although a variety of conditions and variables may account for individual differences in the disfluency of nonstuttering children, none, except for age, has been shown to exert a consistent in-

fluence. References to age-related declines in disfluency can be found in early studies of language development (Adams, 1932; Fisher, 1932; Smith, 1926). In disfluency studies, Davis (1939) found a decline in total repetition from 5.41 per 100 words at age 2 to 4.48 at age 3, and to 3.97 by age 4. She also reported a statistically significant correlation between age and repetition. In Branscom's (1942) study, total repetitions declined from 4.18 at age 3 to 3.42 at age 5. Statistically significant reductions were also found by DeJoy (1975), Wexler (1982), and Yairi (1982). A similar tendency was reported by Bjerkan (1980) but no statistical tests were applied to the data. Only two investigations (Gottfred, 1979; Haynes & Hood, 1977) did not find significant decreases in disfluency with age. In the 1982 Yairi study, thirty-three 2- and 3-year-old children were recorded several times during a one-year period. Their disfluencies peaked in frequency during the latter part of age 2 or near the beginning of age 3, then began a downward slide. Generally, however, these children's third year of life was characterized by large-magnitude, up-and-down alternations in the number of disfluencies. Of special significance was Yairi's finding that the number of part-word repetitions tends to decrease with maturation, even during temporary surges in total disfluencies. Both DeJoy (1975) and Branscom and colleagues (1955) noted that declines in part-word-repetitions are an important feature of normal speech development. Thus, it would appear to me that a rise in part-word repetition at this age is *not* consistent with normal development, and listeners' evaluations of such a rise as abnormal may well be justified.

These findings lead to several conclusions. The overall frequency of disfluency among nonstuttering children is rather low, averaging about 6 to 8 per 100 words. Even lower frequencies result if a syllable metric is used. The average preschool child is likely to produce a rather small number, perhaps 3 per 100 words, of part-word repetitions, monosyllabic word repetitions, and disrhythmic phonations, which are the types of disfluencies found most often in the speech of young stutterers. Although disfluencies are unquestionably a nor-

---

[8]Bjerkan (1980) used handwritten transcripts of speech samples. His "word repetition" also included repetitions of phrases. Floyd and Perkins' "disfluent syllable" included repetitions, prolongations and interjections.

mal speech characteristic of preschool-age children, my analyses lead me to conclude that "normal" should *not* be construed as "frequently occurring" in the majority of children. The popular belief, also held by many speech-language pathologists, that disfluency, especially repetitions, is a pervasive normal phenomenon and that all children go through a "stage" of heightened disfluency is incorrect.[9] The heterogeneity of individual data supports this conclusion and is in accord with both Wingate's (1962) and Yairi's (1981) interpretations.

Additionally, there is consistent evidence that the disfluent speech of nonstuttering preschool children is characterized by a *proportional pattern* in which SLDs are a minor component. This pattern clearly differs from that of children who stutter. From a developmental point of view, there is a general progression from less sophisticated to more sophisticated behaviors and functions. In contrast, disfluency often evidences alternating reversals in frequency during the early years of life. The important question, of course, is what constitutes an *abnormal departure* within such fluctuations in disfluency. According to present developmental data, a sudden rise in SERs constitutes just that, and is, therefore, a valid cause for parental and professional concern.

FREQUENCY OF DISFLUENCIES: CHILDREN WHO STUTTER

Speech-based data on disfluency during early stages of stuttering have been extremely limited until recently. The largest study, reported in 1959 by Johnson and Associates, used recorded speech samples of eighty-nine stuttering children, ages 2 to 8 years, and their matched nonstuttering controls. This study has several shortcomings. First,

the wide age range prevents these data from being viewed as "normative" as was claimed by the authors. Second, the eighteen-month average interval between the onset of stuttering and the recording of speech samples does not permit these data to be viewed as representative of "early stuttering." Third, the likelihood of spontaneous recovery within the first eighteen months after onset is substantial (Andrews & Harris, 1964; Yairi & Ambrose, 1992a; Yairi, Ambrose, & Niermann, 1993), so there is good reason to assume that these data may be heavily weighted by chronic subjects. Furthermore, because speech samples varied in size from 31 to 1158 words, I suspect that most short samples were contributed by younger children whose stuttering may not have been adequately sampled. Fourth, the metric used, disfluencies per 100 words, inflates the measures of older subjects who use many more multisyllable words than do 2-year-old children. Thus, I believe that the group means reported by Johnson and his co-workers should have been lower, a belief that is consistent with data showing higher disfluency levels near stuttering onset (e.g., Yairi & Lewis, 1984). Finally, the interjudge reliabilities reported by the Johnson study, mostly above .90, are questionable because they are based on the counts of two judges for speech samples of adult females, *not* child subjects. It is not known whether these judges analyzed all, or any, of the 178 speech samples used in the study.

In spite of its limitations, the Johnson (1959) data reveal important characteristics that distinguish the disfluencies of young children who stutter from those of normally fluent children. These data show a mean total disfluency of 17.9 per 100 words for sixty-four stuttering boys, nearly two and one-half times larger than the 7.28 disfluencies of nonstuttering controls. Johnson emphasized the extensive overlap between the two groups, noting that one-third of the control subjects had more total disfluencies than one-third of the stutterers. A striking difference, however, emerges from an analysis that focuses on those disfluencies that are typical of stuttered speech. Using the Johnson and Associates data, my calcu-

---

[9]This view was probably influenced by the peculiar way of measuring the number of disfluent words in speech samples used by Branscom, Hughes, and Oxtoby (1955) who counted all of the words in phrase repetitions as disfluencies, which is likely to have inflated their counts to the 23.5 disfluent words per 100 words spoken that they reported.

lation of SLDs found 11.51 per 100 words for stutterers but only 1.88 for nonstutterers, a 6:1 ratio that indicates a greatly reduced overlap between the groups. Furthermore, the percentage of SLDs calculated for each decile rises from 20 percent of all disfluencies in the first decile to 74 percent in the ninth decile. Thus, the more disfluent a stuttering child is, the larger the proportion of SLDs.[10]

The past decade has seen significant progress in obtaining speech samples that meet two important criteria: being close to the onset of stuttering and representing a narrow age range of children. Five studies conducted at the University of Illinois by Yairi and co-workers are easy to compare because of their similarity in procedures, sample sizes (500 to 1000 syllables), and measures (disfluencies per 100 syllables). Yairi and Lewis (1984) obtained tape recordings of ten stuttering and ten nonstuttering control children who were 25 to 39 months old. The stuttering children were within two months of onset (M = 6 weeks) compared to the 18 months for children in the Johnson and Associates study. Their mean total disfluency was 21.46 per 100 syllables while that of controls was 6.18, a ratio of almost 3.5:1. Respective mean SLD measures for the two groups were 16.43 and 3.02, a 5.4:1 ratio. So, again, there was less group overlap for SLD measures. This study provided evidence that large deviations from normal disfluency exist almost from the very beginning of the onset of stuttering, which considerably weakens assertions that the speech of stuttering and nonstuttering children is similar at this time.

Additional investigations by the Illinois group corroborated findings that high levels of disfluency near stuttering onset are markedly different from those of normally fluent children. In 1988, Hubbard and Yairi compared fifteen stutterers, ages 2 to 4 years, who were within five and a half months of stuttering onset, with a like number of nonstuttering subjects who were matched for age, sex, and language development. Although the

group of stutterers was not a random sample—5 disfluencies per 100 syllables were required for selection—their 22.57 disfluencies per 100 syllables indicated that severe stuttering is common during the first six months of stuttering. Later, Yairi and Ambrose (1992a) reported data for twenty-seven preschool-age stutterers that were obtained within one year of onset (M = 6.43 months). A year later, Yairi, Ambrose, and Niermann (1993) presented data from 1000-word samples of sixteen stuttering children, 25 to 39 months of age, which were recorded within twelve weeks of onset (M= 6.88 weeks). A final investigation (Yairi & Ambrose, 1996) reported data from 1000-word samples of 100 stuttering children, sixty-eight boys and thirty-two girls, who were between 25 and 65 months of age (M = 40 months). Maximum post-onset interval was 12 months (M = 5.5 months). Comparison data were obtained from a control group of fifty normally fluent children, thirty-four boys and sixteen girls, having a mean age of 40 months. Selected measures from these studies are presented in Table 3.3, as are data from two additional recent investigations of preschool-aged stuttering children.

Zebrowski (1991) recorded 300-word samples of ten stutterers, ages 32 to 61 months, who were within one year of onset (M = 8.5 months). Meyers (1986) studied twelve stutterers, ages 4 to 5:11 years, with moderate or severe stuttering, using samples of approximately 350 words. Because the samples in these two studies were smaller and used a different metric—percent of disfluent words—direct comparisons are not appropriate. In viewing Table 3.3, recall earlier reservations about wide age ranges and post-onset intervals. Remember, also, that measures using the per-100-word metric tend to overestimate disfluency, whereas those based on percent of disfluent words tend to underestimate its frequency. Adjusting for these biases (and for Meyers' more severe subjects) by increasing or decreasing the respective means, there is a remarkable similarity across these studies. High levels of total disfluency, more than 45 instances per 100 syllables, are found in some preschool-age children who stutter, as is

---

[10]Similar observations of such proportional trends were made by Yairi (1972) with respect to high- and low-disfluent school-age children.

shown in the group ranges in Table 3.3. Of course, some children exhibit low levels of disfluency. As a group, preschool-age children who stutter average around 17 total disfluencies per 100 syllables, or 15 per 100 words. Among very young children near stuttering onset (Hubbard & Yairi, 1988; Yairi, Ambrose, & Niermann, 1993, Yairi & Lewis, 1984), mean disfluency levels tend to be higher, perhaps 19 to 20 instances per 100 syllables. These means are about two and one-half times larger than those of the nonstuttering children that were presented earlier in this chapter. Direct comparisons with control group data (see Table 3.3) yield similar differences.

Of even greater interest are such disfluency measures as SER, which includes part-word as well as monosyllabic word repetitions, and SLD, which consists of short-element repetitions plus disrhythmic phonation and tense pauses. Across the entire age range of the stuttering children represented in Table 3.3, the average number of SERs is 9 per 100 syllables, but 10 to 11 per 100 for the youngest subjects near onset. In comparison, control subjects had only 2 SERs per 100 syllables, on average. SLD measures are even higher, 11 to 12 per 100 syllables for all stuttering preschoolers, and 13 to 16 per 100 for younger subjects. So, children who stutter, on average, had five times as many SERs or SLDs per 100 syllables as did nonstuttering controls. The percentage of SLDs in total disfluency counts ranges from 64 to 88 percent across studies, with an average of 72 percent, almost twice that of normally fluent control subjects. The importance of SLD as a measure of

TABLE 3.3   Range and Means of Total Disfluency, Short-Element Repetition (SER), Stuttering-Like Disfluency (SLD), and Percent of SLD in Total Disfluency for Stuttering (E) and Normally Speaking Children (C)

STUDY	GROUP/N		RANGE OF TOTAL DISFL	MEAN TOTAL	MEAN SER	MEAN SLD	% SLD
Johnson & Associates (1959)	E	68	3.30–46.51 *	17.90	9.72	11.55	64%
	C	68	0.60–18.28	7.28	1.62	1.88	26%
Yairi & Lewis (1984)	E	10		21.54	10.56	16.43	76%
	C	10		6.18	2.24	3.02	49%
Hubbard & Yairi (1988)	E	15	7.72–39.85 **	22.45	10.12	16.88	75%
	C	15	3.40–9.24	5.90	1.9	2.59	43%
Yairi & Ambrose (1992a)	E	27	3.64–32.32 **	16.21	8.79	10.87	73%
Yairi, Ambrose, & Niermann (1993)	E	16	3.90–23.30 **	17.41	10.13	11.99	69%
Yairi & Ambrose (1996)	E	100	4.52–48.59 **	16.05	8.73	10.52	65%
	C	50	0.00–16.96	5.75	1.54	0.87	15%
Zebrowski (1991)	E	10	***	13.00			73%
	C	10		5.00			36%
Meyers (1986)	E	10	13.00–35.00 ***	15.32	9.12	13.52	88%
	C	10		5.12	2.2	3.50	34%

*per 100 words.

**per 100 syllables.

***percent of words stuttered.

early stuttering and its differentiating power should be apparent. Furthermore, its sensitivity as a measure of early childhood stuttering will become even more apparent in relation to developmental aspects of the disorder.

Although the data presented thus far depict general patterns that distinguish the disfluent speech of children who do and do not stutter, the overlap in individual data distributions is important in differential diagnosis, particularly in borderline cases. Yairi and Lewis (1984), for example, reported that group overlap was minimal on both part-word repetition and tense pause. Ninety percent of stutterers had more part-word repetitions and tense pauses than the maximum for nonstutterers. Johnson and Associates (1959) showed that only 10 percent of nonstuttering children had 3 or more SLDs per 100 words, whereas 80 percent of stutterers had at least 2.60 SLDs per 100 words. A sharper cutoff point using the syllable metric was reported in a recent investigation by Yairi and Ambrose (1996). They found that 11 percent of the least disfluent stuttering children had 3 to 4 SLDs per 100 syllables as did 11 percent of the most disfluent nonstuttering children. Thus, children suspected of stuttering exhibited at least 3 SLDs per 100 syllables, although not all children who exhibit 3 to 4 or more SLDs per 100 syllables are stutterers.

DEVELOPMENTAL CHANGES OF DISFLUENCY OF CHILDREN WHO STUTTER

Although it has been consistently demonstrated that disfluencies of normally fluent children decline with age (Davis, 1939; Yairi, 1982), the belief that disfluencies of beginning stutterers most often increase in frequency and severity with time has persisted for many years. A number of developmental models and theoretical positions (Bloodstein, 1960b; Bluemel, 1932; Froeschels, 1921; Johnson & Associates, 1959) have reinforced this belief. One of the more significant developments during the last decade has been the publication of disfluency data that negate, or even reverse, such beliefs. An early indication was the Yairi and Lewis (1984) study, which found very high disfluency

levels near the onset of stuttering (21.54 per 100 syllables), clearly surpassing those reported by Johnson and colleagues (17.90 disfluencies per 100 words) some 18 months after onset. Subsequently, Yairi and Ambrose (1992a) published disfluency data obtained from periodic tape-recorded speech samples of twenty-seven stuttering children who had been followed for three to twelve years. During the first two years, untreated stuttering children evidenced reductions in mean Total Disfluency from 16.21 to 10.35 per 100 syllables, and from 10.47 to 4.80 in mean SLDs. Mean SLD declined further to 2.72 in subsequent recordings. Sixty-five percent of these children recovered within the first two years of onset, and recoveries had climbed to 85 percent by the end of the study. Much of this amelioration, however, occurred during the first fourteen months after stuttering began. In a perceptual study, Finn, Ingham, Yairi, and Ambrose (1994) reported that sophisticated judges were unable to distinguish the speech of these recovered stutterers from that of their normally fluent peers.

In a second longitudinal study, Yairi, Ambrose, and Niermann (1993) recorded sixteen children within three months of stuttering onset, and at three-month and six-month followups. This study again revealed severe stuttering and high disfluency levels during the earliest stage of the disorder and a trend for quick, sharp reductions in disfluency. Mean Total Disfluency declined from 17.41 to 9.49 per 100 syllables during the six-month period. More importantly, mean SLD declined from 11.99 to 4.46 during the same period. Furthermore, these changes were accompanied by reductions in mean facial-head movements from 3.18 to 1.91 per disfluency. Corresponding mean stuttering severity ratings (7-point scale) fell also, from 4.43 to 1.99. Subsequent followups revealed that not a single child who recovered had relapsed and that most continued to stutter less. There was also a tendency for boys' stuttering to persist longer than that of girls. We concluded that stuttering peaks for many children during the first two to three months of onset, usually prior to a sharp decline. In yet another longitudinal study, Yairi, Ambrose, Paden, and Throneburg (1996) reported preliminary data for three groups of preschool stuttering children who had been followed for three years. Two subgroups of Early and Late Recovered subjects (N = 10 in each) had 12.50 SLDs per 100 syllables during initial recordings but only 3.98 and 2.46 SLDs per 100, respectively, thirteen to eighteen months later. The third subgroup of twelve persistent stutterers began and ended the same observation period with 8.27 and 7.07 SLDs per 100 syllables, which rose to 8.16 per 100 in subsequent testing. Rapid declines in the disfluencies of young stutterers have also been reported in unpublished longitudinal studies by Ryan (1990).

Together, the studies of Ryan and Yairi and his colleagues provide objective support of many past reports concerning high rates of spontaneous recovery during early childhood (e.g., Andrews & Harris, 1964). An important byproduct of these longitudinal investigations has been the identification of SLDs as a sensitive measure of changes in stuttering. In the Yairi, Ambrose, and Niermann (1993) study, during the same six-month period when mean SLDs declined from 11.99 to 6.34 to 4.46 per 100 syllables, measures of Other Disfluency[11] remained surprisingly stable (5.42, 6.45, and 5.03) and did not contribute valuable information about time-related changes in stuttering.

ADDITIONAL CHARACTERISTICS OF DISFLUENCIES

In spite of the different disfluency patterns that emerge among children in the early stage of stuttering compared to those of their normally speaking peers, some overlap in frequency of disfluency remains. Therefore, properties such as extent of iterations, duration, and associated physical movements may provide important distinctions.

Extent of Iterations

For repetitive disfluencies, the number of times that a segment is repeated is an important distinction. Both parental reports and objective data indi-

cate that this is an important dimension for identifying early stuttering. Several early sources referred to iterations but overlooked their importance. For example, Johnson (1942) emphasized the normalcy of disfluencies at the time of stuttering onset and characterized two to four iterations per segment as "brief." Van Riper (1971) observed, and Darley (1955) and Yairi (1983) also noted, that repetitions described by parents often consisted of three iterations. As we shall see, objective data indicate that three iterations are considerably above the average for either stuttering or nonstuttering children.

Initial attempts to quantify the extent of repetitions came in early studies of nonstuttering children. Branscom, Hughes, and Oxtoby (1955) reported that 79 percent of word- and syllable-repetitions consisted of one extra iteration, 17 percent had two extra iterations, and 4 percent three or more iterations. Later studies used mean repetition units, the average number of times that segments were repeated, as their metric. In research with nonstuttering children, Wexler (1982) and Yairi (1981) reported means for several groups that averaged 1.10 and 1.13 respectively, indicating that such children typically have slightly more than one extra repetition. Three studies that compared young stutterers and controls (Ambrose & Yairi, 1995; Johnson & Associates, 1959; Yairi & Lewis, 1984) found significant differences in mean repetition units; another did not (Zebrowski, 1991). The two investigations by Yairi and colleagues were conducted with children who were, respectively, within two and three months of onset. Table 3.4 summarizes the findings from these studies in which data presented separately in original sources for gender, words, and syllables have been combined. When needed, data were adjusted to conform with the Johnson study (1959) definition that a single-repetition unit is *one* extra production of the segment (but-but) and a double-unit repetition has *two* extra productions (but-but-but), and so forth. The data show that normally fluent children seldom repeat more than once, but stuttering children repeat, on average, between 1.5 to 1.7 times, and some occasionally repeat more than ten times.

---

[11]Includes combined counts of interjections, phrase repetitions, and revisions-incomplete phrases.

TABLE 3.4   Means and Ranges for Repetition Units for Nonstuttering and Stuttering Children

		MEAN		RANGE	
STUDY		**NONSTUTTERING**	**STUTTERING**	**NONSTUTTERING**	**STUTTERING**
Yairi (1981)		1.13		1–5	
Wexler (1982)	2-yr olds	1.10		1–2.55*	
	4-yr olds	1.06		1–1.92*	
	6-yr olds	1.03		1–1.56*	
Johnson & Associates (1959)		1.09	1.46	1–2	1–3.4*
Yairi & Lewis (1984)		1.11	1.53	1–2	1–11
Zebrowski (1991)		1.15	1.35	1–4	1–4
Ambrose & Yairi (1995)		1.16	1.70	1–4	1–17

*mean range.

Ambrose and Yairi's (1995) study with twenty-nine subjects in each group included a 28,000-word language corpus per group. Among its findings, 67 percent of all syllable repetitions and single-syllable-word repetitions of stuttering children involved one repetition, while 33 percent involved two or more repetitions, a ratio of 2:1. In the nonstuttering control group, the respective figures were 87 percent and 13 percent, and a ratio of 6.6:1. Thus, two or more unit repetitions are three times as prevalent in beginning stutterers as in normally speaking children. Clearly, repetitions longer than 2 units occur infrequently in the speech of nonstutterers but stutterers exhibit many more. The sharpest difference between the two groups was found in the number of long repetition units (2 or more units) per 100 syllables. The mean of the stuttering group was 3.70, but only 0.21 for control children, and only 10 percent of the nonstuttering children's measures were as high as the lower end of those of stuttering children. Thus, even one repetition with 2 or more units per 100 syllables may exceed that observed in most nonstuttering children. Although the mean number of repetition units per instance has an important effect on severity, other measures, such as the frequency and proportion of repetitions containing several units, may be even more revealing, or differentiating characteristics, of the incipient stage of early childhood stuttering.

As Yairi and Lewis (1984) concluded, measures of repetition units better discriminate stuttering from nonstuttering children than do the frequency of disfluency types. Although the difference between repeating once and one and one-half times was viewed by Johnson and Associates (1959) as having no practical significance, I believe that a failure to appreciate the co-effect of frequency and extent of iterations was a serious error. For example, a moderate-to-highly disfluent, nonstuttering child who repeats "and" on three different occasions during a 100-word sample is likely to utter it six times (3 × 2), but a moderately severe stutterer who repeats a word on nine different occasions is likely utter it twenty-three times (9 × 2.5). Such a difference is likely to affect listeners' perceptions and judgments of normalcy. To my knowledge, this co-effect has not been considered in the theoretical or clinical literature. A measure that combines the co-effect of repetition frequency and number of iterations may greatly enhance the usefulness of current disfluency analyses.

Duration of Disfluencies

Efforts to quantify disfluencies more precisely have recently led to studies of duration. Conture and Kelly (1991) counted videotape frames of speech samples of thirty stuttering children, between 2 and 6 years of age (M= 4:5), and measured the duration of 300 instances of stuttering. Their overall mean length was 913 msec, with sound/syllable repetitions being longer than sound prolongations. For the matched group of nonstuttering controls, however, the investigators measured the duration of fluent tokens (M = 342 msec), rather than disfluencies. Louko, Edwards, and Conture (1990) apparently used the same speech samples to compare the duration of disfluencies of twelve stuttering subjects who also exhibited disordered phonology with that of eighteen stuttering subjects having normal phonological development. No statistically significant differences were found. Data from these as well as other studies are presented in Table 3.5.

Several other studies have measured durational aspects of preschoolers' disfluencies using computer-based acoustic analyses. Zebrowski (1991) compared the duration of part-word repetitions and sound prolongations in the speech of ten children with stuttering histories of up to one year post onset with those of ten matched control subjects. She found no between group differences in the length of either disfluency type. Because group means were derived from pooled measures of the entire group, rather than individual subject means, subjects who contributed more disfluencies had greater influence on this study's results. Similarly, Kelly and Conture (1992) reported "virtually identical" durations for within-word disfluencies of thirteen preschool children (M = 4:0) and their matched nonstuttering controls.

TABLE 3.5   Mean Duration (in milliseconds) of Disfluencies of Preschool Stutterering and Nonstuttering Children. Durations of Intervals Between Repetition Units Are Also Presented.

STUDY	DISFLUENCY		STUTTERERS		NONSTUTTS	
Louko and Conture (1990)	within word disfluencies (overall)		Dis. phonol 938 Normal phonol 896			
Conture & Kelly (1991)	sound/syllable repetition prolongation monosyllabic word repetition		1,015 727 870			
Zebrowski (1991)	syllable repetition all size prolongation		556 435		520 404	
Kelly & Conture (1992)	within word disfluencies		650		640	
Yairi & Hall (1993)	single-unit monosyllabic word repetition	interval total	283 840		409 916	
Throneburg & Yairi (1994)	single-unit syllable repetition single-unit monosyllabic word repetition double-unit monosyllabic word repetition	interval total interval total interval total	136 627 161 742 228 1384	195	418 890 495 1024 569 2028	491

An alternate approach by Yairi and his associates assesses several durational components of disfluencies. Yairi, Hilchie, and Hall (1990) measured three segments within the single-unit repetitions of monosyllabic words of children who were within a year of stuttering onset and those of nonstuttering controls. These segments included the duration of the first and second productions of a word and of the intervening silent interval (e.g., but-but). They found that the ratio of the silent interval to the total duration of the disfluency was substantially smaller for stutterers than for nonstuttering controls. In a followup study, Yairi and Hall (1993) measured 55 monosyllabic word repetitions of fifteen stutterers who were within three months of onset and 47 such repetitions of eighteen control subjects. No statistically significant differences in overall duration were found; however, the tendency for stuttering children to exhibit shorter silent intervals between repeated segments than did control subjects clearly warrants further research. Yairi and Hall commented that shorter silent intervals would indicate that children who stutter repeat faster than do normally speaking children, which may prove useful in differentiating the disfluencies of the two groups.

These findings led to a larger study by Throneburg and Yairi (1994) that included part-word repetitions with one repeated unit, monosyllabic whole-word repetitions with one repeated unit, and monosyllabic words with two repeated units. Twenty preschool children having stuttering histories of less than three months contributed a total of 571 disfluent events for analysis. Twenty nonstuttering control subjects contributed 149 episodes. Using visual displays of sound spectrograms, the durations of spoken repetition unit(s), silent interval(s) between units, as well as the duration of the total disfluency were measured. The duration of silent intervals between repeated units was consistently shorter for children who stutter than for control children. Furthermore, the silent interval was the *longest* element in the repetitions of nonstuttering children but the *shortest* element in the repetitions of young beginning stutterers. The consistency of these significant differences is reflected in each of the speech materials analyzed. In part-word repetitions, the mean interval between the two repeated units (bu-but) was 136 msec for stutterers but 418 msec for controls. In single repetitions of whole-words (but-but), the respective mean intervals were 161 and 495 msec. In double repetitions of whole-words (but-but-but), the two mean intervals for stutterers were 228 and 195 msec but 569 and 491 msec for controls. Statistical analyses revealed that silent intervals alone differentiated stuttering from nonstuttering children with 72 to 87 percent accuracy, depending on disfluency type. Also, the overall durations of stutterers' disfluencies were significantly shorter than were those of controls due to their shorter silent intervals. These data are also presented in Table 3.5.

The current body of data on durational characteristics of disfluencies during early stages of stuttering is limited and somewhat inconsistent. Most syllable and monosyllabic word repetitions, as well as sound prolongations, are produced within one-half to one second. Comparisons of the duration data of stuttering and nonstuttering children have yielded contradictory findings. Apparent differences in length among different types of disfluencies in stutterers, such as prolongations and repetitions, or among repetitions containing different numbers of units (see Table 3.5) may have practical significance and deserve further research. For example, double-unit repetitions (but-but-but) were reported by Throneburg and Yairi (1994) as approximately twice as long as single-unit repetitions (but-but). Because multiple unit repetitions of beginning stuttering children occur considerably more frequently than do those of nonstutterers, the number of units and their duration and frequency may have a combined effect on listeners.[12]

The recent work of Yairi and Hall (1993) and Throneburg and Yairi (1994) on the durations of segments within repetitions appears to be a

---

[12]The relation between duration and several speech parameters as well as other factors have been investigated recently by Zebrowski (1994) with school-age children, an age group beyond the scope of this chapter.

promising research approach. Their findings support the assumption that beginning stutterers tend to repeat faster than do normally fluent children but do not support earlier speculations that such repetitions are initially of normal tempo but become faster as the disorder of stuttering progresses (Froeschels, 1921; Van Riper, 1971). These findings also support my contention that many of the disfluencies produced by children near stuttering onset are objectively different than those of normally speaking children.

Other Acoustic Characteristics

Van Riper (1971) suggested that vowels in stutterers' syllable repetitions tend to be neutralized. Although several investigators have studied the acoustic characteristics of vowels in repetitions of adults who stutter (e.g., Howell & Vause, 1986; Montgomery & Cooke, 1976), corresponding data for child stutterers are sparse. Howell and Williams (1992) published what appears to be the only study in this area utilizing data from children. These investigators compared the formant frequency, duration, and intensity of vowels in repetitive productions with those of the final fluent production of the intended segment. Acoustic analyses indicated that formant frequencies in repetitive units did not shift toward neutral vowel positions, that vowels were significantly shorter during disfluent than fluent productions, and that intensity did not differ. Because subjects ranged in age from 5 to 9 years and had exhibited stuttering for five years, on average, this age range exceeds the focus of the present discussion.

Most other investigations of acoustic characteristics of young stutterers' speech have focused primarily on fluent utterances, and it appears that the vocal characteristics of the disfluencies of *preschool-age beginning stutterers* have been examined by only one study. Healey and Bernstein (1991) measured the fundamental frequency of disfluent episodes in recorded conversational speech of five stutterers and five matched nonstuttering subjects, ages 2 to 4 years. No differences in fundamental frequency were found between the groups during part-word, whole-word or phrase repetition.

Associated Physical Phenomena

Studies of parental perceptions of early stuttering included occasional reports of tense physical struggle and body movements associated with stuttering (Johnson & Associates, 1959; Yairi, 1983). Until recently, however, such movements, which are often referred to as "secondary characteristics," have been largely ignored by investigators, perhaps because they were regarded as late developing phenomena in stuttering.

A series of three studies by Conture and his co-workers employed frame-by-frame videotape analyses of ten randomly selected instances of stuttering for each subject. Movements were classified using a modified Facial Action Coding System (Ekman & Friesen, 1978). In the first study, Schwartz and Conture (1988) observed forty-three children who were between 3 and 9 years of age and found that all exhibited such "behaviors" as head, eye, torso, and limb movements while stuttering. Because information about age at onset was lacking, a followup investigation (Schwartz, Zebrowski, & Conture, 1990) was carried out with ten children, ages 3 to 5 years, all of whom were within a year of onset (M = 8.5 months). All exhibited associated physical movements during disfluencies. In 1991, Conture and Kelly compared the nonspeech behaviors of thirty stuttering and thirty nonstuttering children, ages 3 to 7 years. Post-onset interval was not specified. They found that these stutterers had significantly more nonspeech behaviors than did nonstuttering controls (M = 1.48 and .63 per instance of stuttering and fluent word, respectively), that the groups differed in types of movement, and that the two groups of children could be differentiated on the basis of their nonspeech behaviors. The associated movements of the stuttering children were analyzed during episodes of disfluencies, but those of control children during fluent speech, thereby limiting the validity of these comparisons. Subsequently, these findings were corroborated by Yairi, Ambrose, and Niermann (1993) who rated the head and neck movements of each of sixteen child stutterers who were videotaped within three months of onset (M = 6 weeks). The individual children's mean number of movements per disfluency ranged from .8 to 5.9, yielding a group mean of 3.18, twice as many as were reported by Conture and Kelly (1991). We also found that the number of movements decreased as the frequency of disfluency decreased during followup testings.

Spatial Distribution of Disfluencies

In 1982, Van Riper commented that stutterers' repetitions often occur in "volleys or clusters" (p. 95). Two studies (Colburn, 1985; Silverman, 1973) focused on this phenomenon in normally fluent preschool children, reporting that clusters of disfluencies occurred in greater numbers than would have been expected by chance.[13] The percentages of clustered disfluencies were 36 and 38 percent in the two studies, respectively. Wexler (1982) also reported clustering but did not calculate percentages or chances of occurrence. The only published study of this phenomenon in early childhood stuttering was that of Hubbard and Yairi (1988). Their 2- to 4-year-old stutterers (mean post-onset interval = 5.5 months) and nonstuttering controls exhibited clustered disfluencies above chance expectations, but the proportion of clustered disfluencies among stutterers (67%) was significantly higher than that of controls (34%). Stuttering children had more than six times as many clusters as nonstutterers, and their clusters were frequently longer. Indeed, 30 percent of their clusters included more than two disfluencies, compared to only 19 percent among controls.

Subgrouping

The possibility that overt speech characteristics, especially disfluency, can be used to subgroup

young stutterers has been explored both clinically and experimentally (Yairi, 1990). Gender differences are an obvious target for investigation because of the well-documented male-to-female ratio of about 2:1 near onset (Yairi & Ambrose, 1992b), which increases with age (Bloodstein, 1995). Many studies have looked for gender differences with little success for more than fifty-five years. Early studies by Davis (1939) and Branscom, Hughes, and Oxtoby (1955) reported that normally fluent boys had a tendency to be more repetitious than did girls, but such differences were not statistically significant. Later investigators (Yairi, 1981; Yairi & Lewis, 1984) made similar observations and reached identical conclusions. Studies of young stutterers have been similarly consistent in their negative findings (Johnson & Associates, 1959, Yairi & Ambrose, 1992a; 1996; Yairi & Lewis, 1984). Although the most disfluent subjects are often males, and groups of males are somewhat more disfluent than females, no statistically significant differences have been found between the disfluencies of males and females.

Disfluency patterns play an important role in Van Riper's (1971) subgrouping system that differentiates stutterers into four developmental tracks based on age, type of onset (early vs. late, sudden vs. gradual), disfluency patterns (repetitions vs. prolongations and blocks), secondary characteristics, and articulatory skills. In this system, early symptomatology that is dominated by repetitions has a favorable prognosis for recovery, but if blocks and prolongations dominate, chronic stuttering is predicted. Preus (1981) and Daly (1981) reported that these subgroups were useful in classifying older children, but the system is based solely on Van Riper's clinical impressions. Others, including Conture (1990), Cooper and Cooper (1985), Curlee (1993), and Riley (1981), also have commented that the presence of a substantial proportion of sound prolongations in a child's total disfluency, 25 percent or more according to Conture (1990), places the child in a high-risk group for developing chronic stuttering. Such suggestions appear to refer to a broad range

---

[13]Clusters include several disfluencies occurring within the same word, on adjacent words, and in between-word spaces either prior to or after a disfluent word.

of stuttering children, without specific considera-tion of their age or length of stuttering history. Longitudinal data collected in my research show that a substantial number of recovering children exhibited prolongations and blocks during the first few months of their disorders. Prolongations may become a more significant factor after stuttering has persisted for a longer period of time.

Several investigators have used more rigorous scientific methods. Schwartz and Conture (1988) applied cluster analyses to data on disfluency and associated behaviors. They isolated three indices: (1) Sound Prolongation Index (SPI), the ratio of prolongations to the total number of stutterings; (2) Nonspeech Behavior Index (NBI), the average number of nonspeech behaviors per stuttering; and (3) Behavioral Variety Index (BVI), the average number of different behaviors per stuttering. Sort-ing subjects according to these indices ultimately yielded two subgroups of stutterers: young stut-terers who predominantly exhibit repetitions and those who predominantly produce sound prolon-gations. These descriptions are similar to those used in Bluemel's (1932) and Van Riper's (1971) classifications. Currently, however, their diagnos-tic and prognostic significance is unclear, but fur-ther research is warranted.

Differentiating between beginning stutterers who appear likely to develop a chronic disorder and those who are likely to recover is a central objective of past efforts to subgroup childhood stutterers (Yairi, 1990; 1993). This objective prompted two investigations of acoustic proper-ties that focused on second formant dynamics of young stutterers' disfluent utterances. Stromsta (1965) reported that stuttering children whose dis-fluencies contained abnormal formant transitions and terminations of phonation were more likely to exhibit stuttering ten years later than were chil-dren whose stuttering did not contain these char-acteristics. Subject selection, measurements, and followup verification were not clearly described, which raises many questions about the validity of these claims. Yaruss and Conture (1993) used a different strategy to assess the prognostic power of second formant transitions and compared them in

disfluencies of high-risk and low-risk groups of young stutterers who were grouped based on their scores on the Stuttering Prediction Instrument (Riley, 1981). Although findings were negative, longitudinal data were not obtained to verify the validity of their grouping by the Riley scale. Kowalczyk and Yairi (1995) measured second for-mant transitions in fluent segments of sixteen chil-dren near the onset of stuttering. They found significant differences between those whose stut-tering persisted and those who recovered.

Finally, Yairi and his colleagues employed longitudinal studies to provide information con-cerning the early predictive power of disfluency counts. In their first investigation of twenty-seven preschool stuttering children, Yairi and Ambrose (1992a) found that changes in the developmental curves of SLD data reveal a divergence between persistent and recovering stutterers within twenty months of onset. Children who had not shown a decline in disfluency by that time were more like-ly to persist in stuttering. Yairi, Ambrose, Paden, and Throneburg (1996) supported this finding with data from another group of thirty-two preschool-age stuttering children who were followed at six-month intervals from stuttering onset for a three-year period. The twelve chronic subjects maintained consistent levels of SLDs throughout the study, but the twenty recovering subjects ex-hibited sharp declines in SLD by the end of the first year of stuttering and maintained low disflu-ency levels thereafter. In my opinion, the findings of these two studies present some of the most im-portant prognostic data that are currently avail-able, although even earlier prognosis would be more desirable. Incidentally, the Yairi and col-leagues (1996) study also found that persistence of stuttering was significantly related to familial his-tory of chronic stuttering and a number of other speech-language measures.

Clinical Application of Disfluency Measures

Analyses of the research literature have identified several disfluency measures that have practical clin-ical value, especially for initial diagnostic evaluations of young beginning stutterers and subsequent evaluations of their progress. Although such data are essential to evaluations of early childhood stuttering, clinicians should be alert to other aspects of the disorder that can be reasonably assessed.

Keeping in mind the methodological issues I discussed earlier, a minimum 500-syllable speech sample, audio- and video-recorded over two separate days, and the per 100 syllable disfluency metric are recommended. After determining the number of syllables in the sample, the following measures can be used to compare with gross averages of groups of preschool children who stutter:

1. Total number of disfluencies per 100 syllables — Mean of 16

2. Number of SLD per 100 syllables — Minimum of 3; mean of 11

3. Percent of SLD to total disfluency — Range of 60% to 75%

4. Number of SER per 100 syllables — Mean of 6 to 8

5. Number of units per instance of SER — Mean of 1.5

6. Percent of SER containing two or more extra units — Mean of 33%

7. Number of SER containing two or more extra units per 100 syllables — Mean of 3

8. Percent of disfluencies occurring in clusters — Mean of 50%

9. Number of disfluencies per cluster — Mean of 3

10. Number of face and head movement per disfluency — Mean of 1.5 to 3

11. Duration of disfluencies msec — Mean of 750

12. Duration of interval between repetition units — Mean of 200 msec

13. Proportion of silent interval to total duration of SER containing one extra unit — Mean $\frac{1}{4}$ to $\frac{1}{3}$

None of these measures, or combinations of them, have been established as differential diagnostic criteria. They can be used, however, as guidelines for meaningful, comprehensive descriptions of a child's speech relative to that of other children who stutter. Future, perhaps computerized, diagnostic instruments may incorporate many of these features.

SUMMARY

Many investigators, with different backgrounds and at different times and locations, have reported similar data on disfluency in normally fluent children and those who stutter. Such similarity indicates that discrete instances of disfluency are a useful unit of quantification, and recent acoustic-based durational data provide a physical basis for assessing them. Experienced investigators, using large speech samples and repeated listening, have achieved satisfactory to good accuracy, including point-by-point interjudge agreement. It appears that training and experience with this task contribute to higher listener agreement in identifying disfluencies, a point that was also made by Costello and Hurst (1981).[14] Plausibly, reports of listener disagreement in identifying disfluencies and "stuttering" (Curlee, 1981; Onslow et al., 1992) resulted, in part, from laboratory experiments that reduced the full display of all aspects of disfluency discussed in this chapter and the interaction among them. Current data, then, support the use of defined disfluencies as an important measure of childhood stuttering. It is evident, however, that research on speech disfluency has been plagued by inconsistent methodological procedures that must be resolved. Restructuring current disfluency measuring systems, combining and/or eliminating disfluency types, and devising new metrics should be considered and tested experi-

---

[14]The positive influence of training on listeners' agreement was also reported for tasks involving identification of stuttering during time intervals (Ingham, Cordes, & Gow, 1993).

mentally. Additional information on acoustic features of disfluencies and their relation to various aspects of stuttering are likely to increase the usefulness of disfluency data in research as well as their clinical application. It should also enhance the prospects of computer identification and measurement of disfluencies.

Normal Disfluency and Early Stuttering

Analyses of the speech of normally disfluent preschool children, especially at ages 2 and 3 when stuttering onset is most common, have indicated that disfluency is individually variable but ordinarily stays at low levels. Significantly, part-word and word repetitions occur, on the average, at a rate of 2 or fewer per 100 syllables. Developmental data have also shown age-related declines in nonstutterers' disfluencies, primarily in part-word and monosyllabic word repetitions. My data have established that a sudden rise in short-element repetitions constitutes an unusual departure from the typical developmental course of normal disfluency. Such departures can hardly be viewed as "normal" and, in fact, may signify the beginning of abnormal disfluency that emerge at the onset of stuttering.

Scientific interest in the onset of stuttering and of early speech characteristics of this disorder reflects an evolution from the stereotypic concept of inconspicuous, gradually emerging, simple, effortless repetitions to the recognition that heterogeneity of stuttering characteristics at onset, as well as complex, severe symptoms are not uncommon. Findings that approximately one-third of the children who stutter exhibit abrupt onsets of symptoms and that more "gradual" onsets in many others actually take place within two weeks indicate that a fairly rapid onset process, associated with perceptible changes in speech characteristics, is common.

With the growing sophistication of experimental technology and procedures, researchers have begun recording objective speech data much closer to the time of stuttering onset than did past investigators. They have also studied samples of subjects who were more cohesive in age. Analyses of such data have revealed that at, or very near to, stuttering onset, the disfluency of most of these children is markedly different from the disfluency of normally fluent children. The pattern that characterizes their disfluent speech at this early stage of stuttering presents a multidimensional complex. It includes:

1. Quantitative dimension—Frequency of instances, number of iterations or duration
2. Qualitative dimension—Spatial distribution or clustering in speech, ratios of different disfluency categories and of different sizes of iterations
3. Physical dimension—Temporal characteristics, and perhaps other acoustic features
4. Physiologic dimension—Associated tense movements

These dimensions suggest several guidelines that distinguish the disfluent speech of early childhood stuttering. Compared with their nonstuttering counterparts, children who begin stuttering exhibit: (1) two-and-a-half to three times as many total instances of disfluencies, (2) five to six times as many instances of SLDs,[15] (3) proportions of SLDs to total disfluency that are twice as large, (4) proportions of part-word and monosyllabic word repetitions having two or more extra repetition units that are three times larger, (5) six times as many disfluency clusters and, proportionally, at least twice as many clusters, (6) longer clusters, (7) repetitions in which intervals between iterations are shorter, and (8) twice as many head and neck movements accompanying disfluencies.

Interactions among these factors often amplify differences. For example, multiplication of larger numbers of repetitions by larger mean iterations yields a powerful *co-effect* of much larger quantities of repeated speech segments in the verbal output of stutterers compared to that of nonstuttering

---

[15]This surge in disfluency stands out even more, because it occurs at an age when most normally speaking children show a decline in repetitions.

children. Conventional counts of disfluencies fail to capture this co-effect, but multiplying the frequency of repetitions by the average number of iterations per repetition heightens the difference in the number of repeated syllables or words between the two groups on the order of five to seven times. When clustering and duration of disfluencies are considered also, the result is a series of "disfluency concentrations" that are of greater number, often longer in duration, faster in rate, and in more and longer clusters that normally fluent children seldom ever approximate.

Taken together, this objective evidence leaves little doubt that most parents who believe their children are stuttering are reacting to real changes in their speech (Yairi & Lewis, 1984). Although the present analysis has not addressed etiological theories of stuttering, the often abrupt and large departures from normal speech at onset, and their subsequent, frequent diminution appear to reflect neurophysiological changes more than learning processes.

Development of Disfluency

Recent longitudinal studies (Ryan, 1990; Yairi & Ambrose, 1992a; Yairi, Ambrose & Niermann 1993; Yairi et al., 1996) have carefully documented substantial reductions in disfluencies and the eventual recovery of 65 to 85 percent of the children studied, especially during the first two years after onset.[16] These data and the apparent resilience of recovery during early stages of stuttering, particularly among young girls, should be carefully considered when developing a case-selection strategy for treatment and in assessing treatment efficacy of early childhood stuttering.

There are at least three critical implications for future research. First, priority should be given to identifying those children at high risk for developing chronic stuttering so that resources are directed to those with the greatest need. Second, research on treatment efficacy during early stages of stuttering requires extraordinary control measures, such as different treatment groups, no-treatment groups, and a monitored pretreatment period to establish the stability of this disorder. Control of age, gender, and post-onset interval is imperative, as well. In light of the high likelihood of recovery during the first eighteen months after onset, and the appreciable recoveries during the subsequent year, research on treatment efficacy of early childhood stuttering should focus on children who have stuttered at least eighteen months. Reports of high percentages of therapeutic success should be carefully evaluated also. For example, the Fosnot (1993) study reporting 95 percent recovery following treatment falls short in all of the above controls. In addition to lacking a no-treatment control group, the study included children who were only two months post-onset and whose chances for a spontaneous recovery had to be high. Moreover, the sample included 46 percent females (15 subjects), a subgroup having substantially higher chances of recovery than boys. Considering the age span and post-onset interval, the proportion of females in this study was about twice what would be appropriate. Third, research comparisons of data from different age groups of young stutterers on any aspect or measure are comparing subject samples drawn from different populations. For example, differences in speaking rate between younger and older groups may result from the early recovery of fast-talking stutterers, not from age-related changes. This research design, therefore, does not support causal conclusions.

The growing evidence of high recovery rates, lack of effective predictors of stuttering chronicity, and insufficient data on treatment efficacy have combined to create a difficult, double-edged ethical dilemma of waiting to start therapy versus recommending unnecessary, expensive treatment. The view of several investigators that all beginning young stutterers should receive clinical intervention as soon as possible (e.g., Onslow, Costa, & Rue, 1990; Starkweather, Gottwald, & Halfond,

---

[16]I disagree with Ramig's (1993) argument that recovery has been overestimated. The great majority of stutterers in his survey were several years older than the children in my studies and had, therefore, already passed the period in which much spontaneous recovery occurs.

1990) has been questioned by others (Andrews, 1984; Curlee, 1992b; Yairi, 1993). In forming a position about intervention in early childhood stuttering, one should keep in mind that (1) the specific reasons for apparent spontaneous recoveries have not yet been isolated, (2) some children persist in stuttering, and (3) there are indications that the chance for chronicity increases around fourteen to eighteen months after onset. Until better information is accumulated, young beginning stutterers should receive a thorough speech-language evaluation accompanied by basic parent education about childhood stuttering. If therapy is deferred, the child should be monitored through periodic re-evaluations. More aggressive, direct intervention should receive higher priority for those children who have stuttered for more than fourteen to eighteen months without exhibiting substantial improvement.

REFERENCES

Adams, M. (1977). A clinical strategy for differentiating the normally nonfluent child and the incipient stutterer. *Journal of Fluency Disorders, 2,* 141–148.

Adams, S. (1932). A study of the growth of language between two and four years. *Journal of Juvenile Research, 16,* 267–277.

Ambrose, N. & Yairi, E. (1995). The role of repetition units in the differential diagnosis of early childhood incipient stuttering. *American Journal of Speech and Language Pathology, 4,* 82–88.

Andrews, G. (1984). The epidemiology of stuttering. In R. Curlee & W. Perkins (Eds.), *Nature and treatment of stuttering.* San Diego: College Hill.

Andrews, G., & Harris, M. (1964). *The syndrome of stuttering. Clinics in developmental medicine.* No. 17. London: Spastic Society in association with Wm. Heinemann Medical Books.

Bjerkan, B. (1980). Word fragmentations and repetitions in the spontaneous speech of 2-6-yr-old children. *Journal of Fluency Disorders, 5,* 137–148.

Bloodstein, O. (1960a). The development of stuttering: I. Changes in nine basic features. *Journal of Speech and Hearing Disorders, 25,* 219–237.

Bloodstein, O. (1960b). The development of stuttering: II. Developmental phases. *Journal of Speech Disorders, 25,* 366–376.

Bloodstein, O. (1970). Stuttering and normal nonfluency—A continuity hypothesis. *British Journal of Journal of Disorders of Communication, 5,* 30–39.

Bloodstein, O. (1987). *A handbook on stuttering* (Fourth edition). Chicago: Easter Seal Society.

Bloodstein, O. (1995). *A handbook on stuttering* (Fifth edition). San Diego: Singular Publishing Group, Inc.

Bloodstein, O., Jaeger, W., & Tureen, J. (1952). A study of the diagnosis of stuttering by parents of stutterers and nonstutterers. *Journal of Speech and Hearing Disorders, 17,* 308–316.

Bluemel, C. (1913). *Stammering and cognate defects of speech. Vol. 1.* New York: Stecher.

Bluemel, C. (1932). Primary and secondary stuttering. *Quarterly Journal of Speech, 18,* 187–200.

Brandenburg, G. (1915). The language of a three-year-old child. *Pedagological Seminary, 22,* 89–120.

Branscom, M. (1942). The construction and statistical evaluation of a speech fluency test for young children. Master's thesis, University of Iowa.

Branscom, M., Hughes, J., & Oxtoby, E. (1955). Studies of nonfluency in the speech of preschool. In W. Johnson and R. Leutenegger (Eds.), *Stuttering in children and adults.* Minneapolis: University of Minnesota Press.

Campbell, J., & Hill, D. (1987). *Systematic disfluency analysis.* Chicago: Northwestern University.

Colburn, N. (1985). Clustering of disfluency in nonstuttering children's early utterances. *Journal of Fluency Disorders, 10,* 51–58.

Colburn, N., & Mysak, E. (1982). Developmental disfluency and emerging grammar: Disfluency characteristics in early syntactic utterances. *Journal of Speech and Hearing Research, 25,* 421–427.

Conardi, E. (1904). Psychology and pathology of speech development in the child. *Pedagological Seminary, 11,* 328–380.

Conture, E. (1982). *Stuttering* (1st Edition). Englewood Cliffs, NJ: Prentice Hall.

Conture, E. (1990). *Stuttering* (2nd Edition). Englewood Cliffs, NJ: Prentice Hall.

Conture, E., & Caruso, A. (1987). Assessment and diagnosis of childhood disfluency. In L. Rustin, H.

Purser, & D. Rowley (Eds.), *Progress in treatment of fluency disorders*. London: Taylor & Francis.

Conture, E. & Kelly, E. (1991). Young stutterers' non-speech behaviors during stuttering. *Journal of Speech and Hearing Research, 34*, 1041–1056.

Cooper, E., & Cooper, C. (1985). *Cooper personalized fluency control therapy* (revised). Allen, TX: DLM Teaching Resources.

Cordes, A., & Ingham, R. (1994). Reliability of observational data: II. Issues in the identification and measurement of stuttering events. *Journal of Speech and Hearing Research, 37*, 279–294.

Costello, J., & Hurst, M. (1981). An analysis of the relationship among stuttering behaviors. *Journal of Speech and Hearing Research, 24*, 247–256.

Curlee, R. (1980). A case selection strategy for young disfluent children. In W. Perkins (Ed.) *Seminars in speech, language and hearing* (pp. 277–287). New York: Thieme-Stratton.

Curlee, R. (1981). Observer agreement on disfluency and stuttering. *Journal of Speech and Hearing Research, 24*, 595–600.

Curlee, R. (1992a). Comments on "stuttering prevention I". *Journal of Fluency Disorders, 17*, 57–62.

Curlee, R. (1992b). To treat or to prevent: Are those the issues? *Journal of Fluency Disorders, 17*, 107–112.

Curlee, R. (1993). Identification and management of beginning stuttering. In R. Curlee (Ed.), *Stuttering and related disorders of fluency*. New York: Thieme.

Daly, D. (1981). Differentiating stuttering subgroups with Van Riper's developmental tracks: A preliminary study. *Journal of National Student Speech and Hearing Association, 9*, 89–101.

Darley, F. (1955). The relationship of parental attitudes and adjustment to the development of stuttering. In W. Johnson & R. Leutenegger (Eds.), *Stuttering in children and adults*. Minneapolis: University of Minnesota Press.

Davis, D. (1939). The relation of repetitions in the speech of young children to certain measures of language maturity and situational factors: Part I. *Journal of Speech Disorders, 4*, 303–318.

DeJoy, D. (1975). An investigation of the frequency of nine individual types of disfluency and total disfluency in relationship to age and syntactic maturity in nonstuttering males, three and one half years of age and five years of age. Unpublished doctoral dissertation, Northwestern University.

Egland, G. (1955). Repetition and prolongation in the speech of stuttering and nonstuttering children. In W. Johnson & R. Leutenegger (Eds.), *Stuttering in children and adults*. Minneapolis: University of Minnesota Press.

Ekman, P., & Friesen, W. (1978). *Facial Action Coding System* (manual). Palo Alto, CA: Consulting Psychologists Press.

Finn, P., Ingham, R., Yairi, E., & Ambrose, N. (1994). Unassisted recovery from stuttering in preschool children: A perceptual study. A paper presented to the convention of the American Speech-Language-Hearing Association, New Orleans. Abstract published in *Asha, 36*, 52.

Fisher, M. (1932). Language patterns of preschool children. *Experimental Education, 1*, 70–85.

Floyd, S., & Perkins, W. (1974). Early syllable disfluency in stutterers and nonstutterers: A preliminary report. *Journal of Communication Disorders, 7*, 279–282.

Fosnot, S. (1993). Research design for examining treatment efficacy in fluency disorders. *Journal of Fluency Disorders, 18*, 221–252.

Froeschels, E. (1921). Beitrage zur symptomatologie des stotterns. *Monatsschrift fur Ohrenheilkunde, 55*, 1109–1112.

Froeschels, E. (1943). Pathology and therapy of stuttering. *Nervous Child, 2*, 148–161.

Froeschels, E. (1943). The significance of symptomatology for the understanding of the essence of stuttering. *Folia Phoniatrica, 4*, 217–230.

Froeschels, E. (1964). *Selected papers (1940–1964)*. Amsterdam: North-Holland.

Gordon, P., & Luper, H. (1992). The early identification of beginning stuttering I: Protocols. *American Journal of Speech-Language Pathology, 1*, 43–53.

Gottfred, C. (1979). A longitudinal analysis of type and frequency of disfluency, related to communicative pressure and length of utterance, in children twenty-four to thirty months of age. Unpublished doctoral dissertation, Northwestern University.

Gutzmann, H. (1894). *Des kindes sprache und sprachfehler*. Leip ig.

Haynes, W., & Hood, S. (1977). Language and disfluency variables in normal speaking children from discrete chronological age groups. *Journal of Fluency Disorders, 2*, 57–74.

Healey, C., & Bernstein, B. (1991). Acoustic analyses of young stutterers' and nonstutterers' disfluencies. In

H. Peters, W. Hulstijn, & W. Starkweather (Eds.), *Speech motor control and stuttering*. Amsterdam: Elsevier Science Publishers.

Hoefner, T. (1911). Stuttering as associated with aphasia. *Zeitscrift fur Pathgopsychologie, 1*, 448–452.

Howell, P., & Vause, L. (1986). Acoustic analysis and perception of vowels in stuttered speech. *Journal of the Acoustical Society of America, 79*, 1571–1679.

Howell, P., & Williams, M. (1992). Acoustic analysis and perception of vowels in children's and teenagers' stuttered speech. *Journal of the Acoustical Society of America, 91*, 1697–1706.

Hubbard, C., & Yairi, E. (1988). Clustering of disfluencies in the speech of stuttering and nonstuttering preschool children. *Journal of Speech and Hearing Research, 31*, 228–233.

Hughes, J. (1943). A quantitative study of repetition in the speech of two-year-olds and four-year-olds. Unpublished Master's thesis, University of Iowa.

Ingham, R., Cordes, A., & Gow, M. (1993). Time-interval measurement of stuttering: Modifying interjudge agreement. *Journal of Speech and Hearing Research, 36*, 503–515.

Johnson, W. (1942). A study of the onset and development of stuttering. *Journal of Speech Disorders, 7*. 251–257.

Johnson, W., & Associates. (1959). *The onset of stuttering*. Minneapolis: University of Minnesota Press.

Kelly, E., & Conture, E. (1992). Speaking rate, responses time latencies, and interrupting behaviors of young stutterers, nonstutterers, and their mothers. *Journal of Speech and Hearing Research, 37*, 1256–1267.

Kirkpatrick, E. (1891). How children learn to talk. *Science, 18*, 170–178.

Kowalczyk, P., & Yairi, E. (1995). Features of F2 transitions in fluent speech of children who stutter. A paper presented at the national convention of the American Speech-Language-Hearing Association. Abstract published in *Asha, 37* (October issue), 79.

Kully, D., & Boberg, E. (1988). An investigation of the inter-clinic agreement in the identification of fluent and stuttered syllables. *Journal of Fluency Disorders, 13*, 309–318.

Louko, L., Edwards, C., & Conture, E. (1990). Phonological characteristics of young stutterers and their normally fluent peers: Preliminary observations. *Journal of Fluency Disorders, 15*, 191–210.

McCarthy, D. (1930). *The language development of the preschool child*. Minneapolis: The University of Minnesota Press.

McDearmon, J. (1968). Primary stuttering at the onset of stuttering: A reexamination of data. *Journal of Speech and Hearing Research, 11*, 631–637.

Metraux, R. (1950). Speech profiles of the preschool child 18 to 54 months. *Journal of Speech and Hearing Disorders, 15*, 37–53.

Meyers, S. (1986). Qualitative and quantitative differences and patterns of variability in disfluencies emitted by preschool stutterers and nonstutterers during dydactic conversations. *Journal of Fluency Disorders, 11*, 293–706.

Montgomery, A., & Cooke, P. (1976). Perceptual and acoustical analysis of repetitions in stuttered speech. *Journal of Communication Disorders, 9*, 317–330.

Nice, M. (1920). Concerning all day conversations. *Pedagological Seminary, 27*, 166–177.

Onslow, M., Costa, L., & Rue, S. (1990). Direct early intervention with stuttering: Some preliminary data. *Journal of Speech and Hearing Disorders, 55*, 405–426.

Onslow, M., Gardner, K., Bryant, K., Stuckings, C., & Knight, T. (1992). Stuttered and normal speech events in early childhood: The validity of a behavioral data language. *Journal of Speech and Hearing Research, 35*, 79–87.

Oxtoby, E. (1943). A quantitative study of the repetition in the speech of three-year-old children. Unpublished Master's thesis, University of Iowa.

Pindzola, R., & White, D. (1986). A protocol for differentiating the incipient stutterer. *Language, Speech, and Hearing Services in Schools, 17*, 2–11.

Preus, A. (1981). *Identifying subgroups of stutterers*. Oslo: University of Oslo Press.

Ramig, P. (1993). High reported spontaneous recovery rates: Facts or fiction. *Language, Speech, and Hearing in Schools, 24*, 156–160.

Riley, G. (1981). *Stuttering prediction instrument for young children*. Austin, TX: Pro-Ed.

Ryan, B. (1990). Development of stuttering, a longitudinal study, report 4. A paper presented at the convention of the American Speech-Language-Hearing Association, Seattle. Abstract published in *Asha, 32*, 144.

Schwartz, H., & Conture, E. (1988). Subgrouping young stutterers: preliminary behavioral observations. *Journal of Speech and Hearing Research, 31*, 62–71.

Schwartz, H., Zebrowski, P., & Conture, E. (1990). Behaviors at the onset of stuttering. *Journal of Fluency Disorders, 15*, 77–86.

Shames, G., & Sherrick, H. (1963). A discussion of nonfluency and stuttering as operant behavior. *Journal of Speech and Hearing Disorders, 28*, 3–18.

Silverman, E. (1971). Situational variability of preschoolers' disfluency: Preliminary Study. *Perceptual and Motor Skills, 33*, 1021–1022.

Silverman, E. (1972). Generality of disfluency data collected from preschoolers. *Journal of Speech and Hearing Research, 15*, 84–92.

Silverman, E-M. (1973). Clustering: A characteristics of preschoolers' disfluency. *Journal of Speech and Hearing Research, 6*, 576–583.

Smith, M. (1926). An investigation of the development of the sentences and the extent of vocabulary in young children. *University of Iowa, Studies in Child Welfare, 3*, No. 5.

Starkweather, W., Gottwald, S., & Halfond, M. (1990). *Stuttering prevention.* Englewood Cliffs, NJ: Prentice Hall.

Stromsta, C. (1965). A spectographic study of disfluencies labeled as stuttering by parents. *De Therapia Vocis et Loquelae, 1*, 317–318.

Taylor, G. (1937). An observational study of the nature of stuttering at its onset. Unpublished Master's thesis, University of Iowa.

Throneburg, R., & Yairi, E. (1994). Temporal dynamics of repetitions during the early stage of childhood stuttering: An acoustic study. *Journal of Speech and Hearing Research, 37*, 1067–1075.

Van Riper, C. (1971). *The nature of stuttering.* Englewood Cliffs, NJ: Prentice Hall.

Van Riper, C. (1982). *The nature of stuttering* (Second edition). Englewood Cliffs, NJ: Prentice-Hall.

Wexler, K. (1982). Developmental disfluency in 2-, 4-, and 6-year-old boys in neutral and stress situations. *Journal of Speech and Hearing Research, 25*, 229–234.

Williams, D., & Kent, L. (1958). Listener evaluations of speech interruptions. *Journal of Speech and Hearing Research, 1*, 124–131.

Williams, D., Silverman, F., & Kools, J. (1968). Disfluency behavior of elementary-school stutterers and nonstutterers: The adaptation effect. *Journal of Speech and Hearing Research, 11*, 622–630.

Wingate, M. (1962). Evaluation and stuttering, Part I: Speech characteristics of young children. *Journal of Speech and Hearing Disorders, 27*, 106–115.

Wyatt, G. (1969). *Language learning and communication disorders.* New York: Appleton-Century-Crofts.

Yairi, E. (1972). Disfluency rates and patterns. *Journal of Communication Disorders, 5*, 225–231.

Yairi, E. (1974). Personal observations of the onset of stuttering and its early stage: A case report. Unpublished.

Yairi, E. (1981). Disfluencies of normally speaking two-year-old-children. *Journal of Speech and Hearing Research, 24*, 490–495.

Yairi, E. (1982). Longitudinal studies of disfluencies in two-year-old children. *Journal of Speech and Hearing Research, 25*, 155–160.

Yairi, E. (1983). The onset of stuttering in two- and three-year-old children: A preliminary report. *Journal of Speech and Hearing Disorders, 48*, 171–177.

Yairi, E. (1990). Subtyping child stutterers for research purposes. *Asha Reports, 18*, 50–57.

Yairi, E. (1993). Epidemiology and other considerations in treatment efficacy research with children who stutter. *Journal of Fluency Disorders, 18*, 197–220.

Yairi, E., & Ambrose, N. (1992a). A longitudinal study of stuttering in children: A preliminary report. *Journal of Speech and Hearing Research, 35*, 755–760.

Yairi, E., & Ambrose, N. (1992b). Onset of stuttering in preschool children: Selected factors. *Journal of Speech and Hearing Research, 35*, 782–788.

Yairi, E., & Ambrose, N. (1996). Disfluent speech in early childhood stuttering. An unpublished report. Stuttering Research Project, University of Illinois.

Yairi, E., Ambrose, N., & Niermann, R. (1993). The early months of stuttering: A developmental study. *Journal of Speech and Hearing Research, 36*, 521–528.

Yairi, E., Ambrose, N., Paden, E., & Throneburg, R. (In press). Predictive factors of persistence and recovery: Pathways of early childhood stuttering. *Journal of Communication Disorders.*

Yairi, E., & Carrico, D. (1992). Pediatricians' attitudes and practices concerning early childhood stuttering. *American Journal of Speech-Language Pathology, 1*, 54–62.

Yairi, E., & Clifton, N. (1972). Disfluent speech behavior of preschool children, high-school seniors, and geriatric persons. *Journal of Speech and Hearing Research, 15*, 714–719.

Yairi, E., Hilchie, C., & Hall, K. (1990). Dynamics

within repetitions of stuttering and normal preschool children. Proceedings of the 2nd international conference on Stuttering and Speech Motor Control, p. 51.

Yairi, E., & Jennings, S. (1974). Relationship between the disfluent speech behavior of normal speaking preschool boys and their parents. *Journal of Speech and Hearing Research, 17*, 94–98.

Yairi, E., & Lewis, B. (1984). Disfluencies at the onset of stuttering. *Journal of Speech and Hearing Research, 27*, 154–159.

Yairi, E. & Hall (1993). Temporal relations within repetitions of preschool children near the onset of stuttering: A preliminary report. *Journal of Communication Disorders, 26*, 231–244.

Yaruss, S., & Conture, E.(1993). F2 transitions during sound/syllable repetitions of children who stutter and prediction of stuttering chronicity. *Journal of Speech and Hearing Research, 36*, 883–896.

Young, M. (1984). Identification of stutterers and stuttering. In R. Curlee & W. Perkins (Eds.), *Nature and treatment of stuttering: New directions.* San Diego: College Hill.

Zebrowski, P. (1991). Duration of speech disfluencies of beginning stutterers. *Journal of Speech and Hearing Research, 34*, 483–491.

Zebrowski, P. (1994). Duration of sound prolongation and sound/syllable repetition in children who stutter. *Journal of Speech and Hearing Research, 37*, 254–263.

SUGGESTED READINGS

Each of the following publications presents information about the speech disfluencies that characterize childhood stuttering.

Ambrose, N. & Yairi, E. (1995). The role of repetition units in the differential diagnosis of early childhood incipient stuttering. *American Journal of Speech and Language Pathology, 4,* 82–88.

Bloodstein, O. (1960b). The development of stuttering: II. Developmental phases. *Journal of Speech and Hearing Disorders, 25*, 366–376.

Conture, E. & Kelly, E. (1991). Young stutterers' non-speech behaviors during stuttering. *Journal of Speech and Hearing Research, 34*, 1041–1056.

Johnson, W. & Associates (1959). *The onset of stuttering.* Minneapolis: University of Minnesota Press.

Hubbard, C., & Yairi, E. (1988). Clustering of disfluencies in the speech of stuttering and nonstuttering preschool children. *Journal of Speech and Hearing Research, 31*, 228–233.

Throneburg, R., & Yairi, E. (1994). Temporal dynamics of repetitions during the early stage of childhood stuttering: An acoustic study. *Journal of Speech and Hearing Research, 37*, 1067–1075.

Yairi, E. (1981). Disfluencies of normally speaking two-year-old-children. *Journal of Speech and Hearing Research, 24*, 490–495.

Yairi, E., Ambrose, N., & Niermann, R. (1993). The early months of stuttering: A developmental study. *Journal of Speech and Hearing Research, 36*, 521–528.

Yairi, E. & Lewis, B. (1984). Disfluencies at the onset of stuttering. *Journal of Speech and Hearing Research, 27*, 154–159.

CHAPTER 4

LEARNING AND ITS ROLE IN STUTTERING DEVELOPMENT

C. WOODRUFF STARKWEATHER

INTRODUCTION

The purpose of this chapter is to examine the extent to which learning processes may be involved in the development of stuttering. Learning depends on the unique experiences of each person, and as a result, patterns of learning are highly individualized. This suggests that, to the extent that stuttering is learned through experience, it is a different disorder in each individual. Of course, as humans we experience a number of things in similar ways, and many aspects of life experience, including those constrained by genetics, are similar among individuals. As a result, there may be general trends and patterns among stutterers. But it is also possible that there will be patterns of stimulation and responding that are unique to each individual person who stutters. Every person's story is different and uniquely important in determining the nature of that person's stuttering.

This extraordinary variability of stuttering behavior and pattern has been identified by numerous researchers and could be said to be the most robust single finding about stuttering. It means, however, that the identification of learning processes pertinent to stuttering development is applicable only to specific cases.

This chapter, then, will describe learning processes that may operate to produce some of the characteristics of stuttering, and it will also suggest, where possible, how certain processes may be identified. Consequently this chapter is more of a guide for clinicians than it is a theoretical statement of how stuttering is acquired. It seems most likely that stuttering can be acquired in many different ways, ways in which inborn characteristics relating to movement, language, emotion, and cognition interact with experiential processes, including learning, that impact on movement, language, emotion, and cognition. This is the familiar Demands and Capacities model (Starkweather, Gottwald, & Halfond, 1990).

In spite of the great individual variability of stuttering, several general statements can be made about the role of learning in the onset and development of this most troubling disorder. It seems unlikely that learning plays more than a minor role, if any, in the earliest stuttering behaviors. The easily produced whole-word and whole-syllable repetitions that so often characterize the speech of young children at risk for stuttering are seldom individualized, nor are they likely to be attached to specific situations (Bloodstein, 1960). These two characteristics, which are suggestive of a learning process, are absent from the earliest "at-risk" behaviors. However, I don't consider these early behaviors to be stuttering, at least not in the sense that they are a disorder and a problem. I see the problem of stuttering as the extraneous effort (Starkweather, 1987), the reactions, and the struggles that can develop in response to those disfluencies. On the other hand, I don't believe that these early, easy repetitions are normal either. Most normal 2-year-olds do not display such behavior but show typical infantile types of discontinuity, and these discontinuous speech behaviors occur at, or close to, adult levels of frequency (Yairi, 1981). Instead, I believe that whole-word and whole-syllable repetitions in a very young dysfluent child are a sign of risk that the child may become a stutterer. And they do not appear to be learned. Instead, it is in the development of reactions to these behaviors, and later to other behaviors and stimuli—that is, in the process of becoming a stutterer—that learning processes seem to play such an important role.

TYPES OF LEARNING PROCESSES AND SYMBOLIZATION

Two basic types of contingencies—response contingencies and stimulus contingencies—are critical to learning. Response contingencies are based on the dependent relationship between an individual's behavior and the stimulation that follows it. For example, an infant in a highchair often drops things on the floor, after which a parent picks them up and puts them back on the tray in front of the child. Children at this age often find it amusing to watch parents pick things up and often quickly learn that by dropping something on the floor they can produce the amusing show of Mommy or Daddy bending over to pick it up. Sometimes they laugh. When parents catch on and stop picking things up until the child is out of the room or has forgotten them, the behavior soon disappears. In this example, parents' picking up an object is stimulating in a positive way, and it follows as a consequence of the child's behavior, so the child's dropping behavior increases. It is the contingent relationship between the dropping behavior and the amusing show it produces that is the basis of this brief learning. Such behavior lasts as long as the contingency remains and disappears when the contingency is removed.

Stimulus contingencies, or classical learning, are based on the same kind of relationship, but between two stimuli. The same child may begin to drool as soon as she is placed in the highchair, before there is any food on the tray, if the experience of being placed in the highchair has been followed on repeated occasions in the past by food being placed on the tray. The drooling, which was originally stimulated by the food, comes to be stimulated by being placed in the highchair because of the contingent relationship between the two. Here, too, if the child were repeatedly placed in the highchair without being fed, the drooling would slowly decrease and eventually stop. Again, as long as the contingent relationship occurs some of the time, the learned behavior persists, but when it no longer occurs, the contingency is removed, the behavior weakens, and eventually stops.

By "contingent," I mean that one event follows another repeatedly. Often this repeated occurrence results from a consequential, cause-and-effect relationship, but it doesn't have to. If one event follows another repeatedly by accident, a person experiencing the events may also develop learned reactions even though their co-occurrence is accidental. This, too, should be considered a contingent relationship, because it can result in learning, even though the relationship is established only by coincidence. The contingency is, in reality, something that occurs in the subject's perception, although not necessarily with awareness.

A contingency can occur naturally, as in the examples above, or it can be arranged by an experimenter or clinician. Repetition is, however, important. It is the repetition of the two events that signals a person that they are related, even though that may in fact be fortuitous. I use the word "signals" rather than "informs," because it is not necessary for someone to be aware of the contingency or be able to describe it. Learning of this kind often happens without someone being aware of it, which I believe happens frequently in stuttering. For some experiences, however, repetition may not be as important. Most often this occurs when stimulation is strong, and the person is alerted to everything that occurs, of which the contingency is one element. For example, a baby who touches something hot usually learns without further repetition not to touch that object.

It is sometimes asserted that voluntary behavior, such as dropping something on the floor (which is mediated by striated muscles), is learned through response contingencies, whereas involuntary behavior, such as drooling (which is mediated by smooth muscle activity), is learned through stimulus contingencies. In the real world, however, as we shall see, events are rarely so simple. It does seem likely, nevertheless, that there is a tendency for people's emotions to be shaped more by stimulus contingencies, and for the business-like, thinking part of life to be influenced more by response contingencies.

Response Contingencies

There are two basic types of response contingencies—reinforcement and punishment—both of which come in positive and negative versions. Positive reinforcement is symbolized by

$$R \rightarrow S+$$

where R = a response, and S+ indicates a positively valenced stimulus. The arrow is used to symbolize the contingent relationship. The valence of a stimulus indicates whether it is desirable or undesirable. There are various ways of determining the valence of a stimulus, both before and after the fact. Because I am discussing human beings who are generally attracted to the same things, it is not particularly risky to guess about the valence of most stimuli. There are, however, some important exceptions, which will be discussed later. When a behavior is repeatedly followed by a positively valenced stimulus, there is an increased likelihood that the behavior will occur again, all other things being equal. The baby in the highchair who learns to drop objects because her parents keep picking them up is one example of positive reinforcement.

When the contingency is removed, the behavior occurs but the S+ does not. Discontinuation of a reinforcement contingency is called extinction, and it is the process by which behaviors previously learned are dropped from a person's repertoire. Extinction following positive reinforcement can be symbolized by

$$R \rightarrow \phi(S+)$$

where R = a response, and ϕ = the contingent nonoccurrence of the stimulus specified in the parenthetical expression.

Positive punishment is symbolized by

$$R \rightarrow S-$$

where R = a response and S- = a negatively valenced stimulus. If it is a simple situation, which it rarely is in humans, one would expect that the probability of this response occurring again will be decreased. If the parent in the positive reinforcement example says "No!" in a loud voice just as the child picks up an object to drop from the highchair, the child will probably be less likely to drop it on the floor. Discontinuation of punishment—

$$R \rightarrow \phi(S-)$$

will stop the decrease in the response's frequency, but it may not return to previous levels unless a positive contingency is reinstituted.

Negative reinforcement is symbolized by

$$R \rightarrow -S-$$

The symbols are the same as previously defined, but in this case a negative stimulus, S-, which was continuously present, is removed rather than presented. The net effect is a reduction or elimination in undesirable stimulation, so that the contingency is experienced as reinforcing, and the behavior tends to increase. A child with a soiled diaper feels uncomfortable and cries. A parent comes and changes the diaper, removing the discomfort. So, under similar circumstances in the future, the child will be more likely to cry. Removal of this contingency—

$$R \rightarrow \phi(-S-)$$

automatically reinstates a continuously aversive state of affairs, but since aversive stimulation is not contingent on the occurrence of behavior, the effect is simply for the behavior that had increased to return to previous levels.

Negative punishment is symbolized by

$$R \rightarrow -S+$$

Again, the symbols are as previously defined, but in this case, the positive stimulus S+ is removed, rather than presented. The net effect is a reduction or elimination of desirable stimulation, so that the contingency is punishing, which tends to decrease the behavior in question. Suppose the child in the highchair was drinking from a bottle while dropping objects from the highchair (you might as well have some entertainment with lunch). The parent might take the bottle away just as the child picks up an object to drop. After a few repetitions of this contingency, the child would be less likely to drop objects from the tray.

Stimulus Contingencies

The two basic forms of stimulus contingencies are the same as the two types of response contingencies. The first form is symbolized by

$$S_1 \rightarrow S+$$

where S+ is a stimulus (unconditioned) that evokes a particular (unconditioned) response, such as a child's drooling. S_1 is any stimulus[1] that does not evoke the response before learning has taken place, such as placing the child in the highchair. The subscript 1 indicates that there is some specificity to the stimulus; it has to be defined in some way. After S_1 is repeatedly paired with S+,[2] the response formerly evoked by S+ but not by S_1,

comes to be elicited by S_1 before S+ has occurred. At this point, S+ can be removed, at least for a limited time, and S_1 will continue to elicit the response. However, continued occurrences of S_1 without being followed by S+ result in reductions of the learned response.

When a stimulus with a negative valence, S–, which evokes a particular response, is repeatedly paired with a stimulus that does not evoke that response, it is symbolized by

$$S_1 \rightarrow S-$$

The result is an increased probability that the response previously evoked by S– will come to be elicited by S_1, before S– has occurred. For example, when a baby is taken to the pediatrician for a checkup, and as is sometimes necessary, the doctor gives a shot (which may be painful), the baby will cry. If this happens several times, as it usually does, the result is predictable. After a while, the baby will begin to cry as soon as the doctor's face appears, when the child is brought into the doctor's office, or even hears the word "doctor." The reason, of course, is that all of these stimuli have become associated with the pain of the needle.

The S $\rightarrow$ S contingencies of classical conditioning have traditionally been used to explain emotional behavior, although, as we shall see, emotional conditioning occurs in R $\rightarrow$ S contingencies also. When a neutral stimulus,[3] such as a bell or a light is repeatedly followed by a stimulus that has either a negative or a positive emotional significance for the subject, the neutral stimulus

---

[1]The traditional term for this stimulus is the conditioned stimulus (CS), but the term is misleading because conditioning is what takes place during and after the presentation of these events. We could say it is the to-be-conditioned stimulus, but that is quite awkward. The term "conditioned" stimulus is in fact a mistranslation from Pavlov's Russian. It would have been better translated as "conditional," and the response that accompanies it as the "conditional response" because their relationship was dependent on the arbitrary decision of the experimenter. The unconditioned stimulus, similarly, should have been termed the unconditional stimulus, and its corresponding response the unconditional response, because their relationship is predetermined.

[2]The traditional description of classical conditioning suggests that the two stimuli need only be "paired" and that their temporal order is not important. This may be true, but when classical

and operant conditioning are closely compared, it seems as though the necessity for stimulation to follow responding in operant conditioning is true only by virtue of the fact that the response occurs in the organism, while the stimulus occurs in the environment (although of course the important fact of stimulation is what is internally perceived). It seems, therefore, that what is essential about the relationships in both types of conditioning is the repeated association of one with the other, which is how "contingency" has been defined here. In operant conditioning that association is established by having the stimulation follow the response, while in classical condition it may be established in other ways as well. It is the association that is important.

[3]By "neutral" here I mean a stimulus that has no meaning, no emotional significance, for the subject.

tends to acquire the valence of the stimulus that already has significance. If the originally meaningful stimulus is negative in some way, the neutral stimulus, as a result of the repeated contingency, will also become negative. If the originally meaningful stimulus is positive, the neutral stimulus will tend to become positive. Negative and positive valences can be operationally defined by the behavior of the subject. Stimuli that an organism will approach or consume are positive, those that an organism will move away from or avoid are negative. It is through such associations of neutral stimuli with emotionally meaningful stimuli that organisms acquire tendencies to approach or avoid various stimuli that they may encounter throughout life. The tendency to approach or avoid may be inferred to be similar to or associated with likes and dislikes, or positive and negative feelings.

Combinations

I have tried to provide realistic examples, but in reality, it is unusual to encounter such simple examples of either response contingencies or stimulus contingencies. Several realities complicate the picture. First, a response contingency invariably takes place in a setting or circumstance, and this means that there are usually a variety of stimuli associated with the occurrence of a response contingency. My example of positive reinforcement, for instance, in which a child learns to drop objects in order to see the parents bend over and pick them up, only happens when the child is sitting in the highchair. Because learning is typically specific to the circumstances in which it occurs, this child is not likely to drop objects when walking around the room. This tendency for learning to be specific to a situation is symbolized for reinforcement contingencies by

$$S_1 + R_1 \to S+ \text{ (or } -S-)$$

and for punishment contingencies by

$$S_1 + R_1 \to S- \text{ (or } -S+).$$

It should be evident that the contingency is not just between R_1 and $S+$ (or $S-$), but also between S_1 and $S+$ (or $S-$). Consequently, there is a stimulus contingency built into the response contingency. This implies that a person learning a behavior as a result of positive consequences will, in addition to acquiring that behavior, acquire positive emotional associations with the circumstances under which the behavior was learned, all else being equal. An excellent example is a classroom experience that is familiar to most of us. Public speaking is feared by most people. Indeed, someone once claimed that the fear of public speaking was actually greater than the fear of death, to which one wit replied, "Of course, after death you don't have to walk back to your seat." Intense as the fear of public speaking is, most students become less fearful after they have taken a course in public speaking in which they have prepared and presented several speeches to the class. The applause they receive and the grades for good performance surely reinforce their skills at organizing and presenting a speech. In addition, because approval is a positively valenced stimulus, these reinforcing contingencies also associate the emotional reactions to approval with the stimulus circumstances of talking before an audience. As a result, the act of giving a speech becomes a more positive, or at least a less fearful, experience than it was before the class. Those students who do not do well in public speaking courses, of course, would be expected to continue to fear public speaking.

It can also be said that stimulus contingencies are not as pure as they may appear. When we go to the dentist to have cavities filled, the drilling is unpleasant, and so many people learn to feel afraid or uncomfortable at the smell of the dentist's office, or the sound of the drill, or just the thought of having to make an appointment. But more than just a stimulus contingency occurs. We have to perform a number of behaviors to get to the dentist—making an appointment, transporting ourselves, and so on. These behaviors are also followed by the pain and discomfort that occur when our teeth are filled. As a result, some people procrastinate about making the appointment, arrive late, or even cancel the appointment. Of course, in the long run, there should be a positive payoff (i.e., the removal of a negative consequence), so our mature minds usually overrule our learned emotional deterrents and we go anyway. Nevertheless, the procrastination, cancellations, and tardiness based on the response contingencies that are inherent in these circumstances may continue to occur.

Generalization

One effect of co-occurring stimulus and response contingencies is a strong tendency for the behavior learned in one set of stimulus circumstances not to be performed under other circumstances. The baby who dropped objects in order to be amused by a parent picking it up is not likely to drop objects when sitting on the floor, or when a parent is not present. Most speech clinicians know all too well that behaviors learned in the clinic may not occur automatically in clients' everyday talking situations.

Although behavior learned in one set of circumstances will be less likely to occur under different circumstances, it may occur in circumstances that are similar to the one in which the learning took place, which is known as generalization. The rule of generalization is that the more the original learning situation and the new situation resemble each other, the more likely it is that the learned response will occur in the new situation. This tendency for behaviors learned under one circumstance to be performed in different but similar circumstances has important implications for therapy. The tendency to carry over, to utilize behaviors learned in the clinical setting in other, everyday settings, also has implications for the development of stuttering.

Punishment with aversive stimuli can be highly disagreeable, painful, or noxious. Such stimuli naturally evoke strong reactions, one of which is known as generalized inhibition. If a highly aversive stimulus is used to punish a specific response, that response will be less likely to occur again, but other similar or related responses may also be inhibited by this punishing experience. Thus, a child who experiences stuttering as very humiliating may decide not to talk at all, at least for a while. For another child, this experience, although un-

pleasant, may not be so aversive, and the inhibition that is generalized may not be sufficient to make not talking a viable option, because that would also remove other sources of reinforcement.

Another type of contingency combination may have particular significance for the development of stuttering. Sometimes a stimulus and response are combined so that a response must *not* be performed in the presence of the stimulus in order for the consequent positive stimulus to occur. For example, a boy may have been told that when he meets a very important guest, who happens to have a very big nose, at a tea given by the child's mother, under no circumstances is anything to be said about the size of the guest's prominent member. If the boy succeeds in not mentioning this large appendage, the mother promises a special treat after the party. Thus,

$$S_1 - R_1 \rightarrow S+$$

where S_1 = the tea party with the guest having the large nose, and where R_1 = mentioning the guest's nose. This story, which is said to have actually occurred, notes that although the boy said nothing, he stared fixedly at the guest's nose throughout the party. Eventually, the child was sent off to play, and the mother turned to her eminent guest and said, "And now, Mr. P____, would you like cream or lemon in your nose?"

Although this kind of contingency is sometimes used by parents in child-rearing, it is limited by the vagueness of "not doing something." If children are promised a reward for not biting their fingernails, it is necessary to have periodic inspections and a clear understanding of how much time has to pass before the reward is given. Using the nonoccurrence of a response as the basis for a contingency can pose a variety of difficulties. This contingency is a process that will tend to promote a child's recovery from stuttering. Since stuttering is extraneous behavior that delays the reinforcement inherent in communication, its nonperformance provides earlier reinforcement than its performance. It is well documented that earlier contingencies tend to be more powerful than later ones, providing the two stimuli are of equal strength. Consequently, the child who does not repeat or prolong sounds will communicate more easily and thus gain the reinforcement of communication more quickly. Of course, many children do recover from early stuttering, and perhaps this contingency is part of that process.

Another combination of contingencies occurs when the failure to perform a certain response leads to a negative stimulus contingency. This is symbolized by

$$S_1 - R_1 \rightarrow S-$$

and is known as avoidance learning. It is a common learning process and is probably the basis for many human behaviors. For example, when we brake our car as we approach an intersection, we are avoiding the possibility of an exceedingly aversive consequence. Avoidance learning has several interesting properties. Even if the behavior seems to be performed quite coolly, as if there is complete confidence in the ability to avoid an aversive consequence, there may be a residue of fear, a kind of undercurrent of anxiety that emerges if there is any uncertainty that the feared consequence will be avoided successfully. Imagine the emotional reaction, for example, if, when a person presses down on the brake pedal, it goes to the floor.

Avoidance has, of course, been implicated in the development of stuttering in a number of different ways, most notably, as a mechanism by which secondary characteristics can be acquired. I will explore some of these possibilities as we proceed.

Points to Remember

A number of points should be remembered. First, the valence of a stimulus can be affected by experience, and therefore may differ from one person to another. Although there is some possibility of error in assuming that the valence of a stimulus is the same for everyone, there are widespread commonalities, and it would be equally erroneous to assume that such commonalities do not exist.

A second point to remember is that behavior is also a stimulus. When a person stutters, we can see that behavior, but the occurrence of stuttering is also an experience, and serves therefore as a stimulus. Stimulation is anything to which a person responds.

A third point is that many events to which human beings respond are internal—thoughts and feelings. Elsewhere (Starkweather, Gottwald, & Halfond, 1990), I have described this as our "internal environment," a valuable construct when trying to understand the behavior of human beings.

A fourth point to remember is that not all changes are learned. Children develop, and in the years we are most intensely interested in—2 to 6 years of age—they develop rapidly. Many of these changes are a result of maturation, which, it is worth noting, is heavily influenced by genetics. Learning, too, is influenced by genetic constraints and predispositions, so dividing influences into nature or nurture creates an artificial dichotomy. All change combines genetic influences (constraints and predispositions) with environmental influences, including learning. E.O. Wilson (1975) has shown that the interaction among genetic and environmental influences is essentially a universal of animal life, and there is no reason to believe that stuttering may be an exception to this universal rule. Thus, my task here is to discuss the relative roles of genetic and environmental factors in the development of stuttering. Or, put another way, how the development of stuttering emerges as an integral aspect of an individual's development (Peters & Starkweather, 1990). Even more important, in my opinion, is the fact that childhood stuttering usually has a strong impact on the child's family, which, in turn, changes in reaction to the child's disorder. The changed family, then, becomes a source of stimulation for the child. In short, once the child's problem is perceived, the family adapts and begins to develop in a somewhat different direction than before. The child, of course, develops along with them. It seems evident to me that the best way to deal with this situation is for clinicians to become involved in these families and attempt to guide their development in directions that will promote the child's fluency.

A fifth point to remember is that all learned

changes are modifiable. It may be difficult in some cases, but whatever has been learned can be changed. This is not to say that changes that are not learned are immutable. All behavior can be changed. Often, the child's own development will help.

A sixth point to remember is that the acquisition of language is a special case. The evidence suggests that the role of learning in language acquisition is somewhat different from that in other behaviors. Humans are predisposed genetically to develop a symbolic system of communication. As a result, language acquisition in the preschool child happens rather quickly, and it seems evident that there is a critical age range during which development is facilitated (Krashen, 1973). Once past this critical period, further changes in language do not happen with the same facility. This is of some importance for stuttering, because it usually begins and develops rapidly during this same period. And since stuttering is also a behavior that manifests itself in speech, it is possible that the development of language and of stuttering may influence each other. Of particular importance is the possibility that when stuttering is present in the child's speech at the end of this critical period of language development, along with such language behaviors as phonologically based speech gestures, it becomes less plastic, less changeable.[4] It seems likely that such a loss of plasticity, which occurs about the same time that a child enters school, may be responsible, at least partially, for the increased difficulty with which stuttering is treated after this time.

A SUMMARY OF STUTTERING DEVELOPMENT

Stuttering development can best be seen as a dynamic balance between the demands placed on a child to produce fluent speech and the child's capacities, inherent as well as learned, to meet those

---

[4]In the famous longitudinal study of Andrews and Harris (1964), 93 percent of persistent (longer than one year) stutterers could be predicted from the fact that they were stuttering during the 5½ to 6½ year age range.

demands. A child's capacities for fluency lie in four domains: motor skills, language production skills, emotional maturity and stability, and level of cognitive development. In each of these areas, evidence suggests, sometimes clearly and sometimes murkily, that a child who stutters may be lacking in one or more capacities, but that the combination of skills that any individual child lacks will be unique. Some children may stutter because they lack motor skill, others language skill, others emotional stability, and still others cognitive ability.

The demands of the environment can also be categorized according to these same four domains. Thus, a child's environment may be particularly demanding of motor performance. For example, parents who talk rapidly may be putting time pressure on the child. Another child's environment may be demanding in the area of language, another in the emotional area. In each case there is an imbalance between a child's abilities to speak fluently and the environmental demands on the child. It is worth noting that this account of stuttering development suggests why some children brought up in very difficult environments do not stutter; they have strong capacities. It also suggests why children brought up in nondemanding environments may, nonetheless, develop stuttering; they lack one or more of the essential capacities for producing fluent speech.

STUTTERING BEHAVIORS DESCRIBED BY RESPONSE CONTINGENCIES

Behaviors learned by response contingencies have certain characteristics that can help us decide what kind of processes may have been involved in their development. Two laws apply to such behaviors: the Law of Effect and the Law of Least Effort. The Law of Effect basically restates how response contingencies operate—that behaviors tend to increase or decrease in their frequency of occurrence according to the valence of their consequences; punishers ($S_1 + R_1 \rightarrow S-$) tend to decrease frequency, reinforcers ($S_1 + R_1 \rightarrow S+$) tend to increase them.

The extent to which it can be inferred that a

specific behavior has been shaped by the Law of Effect is limited by two considerations. First, as was mentioned before, the valence of a stimulus for an individual may be uncertain. A stimulus that appears to be reinforcing for one person may be punishing for another. Attention is a good case in point. Some children appear to have an unusual need for attention; perhaps because they have not received adequate amounts of it from their parents. Their need for attention is so great that they do things that provide a kind of attention that appears punishing. They engage in behavior their parents disapprove of in order to attract the negative attention that comes with being punished. An interesting experiment illustrates this point (Church, 1963). In a classroom full of teenagers, a teacher would periodically yell "sit down" when students got out of their seats. Systematic observation found that yelling "sit down" actually increased the frequency with which the students got out of their seats. For teenagers in this setting, the positive reactions of peers that followed the teacher's yelling were apparently more important in shaping students' behavior than was the negative attention of the teacher's yelling. This suggests the possibility that stuttering may, in some cases, be reinforced even by the negative attention it generates, such as parental disapproval, concern, or anxiety. It should be noted, however, that a child has to fail to get sufficient attention through other channels in order for this mechanism to function.

A second reason that it is difficult to ascertain that a behavior was acquired through the Law of Effect is that it applies to a wide variety of behaviors, not just those with a history of response contingency. For example, DiCara and Miller (1968) demonstrated that the amount of blood in a rat's ear can be altered by attaching a device that measures blood volume and then rewarding the rat for having more blood in the left than in the right ear, or vice versa. Somehow, the rat learned to do something that altered blood flow so that the sensor detected more blood in the reinforced ear. Blood flow is not a learned behavior, but a reflexive response. So it seems likely that many behaviors, with diverse histories, can demonstrate the

Law of Effect. This makes it nearly useless in analyses for uncovering a response's history.

The Law of Least Effort applies almost exclusively to behaviors acquired through response contingencies. It states that a behavior acquired through a response contingency will be performed in a way that requires the least possible effort but still obtains the reinforcer. For example, as I type this chapter, I am aware that I have learned how to type while resting my wrists on the desk in front of the keyboard. I can do this because my hands are large enough for me to reach all the keys without lifting my wrists from the surface. This saves me only a tiny amount of effort, and probably increases the number of typing errors I make, but the reduction in effort while still hitting most of the keys correctly is a payoff that seems to have been sufficient to alter my method of typing. A laboratory example of this law occurs when rats are reinforced with water for pressing a bar in the cage. After many trials, most rats learn to press the bar with one paw so that their mouth is closer to the water dipper. This saves the rat the effort of moving its head from the bar to the dipper and seems to be acquired only for this reason.

When stuttering behaviors are examined, however, it is clear that they do not follow the Law of Least Effort. Stuttering behaviors typically involve unusual effort. Indeed, this quality is so characteristic that I defined stuttering as the use of excessive effort in speech production (Starkweather, 1987). Stuttering behaviors seem to follow an opposite rule. If the Law of Least Effort applied to stuttering, it would simply disappear as unnecessary efforts in the act of speaking. That, of course, does not happen routinely, but there may be times when it does happen. Many children recover from stuttering, often with no formal treatment. Perhaps in these children the learning processes that shaped the behavior in the first place included enough response contingencies that the Law of Least Effort was helpful in reducing severity. Although it seems unlikely that childhood stuttering is acquired by response contingencies, the possibility remains that it may be reinforced in those children who feel they do not get sufficient attention by more ordinary, less effortful, means.

The Law of Least Effort may also play a role in the reductions in severity that occur in some adults who stutter. When they were children, they may have learned a number of "tricks" to reduce stuttering, devices such as nodding their head rhythmically or clicking the tongue as a way of getting started. As they become more mature, they realize that the effort that goes into using such behaviors is not worth the payoff. They may stutter a little bit less, which may be less important for the adult than it is for the child, because they have become more accepting of their stuttering behavior. So it sometimes seems that adults simply give up these extraneous behaviors. Van Riper (1994) tells the story of meeting an older man who had made such a decision. From that day on, Van Riper vowed to seek an easier way to stutter, and in time, he gave up much of the struggle in his speech. He went on to teach others how to stutter in an easier way.

Response contingencies may play several roles in maintaining stuttering once it is present. One role can best be explained using a concept that Van Riper (1971, p. 209) called the "giant-in-chains" phenomenon. A stutterer may be good-looking or ugly, smart or stupid, affable or dweebish. These qualities are independent of stuttering. When a person who stutters is unattractive, because of appearance or personality, it can be very convenient for him or her to blame the lack of friends on stuttering rather than the real cause. This also relieves the person from feeling the need to make improvements. Similarly, if there are problems at school or on the job, a stutterer has a built-in excuse for performance failures, which may be easier than accepting responsibility for the problems. Although this process does not occur often, in my clinical experience, when it does occur it diminishes a person's motivation to work on developing better speech, because tinkering with an excuse for problems or concerns that are difficult to face threatens anyone's self-esteem. In this way, stuttering may be maintained by the reinforcement gained from its use as a convenient excuse for unrelated problems.

ASPECTS OF STUTTERING DESCRIBED BY STIMULUS CONTINGENCIES

A common stuttering phenomenon that is likely to be acquired through stimulus contingencies is situation dependency—the well-known tendency for stuttering to occur more often in some situations than in others. This tendency also involves certain listeners or types of listeners, such as authority figures, adults, or fit-looking people, and is a subset of the same phenomenon. Situation dependency is seldom present in very young (preschool) children who stutter (Bloodstein, 1960), but it usually develops rather early, typically within the first few years that a child stutters. Thus, the timing of the emergence of situation dependency suggests that it may be based on learning. Furthermore, the pattern of situations in which stuttering occurs is unique to each individual. There are some situations that many stutterers report to be of special difficulty, such as talking on the telephone or talking to strangers, but there are some stutterers who do not participate in these general trends. Consequently, the collection of difficult situations and listeners is, by and large, highly individual. This, too, suggests a role for learning, since each individual's experiences are unique.

The association of stuttering with specific stimulus characteristics seems to happen when a child is talking and also doing a lot of stuttering. For example, a young boy might be asked by his father to explain some misbehavior. Because of guilt or fear the muscles of the boy's speech mechanism may tighten and make the smooth, fluid movements of speech more difficult. A few days or weeks later, in the same kind of situation, the boy has the same or a similar emotional reaction. The internal stimuli associated with talking to the father while defending a behavior under threat of punishment on the previous occasion may reoccur, and frequent stuttering is repeated. Now, some time later, talking to his father, even when he is not being disciplined, may evoke the same reaction. Thus,

$$S_1 \rightarrow S-$$

where S_1 = talking to his father, and $S-$ = the feelings of fear and guilt. Whereas the feelings of fear and guilt evoked stuttering, but talking to his father did not, now, after repeated pairings of these two stimuli, talking to his father comes to elicit stuttering. The tendency for stuttering to occur is only slight at first, but each time the child stutters more severely when talking to his father, the probability increases that the same thing will happen again. Of course, if the child has a number of pleasant (no fear, no guilt) experiences talking to his father, these experiences will decrease the probability of stuttering occurring again in this situation. Nevertheless, if enough negative experiences occur so that an expectation of stuttering develops, either with or without the child's awareness, the development of a specific situation dependency is likely. This same process can occur with any kind of situation, with or without a logical connection between stuttering and the situation. This gives the appearance that stuttering has become "attached" to the specific listener or communicative circumstances.

Just as stuttering can become attached to specific situations through stimulus contingencies, it can also become "detached" from situations through the discontinuation of stimulus contingencies. In the example just given, if the child has enough nonthreatening conversations with his father in which stuttering does not occur, talking to his father will cease to be a situation in which stuttering typically occurs. In other words, just as a stimulus contingency can increase stuttering severity in a situation, the extinction of such a contingency can decrease it in the same situation. Extinction of this kind may play a role in the spontaneous recovery that many children have.

Once there is a specific situation in which stuttering occurs more often than in others, there is a tendency for other situations that resemble the initial one to acquire an increased capacity to evoke stuttering as well. The tendency for stuttering to spread from one situation to another similar situation seems to be based on stimulus generalization. A child who stutters most with his or her father initially will likely stutter more, though perhaps not quite as much, with other men or authority figures who evoke the same emotional response as the father. If the father has some particular characteristic that stands out in the child's experience, generalization to other listeners can occur who have that characteristic. One young man I worked with perceived his father as being highly judgmental and critical. The young man tended not only to stutter most severely with his father but also with other men and anyone else, male or female, whom he perceived as judgmental or critical.

The collection of difficult situations for a stutterer has been called a hierarchy (Brutten & Shoemaker, 1967), because it also has an internal structure. Most stutterers can order situations so that the most difficult ones are at one end of the continuum and the easiest ones are at the other. In addition, most hierarchies have an internal structure of themes—certain categories of situations that share specific features in common. For example, one stutterer I met recalled that his most difficult situations (i.e., when he stuttered the most) were (1) buying tokens in the subway, (2) making long distance telephone calls, and (3) giving the prices of items when working in retail sales. The theme, which was uncovered after a little probing, was saying numbers. Each of the situations he described as difficult involved having to say a specific number, whether it was the number of subway tokens that he wanted to buy, the telephone number he was trying to reach, or the prices of items in the store where he worked.

Another example was a young man who reported four categories of listeners as eliciting severe stuttering: fit-looking men, older men, authority figures, and bright-looking people, male or female. His theme, as it turned out, had to do with his insecurity. Whenever he spoke with listeners in any of these categories, he felt threatened by comparison, which exacerbated his stuttering behavior. A third person was a girl whose stuttering was most severe when she was (1) talking in front of class, (2) saying grace, even though only her mother was usually present, (3) talking to information operators, and (4) reading aloud. The theme here was talking when something specific needs to be said and only a few words can make the same point. Many stutterers who are adept at changing words find their most difficult situations are those in which opportunities to do so are limited.

These themes seem to arise through generalization based on the similarities in the situations as stimuli. Sometimes there is a logical connection, as in the case of the girl described last, but such a connection is not necessary. Thematically related situations need only share common stimulus characteristics. I believe that the common tendency for certain words and sounds to be stuttered more often than others develops in the same way. By chance, certain words are stuttered a few times, and an expectation develops that the word, or the sound that it begins with, is "difficult." Once such an expectation is in place, the necessity for saying the word becomes a stimulus that will elicit more stuttering. In other words,

$$S_1 \rightarrow S-$$

where S_1 = a specific word or sound, and S– = the experience of stuttering, including listener or self-reactions to the stuttering. After a few experiences, a word or sound can come to elicit the same struggle and forcing reactions that were not present originally. Such "word fear" may then spread to other words in several different ways—to those that begin with the same sound or those that are semantically related (e.g., if "cow" elicits stuttering, in time, "pig" and "chicken" may, too). Even syntactic and pragmatic categories can be the basis of generalization. Some people stutter most severely on question words, and because most question words begin with /w/, they may acquire a sound fear as well. Similarly, many stutterers have difficulty saying their names, perhaps because few words can be substituted or because time pressure results from appearing to be unable to recall or say one's own name.

Many times, I have seen stutterers whose sound fears match the first sound of their first or last name. The initiation of a new topic is a pragmatic category that some stutterers find difficult (Bell, 1986).

ASPECTS OF STUTTERING DESCRIBED BY VICARIOUS LEARNING

Vicarious learning is a process that is seldom appreciated or considered when trying to understand human change. Nevertheless, it is a powerful type of learning for humans, because it can often be mediated by language. The process involves a person who is to change, called the observer, who observes another person, called the model, who experiences one of several contingencies. An actual observation is not necessary. If the observer simply believes that the model has experienced such contingencies, the belief can become the force for vicarious learning (Bandura, 1969). In order for vicarious conditioning to occur most effectively, the model has to be someone whom the observer wishes to emulate. If the model's attraction to the observer is particularly powerful, the observer may simply assume that the desired contingencies are in force. For example, there are several individuals who advertise themselves as experts in entrepreneurial activities. These people give workshops to others who are interested in making money. These "experts" take care to look wealthy and to talk about the wealth they have earned. The audience is "sold" on the idea that all they need to do is emulate the person giving the workshop and they will be as successful in their own business. Symbolically,

$$R_1 \text{ -o-> } S+$$

where R_1 = behaviors that the expert claims to have performed, and S+ = the money that is claimed to have been made. The -o-> symbol indicates that the contingency was not directly experienced by the person but was either observed in the model, or inferred from the model's behavior, words, or appearance. This last point is important. An observer does not have to see the model experience the contingency; it can simply be inferred.

In vicarious conditioning it is also important that the observer believe that the rules that apply to the model also apply to the observer. Suppose, for example, that a 60-year-old man, who has lost his retirement nest egg in a failed business, attends a workshop given by a 30-year-old successful entrepreneur. He might come away without believing that he could successfully follow the younger man's program because of age differences. In effect, he would be saying to himself, "Sure, it's all right for you to say that all you have to do is adopt this brand of management. You're still young and can impress people with your dynamic charisma. But people look at me and think I am over the hill." In this situation, the young entrepreneur is not a good model for the older man. The same older man might attend a similar workshop given by someone his age and come away feeling that, "If he can do it, so can I." Age, gender, apparent success, verbal facility, and appearance are model characteristics that lead observers to decide if they can emulate the model.

All types of learning can occur vicariously. Reinforcement, punishment, classical learning, and combinations of these processes can be observed or inferred to have occurred in models, and result in behavior change in an observer. Some psychologists believe, in fact, that vicarious processes are far more important in changing human behavior than are direct conditioning processes (Bandura, 1969). Vicarious processes seem to require, or to be enhanced by, the use of language, which suggests they may be particularly useful for humans.

Several aspects of stuttering seem to be good candidates for vicarious conditioning. Perhaps the most obvious is the situation in which a father and son (or mother and daughter) both stutter. Parents are good models, because they are both higher in status and comparable to their children. A father who stutters and uses various tricks or techniques to escape from or avoid stuttering is modeling these behaviors for his son. Genetic proclivities, of course, also play a role in how similar the son's behavior pattern is to his father's, but the opportunity for vicarious learning processes seems undeniable. Indeed, I have seen a number of parent-

child dyads in which children acknowledged that they had learned certain stuttering behaviors from a stuttering parent.

Of course, nonstuttering parents are also models for their children who stutter, and a number of aspects of stuttering are likely to be acquired this way. A striking example of this is the way in which very young preschool children who either stutter or are at risk for stuttering develop attitudes about stuttering that are modeled by their parents' reactions to stuttering. A parent who feels ashamed when the child stutters in front of another person is modeling that reaction for the child, and the child will likely develop a sense of shame about stuttering. Similarly, parents who show fear when their child stutters (e.g., fear that the child will develop a chronic stuttering problem or be teased in school) are modeling fear for their children. Over and over, in the Temple University Stuttering Prevention Center, I have been struck by the fact that very young children evidence attitudes toward their stuttering that are the same as those of their parents. Guilt, anger, panic, and insecurity are among the reactions to stuttering that a parent may feel and show and which the child may also adopt. Even the common and generally unhelpful advice of parents to slow down, take a breath, or just relax may signal the child that something wrong is happening, even though the advice might be helpful (e.g., slowing down) if the child could follow it. However, such advice also models an attitude about stuttering, often conveyed by nonverbal behaviors that belie the advice to relax, that may lead to struggle and avoidance later on. Finally, parents who never talk to their children about stuttering may be modeling, by their silence, a reaction that leads the child to believe that stuttering is unspeakably awful or shameful.

It seems likely to me that many of the beliefs, perceptions, and attitudes of stutterers are acquired this way, first, and powerfully, from the modeled reactions of their parents to stuttering, then, later, from the reactions of peers and teachers during their school years, and even later from the reactions of friends, spouses, and professionals who interact with them. It is through the reciprocal interactions with those around us that cultural values are acquired, and attitudes about stuttering may be shaped the same way. As with other conditioning processes, many modeling experiences may be beneficial for stutterers. For example, the interactions of stuttering clients with their speech clinicians should provide good vicarious learning processes that lead to improvement of fluency. Also, many parents, with both love and understanding, model attitudes that are helpful to a child—attitudes of self-acceptance, confidence, doing what you want to do whether or not you stutter. But if most experiences, vicarious and otherwise, are negative, the attitudes acquired are most likely to be negative. In all cases, the summation, or net effect, of all such learning processes influences the stutterer's attitude.

SPECIFIC PATTERNS

Avoidance Learning and Defensive Reactions

Avoidance has frequently been described as an especially important aspect of stuttering (Bloodstein, 1987; Brutten & Shoemaker, 1967; Van Riper, 1971; Wischner, 1950). Avoidance behaviors are acquired through avoidance conditioning, which is a particular form of defensive reaction (Bandura, 1969). Avoidance, in particular, and defensive reactions, in general, are well-documented learning patterns that lead to specific types of behaviors. They also have a well-deserved reputation for producing behavior that is tenaciously resistant to change. Symbolically, avoidance learning is represented by

$$S_1 - R_1 \rightarrow S-$$

where S_1 = the stimulus circumstances, or a specific stimulus; R_1 = the avoidance behavior; and $S-$ = an aversive consequence. Thus, an aversive event occurs unless the avoidance behavior is produced. A laboratory example of this process can be arranged by placing a rat or other small animal in a cage that has an electrified floor and is divided by a low barrier. A light is turned on and a few seconds later a mild electric current is sent through the floor. The animal feels uncomfortable and will likely jump around, and in time find its way over the barrier and escape the discomfort. After a few repetitions of this experience, the animal will jump the barrier as soon as the light is turned on and will not experience any of the discomfort caused by the electric current. Once learned, avoidance behavior is very difficult to eliminate through extinction. The experimenter can turn off the electricity to the floor of the cage completely, but each time the light is turned on, the animal will jump the barrier. The animal has, in fact, no way of discovering that the floor of the cage is no longer electrified since it always jumps the barrier when the light is turned on.

The reason that this form of learning produces behavior that is so resistant to change is that the consequence of avoidance behavior prevents the occurrence of an expected negatively valenced stimulus. In short, nothing happens, and it is impossible to know if that was a result of the behavior that was learned or if nothing would have happened anyway. As a result, avoidance behaviors are sometimes performed in a kind of superstitious way, to ward off a feared event that may not happen. We do such things all the time—we throw salt over our shoulders, don't walk under ladders, drink chicken soup when we have a cold, knock on wood. Such behaviors cost little in effort, and there is no way to know what would have happened if they had not been performed. Similarly, when stutterers change a word because of concern about anticipated stuttering, that behavior is reinforced regardless of its actual outcome. Even if they stutter on the substituted word, they still avoided stuttering on the word they changed.

Although changing a word to one less likely to be stuttered is an obvious avoidance behavior, many other stuttering behaviors may be based on this learning process. When the powerful processes of avoidance learning are coupled with differential reinforcement, some of the most difficult stuttering behaviors become understandable. An example is a child who is asked to take a deep breath before trying to speak and who then tries this when expecting to stutter. In the beginning, it seems to work, at least some of the time, perhaps because the delay while taking a breath allows muscle tensions to subside. This brief period, when breath-taking seems to be instrumental in reducing stuttering, reinforces the behavior. Symbolically,

$$S_1 - R_1 \rightarrow S-$$

where S_1 = a perceived difficult word, R_1 = taking a deep breath, and $S-$ = the occurrence of stuttering. However, after a while, taking a deep breath stops working, or it works less often in forestalling stuttering. Just why its effectiveness, and that of many other avoidance behaviors, weakens with repeated use is uncertain and a matter of some interest for researchers to investigate. But most such "tricks" that children learn in efforts to make their speech more fluent become less effective over time.

When this happens, a child may respond with a larger, more effortful version of the same behavior. In the case of a deep breath, this may mean taking a deeper breath or several such breaths. For some reason, this "new" behavior may again seem to have a fluency-enhancing effect, and the child says the word more fluently, as if it were a result of having taken a deeper or several breaths. Unfortunately, this means that when the deeper or several breaths lose their fluency gains, the child has now learned to breathe a little deeper or take more breaths, and the behavior's effectiveness will be restored. This is likely to continue with more and deeper breaths, perhaps joined by throwing back the head or lifting the arms to achieve the desired effect. Eventually, an extremely anomalous behavior pattern may develop, one that is far removed from the original deep breath and that seems unrelated in any logical way to an attempt to speak. Such behavior will have developed and become part of the child's stuttering, even though it had little if any effect in saying a word fluently.

I also recall another child who began to lick his lips, as if to stall for time while momentary panic or excessive muscle tension passed. Of course, it stopped working, and like the breathing pattern just described, lip-licking became more and more extreme, until the tongue was protruded far out of a wide-open mouth. In the end, this child seemed to be gagging, and it was no longer apparent that lip-licking had ever been a part of this pattern.

Such extreme avoidance behaviors arise and can become firmly entrenched in a young stutterer's speech pattern because of the powerful effects of avoidance learning, on the one hand, and differential reinforcement on the other. These behaviors have a compulsive-appearing quality, but I know of no literature that suggests stutterers are more compulsive than nonstutterers. It has been suggested, however, that compulsive behaviors, such as ritualistic hand-washing, have a similar origin in avoidance learning (Bandura, 1969).

The struggle and forcing that is often a common aspect of stuttering behavior can also be seen as a defensive reaction. This view suggests that persons perform such behavior because they think they may have stuttered worse had they not struggled and forced the word out. This way of dealing with word and syllable repetitions is characteristic of a 2- or 3-year-old child. If a child at this age meets an obstacle in play, the natural reaction is to push with increased effort to overcome the obstacle. Such children are too young to understand that some things happen better if they are not forced. So struggle and forcing are used as a way of getting through a repeated word, to hurry it along, and get on with the rest of the message.

It is probably no accident that the earliest emotional reaction of children during the early stages of stuttering for most children, when only easy whole-word or whole-syllable repetitions are produced, is frustration at being unable to complete what they are saying as quickly as they want. This frustration reaction, which is well-documented (Amsel & Roussel, 1952), consists of putting additional effort into a response that previously resulted in a desired reinforcement. So, when children who are just learning to produce sentences that have desirable consequences in their listening environment are frustrated that a word is being repeated, they naturally try to push harder when saying the word in order to get on to the rest of the sentence.

It is my sense that avoidance learning can account for the earliest struggle and forcing behaviors, as well as the later development of such tricks as stalling for time, rhythmic foot-tapping or finger-pinching, pretending to think of a word, and all of the other behaviors that are usually called secondary reactions or accessory behaviors. These are behaviors that occur in reaction to stuttering. Of course, in the earliest stages for most children (there are exceptions), "stuttering" behaviors are repetitions that have little or no struggle or tension. Whether these early behaviors should be called "stuttering" or not is a definitional issue which has not yet been resolved. Some clinicians think of them as stuttering, others as normal nonfluencies. My sense is that they are not normal, since relatively few children exhibit these behaviors at frequencies that exceed normal adult values (Yairi, 1981). At the same time, they seem more like pre-stuttering behaviors in that they lack the struggle and tension that, in my opinion, are definitive of the disorder. I have chosen to call them "at risk" behaviors, since the struggle and forced behavior seems to develop in reaction to them, and because if struggling and forcing is forestalled with

appropriate prevention techniques, easy whole-word repetitions seem to disappear on their own.

SUMMARY

I have tried to describe here some speculations about the possible roles that learning processes may play in the development of stuttering in children. Two basic classes of learning have been described: response contingencies and stimulus contingencies. These two types can be, and usually are, combined in complex forms of learning processes, of which a few specific ones seem to be particularly important in the development of stuttering. In addition, the process of vicarious conditioning was described, which is another method by which learning processes can occur, and one commonly recognized as more important for human beings than the more direct methods that have been explored in such detail by experimental psychologists. Moreover, several aspects of stuttering development are consistent with vicarious learning explanations.

REFERENCES

Amsel, A., & Roussel, J. (1952). Motivational properties of frustration: I. Effect on a running response of the addition of frustration to the motivational complex. *Journal of Experiment Psychology, 43,* 363–368.

Andrews, G., & Harris, M. (1964). *The syndrome of stuttering.* London: Heinemann.

Bandura, A. (1969). *Principles of behavior modification.* New York: Holt.

Bell, H. (1986). Topic change as a predictor of stuttering in young children. Convention presentation, ASHA.

Bloodstein, O. (1960). The development of stuttering I. Changes in nine basic features. *Journal of Speech and Hearing Disorders, 25,* 219–237.

Bloodstein, O., (1987). *The handbook of stuttering* (fourth edition). Chicago: National Easter Seal Society.

Brutten, G.J., & Shoemaker, D. (1967). *The modification of stuttering.* Englewood Cliffs, NJ: Prentice-Hall.

Church, R.M. (1963). The varied effects of punishment on behavior. *Psychological Review, 70,* 369–402.

DiCara, L.V., & Miller, N.E. (1968). Instrumental learning of vasomotor responses by rats: Learning to respond differentially in the two ears. *Science, 159,* 1485–1486.

Krashen, S. (1973). Lateralization, language learning, and the critical period; some new evidence. *Language Learning, 23,* 63–74.

Peters, H.F.M., & Starkweather, C.W. (1990). The development of stuttering throughout life. *Journal of Fluency Disorders, 15,* 107–114.

Starkweather, C.W. (1987). *Fluency and stuttering.* Englewood Cliffs, NJ: Prentice-Hall.

Starkweather, C.W., Gottwald, S.R., & Halfond, M. (1990). *Stuttering prevention: A clinical method.* Englewood Cliffs, NJ: Prentice-Hall.

Van Riper, C. (1971). *Speech correction: Principles and methods* (Fifth edition). Englewood Cliffs, NJ: Prentice-Hall.

Van Riper, C. (1994). A message from Charles Van Riper. In J. Albach & V. Benson (Eds.), *To say what is ours.* San Francisco: National Stuttering Project.

Wilson, E.O. (1975). *Sociobiology: The new synthesis.* Cambridge, MA: The Belknap Press of Harvard University Press.

Wischner, G.J. (1950). Stuttering behavior and learning: A preliminary theoretical formulation *Jour-*nal of Speech and Hearing Disorders*, 15,* 324–335.

Yairi, E. (1981). Disfluencies of normally speaking two-year-old children. *Journal of Speech and Hearing Research, 24,* 490–495.

SUGGESTED READINGS

Ahlbach, J., & Benson, V. (Eds.) (1994). *To say what is ours.* San Francisco: National Stuttering Project. A collection of stories and essays by people who stutter, this book presents the raw data of experience. Every aspiring clinician should read it.

Bandura, A. (1969). *Principles of behavior modification.* New York: Holt. Still the last word on such important principles of learning theory as vicarious conditioning, social learning, reciprocal influence, and defensive behavior, this book is a must for understanding the role of learning in stuttering development.

Bloodstein, O. (1995). *A handbook on stuttering* (Fifth edition). Chicago: Easter Seals Society. Bloodstein is a reference for virtually everything that is known about stuttering, and he has compiled it in a way that is remarkably free of preconceptions.

Bobrick, B. (1995). *Knotted tongues.* New York: Simon and Schuster. A historical and philosophical examination of stuttering, this book makes clear how powerful the drive for an answer to stuttering can be, and demonstrates that stuttering can interfere with the most essentially human function—communication.

Hofstadter, D., (1979). *Gödel, Escher, Bach: An eternal golden braid.* New York: Basic Books. Although writing from the vantage point of artificial intelligence, Hofstadter explains clearly how the process of recursion can operate in human affairs, and recursion is essential to understanding stuttering.

Levelt, W.J.M. (1989). *Speaking: From intention to articulation.* Cambridge, MA: MIT Press. A clear and readable account, from one of the world's foremost psycholinguistics, of the process of speaking.

PART TWO

STUTTERER–NONSTUTTERER DIFFERENCES

Much of what is known about stuttering and people who stutter has come from systematic comparisons of groups of older children, adolescents, and adults who stutter with matched groups of nonstuttering speakers. Such studies have examined how fluent and dysfluent segments of speech of these two groups differ on a variety of perceptual, acoustic, kinematic, aerodynamic, and physiological measures. In spite of its variability and the inconsistency of stuttering from one speaker and one situation to another, stuttering does not occur randomly. It occurs with sufficient regularity in groups and across time for researchers to identify patterns of similarities and differences. This section covers the patterns that have been found in three promising areas of research: psycholinguistic correlates, respiratory and laryngeal function, and cerebral activity.

Any collection of chapters can be organized in a number of ways. We grouped these three chapters together primarily because the data on which they are based were obtained primarily from either adults or children whose stuttering had continued to persist long after onset. The section begins with Bernstein Ratner's discussion of stuttering from a psycholinguistic perspective in which its patterns of occurrence are compared to those of other types of speech errors. As will be seen, advances in our understanding of stuttering are not restricted to those acquired through the use of space-age technology and instrumentation. Indeed, current systems of conceptualization and analysis in linguistics, such as those exemplified in this chapter, also energize and redirect research and theory.

Next, Denny and Smith explore the respiratory and laryngeal control of speech found among stuttering speakers. Their focus on these two components of speech production was not a search for the locus or cause of stuttering. Rather, it was a critical examination of the contributions of these subsystems to a dynamic, multifactorial conceptual framework of speech and stuttering that will be elaborated further in the chapter by Smith and Kelly in the following section.

Watson and Freeman conclude this section with descriptions of the newest methods for imaging the brain and its activity. Recent advances permit systematic comparisons of relative levels of cerebral activity throughout the brain, and such data are now being accumulated from stutterers and nonstutterers while performing various linguistic tasks and during the fluent and stuttered speech of adult stutterers. These fascinating glimpses of cortical architecture and function and the comparisons of stutterers and nonstutterers may even resuscitate the cerebral dominance theory of stuttering. It is interesting to speculate that, as twenty-first century research in this area unfolds, Travis's long-dormant theory of stuttering may assume a new legitimacy. Like old soldiers, old theories of stuttering seem never to die, they just fade away—but then, unlike old soldiers, they reappear wearing freshly laundered uniforms.

CHAPTER 5

STUTTERING: A PSYCHOLINGUISTIC PERSPECTIVE

NAN BERNSTEIN RATNER

INTRODUCTION

The frequency and location of stuttered moments are quite amenable to description within a linguistic framework. Structures (sentence components) that linguistic theory predicts will be more complex for speakers to construct are stuttered on more often by children and adults. Further, the locations (or *loci*) of stutter events are far from random. They occur in disproportionate numbers on the initial portions of linguistic structures. Such phenomena suggest that it may be profitable to consider stuttering to be linguistically conditioned, and therefore a byproduct of some failure in the sentence production process, rather than solely as the result of speech motor execution constraints.

In this chapter, I will briefly review psycholinguistic models of the sentence production process. Next, the relationship of linguistic structure to the frequency and loci of stutter events will be summarized and related to models of speech production. Finally, I will explore the relationship between the process of early language acquisition and stuttering onset, and propose some possible developmental linguistic precipitators of stuttering onset.

ACKNOWLEDGMENTS: I would like to thank Hans-Georg Bosshardt, Ed Conture, Dick Curlee, Barry Guitar, Megan Neilson, Ehud Yairi, and Scott Yaruss for their lively electronic conversations, help, feedback, critiques, suggestions, and support during the preparation of this chapter, and their willingness to bear with me when I threw all sorts of notions against them, much as one tests whether spaghetti is done by throwing it against a wall to see what sticks.

PSYCHOLINGUISTIC MODELS OF NORMAL SPEECH PRODUCTION

There is no single agreed-upon model of the sentence generation process, and speech production has long been an "orphaned" and underexplored domain in psycholinguistic research (O'Connell & Wiese, 1987). Competing models of the speech production process differ in the degree to which they explicitly acknowledge the role of formal linguistic rules in sentence construction as opposed to nonlinguistic probabilities (connectionism). They also differ in the degree to which they can be considered "serial," with discretely ordered stages of syntactic, lexical, and phonological retrieval, or "parallel," in that such processes may occur simultaneously and may interact with one another. Further, as Strand (1992) notes, the majority of work in modeling speech production has focused on adult speech; attempts to model child speech production are rare. This has important consequences for understanding stuttering in children, as I discuss later in this chapter.

It is generally agreed that language production involves two broad processes, those that "create the skeleton of the utterance, and those that flesh the skeleton out" (Bock & Levelt, 1994). The skeleton is built from the selection of appropriate lexical items and the construction of a syntactic frame. "Fleshing out" is done by phonologically encoding the results of these lexical and syntactic processes and specifying the eventual prosody of the utterance as well as its phonological structure.

The product of these two processes is the phonetic plan, a prespeech specification of the utterance that is forwarded for motor encoding and finally, articulation.

"Standard" models of the sentence production process (such as those offered by Garrett, 1975, and Fromkin, 1971) have often been called "frame-and-slot" models (Dell & Juliano, 1991), with syntax and phonology represented by the construction of frames or trees that specify global structure, into which linguistic units are inserted. These models are typically serial and modular, because they propose that syntactic and lexical frames are compiled before phonological frames, and no interactions between levels of representation are presumed. A clear discussion of serial models and other approaches to modeling language production (Table 5.1) can be found in Strand (1992). (See Table 1, Fromkin, 1971).

A representative model of sentence production is shown in Figure 5.1 (Levelt, 1989; Bock & Levelt, 1994). This model is particularly relevant, not only because of its current broad appeal in the psycholinguistic literature, but because it forms the basis for at least one explicit model of stuttering (the Covert Repair Hypothesis, Kolk & Postma, Chapter 9). In this model, three major levels of processing are identified (Jescheniak & Levelt, 1994):

1. **Conceptualization**, during which the concepts to be expressed are specified.
2. **Formulation**, during which concepts are mapped to linguistic form. This level includes the processes of *grammatical encoding* (the selection of lexical items and construction of a syntactic frame or surface structure), and *phonological encoding* (the determination of final phonetic form and phonetic plan). Importantly, in Levelt's model, the phonetic plan, which is a byproduct of phonetic encoding, is inspected for possible errors by an internal monitor before being sent for articulation.
3. **Articulation**, during which the phonetic plan is retrieved from the prearticulatory buffer, initiated, and executed.

TABLE 5.1 Models of Language Formulation and Speech Production

Models of language formulation that focus on the activity included in formulating an utterance, including intent, processes of lexical selection, and syntactic processing.	Models of speech production that focus on how movement of specific range, velocity, and direction occurs to constrict the airstream for a desired acoustic output.
Serial models: Suggest independent levels of linguistic processing. Garrett (1975, 1980); Shattuck-Hufnagel (1979)	**Translation models:** The model assumes a discrete invariant input from the language formulation system. It describes processes of conversion of that linguistic input to movement. (MacNeilage, 1970)
Interactive serial model: Suggests interaction among serially organized levels of linguistic processing. Bock (1982)	
	Action theory: Linguistic units do not exist independent of the motor representation, so there is no conversion process. Groups of muscles perform as a unit to complete a specific task. Fowler et al. (1980)
Connectionist models: Suggest that linguistic processing occurs as a result of a large network of simultaneous and interactive processing elements and their connections. Stemberger (1985); Dell (1988)	

From Strand (1992). In Chapman, R.S. Processes in language acquisition and disorders, 1992, St. Louis, Mosby–Year Book, Inc.

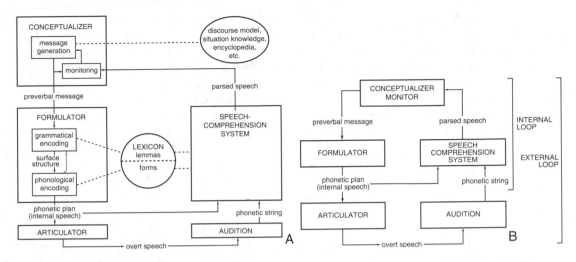

Figure 5.1 (A) A blueprint for the speaker. Boxes represent processing components; circle and ellipse represent knowledge stores. (B) The perceptual loop theory of self-monitoring; illustrates the internal monitoring loops. (From Levelt, W.J.M., Speaking: From intention of articulation. © 1989 MIT Press. Reprinted with permission.)

Levelt (1989, 1992) and others (Garrett, 1991) distinguish two important concepts at the formulation level of language production. The first is the *lemma*, or the semantic properties of words, together with their syntactic specifications (the grammatical environments that they require or permit). Lemmas drive grammatical encoding: Retrieving a noun triggers the system to construct a noun phrase, while retrieving a verb triggers the system to construct an appropriately specified verb phrase. Lemmas are devoid of the phonological information necessary to permit articulation. Such specification of phonological form rests in the *lexeme*, which is accessed after the lemma has been activated. This conceptual distinction between semantic function/syntactic forms (lemmas) and their phonological representation (lexeme) is important for most psycholinguistic theories of fluency breakdown in stuttering.

Models of the speech production process gain large support from errors observed in normal speech production, such as hesitations, fillers, revisions, and "slips of the tongue" (or Spoonerisms) (Fromkin,

1993). A model's strength can be judged by the degree to which it can predict those types of errors that actually appear in spoken language, as well as those that do not. Garrett (1991) conceptualizes the potential loci of language planning failure that can lead to errors and disfluency as follows:

- In going from message to lemma representations
- In going from lemma to word-form representations
- In going from word forms to phonetic representations for connected speech
- In going from speech representations to motor representations

PSYCHOLINGUISTIC MODELS OF STUTTERING: AN OVERVIEW

At least three current models of stuttering suggest that fluency failure arises from disturbance in construction of the prearticulatory plan. The first is Wingate's (1988), whose "fault-line" hypothesis presumes that individuals who stutter have a phonological encoding deficit. The deficit is specified as one in which syllable onsets are retrieved in a timely fashion, while the rimes are not, leading to the speaker's inability to progress past the syllable onset. Though not specified as such, Wingate's model is compatible with a locus of failure at the third of Garrett's four possibilities, the level at which the lexeme is specified and its components retrieved.

The Covert Repair Hypothesis (CRH) of Kolk and Postma (see Chapter 9) attributes the fluency failures of stuttering to efforts to correct phonetic errors prior to their articulation. Their "self-correction hypothesis of stuttering" presumes an underlying impairment—perhaps the slow activation and selection of correct lexemic representations—(Kolk, 1991) that slows phonological encoding. This slowing leads to errors in the compilation of the phonetic plan, which are detected by the internal monitor (Levelt, 1989), and corrected through the responses of postponement and restarting.

Wingate's and Kolk and Postma's models differ in predicting which part of the phonetic plan cannot be fluidly executed. For the CRH, disfluencies reflect problems in accurately encoding the segment that is stuttered, while for Wingate, problems with the word onset reflect difficulty further into the temporal sequence of the phonetic plan.

Perkins, Kent, and Curlee (1991) adopt a somewhat different approach. As with Wingate, their model is strongly based upon frame-and-slot models of speech production in which linguistically defined constituents, such as word and syllable onsets, have psychological reality. Unlike Wingate, Perkins et al. posit that a stuttering speaker is the victim of dissynchrony in the retrieval and integration of frames with their specified segmental content. The Perkins et al. model also posits that the nonlinguistic factor of the speaker's perceived time pressure to continue speaking is crucial in transforming the resulting disfluency into a stuttering event.

Finally, some capacity-demands models of stuttering (Neilson & Neilson, 1987; Starkweather, 1987), can be viewed as psycholinguistic, insofar

as they predict that some children may not be able to simultaneously meet levels of linguistic and motor planning demand. However, specifically defining which level of demand exceeds capacity for individual children who stutter, or for stuttering children as a group, is problematic for such models. Moreover, some examples of child behaviors used to illustrate capacity-demands models (Peters & Guitar, 1991; Starkweather, Gottwald, & Halfond, 1990) appear to require that we distinguish between transient capacity limitations and those that persist indefinitely or cause permanent changes in a child's approach to language production. Later in this chapter, I will propose some specific and developmentally predictable linguistic demands that might suffice to overwhelm a child's speech planning and execution capacities and trigger the evolution of stuttering.

LANGUAGE ABILITY AND STUTTERING

Either explicitly or implicitly, a number of models of stuttering make assumptions about the linguistic capacity of the typical individual who stutters. Usually, it is assumed that the linguistic systems of stutterers are more fragile and subject to encoding error. But is there evidence that children or adults who stutter have atypical or depressed linguistic abilities?

Numerous studies have contrasted the language performance of stuttering and normally fluent children as measured by syntactic complexity of spontaneous speech (Silverman & Williams, 1967a, b; Wall, 1980; Westby, 1979;), sentence imitation ability (Bernstein Ratner & Sih, 1987), scores on standardized tests of language production and comprehension (Byrd & Cooper, 1989; Murray & Reed, 1977; Nippold, Schwarz, & Jescheniak, 1991; Ryan, 1992), receptive vocabulary ability (Murray & Reed, 1977; Ryan, 1992; Westby, 1979), oral and written narrative ability (Nippold, Schwarz, & Jescheniak, 1991), and reading (see Nippold & Schwarz, 1990, for further discussion).

Although Andrews, Craig, Feyer, Hoddinott, Howie, and Neilson's (1983) landmark review of replicated research led them to conclude that "stutterers perform more poorly on some tests of language: the Peabody Picture Vocabulary Test, length and complexity of utterance, and some Illinois Test of Psycholinguistic Ability subtests" (p. 230), the results of many recent studies have, for the most part, suggested that the language capabilities of individuals who stutter do not differ appreciably from those of nonstutterers (Bernstein Ratner & Sih, 1987; Kadi-Hanifi & Howell, 1992; Nippold, Schwarz, & Jescheniak, 1991). Studies that have found diminished language scores for groups of children who stutter usually note that observed differences are of a small magnitude, and are clinically insignificant (Ryan, 1992). Further, some studies suggesting that children who stutter show delayed or deviant speech-language onset and performance failed to exclude children with subnormal intelligence. For example, Andrews and Harris (1964) reported a strong correlation between poor speech-language ability and stuttering in a sample of eighty stuttering children. However, the numbers of children in their stuttering and control groups with frank IQ deficits (32 and 13, respectively) were almost identical to the numbers reported to have deficient language abilities (35 and 14, respectively). Since frank retardation and language ability are correlated (Bernstein Ratner, 1993a), failure to segregate the performance of retarded children from the rest of the cohort when analyzing language factors may yield misleading results.

Nippold (1990), after exhaustive review of the literature, concluded that there was little evidence to support the notion of pervasive or substantive differences between stuttering and nonstuttering children on language tasks. This, in turn, suggests that although stuttering may interact in theoretically and clinically interesting ways with language task requirements, the condition of stuttering cannot clearly be linked to obvious underlying deficiencies in language knowledge or to evidently atypical patterns of language performance.

Nonetheless, some studies and demographic surveys (e.g., Ryan, 1992; St. Louis & Hinzman, 1988) have observed a higher-than-usual incidence of clinically relevant language and/or phonological disturbance in stuttering children.

Phonological deficits are more frequently observed than are language deficits and may in fact be quite pervasive (see Louko, Edwards, & Conture, 1990). Because this pattern is not universal, there is growing sentiment that such co-existing clinical profiles reflect a select subgrouping within the larger population of children who stutter (Nippold, 1990; Schwartz & Conture, 1988).

A research tradition that has emphasized the use of clinical assessment tools in assessing stuttering children's language skills may impede our ability to discern possible subtle forms of linguistic impairment that meaningfully contribute to stuttering. Some research suggests that *subclinically* depressed linguistic skills may be detected in a number of adults who stutter (Watson, Freeman, Chapman, Miller, Finitzo, Pool, & DeVous, 1991; Watson, Freeman, DeVous, Chapman, Finitzo & Pool, 1994; Wingate, 1967, 1988). Recently, Watson et al. (1991, 1994) identified a subgroup of stutterers within their experimental population who were, when compared to other stuttering adults and the fluent controls, impaired in their discourse production abilities, as measured by story grammar coding, and in discourse comprehension, as measured by ability to determine referents for pronouns (anaphoric reference), and ability to disambiguate lexically and grammatically ambiguous sentences.

In an earlier set of reports, Wingate (1967) found that stuttering adults showed decreased ability to reparse Slurvs (e.g., create a meaningful phrase from a semantically anomalous string such as "yearn ever told tool urn"—"you're never too old to learn"), an ability that is probably based in lexical decoding. Wingate (1988) also reported decreased WAIS vocabulary scores in another group of adults who stuttered, even when vocabulary was elicited in written mode. Further, these stuttering subjects provided less common associations on a word association task. Such performance profiles are subclinical and would not be obvious in everyday language interactions.

Additionally, recent and sophisticated studies of linguistic processing have revealed subtle differences in the processing time required by stuttering adults when they are asked to make phonological, semantic and syntactic judgments about experimental stimuli (Bosshardt, 1993, 1994). This is an interesting finding that deserves further investigation. In general, while some variability in adult language proficiency is taken for granted in achievement testing and has been the focus of some psycholinguistic research (e.g., classic work by Gleitman & Gleitman, 1970), relatively little attention has been paid to possible subtle differences in linguistic ability that might distinguish individuals beyond their early language-learning years (Obler, 1993). In this regard, the study of possible differences between the linguistic abilities of adults who stutter and those who are considered normally fluent would chart new territory in a number of research domains.

LINGUISTIC CHARACTERISTICS OF STUTTERED EVENTS

Beyond the question of overt (or subtle) linguistic impairment in the stuttering population, researchers have documented regularities in the frequency and loci of stuttered events that appear to reflect an interaction between linguistic processing and stuttering.

Models of the normal speech production process are based in large part on examination of normal disfluency patterns, and the linguistic regularities that appear to govern speech errors ("slips" or "Spoonerisms"). In fact, few other sources of data are used to construct speech production models (Fromkin, 1993). In many respects, stuttered moments share distributional and situational characteristics with normal disfluencies; however, stuttered moments sound qualitatively distinct from normal disfluencies. The characteristics of normal disfluencies (such as hesitation phenomena, filled pauses, segment repetitions, and retracings) have been rather extensively explored. Unfortunately, much less work has been carried out to specifically examine language production task effects on stuttering, perhaps because of difficulties in compiling adequately large and well-controlled subject samples. Thus, many assumptions about the relationship between syntax and stuttering, particularly in children, have been extrapolated from work with normally fluent speakers, rather than with children who stutter.

In summarizing loci and frequency patterns in stuttering, I will follow a "bottom-up" approach to language production, which is most compatible with frame-and-slot models of the speech production process. Such approaches are intrinsically symbolic and linguistically motivated views of sentence production (Plunkett, 1993), in which linguistic structure and linguistic rules are presumed to play a "psychologically real" role in language functioning. In bottom-up fashion, I will progress from phonetic and phonological properties of stuttered moments, to their lexical properties, followed by successively higher-order properties, such as syntactic regularity and discourse features. In these descriptions, I do not presume a lack of interaction between levels during sentence production, although this is quite likely (Dell, Juliano, & Govindjee, 1993).

In many of the discussions that follow, findings can also be divided into two distinct concepts: loci and frequency constraints. *Loci* analyses ask whether stuttering is randomly dispersed throughout a speaker's output, or follows linguistically relevant topology. Interpretation of loci studies is complicated by the problem of determining whether stuttering or disfluency on a word relates directly to the speaker's difficulty in producing that particular word, or reflects the speaker's inability to move forward in planning and executing sentence elements yet to come. MacWhinney and Osser (1977) take this second, less common view that in normal disfluency, words are repeated not because of uncertainties about their own production, but in order to buy time for other decisions. In contrast, most loci studies of stuttering presume that disfluency patterns are "local" and specifically reflect difficulty in execution of the disfluent word.

Frequency analyses ask whether particular types of tasks that supposedly differ in level of difficulty within phonetic, phonological, lexical, syntactic, or pragmatic domains elicit predictable changes in the numbers of stuttered moments.

It is my own opinion that loci and frequency studies are best conducted with metalinguistically unsophisticated stuttering children. Given the well-documented effects of learning on the evolution of an individual's stuttering profile (Peters & Guitar, 1991; Starkweather, Chapter 4), both loci and frequency of stuttering in adult or older children are probably multiply determined. For this reason, I will focus more closely on studies of stuttering children than those of adults in the sections that follow.

Phonetic Factors in Stuttering

Most work on phonetic factors in stuttering have been loci analyses, with the exception of those (e.g., Brown, 1945; Silverman, 1972; Soderberg, 1966, 1971; Taylor, 1966a, b) that examined phonetic complexity, as defined by word length. In all but a few cases, word length was measured by letter length, rather than length in pronounceable segments, a linguistically odd criterion. It should not be surprising that longer words are stuttered more frequently than are shorter words. For various reasons, however, the well-documented effect that longer words attract more stuttering is currently viewed as an epiphenomenon, because longer words are atypical within a given language not only phonetically, but lexically as well. I will spend more time on loci effects in this area, which can be interpreted much less ambiguously within psycholinguistic framework.

If we put aside instances of what might be called metalinguistic self-fulfilling prophecies, in which an adult speaker is so sure a sound is troublesome that he stutters on a word even when the feared sound isn't actually in the word (e.g., stutters on the p in pharmacy after declaring p to be difficult to articulate fluently), several interesting properties emerge from general patterns of stuttering on the sounds of English. There is a clear inverse relationship between the frequency with which phonemes occur word-initially in English, and the frequency with which stuttering occurs on these phonemes. In short, the most frequent word-initial phones are stuttered least (Wingate, 1988).

This finding can be used to suggest that stuttering does not result from lexical retrieval difficulties, because serial search models of lexical access (e.g., Marslen-Wilson & Tyler, 1980, 1981) predict greater competition among lexical choices when the word-initial phonetic cohort is larger (i.e., when a target word resides in a larger phonological neighborhood). Phonetic factors in stuttering, whether frequency or loci-based, are, unfortunately, difficult to untangle from lexical and syntactic factors, because a phoneme's frequency in word-initial position is determined by lexical frequency, which is in turn driven by the syntax of English. For example, the most frequent words of English are function words, the grammatical "glue" of syntax. Of the top 100 words in Carroll, Davies, and Richman's (1971) *American Heritage Word Frequency Book*, approximately three-fourths are articles, pronouns, verbal auxiliaries and modals, and prepositions.

There is also evidence that function words are stored in the mental lexicon apart from content words, and that their retrieval and phonological encoding is facilitated through a separate look-up system (Bock & Levelt, 1994; Levelt, 1992). Strong evidence of propositionality effects in adult stutterers, in which stuttering occurs more frequently on high-information bearing content words, especially those of lesser frequency or familiarity (see Hubbard & Prins, 1994) additionally leads to the conclusion that any identifiable phonetic profiles of stuttering loci are artifacts of the unequal distribution of phonemes across lexical classes and syntactic functions. Compellingly, in rare cases such as bilingual stuttering, phonetic profiles in stuttering loci differ across the speaker's two languages (Bernstein Ratner & Benitez, 1985), while stutter loci remain constant across syntactic class descriptions.

Phonological Factors in Stuttering

In this section, I distinguish between the ways in which sounds are combined to create phonologically permissible words and the properties of individual sounds themselves. Wingate (1988) presents an excellent discussion of this distinction relevant to analyzing stutter loci. LaSalle and Carpenter (1994) found that children stuttered more when retelling a story that contained vocabulary with varied, as opposed to repetitive, coda structure. This suggests that planning sequences of words with varying phonological structure can tax fluency. Conversely, Throneberg, Yairi, and Paden (1994) did not find increased stuttering on phonologically complex items in the speech of young children.

It is well-known that most stuttered events are word-initial, as are those speech errors that involve consonantal movement (Shattuck-Hufnagel, 1987). As Wingate notes, in phonology, and in many models of sentence production (particularly frame-and-slot models), word and syllable onsets are considered to be distinct phonological constituents that are detachable from their codas and subject to movement and selection errors, such as the classic Spoonerisms, "You have hissed all my mystery lectures," and "She's a queer old dean." Other segments within the word are considered to be more deeply embedded in its hierarchical structure (MacKay, 1972; Meyer, 1992; Shattuck-Hufnagel, 1987). Further, there is speculation that syllable onsets are encoded prior to syllable codas and that this temporal asynchrony explains common "tip-of-the-tongue" phenomena, in which the speaker can identify and sometimes produces the initial phoneme of the target word, but cannot retrieve its full pronunciation. Thus, Wingate's hypothesis that stuttering results from asynchronous and deficient retrieval of syllable rimes is compatible with basic psycholinguistic approaches to phonological encoding. It fails, however, to explain some "higher-order" linguistic regularities in stuttering, especially in children. These sets of regularities will be addressed in a later section that focuses on syntax.

Lexical Factors in Stuttering

Lexical retrieval is a complex task carried out at an extraordinarily rapid rate: The speed of lexical access in normally fluent speech is astoundingly fast: from 2 to 3 words per second at slower rates (Maclay & Osgood, 1959) to 11 or more words per second (Deese, 1984), with relatively few errors of selection (Shallice & Butterworth, 1977).

Lexical Frequency and Stuttering. The frequency with which a word typically appears in a language affects its speed of retrieval (Oldfield & Wingfield, 1962), as well as its pronunciation accuracy (Balota & Chumbly, 1985), so it is not surprising that infrequent or unfamiliar words of a language are also stuttered more often than are frequent words (see Hubbard & Prins, 1994 for discussion). Low frequency/familiarity words are also more susceptible to speech error (Stemberger & MacWhinney, 1986), particularly phonological "slips" such as the Spoonerisms illustrated previously (Dell, 1990).

Frequency appears most strongly to affect production, in contrast to word verification or comprehension tasks (Jescheniak & Levelt, 1994). Bock and Levelt (1994) suggest that the frequency factors operate at the lexeme level, the level at which phonological encoding of words occurs. As with other aspects of linguistic organization, it is difficult to cleanly ascertain how word frequency impacts stuttering in conversational speech, because any effects tend to be masked when syntactic complexity of the target word's carrier phrase or sentence is manipulated (Ronson, 1976; Palen & Peterson, 1982).

Lexical Class and Stuttering. Words of many languages can be readily divided into *content* and *function* words. Content words include nouns, main verbs, and modifiers, while function words include articles, pronouns, verbal auxiliaries and modals, deictics, prepositions, and small numbers of other grammatical elements (e.g., the *by* in "John is loved by Mary"). As mentioned previously, content and function words differ in several ways. Among these are size of class. The content class is large and conceptually open, while the function word class is small and closed to new lexical additions. Other differences include relative frequency in the language (function words are more frequently used by a large factor), phonetic characteristics, and automaticity of retrieval. They may also be processed by different areas of the cerebral cortex, even in children (Kutas & Van Petten, 1994).

In normal speech errors, slips occur more often on open class words (Garrett, 1991; Stemberger, 1989), even when frequency of occurrence is controlled. Stuttering is much more common on content than function words in the speech of adults (e.g., Johnson & Brown, 1935; Brown, 1938a, b; Hejna, 1955). Paradoxically, stuttering in young children appears to gravitate to function words (Bernstein, 1981; Bloodstein & Gantwerk, 1967; Bloodstein & Grossman, 1981; Wall, 1977;). This finding has been widely interpreted as the overriding effect of syntactic encoding on lexical frequency in children's speech. While lexical acquisition is a lifelong process, and a speaker's frequency of lexical usage undergoes constant change, young children face the problem of acquiring the appropriate use of function words within grammatical constituents, a problem they will solve for the most part by age 6 to 8. I will return to this issue later; however, it is important to note that the use of function words is a byproduct of syntax, rather than a self-contained lexical function.

It is probable that lexical access during sentence production may not have been sufficiently well investigated in research on stuttering. A number of methodological issues complicate analysis of lexical access in stuttered speech. The majority of psycholinguistic research on lexical access in normally fluent speakers has used adults, rather than children, and involves analysis of reaction time (RT) to lexical stimuli (for a recent review of psycholinguistic research on the mental lexicon, see Hirsh-Pasek, Golinkoff, & Reeves, 1993). Because a large body of research suggests that both verbal and nonverbal reaction time delays characterize adult stutterers' performance, regardless of task (see Andrews et al., 1983; Bishop, Williams, & Cooper, 1991; and Ferrand, Gilbert, & Blood, 1991 for discussion), use of either manual or vocal RT to estimate efficiency of lexical storage and retrieval in individuals who stutter is complicated. Watson et al. (1991) provide evidence that suggests that longer RTs in adults who stutter may reflect increased motor, rather than linguistic load.

However, the nature of most RT studies limits subjects' expected output to well-rehearsed, nonspontaneous language tasks that are devoid of spontaneous syntactic formulation and lexical retrieval. There is a general lack of RT studies using people who stutter that involve lexical verification (distinguishing words from nonwords), phoneme monitoring (to measure rapidity of receptive lexical access), or other tasks involving the receptive lexicon in people who stutter. Recent work by Bosshardt (1993, 1994), for example, suggests that adults who stutter demonstrate relatively long RTs on tasks requiring them to monitor for rhymes and category membership of target words (phonological and lexical tasks, respectively). The relative paucity of research into the lexical processing skills of both adults and children who stutter is somewhat surprising, given the fact that depressed receptive vocabulary scores (as measured by the Peabody Picture Vocabulary Test) are the most consistently reported differences observed between groups of stuttering and normally fluent children.

Before leaving the areas of phonology and the lexicon, I would like to return to predictions made by Perkins, Kent, and Curlee (1991), whose neuropsycholinguistic model of stuttering presumes assynchronous retrieval of linguistic frames and assembly of their internal constituents. Such a conceptualization is intrinsic to the explanation of most speech errors in otherwise normal speech production. In slips such as "The little girl bugged her hair," or "Stop beating your brick against a head wall" (Fromkin, 1993), errors of phonetic and lexical insertion into pre-established lexical and syntactic frames are presumed to produce the eventual error. Thus, as with other models that implicate linguistic encoding difficulty in stuttering, it is not clear why stuttered speech does not demonstrate a higher frequency of these types of classical speech errors, even under the time pressures hypothesized by the Perkins, Kent, and Curlee model. Speech errors occur relatively infrequently, and there has been little research to ascertain whether they occur more frequently in stuttered speech. Recent work by Yaruss and Conture (1994) suggests that stuttering children do not demonstrate higher rates of speech errors than do their normally fluent peers.

Syntax and Stuttering

A large quantity of data now show rather robust relationships among language task, syntactic complexity, and mastery of linguistic material and the frequency and loci of normal disfluencies and stutters. There are definite timing requirements on sentence planning that should affect the frequency and loci of stuttering when viewed within a syntactic framework. The planning of simple sentences appears to require a prespeech latency of about .75 seconds (Lindsley, 1975, 1976); more complex syntax, such as might be necessary to caption complex pictures, requires as much as 7 to 9 seconds (Cooper, Soares, & Reagan, 1985).

Loci Effects.   It appears that sentence initiation time reflects the complexity of the speaker's intended subject noun phrase, while intrasentence disfluencies arise from the syntactic complexity of objects (Ferreira, 1991). Thus, it is not surprising that both normal disfluencies and stuttering gravitate heavily to sentence-initial position in the speech of both children and adults (Bernstein, 1981; Bloodstein & Gantwerk, 1967; Brown, 1938a, b; Hejna, 1955; Quarrington, 1963). Further, the eventual length and complexity of utterances strongly correlates with the frequency of both stuttered and normal disfluencies at sentence beginnings (Jayaram, 1984).

Once a speaker commits to the initial constituent structure of a sentence, it is difficult to monitor and adjust the planning of later structures (Bates & Devescovi, 1989), which may explain why normal disfluency and stuttering occur so often at utterance- and clause-initial boundaries. Speech errors and disfluency are often thought to reflect constraints of early commitments to sentence structure that sometimes paint the speaker into a virtual corner, and require intrasentential revisions and stalling so that the end of the utterance can be compiled.

One persuasive kind of evidence for postulating a functional relationship between language formulation and stuttering is the predictability of the loci of stuttered moments. For children, such regularities have long been apparent. Children's stuttered moments are much more likely to occur on utterance-initial and clause-initial words, which in child language are likely to be functors (Bernstein, 1981; Wall, Starkweather, & Cairns, 1981; Wingate, 1976). Within major clausal units, stuttering is more likely on the initial words of sentential constituents, such as noun phrases, verb phrases, and prepositional phrases (Bernstein, 1981). For example, Bernstein (1981) found a very high frequency of stuttering on the initiation of verb phrase constituents in children's spontaneous speech. Verb selection is an integral component of the utterance-generation process, because verbs limit or force the possible arguments that may accompany them (functional role assignment) (Bock & Levelt, 1994; Gropen, Pinker, Hollander, & Goldberg, 1991; Gropen, Pinker, Hollander, Goldberg, & Wilson, 1989;). Thus, there is some evidence that verb selection is particularly difficult for stuttering children.

Recent loci research with adults who stutter has been infrequent, possibly because of the previously noted concern about the multiple determinants of the topology of stuttering in adult speech (see also Bloodstein, 1987). Quarrington (1963) and Soderberg (1971) found that adults were likely to stutter on words that were poorly predictable using older psycholinguistic models of sentence production based upon transitional probabilities. Such words also tend to be longer and located at constituent-initial points in an utterance. Bernstein Ratner and Benitez (1985) found statistically regular tendencies for a Spanish-English bilingual adult to stutter at common constituent-initial points in utterances in both languages (i.e., while initiating subject noun phrases or verb phrases), even though regularities in stuttering locus could not be found by using other criteria, such as the initial sounds of words that were stuttered.

Frequency Effects.   In young children, normal disfluency is increased when they attempt to produce difficult or newly mastered grammatical structures (Bernstein Ratner & Sih, 1987; Colburn & Mysak, 1982a, b; Gordon, Luper, & Peterson, 1986; Wijnan, 1990). In recent years, a large amount of research has investigated whether syntactic (grammatical) factors seem to affect the frequency of stuttering in a child's speech. For the most part, such work has examined the fluency characteristics of either children's imitations or of elicited productions following experimental modeling. Bernstein Ratner and Sih (1987) found a highly significant positive correlation (r = .905) between the grammatical complexity of target sentences to be imitated by children (as defined by the developmental course of their typical emergence in spontaneous child language) and children's stuttering on these stimulus sentences. The apparent effects of syntactic complexity on stuttering were much larger than those of sentence length, which evidenced a statistically significant, but lower correlation (r = .727). Although the data are not amenable to classical partial correlation analyses, a post hoc analysis using the obtained Spearman values rather than Pearson values suggests that when length is partialled from sentence complexity, the relationship between stuttering and syntactic complexity falls from .954 to approximately .909. Conversely and strikingly, partialling complexity from length reduces the association of stuttering with sentence length during imitation tasks from .701 to approximately .103, a sizable drop (M. Neilson, 1994, personal communication).

Suggestive but less strong relationships between utterance complexity and stuttering (and normal childhood disfluency) have been found in studies by Gordon (1991) and Kadi-Hanifi and Howell (1992). Gordon (1991), who sampled a fairly narrow range of sentence types, found that children's attempts to parallel a clinician's model utterance resulted in more stuttering than did direct sentence imitation. Stuttering also increased with estimated degree of syntactic complexity, but not significantly, perhaps due to the restricted range of utterance types examined. Length of utterance effects were not addressed in this study. After employing a covariate analysis to separate length and complexity, Kadi-Hanifi and Howell (1992) found particularly strong associations of syntactic complexity with frequency of stuttering in children between 9 and 12 years of age, but also noted a somewhat counterintuitive tendency for their youngest subjects to stutter more on simpler language constructions.

Sentence-imitation and modeling tasks risk either underestimating a child's sentence generation abilities, because it is easier to repeat than to formulate speech (thereby artificially decreasing stuttering), or exceeding a child's current spontaneous language abilities (thereby artificially increasing stuttered moments). Post hoc analyses of grammatical complexity on spontaneous speech are also problematic, because a child may not provide a full array of constructions to appraise, and the development of taxonomies for sentence complexity is a challenging task. However, in a creative study by Gaines, Runyan, and Meyers (1991), the spontaneous language samples of stuttering children were divided into sets of utterances that were produced without disfluency and those containing stuttering. Developmental Sentence Score (DSS) analysis (Lee, 1974) showed a significant tendency for stuttered utterances to be more structurally complex than those that were produced without disfluency. Stuttered sentences were also significantly longer than fluent sentences; however, the relative contributions of length *and* complexity in predicting moments of stuttering were not appraised.

Realistically, the role of syntactic complexity in conversational fluency is difficult to estimate, because of the tendency in English for more syntactically complex structures (those that are later acquired by children and are more difficult for adults to generate and process) to be longer than simpler constructions. The relationship between length of utterance and frequency of stuttering seems transparently logical (the longer the output, the more opportunities to stutter), and has long been used as a tenet of therapy planning, particularly in work with young children who stutter (e.g., therapy approaches such as Gradual Increases in Length and Complexity of Utterance (GILCU; Ryan, 1979) and Extended Length of

Utterance (ELU; Costello, 1983; Costello Ingham, 1993) to name two such programs.

It is theoretically and clinically interesting to try to separate the effects of linguistic planning (i.e., the structure of utterances, or their length in syntactic units, such as morphemes, constituents, or clauses) from what might be considered motor planning or production variables (the length of an utterance in syllables, for instance). As mentioned earlier, Bernstein Ratner and Sih (1987) noted that sentence length was not as highly correlated with the frequency of stuttering as was syntactic complexity when both were used to predict disfluency in a sentence imitation task. Brundage and Bernstein Ratner (1989) also found that an utterance's length as measured in morphemes (a grammatical measure) was more highly predictive of increases in stuttering than was utterance length in syllables (an articulatory measure), in children's spontaneous language samples. In such an analysis, the same utterance and its associated disfluencies are correlated using separate indices of length and complexity (for example, the phrase "unlaced shoes" contains 2 words, 3 syllables, and 5 morphemes). When Brundage and Bernstein Ratner plotted rates of stuttering in children's spontaneous utterances using each of these alternative measures of utterance length, the likelihood of stuttering was highest when morphemic length of utterance was used as the index of prediction.

Recent work by Logan and Conture (1995) suggests a more complicated picture; in their appraisal of the relationships among spontaneous utterance length, grammatical complexity (as measured by DSS), and articulatory rate, utterance length was best associated with the frequency of stuttering, and articulatory rate was the least well correlated, with grammatical complexity having an intermediate level of association with fluency. Logan and Conture propose that length is a macrovariable that encompasses grammatical encoding and other sentence production demands. As the authors also note, neither spontaneous speech nor imitation tasks may clearly resolve the nature of any effect that syntactic complexity has on fluency, since difficult imitative tasks may overstress a child's natural language capacity, while spontaneous speech may not provide a sufficiently broad sampling of possible degrees of complexity to analyze the relationship properly. That is, designing target stimuli that challenge but do not frustrate a group of subject children is difficult, but using children's spontaneous output creates uneven opportunities to assess the association of linguistic complexity with fluency.

Cross-Linguistic Research in Stuttering

Before leaving this discussion of structural constraints on stuttering frequency and locus, it is important to note that cross-linguistic research in this area is quite lacking. In psycholinguistic and child language acquisition research, it has become increasingly evident that predictions about language processing and development that are based only on data from English speakers are not confirmed by the behaviors of speakers whose languages have grammars typologically distinct from English (MacWhinney & Bates, 1989; Slobin, 1985a, b, 1992). For example, to say that very young children have trouble learning third person agreement is to make a statement about children learning English, not children in general. In particular, the degree to which sentence constituents such as initial noun phrases must be overtly expressed or may be omitted (*pro-drop*), the degree to which grammar is conveyed by rich or poor inflectional morphology, and by free or bound grammatical elements, all have the potential to create distinct loci patterns of stuttering that may not coincide with those observed in English. Further, cross-linguistic analysis as well as linguistic analyses of the speech of bilinguals who stutter offer the potential for determining which levels of linguistic description (phonetic, phonological, lexical, or syntactic) seem to exert the strongest influence upon stuttering frequency and loci. Such findings would also have significant implications for the development of more explanatorily adequate models of stuttering.

Pragmatics and Stuttering

The study of pragmatics emphasizes the ways in which an utterance is used, as opposed to its phonological, lexical, or syntactic structure. Thus, "It's eight o'clock" may serve a number of functions, such as responding to a request for information, warning friends that they will be late if they do not hurry, requesting action from someone, or reprimanding (if in fact something was supposed to have been accomplished by that hour, and wasn't). Despite these varied functions, the structure of the utterance remains the same, albeit with possible alterations in its prosody.

Most pragmatic investigations of stuttering have been done with children. A recent summary of such work appears in Weiss (1993), which I will briefly summarize here. Stuttering and normal children do not appear to differ in the degree to which they produce assertive or responsive utterances when in conversation with parents (Weiss & Zebrowski, 1991). Despite longtime concerns about the adverse effects of adult questions on children's fluency, Weiss and Zebrowski (1992) found that stuttering children were more fluent in responding to parents' requests than in making requests of their own.

The study of pragmatic determinants of fluency is still in its infancy. The most thoroughly researched aspect in the stuttering literature is that of dyadic conversational tempo, or the pacing of conversations between speakers, and its relationship to stuttering. The most frequent dyadic interaction examined has been that between stuttering children and their mothers.

Much attention has been focused on documenting the efficacy of indirect stuttering therapy that adjusts the nature and pacing of parent-child verbal interaction. A recent summary of studies on this topic appears in Kelly (1993). Such research has generally, but not completely, supported the older, anecdotal wisdom of assuming that slowing parental speech rate, decreasing linguistic pressure upon children, and increasing inter-speaker latency appears to facilitate fluency in some young children. Such modifications are presumed to induce the child to produce simpler language or exploit greater opportunities to preplan utterance production.

Conversational Tempo. Child language acquisition research clearly suggests that some aspects of timing synchrony in parent-child dyadic interaction are set in motion very early, in fact, well before the appearance of children's expressive language ability. Even young infants entrain their movements and vocalizations to a pace set by their adult conversational partners (Condon & Sanders, 1974; Jasnow & Feldstein, 1986). The entrainment of children's speech rate to that of their parents seems to be a question primarily of interest to researchers in stuttering. Their studies generally find little change in children's speech rate when adults change the rate of speech addressed to the child, even when improvements in fluency are also observed (e.g., Embrechts, Franken, Mugge, & Peters, 1995; but see Marchinkoski & Guitar, 1993; Guitar, Schaefer, Donahue-Kilburg, & Bond, 1992; Savelkoul, Zebrowski & Buizer, 1993; Starkweather, Gottwald, Kaloustian, & Ridener, 1984; Stephenson-Opsal & Bernstein Ratner, 1988). The clinical wisdom of routinely advising parents of stuttering children to slow their speech rate is tempered by findings that some stuttering children's parents appear to talk fairly slowly (Kelly & Conture, 1992). Moreover, Bonvillian, Raeburn, and Horan (1979) noted *decreases* in children's ability to follow an adult model that was more than one word per second faster or *slower* than their own conventional speech rate.

Conversely, children's turn-taking latencies and the temporal regulation of the conversational "dance" between partners appear to be affected by parental models (Bernstein Ratner, 1992; Newman & Smith, 1989; Welkowitz, Bond, Feldman, & Tota, 1990). Such findings are consistent with those of Condon and Sanders (1974). Furthermore, children's early responsiveness to the tempo of parental speech is predictive of the generally documented effectiveness of modifying conversational tempo in the indirect treatment of childhood stuttering.

Dyadic Modeling Effects on Lexical and Syntactic Patterns.   Speech rate and response time latency manipulations and their outcomes stand in direct contrast to the extent to which syntactic characteristics of adult speech predict either the syntactic characteristics of children's speech or their fluency. As I have discussed previously (Bernstein Ratner, 1993b), child language acquisition research has searched for parental syntactic determinants of children's speech output. While a handful of relationships between parental syntax and the use of syntactic structures by children have been reported, such relationships tend to be few in number, limited in scope, and lagged in effect. Children do not appear to readily adjust their syntax to changes made by adults in their environment, although admittedly, most researchers do not ask parents to simplify their speech to children to see what happens. That is something that only researchers in fluency have been interested in doing. However, the premise that children will adopt short, simple, presumably less demanding syntax because their parents do has yet to be supported by basic child language research and was found empirically false in the one laboratory study that investigated children's entrainment to parental syntax (Bernstein Ratner, 1992). In fact, one study indicates that children appear to build selectively from adults' shorter utterances in dyadic interactions to "vault into" attempts at utterances that are more complicated than their typical output (Nelson & Kamhi, 1985).

It is clear that more work needs to be done in this area. There is limited evidence from research on adults that speakers and hearers may adopt a mutual syntactic style in which particular syntactic patterns, such as the passive, recur across turns (Weiner & Labov, 1983). Thus, even if the length and morphological complexity of parental utterances do not condition changes in the length and complexity of children's output (Bernstein Ratner, 1992), it may be that parental modeling of particular syntactic structures results in these same structures being produced with less effort and stuttering by their children. The notion that parental use of particular structures may "scaffold" their

spontaneous use over time (Bernstein Ratner, Parker, & Gardner, 1993; Snow, Perlmann, & Nathan, 1987) may have important ramifications for counseling the parents of young stutterers. Similarly, Streim and Chapman (1987) found that prior lexical mention by adults appears to scaffold more fluent production of these lexical items by 4- to 8-year-old normally developing children. The effects of prior lexical mention by adults on children's stuttering have not yet been investigated and may have similar implications for early intervention.

"Doing What Comes Naturally," or the Problems of Manipulating Discourse Style.   Adult speech to very young children is a universal speech register that is labeled in a variety of ways (Child-Directed Speech or CDS, babytalk, "motherese"). Speech register refers to a system of language use having predictable prosodic, phonological, lexical, syntactic, and pragmatic characteristics. The CDS register varies from other registers of English and other languages along each of these domains, although CDS properties across languages may vary considerably (Bernstein Ratner & Pye, 1984; see Ochs & Schieffelin, 1995;). Among the more salient aspects of English CDS are its significantly slowed rate, shorter and more redundant sentence structure, and lexical redundancy.

Elsewhere, I have speculated that it is not easy to ask parents of 2- to 6-year-old children to adjust their speech to children along one major dimension of CDS without inadvertently eliciting other adjustments (Bernstein Ratner, 1992). Parents in most research studies are either current users of CDS (because their children are still young enough to elicit some form of it, or because siblings in the household elicit it) or have only relatively recently stopped using CDS with their child. Because slowed speech rate may be the most salient and universal aspect of CDS, other than its prosody, slowing rate may precipitate adoption of other CDS characteristics, such as changes in syntax, lexicon, and pragmatics. This phenomenon is seen in "foreigner talk" (Hatch, 1983), when native speakers are prompted to speak more slowly to non-native listeners (they change syntax and vocabulary, shorten utterances, repeat themselves more often, and make some less easily explainable adjustments, such as speaking more loudly). Support for the hypothesis that instructions to adopt part of a register will elicit additional modifications comes from Bernstein Ratner (1992), who found that different instructions to modify maternal speech style in two groups of mothers produced virtually indistinguishable changes in their speech. Telling a mother to produce slower, simpler speech to her 2- to 4-year-old child resulted in speech that was, in fact, slower and simpler. But identical results for both rate and sentence complexity were obtained when mothers were only told to slow their speech rate. Moreover, additional instructions appeared to hamper some mothers' attempts to formulate conversational speech. Their children responded by interrupting them.

Such findings stress the importance of continued research into the effects of parental speech on children's speech and fluency, as well as the outcomes of parent counseling intended to modify child-directed speech style. We do not yet know whether parents can maximize support for children's attempts at fluent language production through specific adjustments in their own use of syntactic forms or lexicon. Nor do we clearly understand the theoretical rationale for improvements in fluency that follow parent counseling (Bernstein Ratner, 1993b). When we obtain clinical success following parent counseling, we cannot be sure exactly how such success was achieved. Finally, we do not yet appreciate the degree to which adjustments along one dimension of child-directed speech may provoke additional adjustments that are unanticipated by the researcher or clinician.

DEVELOPMENTAL PSYCHOLINGUISTICS AND STUTTERING

In this section, I turn to the question of whether patterns of language acquisition in young children may interact meaningfully with the onset and evolution of stuttering in children. If stuttering is lin-guistically mediated, it may emerge as particular aspects of language structure and use are mastered.

The Onset of Stuttering and the Course of Speech and Language Acquisition

One of the riddles of developmental stuttering is its onset. No other developmental communication disorder presents such a profile of ostensibly normal development, followed by a transition into a pattern of disordered production. For example, children with Specific Language Impairment (SLI) come from the larger population of children with SELD (Specific Expressive Language Delay), and have shown a consistent history of delayed linguistic development (see Miller, 1991). Children with phonological delay have, as far as anyone can tell, always lagged behind their peers in the accuracy of their phonetic approximations. But most children who stutter apparently display an early profile of normally fluent expressive communication, only to develop, typically between the ages of 30 to 36 months, the disfluencies characteristic of stuttering (Andrews & Harris, 1964; Yairi, 1983; Yairi & Ambrose, 1992a, b). It should be noted, however, that of the eighty stutterers studied by Andrews and Harris, about one-third were reported by their mothers to have stuttered from the very onset of expressive language. A recent and provocative finding by Yairi, Paden, Ambrose, and Throneburg (1994) indicates that children who are classified as persistent stutterers present with a later onset of stuttering (mean of roughly 38 months) than do children who recover from early periods of stuttering. In their study, the latter group had a mean stuttering onset that was almost six months earlier.

A number of current models of childhood stuttering posit the evolution of some imbalance between a child's linguistic and motor capacities and the demands of fluent speech production. But a capacity-demands model (Starkweather, 1987), while intuitively satisfying, needs to specify what aspects of linguistic or motor demand cannot be met fluently by a stuttering child, and, more importantly, why it could be met previously. What possible changes or shifts in a child's development, or "verbal environment" (Broen, 1972) might either overwhelm the synergy of the child's linguistic, motor, and/or monitoring systems, or evoke such changes in how speech is processed and produced?

Developmental Reorganization of the Relationships between the Lexicon and Syntax

Starting around 2 years of age, there is a transition from a lexically driven, asyntactic production system to the development of a qualitatively different, grammatically governed system capable of generating syntactic plans for speech execution (Bates, Dale, & Thal, 1995; Wanner & Gleitman, 1992). There are a variety of approaches compatible with this view of child language acquisition. While quite different in theoretical and evidentiary bases, all of the accounts that follow converge on a strikingly similar set of predictions regarding when stuttering is most likely to appear in children. Moreover, they generate testable hypotheses about the loci of stuttering in children whose stuttering is of recent onset.

Wijnan (1990) and Elbers and Wijnan (1993) discuss the evolution of sentence planning and acquisition of sentence frames in young children, reasoning from the normal disfluency patterns of a young language-learner. Wijnan's Development of the Formulator Hypothesis predicts that the development of serial order planning and incorporation of closed-class elements into the expressive grammar precipitates developmental patterns of disfluency. Many child language researchers have proposed that children experience a discontinuous increase in the acquisition of vocabulary (the so-called vocabulary "spurt" or "burst"). As I shall discuss later in this section, if such a burst is indeed typical (Bates, Dale & Thal, 1994), it appears to occur too early (18 to 30 months) to explain most onsets of stuttering. However, there is evidence of a subsequent linguistic "burst," as measured by Mean Length of Utterance (MLU), which has a later onset (24 to 26 months) and steep rise until 30

months, the ceiling age for the 1130 children used in the norming study for the MacArthur Communicative Development Inventory:Toddlers (CDI:T) scale. MLU increases are usually thought to reflect the child's acquisition of grammatical, closed-class morphemes. Of particular interest is the degree to which "bursting" in the two domains appears to interact: Grammatical complexity scores on the CDI:T were highly related to the size of children's expressive lexicons. In other words, those children who are acquiring words most rapidly are also making the greatest strides in grammatical development. In the CDI:T sample, this relationship was especially evident in children who had compiled a base vocabulary of roughly 400 words.

Such data prompt the hypothesis that children may begin to experience fluency problems when their vocabularies and grammatical development undergo simultaneously rapid rates of expansion. If we assume that a child's lemma representations must begin to accommodate the newly acquired grammatical projections governing their use, the coexistence of rapid lexical growth with the emergence of inflectional morphology and phrase structure expansion may trigger problems in efficient retrieval of lemmas and their mapping onto lexemes, which are also likely to have nonadultlike and multiple phonological representations (Leonard, 1995).

Locke's more radical dual specialization hypothesis (1993) proposes that the human language capacity is buttressed by two independent but interlocking modules: a Specialization in Social Cognition (SSC) and a Grammatical Analysis Module (GAM). Pertinent to the onset of developmental stuttering, he has suggested an asynchrony in their maturational properties. The SSC enables early vocal turn-taking and the production of expressive vocabulary that is not phonologically, semantically, or syntactically rule-governed, that is, nonlinguistic in the formal sense. At early stages of expressive language development, the GAM is not operational. Locke hypothesizes that when spoken vocabulary approximates fifty words, at about "twenty-eight months (plus or minus a half year), . . . (is) when the GAM first conspicuously operates in the typical case" (p. 354). Thus, 22 to 34 months would encompass the period when a shift from nongrammatical organization of vocal output to an integrated, layered, linguistically governed system occurs. This period of transition happens to coincide with the emergence of linguistically governed speech errors in children's output (Stemberger, 1989), which then tend to follow the same principles of organization seen in adult speech error data.

Finally, using the framework of Universal Grammar, Radford (1995) makes strikingly similar predictions. Radford argues that Early Child English, which is characterized by combinatorial language produced at 20 to 28 months of age, differs significantly from that which the child produces after this stage. Applying government and binding theory to early language production, one might say that Early Child English sentence structures are projections from lexical heads (such as noun, verb, adjective, and preposition), while adult-like sentence structures are projections of functional heads as well (e.g., auxiliaries, determiners, complementizers). Radford argues that evidence of a child's transition to more adultlike grammar around 24 to 28 months can be found in the child's productive use of elements such as modals (e.g., *will, can, may*), verbal auxiliaries (*do, have, be*), and the third person agreement affix on present tense verbs (e.g., *"Mommy takes top off"*). Radford also proposes that development of other features of English, such as complement clause structures, *wh-* words, the expletive pronoun *it* as in *"it's raining,"* determiners and possessive markers mark the child's transition to mature functional grammar. He also notes from his analysis of more than 100,000 child utterances from a large number of young language learners that there is a protracted period of linguistic instability as the child progresses from early acquisition to full mastery.

Such theories suggest that stuttering may evolve as children bridge between primarily presyntactic, lexically driven, and more formulaic productions to a grammatical system more closely governed by adult linguistic principles and processing strategies. The instability that may mark the child's crossing of this bridge also creates some testable predictions about the behavioral profiles of children at the onset of stuttering, and whether such behaviors bear a meaningful relationship to fluency. If stuttering results from an underlying deficiency in acquiring the basic lemma properties necessary to compile a syntactic plan, children who stutter should demonstrate either dissociation between relative lexicon size and the use of early morphological markers, or produce sentences having MLUs that meet age expectations according to norms, but which lack the properties of mature syntax, and show noticeably unstable use of the grammatical elements targeted in Radford's proposal. In the latter case, a stuttering child's output might be as long as his fluent peer's, but by addition of lexical items to the output string rather than morphological elaboration (e.g., "Baby doll ride truck" vs. "Mommy sits down"). Conversely, if stuttering results from competition between two rapidly expanding and interrelated functions, stuttering children's expressive lexicons and grammatical systems might be undergoing "spurt" simultaneously.

Although such hypotheses would be difficult to track longitudinally if one wanted to examine changes between a child's output prior to and subsequent to the onset of stuttering, except in a sample of children at genetic risk for stuttering, they do make predictions that are relatively easier to verify. First, it may be the case that children whose stuttering is persistent or transient may display different patterns of language ability when examined closely for the kinds of linguistic features noted earlier. The finding that persistent stuttering has a relatively later onset suggests that some differences in language profiles might be found, using more syntactically sensitive measures, such as morphological saturation (the degree to which sentential constituents are inflected) and rate of development using growth profiling (Rollins & Snow, 1994), rather than MLU as the language measure of interest. Further, both sets of children may display distinct patterns of linguistic development when compared to children whose speech is relatively fluent.

One locus prediction that arises from these models is that stuttering children should be more likely to stutter on words identified by parents as newly acquired, and more importantly, should be more likely to stutter on grammatically inflected forms or constituents. This approach is compatible theoretically with that of Colburn and Mysak (1982a, b) for examining linguistic environments in early child speech that appear to elicit normal disfluency, but differs in its structural emphasis. If an utterance contains both expanded and unexpanded constituents (e.g., the object noun phrase contains a determiner but the subject noun phrase does not, as in "Man sees the doggie"), one could hypothesize not only should more stuttering occur on such an utterance than on one in which no expanded constituents appear, but also that stuttering should gravitate to a constituent boundary prior to that containing the inflected elements.

If one asks what major transitional events in a child's language acquisition might be associated with the onset of stuttering, one should also consider which ones do *not* appear to trigger stuttering in children. Specific cases in point would be the relatively late onset of stuttering relative to the most rapid period of early lexical attainment (the "vocabulary spurt"), or the transition from single words to combinatorial language. For example, a capacities and demands model might predict significant disfluency during periods of rapid lexical growth or the transition from single words to true combinatorial speech (Branigan, 1979). However, the most obvious early period of rapid lexical acquisition, the so-called "lexical spurt" (Dromi, 1987; Goldfield & Reznick, 1990; Nelson, 1973), occurs earlier in child language acquisition (after the accumulation of a 50 to 100 word vocabulary (usually in the period between 12 and 24 months of age), a time seldom implicated in the onset of stuttering symptoms. Likewise, most children demonstrate productive combinatorial language by approximately 24 months (Rescorla, 1989). That the onset of combinatorial language does not appear to trigger stuttering is somewhat surprising, because the child's initial acquisition of the ability to combine or string multiple lexical items should present significant motor challenges. Therefore, the data on the acquisition of language

and the onset of stuttering lead to the hypothesis that neither early speech efforts nor early lexical acquisition are sufficient to trigger the onset of stuttering. Instead, stuttering appears to be triggered by a child's inability to generate syntactic representations in a timely fashion. While subject to further influences, some of which I discuss below, it seems particularly suspicious that children are able to succeed at the earliest stages of language production, while failing to fluently "bridge" between lexically and grammatically governed strategies for producing utterances.

Interactive Influences on Children's Early Linguistic and Motor Performance

In early child performance, it is especially important to understand the significant trade-offs that may occur between domains of functioning. Strand (1992) discusses the interactions between speech-motor control and language formulation that are especially relevant to the ongoing debate between speech motor and psycholinguistic accounts of stuttering. For example, children's articulation accuracy is affected by syntactic class and syntactic demand (Camarata & Leonard, 1986; Kamhi, Catts, & Davis, 1984; Panagos, Quine, & Klich, 1979), and a child's phonological inventory may affect acquisition of lexical items (Schwartz, 1988). This information, when combined with information about associations between linguistic phenomena and fluency, emphasizes the need for researchers to search for additional interactions, rather than for isolated domains of impairment that predict fluency failure, a call voiced by Strand (1992) to child language researchers. Such work would be more informative if abilities of the same subjects were assessed under varying levels of motoric and linguistic demand.

Development of Speech-Language Feedback and Monitoring Mechanisms

Significant changes in children's abilities to monitor their expressive output are also occurring during the period most commonly identified with the onset of stuttering. Some readers might be surprised that I discuss feedback and monitoring within a psycholinguistic context. It is true that these terms have a particular significance and interpretation when motor activity is analyzed. However, for accounts of sentence production, there are clear linguistic constraints on the probable nature and ouput of speech monitoring systems. For example, although speech errors occur infrequently in spontaneous speech, they exhibit a characteristic that reveals a possible strategy used by the language system's internal monitor. Speech errors are almost always phonotactically regular (they follow the phonological rules of the language and could be real words in terms of phonological structure). Moreover, and more strikingly, speech errors are overwhelmingly likely to be acceptable words of the language, albeit the wrong ones (see Fromkin, 1973; Carroll, 1994 for discussion). Consider the case of this famous Spoonerism (its fame partially due to the fact that Reverend Spooner produced it):

"You have hissed all my mystery lectures"

Note that while the [h] and [m] exchange (a very common type of slip), the result is two real English words. This is not an isolated example. Dell and Reich (1981) note that the majority of speech errors result in real words. Given a target sentence such as, "The little girl hugged and kissed her bear," a slip such as "The little girl bugged her hair" is statistically likely, while "The little girl [bIst] her care" is not. There is no reason to expect such an outcome, unless an internal monitor blocks slips that would fail a "language test." In this sense, the internal monitor proposed by Levelt and his colleagues functions in much the same way as a "spell checker" in a word processing program: It will quickly reject "teh" for "the," but will unfortunately approve a phrase such as, "Its (it's) two (too) bad," or "I'd just assume (as soon) do that." That this is likely to be the case is borne out by experimental studies in which subjects are provoked into generating slips through repetitive word-pair readings that function as sophisticated tongue twisters. Such "phonetic bias" techniques

(Baars, Motley, & MacKay, 1975) support the notion that speakers selectively inhibit nonword slip outcomes, while allowing slips that "masquerade as real words" to be produced. These and other behaviors too numerous to discuss here (see Levelt, 1989; Motley, Baars, & Camden, 1983), provide compelling evidence that there is a monitor whose functional criteria include assessing the linguistic integrity of the speaker's output.

When does the internal monitor begin to function in children? The onset of stuttering usually occurs too late to attribute it to the very onset of speech self-awareness, if we accept that some sort of "metalinguistic" awareness governs infant vocal behaviors such as routinized babble, crib speech word plays, or, in fact, the very young child's progressive approximation of adult speech models. Children appear to be listening to themselves at a very early age; however, a fully developed "comparator" system may not underlie such early vocal behaviors. In particular, some aspects of phonological maturation have been accounted for by "dual lexicon" hypotheses, in which the child's perception and production are mediated by separate sets of lexical representations. Dual lexicon accounts explain such time-honored yet confusing child behaviors as regressive idioms (in which production accuracy for an individual word regresses under the acquisition of phonological rules) and the "fis/fish" phenomenon, in which a child rejects adult imitations of the child's speech error as poorly formed, while continuing to produce the error without evident awareness.

The question of when effective speech feedback (on-line self-monitoring and adjustment) evolves in children is problematic. DAF studies, which were common at earlier stages of stuttering research, have also been used to assess the feedback behaviors of young children (Belmore, Kewley-Port, Mobley, & Goodman, 1973; Chase, Sutton, First, & Zubin, 1961; MacKay, 1968; Ratner, Gawronski, & Rice, 1964; Yeni-Komshian, Chase, & Mobley, 1968). The results of these relatively old studies are not entirely clear, probably due to significant differences in study methodology (Belmore et al., 1973). However, Yeni-Komshian et al.

(1968), who used some of the youngest experimental subjects in DAF research, suggest that only children above 2 and 3 years of age typically show speech perturbations under DAF conditions and that the strongest effects are seen in children between 2 and 6 years of age. The evolution of speech monitoring ability may contribute to late onsets of stuttering symptoms, especially if one posits a differential threshold for individual children's attendance to and tolerance of their own speech output. In this respect, the Covert Repair Hypothesis may partially explain the development of stuttering in young children; however, the CRH does not specify whether the internal speech monitor is hyperfunctional or legitimately concerned by speech output that is poorly or incompletely specified. The fact that children with clearly deficient speech (i.e., children with phonetic or phonological disturbance, children with grammatical impairment) often do not show symptoms of stuttering suggests that the well-formedness of output is less important to some children than to others and that children who stutter are, for whatever reason, more likely to "check" their output.

The Growth of Metalinguistic Ability and Stuttering

Metalinguistic ability can be defined in many ways. In this discussion, I wish to center on the child's evolving ability to detect the structure of spoken language, specifically, to understand that the auditory signal contains representations of phonemes, syllables, and words. Furthermore, metalinguistic ability can refer to a child's appreciation of his or her own output as linguistically well-formed. Both of these abilities change significantly during the period associated with the onset of stuttering.

Phonological Segmentation Ability.   Because a defining characteristic of stuttering is within-word disfluency, specifically initial sound and syllable repetitions, it is of interest to note that children under the age of 3 do not appear able to identify that words are composed of individual phonemes. Such ability evolves between 3 and 6 years of age (Fox &

Routh, 1975; Zhurova, 1973). Moreover, 3-year-old children begin to evidence awareness of phonological errors in the speech of others, particularly those that appear in word-initial position (Smith-Lock & Rubin, 1993). It would appear that changes in the operation of the internal monitor should accompany a child's growing appreciation of the internal structure of words, a change that might have ramifications for how a child responds to slow or inaccurate compilation of the phonetic plan.

Speech Repair Behaviors.   Another type of evidence for children's growing sensitivity to the well-formedness of their productions can be found in the evolution of self-repairs, speakers' detection, and attempts to correct fully produced errors or slips. While isolated examples of self-repair have been noted in children as young as 1 year of age (Jaeger, 1992; Scollon, 1976), Jaeger's data show a clear increase in self-repairs by age, with a surprising bell-shaped function of highest phonological repairs between 3 and 4 years of age. Thus, at least in Jaeger's sample of thirty-two children, children were most attentive to errors in their phonological output between these ages.

I am aware of only two studies of the self-repair behaviors of children who stutter. Yaruss and Conture (1994) found no difference in the self-repair rates of stuttering children with and without accompanying phonological disorder. A normally fluent control group was not studied. In a study of normally fluent and stuttering children ages 3 to 11 (M = 8) years of age, Howell, Kadi-Hanifi, and Young (1991) found that one type of self-repair—phrase revisions—was half as frequent in the speech of stuttering children than in the speech of their controls. However, it is difficult to tell whether these data are proportioned for sample size, or whether phrasal errors were made in either group that might have elicited revision, but did not. Phrase-based errors requiring revision are the least frequent type of speech error behavior seen in children (Jaeger, 1992).

The relationship between self-repair and the functions of an internal monitor is not entirely clear, but one can predict that, if the internal monitor hyperfunctions and devotes disproportionate effort to scrutinizing phonetic plans, as predicted by the CRH, then stuttering children should be expected to make fewer speech errors and self-repairs, since both result from lapses in the ability of the internal monitor to reject a deficient phonetic plan.

Dissociation between Levels of Functioning in Children Who Stutter

The issue of potential imbalance between stuttering children's levels of linguistic development and speech motor control has long been a matter of discussion (see Starkweather, 1987). Dissociation between levels of competence across domains of language functioning are fairly typical. For example, children with Expressive Language Impairment or Specific Expressive Language Delay usually demonstrate a profile of normal receptive language capacity, despite their inability to generate age-appropriate language ouput. Dissociations between grammatical and phonological impairment are common as well.

These are not novel notions; however, relevant to the issues discussed in this chapter, one could ask whether self-monitoring, as defined by responses to perturbed speech feedback or self-correction, can be asynchronously mature for a child's level of achievement in other domains. If so, children who stutter might demonstrate atypically attentive self-monitoring that turns normal speech planning problems into stutter behaviors. Such a dissociation between output and "tolerance" would be especially troublesome if the expressive output were deficient grammatically or phonologically because of less mature capacity in these domains, or a child's vulnerability to escalating levels of complexity in them.

SUMMARY

Stuttering occurs during spoken language. Thus, attempts to place stuttering within a language formulation framework appear well-motivated. In this chapter, I have integrated data from a number of disparate sources to show that stuttering, particularly in children, follows linguistically lawful patterns of frequency and location within conversational speech. Such patterns suggest that, in order to fully understand stuttering, we must understand how the normal process of going from "intention to articulation" (Levelt, 1989) is disrupted to produce stuttering behaviors.

Data on the language abilities of individuals who stutter are somewhat equivocal. Obvious differences between stuttering and nonstuttering children and adults are difficult to obtain, although more sophisticated measures may detect nonclinical depression of comprehension and production ability in both children and adults who stutter. More data are needed to resolve this issue, and there is growing awareness that mere administration of standardized assessment devices that were developed to diagnose clinical impairment (e.g., throwing test batteries at subject populations) will probably not provide an adequate answer to the question of comparability of language proficiency in stuttering and nonstuttering individuals.

If data from an array of sources on stuttering loci and frequency patterns are considered as a group, children's stuttering appears more heavily constrained by grammatical and syntactic factors, while adults show a pattern of stuttering locus and frequency that seems to be determined by a combination of linguistic factors and experiential learning (Starkweather, Chapter 4). This area is in significant need of further investigation that examines cross-linguistic commonalities (or differences) in stuttering locus and frequency across languages of varying linguistic typology.

In addition, while children's stuttering may fluctuate as a function of the conversational tempo and style used by their parents, the mechanisms by which such changes in fluency occur are not well-understood and deserve further research attention. In particular, there is need for research into parental speech that goes beyond speech rate and turn-taking and targets specific lexical, syntactic, and pragmatic behaviors that may scaffold or impede children's linguistic performance and fluency.

The onset of stuttering in children is problematic for most theories of stuttering. In this chapter, I have attempted to identify some of the major transitional phenomena in early child language that could seriously impair a child's ability to develop fluent language production capacity. Models of the qualitative changes that occur in children's language development between 2 and 4 years of age differ in their specificity and emphasis, but converge on the notion that early child language is lexically driven, and that children between 2 and 4 years of age must reconfigure the language production process to reflect the primacy of planning the grammar of an intended utterance. Further, the process of lexical acquisition and the deepening of lexical representations also present opportunities for the language production system of a young child to experience fluency failure. Many of the models of this lexical-grammatical "shift" permit specific predictions about the onset and early loci characteristics of stuttering in children.

Last, concurrent with the process of language production, children are experiencing changes in their own abilities to monitor and adjust their speech in the face of erred production or distorted auditory feedback. Possible dissociations between monitoring and language production abilities may explain the onset of stuttering in some children.

The issues of dyadic interactions and stuttering, onset of stuttering relative to the course of language acquisition, and dissociation among language domains in children who stutter also suggest that group profiles are likely to be less informative than detailed examination of individual children and how these children's patterns of performance and development may be combined to yield a coherent picture (Bates, Dale, & Thal, 1995). Because of the limitations of any individual researcher's ability to analyze data from varying theoretical perspectives, it will probably be fruitful for stuttering research to adopt a philosophy of shared data resources such as that recently developed in child language acquisition. The Child Language Data Exchange System (CHILDES) (MacWhinney, 1989, 1995; MacWhinney & Snow, 1990) has enabled great progress in the understanding of language acquisition specifically because a large number of children's records can be analyzed from a variety of theoretical positions to determine which account explains the data more fully. Recent publications in child language attest to the widespread impact that this electronic database and its associated computational capacity has had on the development and defense of accounts of language development and disorder (Sokolov & Snow, 1994; Fletcher & MacWhinney, 1995). Because the incidence of stuttering is relatively low, data pooling for statistical purposes and data reanalysis from alternative theoretical frameworks should further our understanding of the nature of stuttering in children.

REFERENCES

Andrews, G., Craig, A., Feyer, A.-M., Hoddinott, S., Howie, P., & Neilson, M. (1983). Stuttering: A review of research findings and theories circa 1982. *Journal of Speech and Hearing Disorders, 48,* 226–246.

Andrews, G., & Harris, M. (1964). *The syndrome of stuttering.* Clinics in Developmental Medicine, No 17. London: The Spastics Society Medical Education and Information Unit in Association with William Heinemann Medical Books Ltd.

Baars, B., Motley, M., & MacKay, D. (1975). Output editing for lexical status in artificially elicited slips of the tongue. *Journal of Verbal Learning and Verbal Behavior, 14,* 382–391.

Balota, D. & Chumbly, J. (1985). The locus of word-frequency effects in the pronunciation task: Lexical access and/or production? *Journal of Memory and Language, 24,* 89–106.

Bates, E., Dale, P. & Thal, D. (1995). Individual differences and their implications for theories of language development. In P. Fletcher & B. MacWhinney (Eds.), *The handbook of child language* (pp. 96–151). Oxford: Basil Blackwell.

Bates, E., & Devescovi, A. (1989). Crosslinguistic studies of sentence production. In B. MacWhinney & E. Bates (Eds.), *The crosslinguistic study of sentence processing* (pp. 225–253). Cambridge: Cambridge University Press.

Belmore, N., Kewley-Port, D., Mobley, R., & Goodman, V. (1973). The development of auditory feedback monitoring: Delayed auditory feedback studies on the vocalizations of children aged six months to 19 months. *Journal of Speech and Hearing Research, 16,* 709–720.

Bernstein, N.E. (1981). Are there constraints on childhood disfluency? *Journal of Fluency Disorders, 6,* 341–350.

Bernstein Ratner, N. (1992). Measurable outcomes of instructions to modify normal parent-child verbal interactions: Implications for indirect stuttering therapy. *Journal of Speech and Hearing Research, 35,* 14–20.

Bernstein Ratner, N. (1993a). Parents, children, and stuttering. *Seminars in Speech and Language, 14,* 238–250.

Bernstein Ratner, N. (1993b). Atypical language development. In J. Berko Gleason (Ed.), *The development of language* (Third edition) (pp. 325–368). Columbus: Merrill.

Bernstein Ratner, N., & Benitez, M. (1985). Linguistic analysis of a bilingual stutterer. *Journal of Fluency Disorders, 10,* 211–219.

Bernstein Ratner, N., Parker, B., & Gardner, P. (1993). Joint bookreading as a language scaffolding activity for communicatively impaired children. *Seminars in Speech and Language, 14,* 296–313.

Bernstein Ratner, N., & Pye, C. (1984). Higher pitch in BT is not universal: Acoustic evidence from Quiche Mayan. *Journal of Child Language, 11,* 515–522.

Bernstein Ratner, N., & Sih, C.C. (1987). Effects of gradual increases in sentence length and complexity on children's dysfluency. *Journal of Speech and Hearing Disorders, 52,* 278–287.

Bishop, J.H., Williams, H.G., & Cooper, W.A. (1991). Age and task complexity variables in motor performance of children with articulation-disordered, stuttering, and normal speech. *Journal of Fluency Disorders, 16,* 219–228.

Bloodstein, O. (1987). *A handbook on stuttering* (Fourth edition). Chicago: National Easter Seal Society.

Bloodstein, O., & Gantwerk, B.F. (1967). Grammatical function in relation to stuttering in young children. *Journal of Speech and Hearing Research, 10,* 786–789.

Bloodstein, O. & Grossman, M. (1981). Early stutterings: Some aspects of their form and distribution. *Journal of Speech and Hearing Research, 24,* 298–302.

Bock, K., & Levelt, W. (1994). Language production: Grammatical encoding. In M. Gernsbacher (Ed.), *Handbook of psycholinguistics* (pp. 945–978). San Diego, CA: Academic Press.

Bonvillian, J.D., Raeburn, V.P., & Horan, E.A. (1979). Talking to children: The effects of rate, intonation, and length on children's sentence imitation. *Journal of Child Language, 6,* 459–467.

Bosshardt, H-G. (1993). Differences between stutterers' and nonstutterers' short-term recall and recognition performance. *Journal of Speech and Hearing Research, 36,* 286–293.

Bosshardt, H-G. (1994). Temporal coordination between pre-motor and motor processes in speech production. *Journal of Fluency Disorders, 19,* 157 (abs).

Branigan, G. (1979). Some reasons why successive single word utterances are not. *Journal of Child Language, 6,* 411–421.

Broen, P. (1972). The verbal environment of the language learning child. *ASHA Monographs, 17.*

Brown, S. F. (1938a). Stuttering with relation to word accent and word position. *Journal of Abnormal and Social Psychology, 33,* 112–120.

Brown, S.F. (1938b). A further study of stuttering in relation to various speech sounds. *Quarterly Journal of Speech, 24,* 390–397.

Brown, S.F. (1945). The loci of stutterings in the speech sequence. *The Journal of Speech Disorders, 10,* 181–192.

Brundage, S., & Bernstein Ratner, N. (1989). The measurement of stuttering frequency in children's speech. *Journal of Fluency Disorders, 14,* 351–358.

Byrd, K., & Cooper, E.B. (1989). Expressive and receptive language skills in stuttering children. *Journal of Fluency Disorders, 14,* 121–126.

Camarata, S., & Leonard, L. (1986). Young children pronounce object words more accurately than action words. *Journal of Child Language, 13,* 51–65.

Carroll, D. (1994). *Psychology of language* (Second edition). Belmont, CA: Wadsworth.

Carroll, J.B., Davies, P., & Richman, B. (1971). *The American Heritage word frequency book.* Boston: Houghton Mifflin.

Chase, R., Sutton, S., First, D., & Zubin, J. (1961). Developmental study of changes in behavior under delayed auditory feedback. *Journal of Genetic Psychology, 99,* 101–112.

Colburn, N., & Mysak, E.D. (1982a). Developmental disfluency and emerging grammar I. Disfluency characteristics in early syntactic utterances. *Journal of Speech and Hearing Research, 25*, 414–420.

Colburn, N., & Mysak, E.D. (1982b). Developmental disfluency and emerging grammar II. Co-occurrence of disfluency with specified semantic-syntactic structures. *Journal of Speech and Hearing Research, 25*, 421–427.

Condon, W., & Sanders, L. (1974). Neonate movement is synchronized with adult speech: Interactional participation and language acquisition. *Science, 183*, 99–101.

Cooper, W., Soares, C., & Reagan, R. (1985). Planning speech: A picture's word's worth. *Acta Psychologia, 58*, 107–114.

Costello, J.M. (1983). Current behavioral treatments for children. In D. Prins & R.J. Ingham (Eds.), *Treatment of stutterers in early childhood*. San Diego: College-Hill Press.

Costello Ingham, J. (1993). Behavioral treatment of stuttering children. In R. Curlee (Ed.), *Stuttering and related disorders of fluency* (pp. 68–100). New York: Thieme.

Deese, J. (1984). *Thought into speech: The psychology of a language*. Englewood Cliffs, NJ: Prentice-Hall.

Dell, G.S. (1990). Effects of frequency and vocabulary type on phonological speech errors. *Language and Cognitive Processes, 5*, 313–349.

Dell, G.S., & Juliano, C. (1991). Connectionist approaches to the production of words. In H.F.M. Peters, W. Hulstijn, & C.W. Starkweather (Eds.), *Speech motor control and stuttering*. Amsterdam: Elsevier Science Publishers.

Dell, G.S., Juliano, C., & Govindjee, A. (1993). Structure and content in language production: A theory of frame constraints in phonological speech errors. *Cognitive Science, 17*, 149–195.

Dell, G.S., & Reich, P.A. (1981). Stages in sentence production: An analysis of speech error data. *Journal of Verbal Learning and Verbal Behavior, 20*, 611–629.

Dromi, E. (1987). *Early lexical development*. Cambridge: Cambridge University Press.

Elbers, L., & Wijnan, F. (1993). Effort, production skill, and language learning. In C.A. Ferguson, L. Menn, & C. Stoel-Gammon (Eds.), *Phonological development: Models, research, implications*. Timonium, Maryland: York Press.

Embrechts, M., Franken, M.C., Mugge, A., & Peters, H. (1995). *The effect of a fluency enhancing environment on speech and language variables in stuttering children*. In C.W. Starkweather & H. Peters, (Eds.), *Stuttering: Proceedings of the First World Congress on Fluency Disorders* (pp. 185–188). Nijmegen: University Press.

Ferreira, F. (1991). Effects of length and syntactic complexity on initiation times for prepared utterances. *Journal of Memory and Language, 30*, 210–233.

Ferrand, C., Gilbert, H., & Blood, G. (1991). Selected aspects of central processing and vocal motor function in stutterers and nonstutterers. *Journal of Fluency Disorders, 16*, 101–116.

Fletcher, P. & MacWhinney, B. (1995). *The handbook of child language*. Oxford: Basil Blackwell.

Fox, B., & Routh, D.K. (1975). Analyzing spoken language into words, syllables, and phonemes: A developmental study. *Journal of Psycholinguistic Research, 4*, 331–342.

Fromkin, V. (1971). The non-anomalous nature of anomalous utterances. *Language, 47*, 27–52.

Fromkin, V. (Ed.) (1973). *Speech errors as linguistic evidence*. The Hague: Mouton.

Fromkin, V. (1993). Speech production. In J. Berko Gleason & N. Bernstein Ratner (Eds.), *Psycholinguistics* (pp. 272–300). Austin, TX: Harcourt, Brace & Jovanovich.

Gaines, N.D., Runyan, C.M., & Meyers, S.C. (1991). A comparison of young stutterers' fluent versus stuttered utterances on measures of length and complexity. *Journal of Speech and Hearing Research, 34*, 37–42.

Garrett, M. (1975). The analysis of sentence production. In G. Bower (Ed.), *The psychology of learning and motivation. Vol. 9* (pp. 133–177). New York: Academic Press.

Garrett, M. (1991). Disorders of lexical selection. In J.M. Levelt (Ed.), *Lexical access in speech production* (pp. 143–180). Cambridge, MA: Blackwell.

Gleitman, L., & Gleitman, H. (1970). *Phrase and paraphrase: Some innovative uses of language*. New York: Norton.

Goldfield, B.A., & Reznick, J.S. (1990). Early lexical acquisition: Rate, content, and the vocabulary spurt. *Journal of Child Language, 17*, 171–183.

Gordon, P.A. (1991). Language task effects: A comparison of stuttering and nonstuttering children. *Journal of Fluency Disorders, 16*, 275–287.

Gordon, P.A., Luper, H.L., & Peterson, H.A. (1986). The effects of syntactic complexity on the occurrence of disfluencies in 5-year-old nonstutterers. *Journal of Fluency Disorders, 11*, 151–164.

Gropen, J., Pinker, S., Hollander, M., & Goldberg, R. (1991). Syntax and semantics in the acquisition of locative verbs. *Journal of Child Language, 18*, 115–151.

Gropen, J., Pinker, S., Hollander, M., Goldberg, R., & Wilson, R. (1989). The learnability and acquisition of the dative alternation in English. *Language, 65*, 203–257.

Guitar, B., Schaefer, H.K., Donahue-Kilburg, G., & Bond, L. (1992). Parent verbal interactions and speech rate: A case study in stuttering. *Journal of Speech and Hearing Research, 35*, 742–754.

Hatch, E. (1983). *Psycholinguistics: A second language perspective.* New York: Newbury House.

Hejna, R.F. (1955). *A study of the loci of stuttering in spontaneous speech.* Unpublished doctoral dissertation, Northwestern University.

Hirsh-Pasek, K., Golinkoff, R., & Reeves, L. (1993). Words and meaning: From primitives to complex organization. In J. Berko Gleason & N. Bernstein Ratner (Eds.), *Psycholinguistics* (pp. 134–199). Austin, TX: Harcourt, Brace & Jovanovich.

Howell, P., Kadi-Hanifi, K., & Young, K. (1991). Phrase revisions in fluent and stuttering children. In H. Peters, W. Hulstijn, & C.W. Starkweather (Eds.), *Speech motor control and stuttering* (pp. 415–422). New York: Elsevier.

Hubbard, C.P., & Prins, D. (1994). Word familiarity, syllabic stress pattern, and stuttering. *Journal of Speech and Hearing Research, 37*, 564–571.

Jaeger, J.J. (1992). "Not by the chair of my hinny hin hin": Some general properties of slips of the tongue in young children. *Journal of Child Language, 19*, 335–366.

Jasnow, M. & Feldstein, S. (1986). Adult-like temporal characteristics of mother-infant vocal interactions. *Child Development, 57*, 754–761.

Jayaram, M. (1984). Distribution of stuttering in sentences: Relationship to sentence length and clause position. *Journal of Speech and Hearing Research, 27*, 329–338.

Jescheniak, J.D., & Levelt, W.J.M. (1994). Word frequency effects in speech production: Retrieval of syntactic information and of phonological form. *Journal of Experimental Psychology: Learning, Memory, and Cognition, 20*, 824–843.

Johnson, W., & Brown, S.F. (1935). Stuttering in relation to various speech sounds. *Quarterly Journal of Speech, 21*, 481–496.

Kadi-Hanifi, K., & Howell, P. (1992). Syntactic analysis of the spontaneous speech of normally fluent and stuttering children. *Journal of Fluency Disorders, 17*, 151–170.

Kamhi, A.G., Catts, H.W., & Davis, M.K. (1984). Management of sentence production demands. *Journal of Speech and Hearing Research, 27*, 329–338.

Kelly, E. (1993). Speech rates and turn-taking behaviors of children who stutter and their parents. *Seminars in Speech and Language, 14*, 203–214.

Kelly, E.M., & Conture, E.G. (1992). Speaking rates, response time latencies, and interrupting behaviors of young stutterers, nonstutterers, and their mothers. *Journal of Speech and Hearing Research, 35*, 1256–1267.

Kolk, H. (1991). Is stuttering a symptom of adaptation or of impairment? In H.F.M. Peters, W. Hulstijn, & C.W. Starkweather (Eds.), *Speech motor control and stuttering.* Amsterdam: Elsevier Science Publishers.

Kutas, M., & Van Petten, C.K. (1994). Psycholinguistics electrified. In M. Gernsbacher (Ed.), *Handbook of psycholinguistics* (pp. 83–143). San Diego, CA: Academic Press.

LaSalle, L., & Carpenter, L. (1994). The effect of phonological simplification on children's fluency. Presentation at American Speech Language Hearing Association Convention, New Orleans.

Lee, L. (1974). *Developmental sentence analysis.* Evanston, IL: Northwestern University Press.

Leonard, L. (1995). Phonological impairment. In P. Fletcher & B. MacWhinney (Eds.), *Handbook of child language* (pp. 573–602). Oxford: Blackwell.

Levelt, W.J.M. (1989). *Speaking: From intention to articulation.* Cambridge, MA: MIT Press.

Levelt, W.J.M. (1992). Accessing words in speech production: Stages, processes and representations. *Cognition, 42*, 1–22.

Lindsley, J. (1975). Producing simple utterances: How far ahead do we plan? *Cognitive Psychology, 7*, 1–19.

Lindsley, J. (1976). Producing simple utterances: Details of the planning process. *Journal of Psycholinguistic Research, 5*, 331–353.

Locke, J. (1993). *The child's path to spoken language.* Cambridge, MA: Harvard University Press.

Logan, K., & Conture, E.G. (1995) Length, grammatical complexity, and rate differences in stuttered and fluent conversational utterances of children who stutter. *Journal of Fluency Disorders, 20,* 35–62.

Louko, L.J., Edwards, M.L., & Conture, E.G. (1990). Phonological characteristics of young stutterers and their normally fluent peers: Preliminary observations. *Journal of Fluency Disorders, 15,* 191–210.

MacKay, D.G. (1968). Metamorphosis of a critical interval: Age-linked changes in the delay in auditory feedback that produces maximal disruption of speech. *The Journal of the Acoustic Society of America, 43,* 811–821.

MacKay, D.G. (1972). The structure of words and syllables: Evidence from errors in speech. *Cognitive Psychology, 3,* 210–227.

Maclay, H., & Osgood, C.E. (1959). Hesitation phonomena in spontaneous English speech. *Word, 15,* 19–44.

MacWhinney, B. (1991). *The CHILDES Project: Tools for analyzing talk.* Hillsdale, NJ: Erlbaum.

MacWhinney, B. (1995). *The CHILDES Project* (Second edition). Hillsdale, NJ: Erlbaum

MacWhinney, B., & Bates, E. (1989). *The cross-linguistic study of sentence processing.* Cambridge: Cambridge University Press.

MacWhinney, B., & Osser, H. (1977). Verbal planning functions in children's speech. *Child Development, 48,* 978–985.

MacWhinney, B., & Snow, C. (1990). The child language data exchange system: An update. *Journal of Child Language, 17,* 457–472.

Marchinkoski, L., & Guitar, B. (1993). When mothers speak more slowly. Paper presented at American Speech-Language-Hearing Association annual convention, Anaheim.

Marslen-Wilson, W., & Tyler, L. (1980). The temporal structure of spoken language understanding. *Cognition, 8,* 1–71.

Marslen-Wilson, W., & Tyler, L. (1981). Central processes in speech understanding. *Philosophical Transactions of the Royal Society of London, B 295,* 317–332.

Meyer, A. (1991). Investigation of phonological encoding through speech error analyses: achievements, limitations and alternatives. In W. Levelt (Ed.), *Lexical access in speech production* (pp. 181–212). Cambridge, MA: Basil Blackwell.

Miller, J. (Ed.) (1991). *Research on child language disorders: A decade of progress.* Austin, TX: Pro-Ed.

Motley, M.T., Baars, B.J., & Camden, C.T. (1983). Experimental verbal slips studies: A review and an editing model of language encoding. *Communication Monographs, 50,* 79–101.

Murray, H.L., & Reed, C.G. (1977). Language abilities of preschool stuttering children. *Journal of Fluency Disorders, 2,* 171–176.

Neilson, M., & Neilson, P. (1987). Speech motor control and stuttering: A computational model of adaptive sensory-motor processing. *Speech Communication, 6,* 325–333.

Nelson, K. (1973). Structure and strategy in learning to talk. *Monograph of the Society for Research in Child Development, 38,* No. 149.

Nelson, L.K., & Kamhi, A.G. (1985). Discourse information as a factor in preschool children's sentence production. Paper presented at the meeting of the Society for Research in Child Development, Toronto, Canada, April.

Newman L., & Smith, A. (1989). Some effects of variations in response time latency on speech rate, interruptions and fluency in children's speech. *Journal of Speech and Hearing Research, 32,* 635–644.

Nippold, M.A. (1990). Concomitant speech and language disorders in stuttering children: A critique of the literature. *Journal of Speech and Hearing Disorders, 55,* 51–60.

Nippold, M.A., & Schwarz, I.E. (1990). Reading disorders in stuttering children. *Journal of Fluency Disorders, 15,* 175–189.

Nippold, M.A., Schwarz, I.E., & Jescheniak, J. (1991). Narrative ability in school-age stuttering boys: A preliminary investigation. *Journal of Fluency Disorders, 16,* 289–308.

Obler, L. (1993). Language beyond childhood. In J. Berko Gleason (Ed.), *The development of language* (Third edition) (pp. 421–450). Columbus: Merrill.

Ochs, E., & Schieffelin, B. (1995). The impact of language socialization on grammatical development. In P. Fletcher & B. MacWhinney (Eds.), *The handbook of child language* (pp. 73–94). Oxford: Basil Blackwell.

O'Connell, D., & Weise, R. (1987). The state of the art: the fate of the start. In H. Dechart & M. Raupach (Eds.), *Psycholinguistic models of production* (pp. 3–16). Norwood, NJ: Ablex.

Oldfield, R., & Wingfield, A. (1962). Response latencies in naming objects. *Quarterly Journal of Experimental Psychology, 17,* 273–281.

Palen, C., & Peterson, J.M. (1982). Word frequency and children's stuttering: The relationship to sentence structure. *Journal of Fluency Disorders, 7,* 55–62.

Panagos, J., Quine, M., & Klich, R. (1979). Syntactic and phonological influences on children's articulation. *Journal of Speech and Hearing Research, 22,* 841–848.

Perkins, W., Kent, R.D., & Curlee, R.F. (1991). A theory of neurolinguistic function in stuttering. *Journal of Speech and Hearing Research, 34,* 734–752.

Peters, T., & Guitar, B. (1991). *Stuttering: An integrated approach to its nature and treatment.* Baltimore: Williams & Wilkins.

Plunkett, K. (1993). Lexical segmentation and vocabulary growth in early language acquisition. *Journal of Child Language, 20,* 43–60.

Quarrington, B. (1963). Stuttering as a function of the information value and sentence position of words. *Journal of Abnormal Psychology, 70,* 221–224.

Radford, A. (1995). Phrase structure and functional categories. In P. Fletcher & B. MacWhinney (Eds.), *The handbook of child language* (pp. 483–507). Oxford: Basil Blackwell.

Ratner, S., Gawronski, J., & Rice, F. (1964). The variable of concurrent action in the language of children: Effects of delayed speech feedback. *Psychological Record, 14,* 47–56.

Rescorla, L. (1989). The language development survey: A screening tool for delayed language in toddlers. *Journal of Speech and Hearing Disorders, 54,* 587–599.

Rollins, P., & Snow, C. (1994). Determinants of mean length of utterance. Paper presented at American Speech-Language-Hearing Association annual convention, New Orleans.

Ronson, I. (1976). Word frequency and stuttering: The relationship to sentence structure. *Journal of Speech and Hearing Research, 19,* 813–819.

Ryan, B. (1979). Stuttering therapy in a framework of operant conditioning and programmed learning. In H.H. Gregory (Ed.), *Controversies about stuttering therapy.* Baltimore: University Park Press.

Ryan, B.P. (1992). Articulation, language, rate and fluency characteristics of stuttering and nonstuttering preschool children. *Journal of Speech and Hearing Research, 35,* 333–342.

Savelkoul, E.M., Zebrowski, P.M., & Buizer, A. (1993). *Reduced maternal speech rate and stuttering.* Unpublished manuscript.

Schwartz, H., & Conture, E. (1988). Subgrouping young stutterers: Preliminary behavioral observations. *Journal of Speech and Hearing Research, 31,* 62–71.

Schwartz, R. (1988). Phonological factors in early lexical acquisition. In M. Smith & J. Locke (Eds.), *The emergent lexicon: The child's development of a linguistic vocabulary* (pp. 185–224). New York: Academic.

Scollon, R. (1976). *Conversations with a one-year old.* Honolulu, HI: University Press of Hawaii.

Shallice, T. & Butterworth, B. (1977). Short-term memory impairment and spontaneous speech. *Neuropsychologia, 15,* 729–735.

Shattuck-Hufnagel, S. (1987). The role of word-onset consonants in speech production planning: New evidence from speech error patterns. In E. Keller and M. Gopnik (Eds.), *Motor and sensory processes of language.* Hillsdale, NJ: Lawrence Erlbaum Associates.

Silverman, F.H. (1972). Disfluency and word length. *Journal of Speech and Hearing Research, 15,* 788–791.

Silverman, F.H., & Williams, D.E. (1967a). Loci of disfluencies in the speech of stutterers. *Perceptual and Motor Skills, 24,* 1085–1086.

Silverman, F.H., & Williams, D.E. (1967b). Loci of disfluencies in the speech of nonstutterers during oral reading. *Journal of Speech and Hearing Research, 10,* 790–794.

Slobin, D. (1985a). *The cross-linguistic study of language acquisition. Volume 1: The data.* Hillsdale, NJ: Erlbaum.

Slobin, D. (1985b). *The cross-linguistic study of language acquisition. Volume 2: Theoretical issues.* Hillsdale, NJ: Earlbaum.

Slobin, D. (1992). *The cross-linguistic study of language acquisition . Volume 3.* Hillsdale, NJ: Earlbaum.

Smith-Lock, K., & Rubin, H. (1993). Phonological and morphological analysis skills in young children. *Journal of Child Language, 20,* 437–454.

Snow, C., Perlmann, R., & Nathan, D. (1987). Why routines are different: Toward a multiple factors model of the relation between input and language acquisition. In K. Nelson & A. van Kleeck (Eds.), *Children's language, Volume 6.* Hillsdale, NJ: Lawrence Erlbaum.

Soderberg, G.A. (1966). The relations of stuttering to word length and word frequency. *Journal of Speech and Hearing Research, 9,* 584–589.

Soderberg, G.A. (1967). Linguistic factors in stuttering.

Journal of Speech and Hearing Research, 10, 801–810.

Soderberg, G.A. (1971). Relations of word information and word length to stuttering disfluencies. *Journal of Communication Disorders, 4,* 9–14.

Sokolov, J., & Snow, C. (1994). *Handbook of research in language development using CHILDES.* Hillsdale, NJ: Erlbaum.

St. Louis, K., & Hinzman, A. (1988). A descriptive study of speech, language and hearing characteristics of school-aged stutterers. *Journal of Fluency Disorders, 13,* 331–355.

Starkweather, C.W. (1987). *Fluency and stuttering.* Englewood Cliffs, NJ: Prentice-Hall.

Starkweather, C.W., Gottwald, C., & Halfond, M (1990). *Stuttering prevention: A clinical method.* Englewood Cliffs, NJ: Prentice Hall.

Starkweather, C.W., Gottwald, C., Kaloustian, H., & Ridener, C. (1984). Parents' rate and children's fluency. Paper presented at annual American Speech-Language-Hearing Association Convention, San Francisco.

Stemberger, J.P. (1989). Speech errors in early child language production. *Journal of Memory and Language, 28,* 164–188.

Stemberger, J.P., & MacWhinney, B. (1986). Frequency and the lexical storage of regularly inflected forms. *Memory and Cognition, 14,* 17–26.

Stephenson-Opsal, D., & Bernstein Ratner, N. (1988). Maternal speech rate modification and childhood stuttering. *Journal of Fluency Disorders, 13,* 49–56.

Strand, E.A. (1992). The integration of speech motor control and language formulation in process models of acquisition. In R.S. Chapman (Ed.), *Processes in language acquisition and disorders.* St. Louis: Mosby–Year Book.

Streim, N.W., & Chapman, R.S. (1987). The effects of discourse support on the organization and production of children's utterances. *Applied Psycholinguistics, 8,* 55–66.

Taylor, I.K. (1966a). What words are stuttered? *Psychological Bulletin, 65,* 233–242.

Taylor, I.K. (1966b). The properties of stuttered words. *Verbal Learning and Verbal Behavior, 5,* 112–118.

Throneberg, R., Yairi, E., & Paden, E. (1994). Relation between phonologic difficulty and the occurrence of disfluencies in the early stage of stuttering. *Journal of Speech and Hearing Research, 37,* 504–509.

Wall, M. (1977). The location of stuttering in the spontaneous speech of young child stutterers. Unpublished doctoral dissertation, City University of New York.

Wall, M.J. (1980). A comparison of syntax in young stutterers and nonstutterers. *Journal of Fluency Disorders, 5,* 345–352.

Wall, M.J., Starkweather, C.W., & Cairns, H.S. (1981). Syntactic influences on stuttering in young child stutterers. *Journal of Fluency Disorders, 6,* 283–298.

Wanner, E., & Gleitman, L. (1982). *Language acquisition: The state of the art.* Cambridge: Cambridge University Press.

Watson, B.C., Freeman, F.J., Chapman, S.B., Miller, S., Finitzo, T., Pool, K.D., & DeVous, M.D. (1991). Linguistic performance deficits in stutterers: Relation to laryngeal reaction time profiles. *Journal of Fluency Disorders, 16,* 85–100.

Watson, B.C., Freeman, F.J., DeVous, M.D., Chapman, S.B. Finitzo, T., & Pool, K.D. (1994). Linguistic performance and regional cerebral blood flow in persons who stutter. *Journal of Speech and Hearing Research, 37,* 1221–1228.

Weiner, E., & Labov, W. (1983). Contraints on the agentless passive. *Journal of Linguistics, 19,* 29–58.

Weiss, A. (1993). The pragmatic context of children's disfluency. *Seminars in Speech and Language, 14,* 215–226.

Weiss, A.L., & Zebrowski, P.M. (1991). Patterns of assertiveness and responsiveness in parental interactions with stuttering and fluent children. *Journal of Fluency Disorders, 16,* 125–141.

Weiss, A.L., & Zebrowski, P.M. (1992). Disfluencies in the conversations of young children who stutter: Some answers about questions. *Journal of Speech and Hearing Research, 35,* 1230–1238.

Welkowitz, J., Bond, R., Feldman, L., & Tota, M. (1990). Conversational time patterns and mutual influence in parent-child interaction. *Journal of Psycholinguistic Research, 19,* 221–243.

Westby, C.E. (1979). Language performance of stuttering and nonstuttering children. *Journal of Communication Disorders, 12,* 133–145.

Wijnan, F. (1990). The development of sentence planning. *Journal of Child Language, 17,* 651–675.

Wingate, M.E. (1967). Stuttering and word length. *Journal of Speech and Hearing Research, 10,* 146–152.

Wingate, M.E. (1976). *Stuttering: Theory and treatment*. New York: Irvington.

Wingate, M.E. (1988). *The structure of stuttering: A psycholinguistic analysis*. New York: Springer-Verlag.

Yairi, E. (1983). The onset of stuttering in two- and three-year-old children: A preliminary report. *Journal of Speech and Hearing Disorders, 48,* 171–177.

Yairi, E., & Ambrose, N. (1992a). A longitudinal study of stuttering in children: A preliminary report. *Journal of Speech and Hearing Research, 35,* 755–760.

Yairi, E., & Ambrose, N. (1992b). Onset of stuttering in preschool children: Selected factors. *Journal of Speech and Hearing Research, 35,* 782–788.

Yairi, E., Paden, E., Ambrose, N., & Throneburg, R. (1994). Pathways of chronicity and recovery: Longitudinal studies of early childhood stuttering. Presentation at American Speech-Language-Hearing Association annual convention, New Orleans.

Yaruss, S., & Conture, E. (1994). Stuttering and phonological disorders in children: Examination of the Covert Repair Hypothesis. Manuscript in review.

Yeni-Komshian, G., Chase, R.A., & Mobley, R.L. (1968). The development of auditory feedback monitoring: II. Delayed auditory feedback studies on the speech of children between two and three years of age. *Journal of Speech and Hearing Research, 11,* 301–306.

Zhurova, L.Y. (1973). The development of analysis of words into their sounds by preschool children. In C. Ferguson & D. Slobin (Eds.), *Studies of child language development* (pp. 141–154). New York: Holt, Rinehart & Winston.

SUGGESTED READINGS

Bernstein Ratner, Nan (Ed.) (1993). Stuttering and parent-child interaction. *Seminars in Speech and Language, 14.* This volume contains articles that examine pragmatic and discourse factors in childhood stuttering.

Fletcher, P. & MacWhinney, B. (1995). *The handbook of child language.* Cambridge: Basil Blackwell. This edited volume brings together current perspectives on the development of communicative ability in children; a number of its contributed articles are used in this chapter to develop hypotheses about possible factors in the development of stuttering.

Gernsbacher, M.A. (1994). *Handbook of psycholinguistics.* San Diego, CA: Academic Press. This edited volume is a broad and detailed compendium of current work in the psychology of language, including current models of the speech production process.

Wingate, M. (1988). *The structure of stuttering: A psycholinguistic analysis.* New York: Springer-Verlag. This unique book thoroughly evaluates linguistic analyses of stuttering and develops a model of the underlying deficit that leads to stuttering. Its particular strengths include its critiques of past study designs, thorough scope, and the integration of research into the proposed model.

CHAPTER 6

RESPIRATORY AND LARYNGEAL CONTROL IN STUTTERING

MARGARET DENNY
ANNE SMITH

INTRODUCTION

The purpose of this chapter is to review respiratory and laryngeal function in stuttering. These two systems are being reviewed together in one chapter because, as is well known, the phonatory and respiratory systems must be closely coordinated to produce acceptable speech. The idea that a discoordination of these systems may be an important feature of stuttering is a familiar one (e.g., Perkins, Rudas, Johnson, & Bell, 1976). This chapter draws on recent research in normal respiratory physiology to show that there are other compelling reasons to consider these two systems simultaneously.

Although we emphasize the close cooperation among systems, it is intuitively reasonable to partition speech production into three major tasks: generation of an airstream (the power supply), which is the functional role of the chest wall; phonatory valving of that airstream, accomplished by the larynx; and filtering of the laryngeal output plus addition of sounds such as frication, as accomplished by the articulators. In this partitioning, respiration may be assigned to the chest wall, and phonation to the larynx. Although this partitioning serves well for consideration of the normally functioning system, it may be less useful when speech motor control breaks down, or is inadequate, for reasons discussed below.

One striking aspect of the control and coordination of the neuromuscular systems that produce speech has received relatively little attention from theorists of speech production. This is the fact that virtually all of the motoneuron pools[1] that are active in speech production also at times receive controlling inputs from other neural sources concerned with the regulation of quite different behaviors. Normal speakers are able to manage the relationships among different neural controllers, but in disordered speakers, including those who stutter, the normal processes by which respiratory, emotional-vocal, and speech motor control are integrated may be impaired. Neural centers that should be responding to inputs related to phonatory or articulatory aspects of speech may also be receiving competing inputs from the neural circuitry that regulates metabolic breathing, emotional vocalization, or both.

TWO DISTINCT NEURAL CENTERS THAT MAY PROVIDE COMPETING INPUTS TO SPEECH MOTOR PROCESSES

The neural circuitry that constitutes the dominant controller for normal speech production includes areas of the cerebral cortex and other components of the voluntary motor system. Here we will briefly introduce two other neural controllers that may provide inputs to speech muscle systems, and explain why we consider that their output could potentially be disruptive to speech.

---

[1]The cell bodies of the motoneurons that supply a given muscle lie together in the brainstem or the spinal cord and are collectively known as a motoneuron pool.

The metabolic respiratory controller: The neural centers essential for the generation of the basic respiratory rhythm are located in the brainstem. We will use the term "metabolic controller" to designate this system. The metabolic controller integrates a great deal of information: It is responsive to variations in wakefulness, emotional state, posture, and variations in blood gases sensed by central and peripheral chemoreceptors. It receives information from sensory receptors throughout the airway; these include muscle spindles, Golgi tendon organs, joint receptors, pulmonary stretch receptors, and laryngeal receptors sensitive to flow, temperature, and pressure. Respiratory pattern is continuously adjusted for variations in these variables, and a multitude of automatic responses such as coughing and gagging protect us from challenges to respiratory function (for review, see Bartlett, 1986; Feldman, 1986).

Because the functional requirements of speech production are in many ways quite different from those of breathing for life support, it is reasonable to hypothesize that the dominant locus of neural control must shift from the metabolic respiratory controller to the speech controller when one prepares to speak. There is substantial experimental confirmation that this does occur in normal speakers. The respiratory pattern changes with respect to the typical ranges of lung volumes employed, and the timing of both phases of the respiratory cycle (Hixon, 1987; Winkworth, Davis, Adams, & Ellis, 1995; Winkworth, Davis, Ellis, & Adams, 1994); inspirations are timed to occur at major linguistic boundaries (Goldman-Eisler, 1968); blood gases are altered after a period of reading, indicating that speakers tend to hyperventilate (Bunn & Mead, 1971). During quiet resting breathing, even small increases in carbon dioxide (CO_2) are a powerful stimulus to increase the volume and frequency of breathing. However, this response to CO_2 is dramatically reduced when subjects are reading aloud (Phillipson, McClean, Sullivan, & Zamel, 1978). This suggests that the speech controller is to some extent able to "ignore" or suppress the metabolic controller's responses to deviations from normal blood gas values. Certain features of respiratory-related EMGs, believed to be indicators of participation by the metabolic respiratory controller, are typically reduced during reading (Smith & Denny, 1990).

Emotional vocalization and the periaqueductal gray matter (PAG): This neural controller is located in the midbrain and is essential for the coordination of a variety of emotional responses, including vocalization (Depaulis & Bandler, 1991). In experimental animals, stimulation of the appropriate area within the PAG produces strongly and consistently patterned motor programs that effectively "take over" muscles of the chest wall, larynx, and face (e.g., Davis, Zhang, & Bandler, 1993; Depaulis & Bandler, 1991; Larson, 1991; Zhang, Davis, Bandler, & Carrive, 1994). It is likely that the PAG contributes strongly to emotional vocalizations, such as laughing and crying, in humans. It is not known whether the PAG is normally active only during states of strong emotional arousal, or whether it contributes inputs modulated by a broader range of emotional states. At present, little is known about whether or how much the PAG contributes to speech in normal humans (for interesting discussion, see Davis & Zhang, 1991; Zhang et al., 1994). For example, we do not know whether the normal modulation of speech that contributes information about emotional state is mediated in part by the PAG.

Figure 6.1 gives a schematic overview of the control systems that we have discussed. It illustrates the three controllers with their access to the motoneuron pools that are active in speech, and shows that both the speech controller and the PAG are capable of affecting the metabolic controller. The dashed arrows and question marks emphasize the limits of our knowledge about the interactions of these systems. We do not know whether, or to what extent, the PAG may influence, or be influenced by, the speech controller. In addition, we have little precise knowledge of the interaction between the speech and metabolic respiratory controllers; this is symbolized by the question mark at the junction

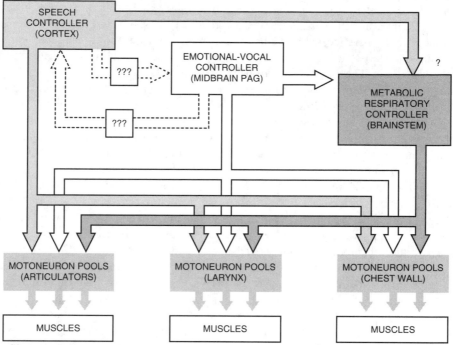

Figure 6.1 This is a schematic diagram of three neural controllers, all having access to the same group of muscles. Dashed arrows and question marks indicate relationships among controllers that are not well understood.

of these two systems. For example, we do not know whether the speech controller simply suppresses the output of the metabolic respiratory controller or whether the interaction is more complex.

The metabolic respiratory controller is especially attractive as a candidate for a source of disruptive inputs during stuttering because:

1. It has broadly distributed outputs that overlap considerably with the outputs that control speech production. It is thus well suited to produce disturbances at any or all levels of the system, as seen in stuttering.

2. It is exquisitely responsive to changes in state, mood, and arousal generated at many levels of the central nervous system (for review see Hugelin, 1986). Emotional state contributes to the variability of speech breathing in normal subjects (Winkworth et al., 1995), and high autonomic arousal is associated with in-creases in both frequency and severity of stuttering (Peters & Hulstijn, 1984; Weber & Smith, 1990).

3. The metabolic controller is always active, and is thus "available" to contribute destabilizing inputs at any time.

The potential importance of the PAG for stuttering is that, like the metabolic respiratory controller, it can influence the entire speech musculature. Second, it is essential for the organization of emotional expression; the significance of this was reviewed in the previous paragraph. The possibility that the PAG may contribute disruptive inputs to motoneuron pools in disordered speakers remains to be studied.

To summarize, the hypothesis we wish to examine is this: During normal speech, there is a reduction of inputs to motoneuron pools that originate from the brainstem circuitry responsible for metabolic (life support) breathing and/or the

PAG, which is active for emotional vocalization. Respiratory and laryngeal function is taken over and managed primarily by the speech controller. In contrast, in individuals who stutter, the metabolic and emotional-vocal centers, for a variety of reasons, may compete with the speech control system. The interaction and competition of these control systems may be a source of instability in speech motor output for individuals who stutter. Because so little is presently known of the role of the PAG in normal or disordered speech production, we will elaborate this hypothesis with respect to the metabolic respiratory controller.

We will begin with a brief review of the respiratory functions of the upper airway (i.e., the larynx and vocal tract) to illustrate that respiratory control is a potentially potent factor affecting the entire speech musculature. We will then point out the ways in which fluent and disfluent speech constitute potential challenges to the metabolic respiratory controller; review findings that suggest voluntary control of respiration may be aberrant in some individuals who stutter; and review recent work in laryngeal control in normal and stuttering subjects. We will argue that consideration of respiratory control is very important in understanding stuttering; that the investigation of its potential importance needs to be framed in terms that extend beyond consideration of chest wall movements; and that it may well be useful to consider respiratory influences on the larynx when theorizing about stuttering.

Like all of our work in stuttering, the viewpoint offered here derives from a multifactorial, dynamic model of stuttering. This has been extensively defined elsewhere (Smith, 1990; Smith & Weber, 1988; Smith & Kelly, Chapter 10), so we will only briefly outline its major features here. Many factors at many levels (e.g., genetic, linguistic, physiological, psychosocial) contribute to the development and maintenance of stuttering. The relative importance of these factors may vary from one stuttering individual to the next. An important challenge, then, is to discover which factors are most important in which stuttering speakers, both for understanding the nature of the disorder and for designing more effective treatment strategies.

In context of this multifactorial model, we hope it will be obvious that to assert that it is important to explore respiratory/laryngeal control in no way asserts or even implies that "respiration is the cause of stuttering," or that inadequate coordination of respiratory or emotional-vocal control plays a role in all individuals who stutter. Rather, difficulties with respiratory and emotional-vocal control are offered as likely candidates for factors that may be influential in a clinically significant number of stuttering speakers.

Another question we have frequently encountered in this context is whether aberrant respiratory behaviors cause stuttering, or stuttering causes the aberrant respiratory behaviors. We suggest that treating these as opposing alternatives is unnecessary and distracting. We believe that it will be more productive to inquire into the hypothesis that individuals who stutter may have difficulties in general voluntary or speech-related control of the respiratory system; that the aerodynamic and ventilatory requirements of speech may be particularly challenging to this already vulnerable system; and that once speech breaks down, the form of the breakdown may exacerbate the control problems even further.

RESPIRATORY INFLUENCES ON THE UPPER AIRWAY

A striking feature of stuttering is that it can affect any or all of the speech muscle systems. Recent work in our laboratory has indicated that some concomitants of stuttering, such as high-amplitude tremor, can occur simultaneously across speech subsystems (e.g., muscles of the larynx and the lip) (Denny & Smith, 1992; Smith, 1989; Smith, Denny, & Wood, 1991; Smith, Luschei, Denny, Wood, Hirano, & Badylak, 1993). This observation motivated us to search for neural controllers that have similar widely distributed outputs, and that might be activated during speech. The following review demonstrates the widespread, powerful influence of the metabolic respiratory controller on all speech subsystems.

Much recent research in respiratory physiology has focused on the role of the upper airway musculature in maintaining a patent airway as well as finely regulating airway resistance. A number of excellent reviews of this literature have been published (Bartlett, 1986; Mathew & Sant'Ambrogio, 1988). What follows here will be relatively brief and focused on work most relevant to speech production.

Inspiratory expansion of the lungs and thorax creates negative (collapsing) pressures in the upper airways that are normally opposed by muscular effort (Brouillette & Thach, 1979; Remmers, de Groot, Sauerland, & Anch, 1978; Schwab, Gefter, Pack, & Hoffman, 1993). In experimental animals, phasic inspiratory activity has been recorded in airway dilating muscles of the larynx, pharynx, tongue, and velum during quiet breathing (Rothstein, Narce, de Berry-Borowiecki, & Blanks, 1983). In human subjects, inspiratory-related EMG activity has been recorded from the genioglossus, which dilates the airway by depressing and protruding the tongue (Sauerland & Harper, 1976; Sauerland & Mitchell, 1970, 1975); tensor veli palatini and mylohyoid (Hairston & Sauerland, 1981); levator palatini and palatoglossus (Tangel, Mezzanote, & White, 1995); and pharyngeal dilators (Hill, Guilleminault, & Simmons, 1978).

On quiet expiration, the laryngeal dilator, posterior cricoarytenoid (PCA), is less active than during inspiration, resulting in a narrower laryngeal aperture. Thus, the vocal folds move with each respiratory cycle; they are widely abducted for inspiration and somewhat less abducted in expiration (e.g., Bartlett, Remmers, & Gautier, 1973; Green & Neil, 1955). These respiratory-related movements may involve abductor, adductor, and tensor muscles of the larynx in humans (Brancatisano, Dodd, & Engel, 1984; Insalaco, Kuna, Cibella, & Villeponteaux, 1990; Kuna, Day, Insalaco, & Villeponteaux, 1991; Kuna, Insalaco, & Woodson, 1988; Kuna, Smickley, & Insalaco, 1990; Wheatley, Brancatisano, & Engel, 1991). However, there appears to be considerable inter-subject variability in the pattern and extent of activation, and some investigators have reported seeing little or no respiratory-related activity in human laryngeal muscles (Chanaud & Ludlow, 1992; Smith, Denny, Shaffer-Westwood, & Hirano, 1995).

In short, resting breathing is associated with a continuously modulated stream of motor inputs from the metabolic respiratory controller to many muscles involved in speech. The metabolic respiratory controller is also highly effective in defending respiration against a variety of challenges. This has strong implications for the study of speech production because speech may be thought of as a set of self-imposed challenges to the respiratory system as it functions in its life support mode. Two common self-imposed perturbations associated with speech are stopping of expiratory airflow, as in stop consonant production, and imposing a sudden high resistance to airflow, as in frication. The response of the metabolic respiratory controller to this type of perturbation can have significant consequences for respiratory control that are interesting in light of the demands of speech production.

Zhou et al. (Zhou, Denny, Bachir, & Daubenspeck, 1995) imposed small but detectable resistance loads (3 cm H_2O/LPS) on single inspirations or expirations in naive normal subjects (an example of a high resistance load is breathing through a straw; a load of 3 cm H_2O/LPS feels like breathing through slightly pursed lips). Glottal area was estimated noninvasively using an acoustic reflection technique (Zhou & Daubenspeck, 1995). When the load was imposed during inspiration, subjects responded by dilating their glottal apertures. That is, they compensated for an imposed restriction of airflow by opening up their own airways at the level of the larynx. However, imposing the same resistive load on expiration elicited a surprising result: The laryngeal aperture narrowed, further *increasing* airway resistance. Thus, it appears that during quiet breathing, when the metabolic controller is the dominant locus of respiratory control, the type of obstruction that speech imposes for consonant production elicits a motor command to adduct the vocal folds. If not suppressed, such a command could easily be disruptive to speech production.

RESPIRATORY PERTURBATION IN STUTTERING

It may be that some of the known overt manifestations of stuttering, in and of themselves, perturb respiratory control. The metabolic respiratory controller acts to maintain aerodynamic variables within preferred ranges at all levels of the airway, and compensates for perturbations to the target levels (for review, see Milic-Emili & Zin, 1986). Failure of stuttering subjects to control both subglottal and transdiaphragmatic pressure during disfluent speech has been reported by Zocchi, Estenne, Johnston, del Ferro, Ward, and Macklem (1990). These investigators used esophageal and gastric balloons to estimate subglottal and transdiaphragmatic pressures during severely disfluent speech in ten stuttering subjects. While both of these pressures were maintained at relatively constant levels during fluent speech in normal subjects, they fluctuated dramatically and unpredictably during stuttered speech.

Even perceptually fluent speech in stuttering subjects may be problematic for an unstable control system. There is evidence that stuttering subjects, compared to normals, initiate voicing more abruptly (which may be in part due to use of higher subglottal air pressure) and generate higher intraoral air pressures during perceptually fluent (Adams, 1974; Agnello, 1975) and stuttered speech (Hutchinson & Navarre, 1977).

Instabilities in control of respiratory-related pressures have even been demonstrated to occur before the onset of perceptually fluent speech. Peters and colleagues (Peters & Boves, 1988; Peters, Hietkamp, & Boves, 1993) studied the buildup of subglottal pressure (P_{SG}) prior to perceptually fluent speech production in normal and stuttering subjects. Patterns of P_{SG} buildup successfully differentiated the two groups. Normal speakers tend-

ed to use smooth, monotonic patterns of P_{SG} buildup, with phonation initiated at or near maximum pressure. In contrast, the stuttering subjects frequently employed patterns that were rarely seen in normals. These included a normal smooth buildup of pressure, but a delayed onset of phonation; non-monotonic patterns of pressure buildup; and initial excessive P_{SG} buildup that dropped noticeably before phonation began. Unusual patterns of P_{SG} buildup preceded both fluent and disfluent speech, but disfluent speech was associated with more frequent and severe departures from the normal patterns.

Lung volume is another variable that is closely regulated by the metabolic respiratory controller. Johnston, Watkin, and Macklem (1993) have reported that four stuttering subjects employed highly unusual ranges of lung volumes during "relatively fluent" speech, compared to four normal subjects. Gastric and esophageal balloons were used to estimate subglottal and transdiaphragmatic pressures; linearized magnetometers provided an estimate of lung volume. The subjects engaged in reading and conversational speech. During spontaneous speech, two of the stuttering subjects employed lung volumes that tended to remain entirely above functional residual capacity (FRC); for the other two, lung volumes tended to remain entirely below FRC. For the reading task, the stuttering subjects did not behave differently from the normal subjects with respect to lung volume, but no comparisons in fluency were made between reading and speech, so we do not know whether the changes in lung volume were associated with any changes in fluency. The stuttering subjects were also more variable in the sizes of the breaths that they took. Johnston et al. suggested that this variability might reflect inadequate coordination of the respiratory muscles during speech.

In summary: Relative to resting breathing, normal speech necessitates rapid changes in volume, pressure, and flow that would be challenges to the normal metabolic control system. The overt manifestations of stuttering commonly include increased variability in these variables, and thus may constitute a further perturbation to a vulnerable speech motor control system.

VOLUNTARY CONTROL OF BREATHING IN STUTTERING

Investigators have long sought clues to the nature of stuttering by examining other motor capabilities of individuals who stutter, but attempts to demonstrate a more general movement disorder have had mixed results (For review, see Bloodstein, 1987). Interestingly, several studies done in the 1930s consistently suggested that stuttering subjects have difficulty in producing voluntarily controlled respiratory movements.

Blackburn (1931) and Seth (1934) tested the ability of stuttering and normal speakers to produce rapid, rhythmic, self-paced movements of the lips, tongue, jaw, chest wall, and fingers. The number of movements per second was measured, and means, standard deviations, and coefficients of variation (CVs) were calculated for each subject (The CV is a measure of variability that is normalized by the mean; $CV = 100 \times$ standard deviation/ mean). Both investigators found that the CVs were higher for the stuttering than the nonstuttering subjects for movements of the chest wall. In addition, both investigators reported the presence of "tonic blocks" (prolonged cessations of movement) in the chest walls of their stuttering, but not their normal, subjects.

Hunsley (1937) tested the ability of stuttering and nonstuttering subjects to reproduce a temporal pattern of clicks with the effectors used in speech (lips, jaw, tongue, and chest wall). The click pattern was presented at twelve speeds ranging from 30.7 to 91.3 RPM. Hunsley devised a measure of ability to reproduce the click pattern that reflected both speed and accuracy of performance. Comparisons between stuttering and normal subjects were computed for each speed of presentation. In general, stuttering subjects performed more poorly than normals at all but the highest speeds, at which error rates were high for both groups. This difference was demonstrated for all effectors.

Hunsley also analyzed her data qualitatively.

She classified possible errors as: (1) breaks; (2) reversals of temporal intervals; (3) extra movements; (4) not enough movements; (5) small movements imposed on larger movements; and (6) blocks, both tonic and clonic. While stuttering and normal subjects did not differ in the number of errors classified as "too few movements," stuttering subjects made significantly more errors than normals in the other categories. With respect to respiratory movements, breaks, small movements imposed on larger ones, and blocks showed the largest differences between stuttering and normal subjects.

COMPARISONS BETWEEN SPEECH AND NONSPEECH BREATHING

In order to evaluate the hypothesis that different levels of control may be competing in stuttering, it would be helpful to have a marker for one or another of these levels. In other words, if the metabolic respiratory controller possessed some unique and measurable property, a reduction in or absence of that property during speech would enable us to draw conclusions about the underlying control processes that contribute to speech. Such a marker apparently exists for the metabolic respiratory controller.

During inspiration, the metabolic respiratory controller, or neurons closely associated with it, produces rhythmic bursts of activity at 80 to 110 Hz (Christakos, Cohen, See, & Barnhardt, 1988; Mitchell & Herbert, 1974). These high-frequency oscillations (HFOs) are distributed to the many motoneuron pools involved in respiration. HFOs have been observed in recordings from motor nerves supplying the tongue, larynx, and diaphragm in experimental animals (Bruce, 1988; Christakos et al., 1988). The amplitudes of the oscillations in the different nerve recordings are highly correlated, presumably because they are all driven by the same source. The coherence statistic is used to measure the strength of the correlation. Coherence ranges from 0.0 to 1.0, and may be thought of as a correlation of the amplitudes of two signals, defined for each frequency in the signals (Bendat & Piersol, 1986).

A similar phenomenon has been demonstrated in human subjects, that is, inspiratory-related EMGs recorded from right and left rib cage sites show correlated oscillations in the frequency band typical of HFOs. This was true whether subjects breathed CO_2, or performed a deep breathing task (Ackerson & Bruce, 1983; Bruce & Ackerson, 1986; Bruce & Goldman, 1983). EMGs recorded from the same electrode sites during voluntary maneuvers did not show evidence of HFOs (Bruce & Ackerson, 1986). A reasonable conclusion is that a significant, well-defined peak in the coherence function, in the 60 to 110 Hz band, between inspiratory-related EMGs recorded from right and left sides of the chest wall, is an indicator that the metabolic respiratory controller is contributing significant inputs to motoneuron pools.[2] As the metabolic controller becomes a less dominant source of controlling inputs, coherence in that frequency band should decrease.

Smith and Denny (1990) reasoned that if the HFO is a marker of the metabolic controller in humans, and that controller is a less powerful influence on motoneuron pools in speech, then the measure of HFO activity, maximum coherence in the 60 to 110 Hz band, should be less for speech than for a deep breathing task such as that used by Bruce and colleagues. The deep breathing task was used to generate EMGs of sufficient amplitude for analysis; the speech task consisted of reading standard passages composed of long sentences. This sentence structure, plus instructions to read moderately loudly, generated comparable levels of respiratory drive for the two tasks. In addition, subjects performed a "speechlike" breathing task, in which they mimicked the ramplike pattern of speech breathing, but did not vocalize.

All subjects showed reduced maximum coherence in the 60 to 110 Hz band for speech compared to a nonspeech voluntary breathing task, suggesting that these subjects did reduce inputs from the meta-

bolic controller during reading aloud. Maximum coherence was comparable for the speech and speechlike tasks, indicating that this change in controlling inputs was not speech-specific.

A subsequent study (Denny & Smith, 1993) used the same methodology to compare respiratory control in ten stuttering subjects and ten normals matched for sex, age, and educational background. A greater variety of speech strategies was seen in this group of normal subjects. Although maximum coherence was reduced for speech compared to deep breathing in five subjects, four showed no difference in maximum coherence for the two tasks (data from the speech task were not available for one normal subject). Six of the ten stuttering subjects reduced maximum coherence in the 60 to 110 Hz band for speech as compared to deep breathing, but the other four showed higher maximum coherence for speech than for deep breathing.

In attempting to interpret this finding, it is important to recall that the deep breathing task was a voluntary one; yet in normal subjects it was characterized by high levels of inputs from the metabolic respiratory controller. This observation suggests that voluntary control of breathing can make use of the metabolic respiratory control circuitry for some tasks. Thus, human respiratory control is apparently not dichotomous between voluntary and automatic, but forms a continuum. Other researchers have suggested that this is true; they have observed that asking subjects to breathe harder (a voluntary task) elicits a patterned motor response that is virtually indistinguishable from more metabolically driven tasks, such as exercise or exposure to CO_2 (Bartlett & Knuth, 1984; England & Bartlett, 1982; England, Bartlett, & Daubenspeck, 1982; Insalaco et al., 1990).

This leaves open the question of how best to characterize the behavior of the four stuttering subjects whose pattern of results departed from that of normals. Did they have low participation of the metabolic controller for the deep breathing task—indicating that they suppressed inputs from the metabolic controller in a situation where normals made use of them? Or did they have unusu-

---

[2]There are experimental manipulations, such as sagittal section of the medulla, that can abolish the HFO, although the animal continues to breathe. Thus, it does not appear that HFOs are a necessary property of the respiratory controller, although they accompany its operation during normal breathing (Davies, Kirkwood, Romaniuk, & Sears, 1986).

ally high levels for speech, indicating that they failed to suppress the inputs when necessary? At present, we cannot answer these questions. It seems most accurate to suggest that some individuals who stutter do not manage relations among controllers as normally fluent speakers do.

Denny and Smith also measured fluency behaviors for their stuttering subjects. After a speech-related inspiration had been identified as suitable for analysis, the fluency of the entire breath group following that inspiration was rated from 0 (no detectable disfluency) to 7 (maximally severe stuttering). All ratings were based on videotapes of the experimental sessions. An unexpected finding was that the four subjects who showed evidence of abnormal respiratory control strategies included the two most disfluent, and two of the most fluent, in the study. This, plus the fact that some of the normal subjects did not reduce HFOs for speech, suggests that there is considerable variation in the strategies that can underlie successful speech, and that participation of the HFO-producing circuitry alone is not sufficient to precipitate disfluency.

LARYNGEAL CONTROL IN STUTTERING

During breathing for life support, the larynx acts as a respiratory effector. If the metabolic respiratory controller contributes destabilizing inputs to speech in stuttering individuals, we would expect laryngeal function to be disrupted; thus, inadequate respiratory control is a potential candidate as a source of the aberrant laryngeal functioning that we review here.

The occurrence of abnormal laryngeal behaviors in stuttering has often been inferred from clinical evaluations of how disfluencies sound (e.g., Van Riper, 1982). Aspects of stuttered speech that have been attributed to faulty laryngeal control include overall vocal quality, prosody, and timing (Bloodstein, 1987; Van Riper, 1982). During their fluent speech, stuttering subjects may employ a restricted range of fundamental frequencies (Healey, 1982). Voice onset and termination times are longer in the perceptually fluent speech of stut-

tering subjects than in the speech of normal subjects (Agnello, 1975).

Vocal reaction times (RTs) have been shown to be longer in stuttering than in normal subjects (Adams, Freeman, & Conture, 1984), but the acoustic measures used in these studies did not allow the estimation of premotor RT. Premotor RT is measured as the time from the presentation of a signal to the first physiological manifestation of a response to that signal, and is assumed to represent the time required for programming the motor response. Peters and Hulstijn (1987) compared premotor RTs for the initiation of speech in stuttering and normal subjects. Comparisons of premotor RTs were based only on fluently produced responses. Stuttering subjects' premotor RTs were significantly longer for both single words and sentences. This was true whether or not the subject was given time to read the words or sentences silently before the signal was given to read them aloud.

Watson and Alfonso (1987) studied four stuttering and four normal speakers in a vocal RT paradigm. They found that normal and mildly stuttering speakers took advantage of the foreperiod to posture the chest wall appropriately for sudden phonation, but that severely stuttering subjects used this strategy less frequently.

More direct observations of laryngeal behavior during speech and stuttering are relatively invasive, so there are not many available. Conture and colleagues, using fiberoptic laryngoscopy, were able to rule out the hypothesis that the larynx may simply "squeeze shut" during disfluency, blocking attempts to speak. They did find an increased incidence of abnormal positioning of the vocal folds in stuttering subjects (Conture, McCall, & Brewer, 1977; Conture, Schwartz, & Brewer, 1985).

Two studies of laryngeal EMGs recorded in stuttering subjects have been widely cited as indicating that stuttering is accompanied by excessive activation of laryngeal muscles. Freeman and Ushijima (1978) recorded EMGs from intrinsic laryngeal muscles in four stuttering subjects. They compared amplitude of EMG activity between initial (stuttered) productions, and later, fluent utterances. The fluent utterances were produced using various fluency enhancing techniques. Quantitative analysis of these data showed higher levels of muscle activity in the stuttered productions. In addition, Freeman and Ushijima observed coactivation of antagonistic muscle pairs in stuttered speech. They suggested that laryngeal muscle activity in stuttered speech was clearly excessive and that coactivation of antagonists was abnormal. Their observations were generally confirmed by Shapiro (1980), who did no quantitative analysis but reported observing excessive activity.

These are crucial findings because they suggest that highly invasive treatments designed to reduce laryngeal muscle activation may be beneficial in treating people who stutter. Specifically, injection of botulinum toxin into the vocal folds has recently been used to treat stuttering (Brin, Stewart, Blitzer, & Diamond, 1994; Ludlow, 1990; Stager & Ludlow, 1994). The rationale for such treatment has been derived specifically from reports of excessive activity in the laryngeal muscles of stuttering subjects.

Smith and colleagues have reported a strikingly different view of laryngeal muscle activity in stuttering (Smith et al., 1995). These investigators analyzed laryngeal EMGs recorded from cricothyroid (CT) and thyroarytenoid (TA) muscles in four stuttering and three normal subjects. Experimental tasks included quiet breathing, conversation, singing scales, forceful exhalation against a closed airway (Valsalva maneuver), phonating the vowel /i/ for as long as possible, and sentence repetition. To evaluate the possibility of excessive activation, both qualitative and quantitative methods were used.

They found that maximal activity usually occurred for singing (CT, TA) or the Valsalva maneuver (TA). For typical conversational intervals in normal speakers, the operating range for TA was approximately 20 to 50 percent of maximum; for CT, the operating range was approximately 30 to 100 percent of maximum. Typical records for the stuttering subjects showed reduced or comparable operating ranges for TA and CT during both fluent and disfluent speech, as compared to maximal activation. When fluent and disfluent intervals were compared within stuttering speakers, it was

seen that stuttered speech could be associated with greater, equal, or lesser activation of laryngeal muscles than fluent speech.

A fluency-enhancing task, repeated readings of a sentence, had no effect on amplitudes of laryngeal EMGs in the normal speakers. In contrast, three of the four stuttering subjects clearly reduced the amplitudes of their laryngeal EMGs in the course of repeated readings. This finding probably explains the different conclusions reported by Freeman and Ushijima (1978) and Smith et al. Freeman and Ushijima compared disfluent intervals to later adapted intervals. Had Smith and colleagues made only that comparison, they might have arrived at similar conclusions. Instead they chose to expand their methods to include a normal control group, conversational speech and reading of a passage, nonspeech activities, and a fluency-enhancing task.

Inclusion of a normal control group provided data against which to evaluate the amplitude of stuttering subjects' EMGs in speech compared to nonspeech tasks. Similarly, data recorded from normal subjects can help evaluate the claim that simultaneous activity in adductors and the abductor of the larynx is an abnormal event that contributes to stuttering. Although other investigators have reported reciprocal activation in laryngeal muscles during speech (Hirose & Gay, 1972, 1973; Hirose & Ushijima, 1974), there is disagreement on this point. Ludlow and co-workers recorded EMGs from PCA, TA, and CT in five normal adults (Ludlow, Yeh, Cohen, Van Pelt, Rhew, & Hallett, 1994). Experimental tasks included production of sustained vowels and syllable repetition. They reported observing activity in all laryngeal muscles throughout speech gestures. Thus it seems premature to regard coactivation of adductors and abductors as abnormal until this question has been explored by analyzing abductor/adductor relationships during a variety of speech and nonspeech tasks in normal subjects.

The major finding of Smith et al. (1995) is clear: It does not support the position that excess activation of laryngeal muscles is a necessary concomitant of stuttering. Rather, stuttered speech could be associated with lower, higher, or equal activation of laryngeal muscles when compared to the same subject's perceptually fluent speech. In light of these findings, it appears that the use of botulinum toxin to reduce activity in laryngeal muscles is a questionable treatment for stuttering.

These investigators have also reported spectral analyses of laryngeal EMGs from normal and stuttering subjects (Smith et al., 1993); these include the three normal and four stuttering subjects discussed above. Data from three additional stuttering subjects were provided by Dr. Christy Ludlow. EMGs recorded from facial and jaw muscles were analyzed as well. These investigators have previously reported that abnormal, tremorlike oscillations in the range of 5 to 15 Hz are part of a neuromuscular pattern that is characteristic of stuttering, although not all individuals who stutter show it. These reports were based on analyses of EMGs recorded from muscles of the face, jaw, and neck.

Smith and co-workers (1993) showed that in disfluent speech, neuromuscular oscillations in the 5 to 15 Hz range were characteristic of laryngeal muscles as well. There were a total of twelve laryngeal EMG channels recorded from the seven subjects (TA and CT in five subjects; CT only in one subject; TA only in one subject). Averaged power spectra showed their maximum values between 5 and 15 Hz for six of these EMG signals. In contrast, of six laryngeal EMG signals recorded from the three normal subjects, no spectra showed a maximum value in the 5 to 15 Hz range.

In addition, Smith et al. (1993) tested the hypothesis that a common driving source might be responsible for producing the abnormal oscillations. If this were so, the amplitudes of the oscillations should have been correlated. To test this, the coherence function was computed for all pairs of EMGs within each subject. (Recall that coherence is mathematically equivalent to a squared cross-correlation of the power in two signals). The results of the analyses of laryngeal activity were similar to those seen for muscles of the face, jaw, and neck: six of the seven stuttering subjects had significant coherence in the 5 to 15 Hz range in at least one muscle pair. Interestingly, the highest coherence could occur within systems (e.g., TA and CT) or across systems (e.g., CT and a lip muscle). Smith and colleagues suggested that while independent mechanisms might drive oscillations in different muscles, those mechanisms could become entrained, possibly by means of neural circuitry subserving autonomic arousal.

Laryngeal muscles appear to behave like facial, jaw, and neck muscles in these respects: Activity for stuttered speech may be higher, lower, or equal to that observed in the same subject for perceptually fluent speech. Tremorlike oscillations may characterize stuttering; and the amplitude of those oscillations may or may not be correlated across muscles and systems.

SUMMARY

The working hypothesis of this review has been that control systems for metabolic breathing and emotional vocalization may compete with speech motor control systems in stuttering individuals. We have suggested that normal speech production may constitute a challenge to respiratory control processes, that certain features of disfluent speech may further contribute to a destabilization of speech motor control, and that difficulties with respiratory control may well have consequences that range over the entire speech effector system.

Our findings with respect to laryngeal activity in stuttering are consistent with an emphasis on the importance of factors that may have broadly distributed effects. We have found that muscles of the face, jaw, and larynx behave in similar ways in stuttered and in fluent speech (Denny & Smith, 1992; Smith, 1989; Smith, Denny, & Wood, 1991; Smith et al., 1993). Of particular importance to the current discussion is the finding that tremorlike oscillations, in some subjects, are correlated between facial and laryngeal muscles, suggesting common influences operating across muscle groups.

In the future, we hope to see many more explorations of the rich interactions among motor systems that coordinate respiration, emotional vocalization, and speech in both normal and stuttering speakers.

REFERENCES

Ackerson, L.M., & Bruce, E.N. (1983). Bilaterally synchronized oscillations in human diaphragm and intercostal EMGs during spontaneous breathing. *Brain Research, 271*, 346–348.

Adams, M.R. (1974). A physiologic and aerodynamic interpretation of fluent and stuttered speech. *Journal of Fluency Disorders, 1*, 35–47.

Adams, M.R., Freeman, F.J., & Conture, E.G. (1984). Laryngeal dynamics of stutterers. In R.F. Curlee & W.H. Perkins (Eds.), *Nature and treatment of stuttering: New directions* (pp. 89–130). San Diego, CA: College-Hill Press.

Agnello, J.C. (1975). Voice onset and termination features of stutterers. In L.M. Webster & L. Furst (Eds.), *Vocal tract dynamics and dysfluency* (pp. 40–54). New York: Speech and Hearing Institute.

Bartlett, D., Jr. (1986). Upper airway motor systems. In A.P. Fishman (Ed.), *Handbook of physiology: Sec. 3. The respiratory system: Vol. II. Control of breathing, Part 1* (pp. 223–245). Bethesda, MD: American Physiological Society.

Bartlett, D., Jr., & Knuth, S.L. (1984). Human vocal cord movements during voluntary hyperventilation. *Respiration Physiology, 58*, 289–294.

Bartlett, D., Jr., Remmers, J.E., & Gautier, H. (1973). Laryngeal regulation of respiratory airflow. *Respiration Physiology, 18*, 194–204.

Bendat, J.S., & Piersol, A.G. (1986). *Random data: Analysis and measurement procedures* (2nd ed.). New York: Wiley.

Blackburn, B. (1931). Voluntary movements of the organs of speech in stutterers and non-stutterers. *Psychological Monographs, 41*, 1–13.

Bloodstein, O. (1987). *A handbook on stuttering*. Chicago: Easter Seal Society.

Brancatisano, T., Dodd, D.S., & Engel, L.A. (1984). Respiratory activity of posterior cricoarytenoid muscle and vocal cords in humans. *Journal of Applied Physiology, 57*, 1143–1149.

Brin, M.F., Stewart, C., Blitzer, A., & Diamond, B. (1994) Laryngeal botulinum toxin injections for disabling stuttering in adults. *Neurology, 44*, 2262–2266.

Brouillette, R.T., & Thach, B.T. (1979). A neuromuscular mechanism maintaining airway patency. *Journal of Applied Physiology, 46*, 772-779.

Bruce, E.N. (1988). Correlated and uncorrelated high-frequency oscillations in phrenic and recurrent laryngeal neurograms. *Journal of Neurophysiology, 59*, 1188–1203.

Bruce, E.N., & Ackerson, L.M. (1986). High-frequency oscillations in human electromyograms during voluntary contractions. *Journal of Neurophysiology, 56*, 542–553.

Bruce, E.N., & Goldman, M.D. (1983). High-frequency oscillations in human respiratory electromyograms during voluntary breathing. *Brain Research, 269*, 259–265.

Bunn, J.C., & Mead, J. (1971). Control of ventilation during speech. *Journal of Applied Physiology, 31*, 870–872.

Chanaud, C., & Ludlow, C. (1992). Single motor unit activity of human intrinsic laryngeal muscles during respiration. *Annals of Otology, Rhinology & Laryngology, 101*, 832–840.

Christakos, C.N., Cohen, M.I., See, W.R., & Barnhardt, R. (1988). Fast rhythms in the discharges of medullary inspiratory neurons. *Brain Research, 463*, 362–367.

Conture, E.G., McCall, G.N., & Brewer, D.W. (1977). Laryngeal behavior during stuttering. *Journal of Speech and Hearing Research, 20*, 661–668.

Conture, E.G., Schwartz, H.D., & Brewer, D.W. (1985). Laryngeal behavior during stuttering: A further study. *Journal of Speech and Hearing Research, 28*, 233–240.

Davies, J.G. McF., Kirkwood, P.A., Romaniuk, J.R., & Sears, T.A. (1986). Effects of sagittal medullary section on high-frequency oscillation in rabbit phrenic neurogram. *Respiration Physiology, 64*, 277–287.

Davis, P.J., & Zhang, S.P. (1991). What is the role of the midbrain periaqueductal gray in respiration and vocalization? In A. Depaulis & R. Bandler (Eds.), *The midbrain periaqeductal gray matter: Functional, anatomical, and neurochemical organization* (pp. 57–66). New York: Plenum, in cooperation with NATO Scientific Affairs Division.

Davis, P.J., Zhang, S.P., & Bandler, R. (1993). Pulmonary and upper airway afferent influences on the motor pattern of vocalization evoked by excitation of the midbrain periaqueductal gray of the cat. *Brain Research, 607*, 61–80.

Denny, M., & Smith, A. (1992). Gradations in a pattern of neuromuscular activity associated with stuttering. *Journal of Speech and Hearing Research, 35*, 1216–1229.

Denny, M., & Smith, A. (1993). Interaction of voluntary and metabolic respiratory control in stuttering. *Asha, 35,* 168.

Depaulis, A., & Bandler, R. (Eds.). (1991). *The midbrain periaqueductal gray matter: Functional, anatomical, and neurochemical organization.* New York: Plenum, in cooperation with NATO Scientific Affairs Division.

England, S.J., & Bartlett, D., Jr. (1982). Changes in respiratory movements of the human vocal cords during hyperpnea. *Journal of Applied Physiology, 52,* 780–785.

England, S.J., Bartlett, D., Jr., & Daubenspeck, J.A. (1982). Influence of human vocal cord movements on airflow and resistance during eupnea. *Journal of Applied Physiology, 52,* 773–779.

Feldman, J.L. (1986). Neurophysiology of breathing in mammals. In F.E. Bloom (Ed.), *Handbook of physiology: Sec. 1. The nervous system: Vol. IV.* (pp. 463–524). Bethesda, MD: American Physiological Society.

Freeman, F., & Ushijima, T. (1978). Laryngeal muscle activity during stuttering. *Journal of Speech and Hearing Research, 21,* 538–562.

Goldman-Eisler, F. (1968). *Psycholinguistics: Experiments in spontaneous speech.* London: Academic Press.

Green, J.H., & Neil, E. (1955). The respiratory function of the laryngeal muscles. *Journal of Physiology (London), 129,* 134–141.

Hairston, L.E., & Sauerland, E.K. (1981). Electromyography of the human palate: Discharge patterns of the levator and tensor veli palatini. *Electromyography and Clinical Neurophysiology, 21,* 287–297.

Healey, E.C. (1982). Speaking fundamental frequency characteristics of stutterers and nonstutterers. *Journal of Communication Disorders, 15,* 21–29.

Hill, M.W., Guilleminault, C., Simmons, F.B. (1978). Fiber-optic and EMG studies in hypersomnia-sleep apnea syndrome. In C. Guilleminault & W.C. Dement (Eds.), *Sleep apnea syndromes* (pp. 249–258). New York: Alan R. Liss, Inc.

Hirose, H., & Gay, T. (1972). The activity of the intrinsic laryngeal muscles in voicing control: An electromyographic study. *Phonetica, 25,* 140–164.

Hirose, H., & Gay, T. (1973). Laryngeal control in vocal attack: An electromyographic study. *Folia Phoniatrica, 25,* 203–213.

Hirose, H., & Ushijima, T. (1974). The function of the posterior cricoarytenoid in speech articulation. *Haskins Laboratory Status Reports on Speech Research, SR-37/38,* 99–107.

Hixon, T.J. (1987). *Respiratory function in speech and song.* San Diego: College-Hill Press.

Hugelin, A. (1986). Forebrain and midbrain influence on respiration. In A.P. Fishman (Ed.), *Handbook of physiology: Sec. 3. The respiratory system: Vol. II. Control of breathing, Part 1* (pp. 69–91). Bethesda, MD: American Physiological Society.

Hunsley, Y.L. (1937). Dysintegration in the speech musculature of stutterers during the production of a non-vocal pattern. *Psychological Monographs, 49,* 32–49.

Hutchinson, J.M., & Navarre, B.M. (1977). The effect of metronome pacing on selected aerodynamic patterns of stuttered speech. *Journal of Fluency Disorders, 2,* 189–204.

Insalaco, G., Kuna, S.T., Cibella, F., & Villeponteaux, R.D. (1990). Thyroarytenoid muscle activity during hypoxia, hypercapnia, and voluntary hyperventilation in humans. *Journal of Applied Physiology, 69,* 268–273.

Johnston, S.J., Watkin, K.L., & Macklem, P.T. (1993). Lung volume changes during relatively fluent speech in stutterers. *Journal of Applied Physiology, 75,* 696–703.

Kuna, S.T., Day, R.A., Insalaco, G., & Villeponteaux, R.D. (1991). Posterior cricoarytenoid activity in normal adults during voluntary and involuntary hyperventilation. *Journal of Applied Physiology, 70,* 1377–1385.

Kuna, S.T., Insalaco, G, Woodson, G.E. (1988). Thyroarytenoid muscle activity during wakefulness and sleep in normal adults. *Journal of Applied Physiology, 65,* 1332–1339.

Kuna, S.T., Smickley, J.S., & Insalaco, G. (1990). Posterior cricoarytenoid muscle activity during wakefulness and sleep in normal adults. *Journal of Applied Physiology, 68,* 1746–1754.

Larson, C.R. (1991). On the relation of PAG neurons to laryngeal and respiratory muscles during vocalization in the monkey. *Brain Research, 552,* 77–86.

Ludlow, C.L. (1990) Treatment of speech and voice disorders with botulinum toxin. *The Journal of the American Medical Association, 264,* 2671–2675.

Ludlow, C.L., Yeh, J., Cohen, L.G., Van Pelt, F., Rhew, K., & Hallett, M. (1994) Limitations in electromyography and magnetic stimulation for assessing laryngeal muscle control. *Annals of Otology, Rhinology & Laryngology, 103*, 16–27.

Mathew, O., & Sant'Ambrogio, G. (Eds.). (1988). *Respiratory function of the upper airway.* New York: Marcel Dekker, Inc.

Milic-Emili, J., & Zin, W.A. (1986). Breathing responses to imposed mechanical loads. In A.P. Fishman (Ed.), *Handbook of physiology: Sec. 3. The respiratory system: Vol. II. Control of breathing, Part 1* (pp. 1–68). Bethesda, MD: American Physiological Society.

Mitchell, R.A., & Herbert, D.A. (1974). Synchronized high frequency synaptic potentials in medullary respiratory neurons. *Brain Research, 75*, 350–355.

Perkins, W., Rudas, J., Johnson, L., & Bell, J. (1976). Stuttering: Discoordination of phonation with articulation and respiration. *Journal of Speech and Hearing Research, 19*, 509–522.

Peters, H.F.M., & Boves, L. (1988). Coordination of aerodynamic and phonatory processes in fluent speech utterances of stutterers. *Journal of Speech and Hearing Research, 31*, 352–361.

Peters, H.F.M., & Hietkamp, R.K., & Boves, L. (1993). Aerodynamic and phonatory processes in dysfluent speech utterances of stutterers. *ASHA, 35*, 144.

Peters, H.F.M., & Hulstijn, W. (1984). Stuttering and anxiety: The difference between stutterers and non-stutterers in verbal apprehension and physiologic arousal during the anticipation of speech and non-speech tasks. *Journal of Fluency Disorders, 9*, 67–84.

Peters, H.F.M., & Hulstijn, W. (1987). Programming and initiation of speech utterances in stuttering. In H.F.M. Peters & W. Hulstijn (Eds.), *Speech motor dynamics in stuttering* (pp. 185–196). New York: Springer-Verlag.

Phillipson, E.A., McClean, P.A., Sullivan, C.E., & Zamel, N. (1978). Interaction of metabolic and behavioral respiratory control during hypercapnia and speech. *American Review of Respiratory Disease, 117*, 903–909.

Remmers, J.E., DeGroot, W.J., Sauerland, E.K., & Anch, A.M. (1978). Pathogenesis of upper airway occlusion during sleep. *Journal of Applied Physiology, 44*, 931–938.

Rothstein, R.J., Narce, S.L., deBerry-Borowiecki, B., & Blanks, R.H.I. (1983). Respiratory-related activity of upper airway muscles in anesthetized rabbit. *Journal of Applied Physiology, 55*, 1830–1836.

Sauerland, E.K., & Harper, R.M. (1976). The human tongue during sleep: Electromyographic activity of the genioglossus muscle. *Experimental Neurology, 51*, 160–170.

Sauerland, E.K., & Mitchell, S.P. (1970). Electromyographic activity of the human genioglossus muscle in response to respiration and to positional changes of the head. *Bulletin of the Los Angeles Neurological Societies, 35*, 69–73.

Sauerland, E.K., & Mitchell, S.P. (1975). Electromyographic activity of intrinsic and extrinsic muscles of the human tongue. *Texas Reports on Biology and Medicine, 33*, 445–455.

Schwab, R.J., Gefter, W.B., Pack, A.I., & Hoffman, E.A. (1993). Dynamic imaging of the upper airway during respiration in normal subjects. *Journal of Applied Physiology, 74*, 1504–1514.

Seth, G. (1934). An experimental study of the control of the mechanism of speech, and in particular that of respiration, in stuttering subjects. *British Journal of Psychology, 24*, 375–388.

Shapiro, A.I. (1980). An electromyographic analysis of the fluent and dysfluent utterances of several types of stutterers. *Journal of Fluency Disorders, 5*, 203–232.

Smith, A. (1989). Neural drive to muscles in stuttering. *Journal of Speech and Hearing Research, 32*, 252–264.

Smith, A. (1990). Factors in the etiology of stuttering. *American Speech-Language-Hearing Association Reports, Research Needs in Stuttering: Roadblocks and Future Directions, 18*, 39–47.

Smith, A., & Denny, M. (1990). High-frequency oscillations as indicators of neural control mechanisms in human respiration, mastication, and speech. *Journal of Neurophysiology, 63*, 745–758.

Smith, A., Denny, M., & Wood, J. (1991). Instability in speech muscle systems in stuttering. In H.F.M. Peters, W. Hulstijn, & W. Starkweather (Eds.), *Speech motor control and stuttering* (pp. 231–242). New York: Elsevier.

Smith, A., Denny, M., Shaffer-Westwood, L., & Hirano, M. (1995). Activity of intrinsic laryngeal muscles in normally fluent and stuttering adults. Manuscript submitted to *Journal of Speech and Hearing Research*.

Smith, A., Luschei, E., Denny, M., Wood, J., Hirano, M., & Badylak, S. (1993). Spectral analysis of activity of laryngeal and orofacial muscles in stutterers. *Journal of Neurology, Neurosurgery, & Psychiatry*, *56*, 1303–1311.

Smith, A., & Weber, C.M. (1988). The need for an integrated perspective on stuttering. *Asha*, *30*, 30–32.

Stager, S.V., & Ludlow, C.L. (1994) Responses of stutterers and vocal tremor patients to treatment with botulinum toxin. In J. Jankovic & M. Hallett (Eds.), *Therapy with botulinum toxin* (pp. 481–490). New York: Marcel Dekker, Inc.

Tangel, D.J., Mezzanotte, W.S., & White, D.P. (1995). Respiratory-related control of palatoglossus and levator palatini muscle activity. *Journal of Applied Physiology*, *78*, 680–688.

Van Riper, C. (1982). *The nature of stuttering* (2nd ed.). Englewood Cliffs, NJ: Prentice-Hall.

Watson, B.C., & Alfonso, P.J. (1987). Physiological bases of acoustic LRT in nonstutterers, mild stutterers, and severe stutterers. *Journal of Speech and Hearing Research*, *30*, 434–447.

Weber, C.M., & Smith, A. (1990). Autonomic correlates of stuttering and speech assessed in a range of experimental tasks. *Journal of Speech and Hearing Research*, *33*, 690–706.

Winkworth, A.L., Davis, P.J., Adams, R.D., & Ellis, E. (1995). Breathing patterns during spontaneous speech. *Journal of Speech and Hearing Research*, *38*, 124–144.

Winkworth, A.L., Davis, P.J., Ellis, E., & Adams, R.D. (1994). Variability and consistency in speech breathing during reading: Lung volumes, speech intensity, and linguistic factors. *Journal of Speech and Hearing Research*, *37*, 535–556.

Wheatley, J.R., Brancatisano, A., & Engel, L.A. (1991). Respiratory-related activity of cricothyroid muscle in awake normal humans. *Journal of Applied Physiology*, *70*, 2226–2232.

Zhang, S.P., Davis, P.J., Bandler, R., & Carrive, P. (1994). Brain stem integration of vocalization: Role of the midbrain periaqueductal gray. *Journal of Neurophysiology*, *72*, 1337–1356.

Zhou, Y., & Daubenspeck, J.A. (1995). Measurement of upper airway movement by acoustic reflection. *Annals of Biomedical Engineering*, *23*, 85–94.

Zhou, Y., Denny, M., Bachir, N.M., & Daubenspeck, J.A. (1995). Laryngeal responses to single-breath expiratory and inspiratory resistance loads. *FASEB Journal*, A567.

Zocchi, L., Estenne, M., Johnston, S., del Ferro, L., Ward, M.E., & Macklem, P.T. (1990). Respiratory muscle incoordination in stuttering speech. *American Review of Respiratory Disease*, *141*, 1510–1515.

SUGGESTED READINGS

Bartlett, D., Jr. (1986). Upper airway motor systems. In A.P. Fishman (Ed.), *Handbook of physiology: Sec. 3. The respiratory system: Vol. II. Control of breathing*, Part 1 (pp. 223–245). Bethesda, MD: American Physiological Society.

Bartlett, D., Jr. (1989). Respiratory functions of the larynx. *Physiological Reviews*, *69*, pp. 33–57.

Milic-Emili, J., & Zin, W.A. (1986). Breathing responses to imposed mechanical loads. In A.P. Fishman (Ed.), *Handbook of physiology: Sec. 3. The respiratory system: Vol. II. Control of breathing*, Part 1 (pp. 1–68). Bethesda, MD: American Physiological Society.

Smith, A., & Denny, M. (1990). High-frequency oscillations as indicators of neural control mechanisms in human respiration, mastication, and speech. *Journal of Neurophysiology*, *63*, 745–758.

CHAPTER 7

BRAIN IMAGING CONTRIBUTIONS

BEN C. WATSON
FRANCES J. FREEMAN

INTRODUCTION

A neurological perspective appears in stuttering theory throughout recorded history. However, the specifics of this approach have changed with the contemporary scientific zeitgeist. Several of these changes are reflected in the historical review of stuttering theory compiled by Reiber and Wollock (1977). The following examples are taken from that review. A neurological approach appeared in the writings of Aristotle (circa 350 B.C.) in the guise of a mind/body dyssynchrony in which "the instruments of the tongue itself are weak and cannot exactly follow the concept of the mind." Jumping forward a millennium or so, Hartley (circa 1749) echoed Aristotle's view and described stuttering as a consequence of confusion that disrupts vibrations traveling neural pathways to the peripheral speech mechanism.

The nineteenth century saw an increased emphasis on relations between speech, language, and thought. Combe (circa 1826), a phrenologist and stutterer, claimed that stuttering was not due to a physical malformation in the brain, but to irregular nervous impulses from the brain. He believed these irregular impulses produced a breakdown of synchronization between language and thought. Kussmaul (1887) noted the similarity between stuttering as a motor control disorder and aphasia as a language disorder. Kussmaul described stuttering as an aphasia that produced a syllabic dysarthria characterized by a lack of coordination of voice, respiration, and articulation.

The hemispheric dominance/laterality hypotheses advanced by Orton (1927) and Travis (1931) influenced neurologic approaches to stuttering in the early and mid twentieth century. The development and application of neuropsychologic tasks (for example, dichotic listening and tachistoscopic viewing), while indirect and inferential, provided the first entree into systematic studies of brain function and revealed interhemispheric processing differences between stutterers and nonstutterers. Unfortunately, the cortical and subcortical regions involved were not identified unambiguously. On another front, clinicians sometimes observed stuttering-like behaviors as sequelae of stroke or head trauma. Together, these laboratory findings and clinical observations reinforced the relevance of a neurologic approach to stuttering at a time when behaviorism and other forms of learning theory were moving theorists away from a neurophysiologic orientation.

In the first edition of this text, Moore (1984) offered a comprehensive review and integration of neuropsychologic research in stuttering, while Rosenbeck (1984) addressed the topic of acquired stuttering following nervous system damage. These chapters represent accurately the schism in neurologic approaches to stuttering in the recent past: There are neurologic theories of developmental stuttering and there are theories of neurologic (acquired) stuttering, and "never the twain shall meet."

The present chapter reviews findings obtained from direct imaging of brain structure and function in adults. Following this review, we will argue that the historically divergent neurological approaches to developmental and acquired stuttering are counterproductive. We will propose a theory of fluency as an alternative to a neurologic approach to stuttering. This theory recognizes stuttering as one of many possible forms of fluency failure. Finally, we will conclude with a glimpse into the future of brain imaging techniques as they may apply to advancing understanding of brain, fluency, and stuttering.

A neurologic perspective on stuttering in this day and age requires a multi-disciplinary approach to research. Technologies presently used to study brain structure and brain function necessitate collaborations among speech and language scientists and professionals in neurology, neuroradiology, electrophysiology, and nuclear medicine. Current technologies provide several approaches to neurologic studies. Computerized tomography (CT) and magnetic resonance imaging (MRI) reveal brain structure. Imaging techniques that reflect electrical, biochemical, or physiologic properties of the central nervous system (CNS) reveal brain function (Devous, 1995).

Several functional measures are now well developed for research. Topographic mapping of electroencephalographic (EEG) spectra and various event-related potentials permit investigation of electrical properties of brain function. Evoked potentials document the CNS response to auditory, visual, or somatosensory stimuli. Readiness potentials (for example, contingent negative variation, Bereitschaft, and event-related desynchronization) document CNS antecedents of a specific volitional response. Single-photon emission computed tomography (SPECT) and positron emission tomography (PET) reveal biochemical and physiologic properties of brain, including perfusion, metabolism, and receptor function (Devous, 1992). These techniques trace the distribution of a radiopharmaceutical throughout the brain. Biochemical and neurophysiologic properties of brain function are tightly coupled because active neurons alter metabolism, which, in turn, requires increased perfusion to transport nutrients to the nerve cells. The following sections summarize contemporary findings from the application of structural and functional brain imaging technologies in stuttering research.

STRUCTURAL IMAGING FINDINGS

Computerized Tomography

Computerized tomography (CT) combines principles of planar X-ray methods with computerized reconstruction techniques to produce images of cross-sections of the body (Office of Technology Assessment, 1978). X-ray (transmission) images display structures that are differentiated by their absorption of energy from X rays. A structure's image is linked to its density. For example, bone, being denser than soft tissue, absorbs more energy and produces a lighter image on X-ray film. Construction of a CT image of the brain requires obtaining numerous scans as the X-ray source and detector rotate around the subject's head. A computer then uses the complete set of scans to construct an image of a cross-section (or slice) for display. CT scans overcome two major limitations of planar X rays: (1) Production of cross-sectional slices prevents images of adjacent organs from overlapping, and thus obscuring one another, and (2) CT images provide better resolution of adjacent structures with similar densities because cross-sections are obtained from scans taken at several different angles. Applied to images of the head, CT scans reveal structural characteristics of cortical and immediate subcortical regions. Typically, CT scans are used to diagnose mass lesions (for example, tumors), cerebrovascular disease, head trauma, and disease processes that alter the ventricular space (for example, hydrocephalus or cerebral atrophy).

Strub, Black, and Naeser (1987) presented CT and neuropsychological findings for two adult developmental stutterers (brother and sister). Neuropsychological findings for the sister "suggested mild relative deficits in functions hypothesized to be subsumed by both hemispheres, with somewhat greater impairment of the language dominant hemisphere" (p. 341), although the patient had a normal electroencephalogram. The CT scan showed no focal lesions, but enlargement of the anterior horns of the ventricles was evident. Measures of brain symmetries revealed a focal anatomical asymmetry (right wider than left) in the occipital lobe at a slice presumed to traverse Wernicke's area. Dichotic testing (consonant+vowel syllable stimuli) revealed a small right ear advantage.

Neuropsychological findings for the brother revealed mild impairment of visual motor integration and better manual dexterity and grip strength with the nondominant hand. His evaluation was generally normal in other respects. Although he wrote with his left hand, his handedness score indicated ambidexterity. The authors reported a normal electroencephalogram, a CT scan with no focal lesions, and, again, enlargement of the anterior horns of the ventricles. Measures of brain symmetries revealed an atypical left frontal asymmetry (left longer and/or wider than right) on slices presumed to traverse Broca's and Wernicke's areas. The brother also showed the occipital asymmetry seen in his sister (right wider than left); however, his asymmetry was noted in slices presumed to traverse both Wernicke's area and the supramarginal gyrus. Dichotic testing (CV syllable stimuli) revealed a small left ear advantage.

Strub et al. (1987) concluded that their findings provide additional neuropsychologic and anatomic support for anomalous hemispheric dominance as an etiologic factor in stuttering as proposed by Orton (1927) and Travis (1931). Neuropsychologic findings suggest mild bilateral cortical dysfunction for both patients. However, the anatomic asymmetries they observed are often difficult to interpret and may not be replicable with higher-resolution scans.

Magnetic Resonance Imaging

Magnetic resonance imaging (MRI) uses electromagnetic principles to construct images of brain structure. Details of MRI scanning are beyond the scope of this chapter, but Newhouse and Wiener (1991) provide a clear and detailed discussion of its principles. Briefly, the magnetic dipoles of molecules in a tissue are normally oriented randomly. During an MRI scan, the tissue is placed within a strong magnetic field and the molecules align in polarity with the field. This alignment is then perturbed by a radio frequency. An image is obtained from energy (radio waves) released by the perturbed molecules as they return to alignment. Different tissue types emit signals with different amplitudes and decay constants. The signals emitted are used to construct an image of the tissues scanned.

We are not aware of any published MRI data for stutterers; however, our research team obtained MRI scans for twenty adult developmental stutterers. Scans for thirteen of the twenty stutterers were interpreted as normal by a neuroradiologist. No abnormalities were found in the normal controls. Small, questionable periventricular signal changes were noted for six stutterers. Finally, the left cervical and intracavernous internal carotid artery could not be visualized for a mild stutterer. Failure to visualize these structures could be due to occlusion, dissection, or severe hypoplasia. At this point, we can conclude that there is little evidence of gross structural abnormalities by MRI in adult developmental stutterers.

FUNCTIONAL BRAIN IMAGING

As noted earlier, functional brain imaging technologies reflect electrical, chemical, or physiologic properties of the CNS (Devous, 1995). Established technologies for functional brain imaging include electroencephalography (EEG), positron emission tomography (PET), and single photon emission computed tomography (SPECT).

EEG Studies

At every moment in time, the brain is in a unique electrophysiologic functional state. This state is a product of the interaction between the reception of new information and spontaneous activity (Lehmann, 1989). Spontaneous activity reflects brief epochs of different functional electrophysiologic states and produces the electroencephalographic signal (EEG) that is typically recorded at rest

(Lehmann, 1989). Newly arriving information produces a series of different, brief electrophysiologic states that reflect the processing of this information. These states are analyzed as components of an evoked potential (EP) response.

A specific class of EP response occurs prior to a discrete motor behavior. This event takes the shape of a slow negativity that is superimposed on the background EEG signal. It is called the Bereitschaft potential (BP) when the motor behavior is produced without an external cue. It is called the Contingent Negative Variation (CNV) when a motor act occurs (with or without antecedent cognitive processing) in response to an external stimulus. Amplitudes of BP and CNV are sensitive to characteristics of the motor response, such as speed, force, and complexity.

The stuttering literature contains numerous references to EEG and EP studies (see reviews by Van Riper, 1982; Bloodstein, 1983; Moore, 1984, 1990). Studies of event related potentials in stutterers include those of Zimmerman and Knott (1974), Pinsky and McAdam (1980), Prescott and Andrews (1984), and Prescott (1988). To date, neither EEG or EP studies have revealed systematic or compelling differences between stutterers and nonstutterers. Inconclusive findings from EEG studies may be due, in part, to limitations of traditional visual analysis of EEG data. Subtle between-group differences may not be discernible on visual inspection of EEG recordings from multiple sites.

Quantitative electroencephalographic (QEEG) techniques provide an approach to examining cortical electrophysiology and investigating the spatial pattern of neuronal activity at discrete time intervals (Pool, Freeman, & Finitzo, 1985). Digital acquisition and processing of electrophysiologic data overcome many previous technical limitations by providing increased resolution in the spectral, temporal, and amplitude domains. Digital recording also facilitates sampling CNS activity from a larger number of scalp recording sites and permits topographic "mapping" of events recorded from those sites. We are aware of only one study that applied QEEG techniques to study brain electrophysiology in stutterers.

Finitzo, Pool, Freeman, Devous, and Watson (1991) reported resting EEG (eyes open and eyes closed conditions) and auditory EP data for twenty adult developmental stutterers. EEG electrodes were placed at twenty sites over the scalp. Additional electrodes served as extracerebral monitors and linked earlobe references.

Analysis of EEG spectra revealed a significant reduction in the amplitude of Beta1 (12.0–15.5 Hz) for the stutterers relative to a group of twelve adult male normal speakers. Figure 7.1 shows topographic maps (BEAM, Nicolet Instruments Corp.) of group-averaged absolute Beta amplitude for the stutterers (left panel) and normal speakers (center panel). The right panel in this figure maps the significance of t test comparisons at each recording site. Significance levels were corrected for multiple frequency band comparisons, but not for multiple electrode site comparisons. Consequently, findings from this analysis are exploratory. With that caution in mind, group differences were most pronounced (significant at $p< 0.01$) over right posterior temporal and bi-occipital sites. Similar amplitude differences occurred at adjacent paramedian central and parietal sites. Beta2 amplitudes were also reduced in the stutterer group. The significance of a group difference over occipital sites is not clear; however, recall that Strub et al. (1987) observed structural asymmetry of the occipital cortex in CT scans of their two subjects.

Auditory EP (AEP) data were recorded in the same session and with the same electrode configuration. Auditory stimuli were 103 dB SPL tone bursts with a 10 ms rise/fall time and were presented binaurally through headphones. EEG was monitored continuously during the AEP study to ensure that subjects remained alert and to monitor for artifacts. Salient landmarks of a cortical evoked potential are peaks identified by their direction (positive or negative) and order of latency. Finitzo and colleagues (1991) reported AEP data for three major peaks: P1, N1, and P2. These peaks were selected because they originate, at least in part, from tempo-

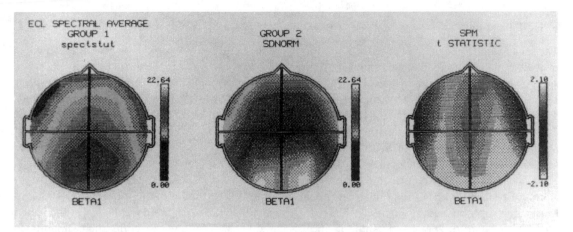

Figure 7.1 Topographic brain maps of group average absolute Beta amplitude. The map on the left is the stutterers' data. The map in the center is the nonstutterers' data. The image on the right is the significance probability map for the *t* test set to a *p* value of 0.02. The authors recognize that brain images produced by quantitative electrophysiologic and tomographic technologies are usually scaled in color but publication costs prohibited inclusion of color images. (From Finitzo, T., Pool, K.D., Freeman, F.J., Devous, M.D., Sr., & Watson, B.C. (1991). Cortical dysfunction in developmental stutterers. In H.F.M. Peters, W. Hulstijn, & C.W. Starkweather (Eds.), *Speech motor control and stuttering* (pp. 251–262). Copyright 1991 by Elsevier Science. Reprinted by permission.)

ral cortex (Hari, 1983; Scherg & Von Cramon, 1985), a region associated with language processing.

AEP analysis revealed significant amplitude reductions at all three latencies for the stuttering group; however, these differences occurred at different electrode sites. P1 and N1 group differences were significant for the left temporal recording site (T3), whereas P2 group differences were significant for the mesial frontal recording sites (F3, Fz, and F4). In addition, Finitzo and colleagues (1991) reported several systematic relations between AEP findings and clinical ratings of stuttering severity. Mild to moderate stutterers showed significant amplitude reductions at all three latencies compared to normal speakers at the Cz recording site. However, amplitudes of these components were not reduced for the severe stutterers. P1 and N1 amplitudes were reduced for all stutterers at the left temporal (T3) recording site, whereas amplitude of P2 was not reduced for severe stutterers at this site.

To summarize, QEEG findings in these twenty stutterers revealed: (1) global reduction of EEG amplitude in the Beta frequency region; (2) AEP differences for P1 and N1 that may implicate temporal cortex dysfunction; (3) AEP differences for P2 that may implicate cingulate cortex dysfunction; and (4) AEP differences that are related to stuttering severity. Although the location of P2 AEP generators is largely unknown, there is evidence for temporal and frontal contributions as well as possible thalamic involvement (Pool & Finitzo, 1989). Finally, these QEEG findings are noteworthy because resting EEG and AEP data are not contaminated by elicitation of a behavioral response and because observation of abnormalities in the processing of an auditory stimulus in a population whose salient characteristic is a motor impairment suggests that there may be something fundamentally different about the brains of persons who stutter. Neurophysiologic bases of abnormalities identified by QEEG are not clear. Further insights may arise from studies of brain blood flow and metabolism that use two other functional imaging techniques: SPECT and PET.

SPECT Findings

The success of CT techniques led to its application in nuclear medicine and the development of Emission Computed Tomography (ECT) (Chandra, 1987). Instead of detecting X rays, ECT uses radionuclides that emit single photons (SPECT) or the photons from positron annihilation (PET). The principles and technology of SPECT and PET scans are described in Chandra (1987). Briefly, a SPECT or PET image is constructed by recording gamma rays emitted by a radiopharmaceutical. Recordings are obtained by scanning thin cross-sectional areas of the brain from multiple directions. Data obtained from multiple directions are combined to produce a cross-sectional image of the scanned region. The stuttering literature contains two reports of SPECT brain imaging and two of PET imaging.

The first use of SPECT imaging to investigate brain function in stutterers of which we are aware was reported by Wood, Stump, McKeehan, Sheldon, and Proctor (1980). Two subjects were studied in resting and reading aloud conditions. These studies were repeated after the subjects received a 2-week trial of Haloperidol, a psychoactive medication that acts as a central nervous system depressant (Physicians' Desk Reference, 1991) and is used in the treatment of certain neurogenic motor control and psychiatric disorders. Wood and colleagues (1980) used SPECT imaging to test the hypothesis that stutterers have inadequate left hemisphere dominance for speech production. This hypothesis has its origins in the work of Orton and Travis. One of the subjects was a female who began stuttering after sustaining head trauma at age 13. The other subject was a male who began stuttering before age 4. Resting SPECT findings were not reported.

In the unmedicated reading-aloud condition, the female subject reportedly showed severe stuttering and higher blood flow to all right hemisphere anterior regions than to the homologous left hemisphere regions. A small left hemisphere > right hemisphere flow occurred in the region of Wernicke's area. In the medicated reading-aloud condition, this subject reportedly stuttered less and showed left hemisphere blood flow greater than right for all anterior regions as well as lower overall blood flow. The male subject did not show the same pattern of diffuse hemispheric flow asymmetries. However, he demonstrated right hemisphere > left hemisphere flow in the region of Broca's area in the unmedicated reading-aloud condition and left hemisphere > right hemisphere flow in this region during the medicated reading-aloud condition. Wood and colleagues (1980) concluded that their findings reveal "regionally specific evidence of brain mechanisms implicated in stuttering" in anterior cortex that support the proposition that stuttering "involves a lack of the expression of normal left hemisphere dominance for speech production" (Wood et al., 1980, p. 144).

Pool, Devous, Freeman, Watson, and Finitzo (1991) reported resting regional cerebral blood flow (rCBF), an index of brain metabolic activity, in twenty adult developmental stutterers. These were the same twenty adult stutterers who participated in the QEEG study reported by Finitzo and colleagues (1991). RCBF was determined by measuring the cerebral transit of ^{133}Xenon in three tomographic cross-sections oriented parallel to the canthomeatal line. Figure 7.2 shows the orientation and approximate location of these SPECT cross-sections with respect to a sagittal view of the cortex. Spatial resolution of the scans is 1.7 cm in the transverse dimension and 1.9 cm in the axial dimension. Details of data acquisition and processing can be found in Devous, Stokely, Chehabi, and Bonte (1986) and Pool and colleagues (1991). Figure 7.3 shows a SPECT cross-section obtained 6 cm above the canthomeatal line. A graphic of the standard brain outline and regions of interest (ROIs) is superimposed on the image. The 6-cm slice includes ROIs for frontal, parietal, superotemporal, occipital, and central gray matter and white matter for both hemispheres and was analyzed by Pool and colleagues (1991).

RCBF data showed absolute blood flow reductions in stutterers compared to age- and gender-matched normal controls in twenty of twenty (ten in each hemisphere) ROIs. A subsequent

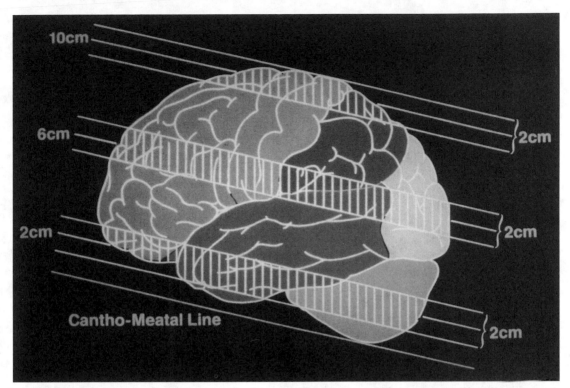

Figure 7.2 Approximate orientation and location of SPECT tomographic cross-sections superimposed on a sagittal perspective of the cortex. (Figure courtesy of Dr. M.D. Devous, Sr., University of Texas Southwestern Medical Center, Dallas, TX.)

analysis sought to identify focal rCBF reductions in the stuttering group relative to normal controls by examining relative rCBF asymmetries (left ROI/left hemisphere – right ROI/right hemisphere) as a function of ROI. Relative rCBF ratios are not gender sensitive, so a larger control group (N=78) was used for these analyses. Significant ($p < .005$, t tests corrected for multiple comparisons) relative blood flow asymmetries (left less than right) were found for the anterior cingulate, superior temporal, and middle temporal ROIs (see Figure 7.4). A similar, but not significant, asymmetry was noted for the inferior frontal ROI. Individual subject data revealed that all stutterers showed relative flow asymmetries below the normal median for the left anterior cingulate or the left middle temporal ROIs. A reduction in relative blood flow could result from cerebrovascular disease, primary alterations in neuronal activity, or both. MRI scans

of these twenty stutterers revealed no *significant* vascular anomalies. Consequently, globally reduced absolute blood flow and focal reductions in relative blood flow may reflect metabolic, or functional, anomalies in these subjects. To summarize, these twenty adult developmental stutterers showed a global reduction in absolute blood flow and focal asymmetries in relative blood flow when compared with matched normal controls. The focal rCBF asymmetries observed in these stutterers are consistent with presumed cortical centers for speech motor control (inferior frontal), language processing (middle temporal), and motor initiation (the region of anterior cingulate) and with findings reported by Wood and colleagues (1980).

RCBF asymmetries were examined (Pool et al., 1991) in the context of clinical/behavioral evaluations of stuttering severity (Riley, 1980; Ryan, 1974). Figure 7.5 shows average relative

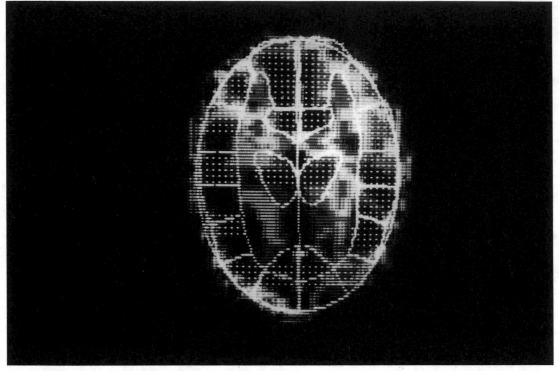

Figure 7.3 SPECT cross section at 6 cm above the canthomeatal line with graphic overlay of the standard brain outline including regions of interest. (Figure courtesy of Dr. M.D. Devous, Sr., University of Texas Southwestern Medical Center, Dallas, TX.)

rCBF asymmetry in anterior cingulate, middle temporal, and superior temporal ROIs for mild, moderate, and severe stutterers. All stutterer subgroups showed average flow asymmetries (left < right) in superior and middle temporal ROIs. However, average flow asymmetry in the anterior cingulate ROI increases with stuttering severity. Nine of ten severe stutterers showed relative flow asymmetry below the normal median value in the anterior cingulate ROI.

It is informative to consider rCBF findings for these twenty stutterers in the context of their QEEG findings described earlier. Recall that reduced Beta amplitude was observed in resting EEG spectra, whereas globally reduced blood flow was noted on rCBF analyses. Sugar and Gerard (1938) and Lennox, Gibbs, and Gibbs (1938) described the positive relationship between decreased Beta

amplitude and reduced rCBF. Thus, the global reduction in blood flow in these subjects is consistent with their reduced Beta amplitudes. Recall as well that QEEG for these twenty stutterers revealed differential brain imaging findings as a function of stuttering severity. QEEG and rCBF findings are congruent in suggesting a primarily temporal region anomaly in the mild and moderate stutterers.

The finding of anomalous cortical activity in stuttering adults in temporal, inferior frontal, and anterior cingulate regions is of particular interest because these regions are hypothesized centers for motor control and for speech and language production. Motor initiation is localized to the mesiofrontal cortex in the region of the cingulate or supplementary motor area (Goldberg, 1985), whereas motor programming for speech is localized to the left perisylvian (inferior frontal) cortex.

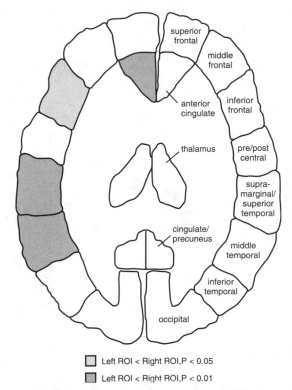

Left ROI < Right ROI, P < 0.05

Left ROI < Right ROI, P < 0.01

Figure 7.4 Schematic representation of ROIs for the SPECT scan 6 cm above the canthomeatal line. Shaded ROIs indicate loci of relative rCBF asymmetry for the stuttering group. (Adapted from Pool, K.D., Devous, M.D., Sr., Freeman, F.J., Watson, B.C., & Finitzo, T. Regional cerebral blood flow in developmental stutterers. *Archives of Neurology, 48*, 509–512. Copyright 1991, American Medical Association. Used with permission.)

Thus, one can hypothesize that those stutterers who demonstrate deficits in speech motor performance will also evidence anomalous cortical activity in regions classically related to speech motor control (anterior cingulate and inferior frontal).

With respect to anomalous temporal region findings, two hypotheses can be formulated with respect to language functioning for these stuttering subjects. First, a subgroup of stuttering individuals should exhibit linguistic performance deficits. Second, linguistic performance deficits should co-occur with rCBF asymmetry (left <

right) in those regions classically related to language processing (superior/middle temporal and inferior frontal).

Ingham, Fox, and Ingham (1994) presented preliminary PET rCBF findings for four adult stutterers and four normal speakers. PET images were obtained for resting, solo reading, and choral reading conditions. This study is part of a larger effort by Ingham and his colleagues to "use a variety of known fluency-inducing procedures to identify systematically neural regions that might be functionally associated with the presence and absence of stuttering" (Ingham et al., 1994, p. 2). All stuttering subjects demonstrated stuttering (7 to 49 stuttered events) during the solo reading condition and no stuttering during the choral reading condition. PET data were presented as the differences between neural activity recorded during each of the reading conditions and the resting condition. Normal speakers showed bilateral (left > right) activation of the primary sensorimotor cortex during both reading conditions. The stutterers showed increased neural activity in the supplementary motor area (left > right) and the superior lateral premotor cortex (right > left) during the solo reading condition. Activation of these regions was "substantially reduced or removed" during the choral reading condition. In sum, Ingham and colleagues (1994) found preliminary evidence of differences in neural activity associated with stutterers' perceptually fluent and dysfluent speech.

Wu, Maguire, Riley, Fallon, LaCasse, and colleagues (1995) also report a PET study of stutterers during solo and choral reading tasks. These investigators sought to identify alterations in brain metabolism in stutterers that could be considered "nonreversible trait differences" as well as alterations that were "state-dependent" upon the occurrence of stuttering. Wu and colleagues (1995) identified multiple regions of metabolic change and suggested that stuttering may arise from a "functional neuroanatomical circuit." A trait characteristic of this circuit appears to be a left caudate hypometabolism observed during stuttering and induced fluency. State-dependent characteristics

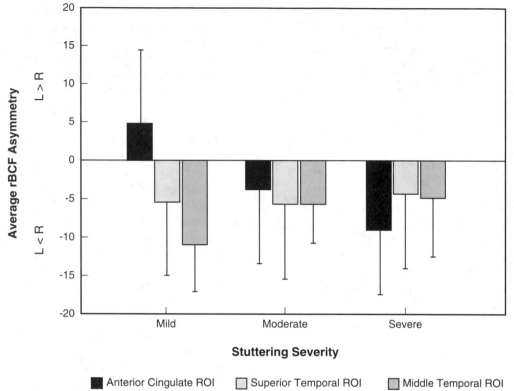

Figure 7.5 Average rCBF asymmetry for anterior cingulate, middle temporal, and superior temporal ROIs for stutterers grouped by clinical ratings of severity. Error bars represent one standard deviation. (Adapted from Pool, K.D., Devous, M.D., Sr., Freeman, F.J., Watson, B.C., & Finitzo, T. Regional cerebral blood flow in developmental stutterers. *Archives of Neurology*, *48*, 509–512. Copyright 1991, American Medical Association. Used with permission.)

include: (1) hypoactivity in Broca's area, Wernicke's area, superior frontal cortex, and the right cerebellum that normalized during induced fluency and (2) hyperactivity in substantia nigra/ventral tegmental areas and the limbic system (that is, posterior cingulate) during induced fluency. In sum, Wu and colleagues (1995) present metabolic evidence in support of a functional neurophysiologic system underlying the production of fluency that implicates cortical regions associated with speech motor control, language, and affect.

QEEG and SPECT rCBF findings reviewed above were obtained while subjects were seated quietly and not actively engaged in speech or language production tasks; conversely, PET findings revealed differences in neural activity when stutterers spoke fluently versus dysfluently. The potential significance of the QEEG and rCBF findings rests on their correlation with speech and language performance in stutterers. This correlation is considered in the following sections.

BRAIN FUNCTION AND BEHAVIORAL MEASURES OF SPEECH MOTOR AND LANGUAGE PERFORMANCE

RCBF Related to Speech Motor Performance

Watson, Pool, Devous, Freeman, and Finitzo (1992) examined rCBF findings in the context of speech motor performance. The measure of performance was acoustic laryngeal reaction time (LRT) as a function of the linguistic complexity of the required response. The theoretical framework for this analysis is a model of motor control described by Goldberg (1985). This model includes two premotor systems. The lateral system is hypothesized to be a control center for nonpropositional, repetitive speech and to function in a responsive mode to external input. This system has connections to auditory association areas in temporal cortex. The medial system is hypothesized to control extended, spontaneous speech and to function in a projectional mode with input from a predictive model. This system has connections to the cingulate cortex. Watson and colleagues (1992) reasoned that the stimulus-dependent nature of the LRT task and their manipulation of response complexity preferentially involved the lateral premotor system in Goldberg's model. Specifically, they expected stutterers with relative flow asymmetries (left < right) below the normal median in both left superior and middle temporal ROIs to show significantly longer LRT for the linguistically complex response than normal speakers and stutterers having relative flow asymmetries above the normal median value in at least one of these temporal ROIs. Goldberg's model predicts that asymmetric flows to the cingulate ROI do not affect LRT values.

RCBF and speech motor performance findings were reported for sixteen adult male developmental stutterers who were a subgroup of the twenty described by Pool and co-workers (1991). All were native speakers of American English who completed both SPECT and LRT studies. Normally fluent control subjects were drawn from published databases in the SPECT (Devous et al., 1986) and speech motor (Watson, Freeman, & Dembowski, 1991) laboratories. Stutterers' rCBF data were compared to those of seventy-eight normal controls, while their LRT data were compared to those of thirty normal controls. Stutterer and normal control groups were matched for age.

Resting rCBF and LRT data were obtained during separate sessions within a 48-hour period. RCBF procedures were described above. The LRT reaction signal was a 1-inch square light-emitting diode (LED) that was mounted at eye level approximately 1 meter from the subject. Onset of the LED served as the warning cue, and its offset was the respond cue. Variable duration preparatory intervals separated the warning and respond cues. Three response-types were studied: isolated vowel (/a/), single word (Oscar), and short sentence (Oscar took Pete's cat). The vowel is nonlinguistic because no prosodic contour is applied during its production. The word is a linguistically simple response because it requires only phonologic and semantic processes. The sentence is linguistically complex because it requires phonologic, morphophonemic, semantic, and syntactic processes. All LRT responses analyzed met perceptual criteria for fluency and were fluent by subject report.

The sixteen stutterers were divided into two subgroups: those with low relative blood flow to superior and middle temporal ROIs, and those with low relative blood flow only to either the superior or the middle temporal ROIs. Figure 7.6 shows LRT values as a function of response complexity for normal controls and these two stutterer subgroups. Significant LRT differences were found between normal controls and those stutterers with low flow to both temporal ROIs for both the word and sentence responses. Significant differences were also found between those stutterers having low flow to only one temporal ROI and those with low flow to both temporal ROIs for the sentence response. Thus, only those stutterers with low blood flow to both superior and middle temporal ROIs show a pronounced response complexity effect on LRT values. Patterns of LRT as a function of response complexity did not change when reduced blood flow to the cingulate ROI was considered in combination with temporal flow findings for the stutterer groups.

The relation between rCBF and speech motor performance reported by Watson et al. (1992) is consistent with predictions of Goldberg's (1985) model regarding defects in the lateral premotor system (see also Dembowski & Watson, 1991). Goldberg's model has been invoked by others to explain stuttering behaviors (Caruso, Abbs, & Gracco, 1988; Webster, 1988); however, they hypothesized that abnormality of the medial premotor system was the mechanism underlying stuttering. The discrepancy

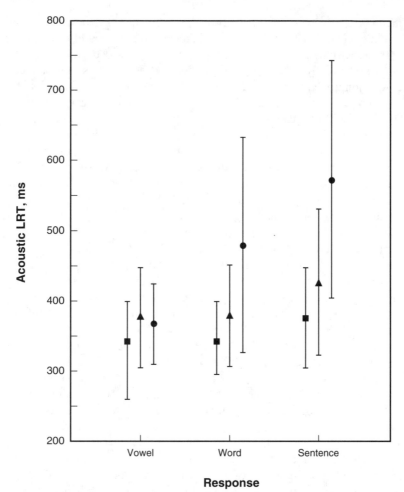

Figure 7.6 Acoustic laryngeal reaction time as a function of response complexity for nonstutterers (■), stutterers with reduced relative rCBF to left superior *or* middle temporal ROIs (▲), and stutterers with reduced relative rCBF to left superior *and* middle temporal ROIs (●). Values are shown as means ± one standard deviation. (From Watson, B.C., Pool, K.D., Devous, M.D., Sr., Freeman, F.J., & Finitzo, T. (1992). Brain blood flow related to acoustic laryngeal reaction time in adult developmental stutterers. *Journal of Speech and Hearing Research*, *35*, 555–561. Reprinted by permission of the American Speech-Language-Hearing Association.)

among these conclusions can be resolved if one considers the differential functions of the two premotor systems in Goldberg's model. Specifically, reaction time tasks may preferentially tap processes mediated by the lateral system (as noted above), whereas spontaneous speech tasks may preferentially tap the medial system. The concept of functionally specific

motor systems embodied in Goldberg's model suggests that the well-documented heterogeneity of the stuttering population may result from differences in the presence, loci, and relative magnitude of neurophysiolgic abnormalities in multiple CNS regions (cortical, subcortical, or both) subserving speech motor control.

RCBF Related to Linguistic Performance

Watson, Freeman, Devous, Chapman, Finitzo, and Pool (1994) tested the hypothesis that a subgroup of linguistically impaired adults who stutter will also demonstrate cortical blood flow asymmetries in cortical regions classically related to language processing (that is, superior temporal, middle temporal, and inferior frontal). RCBF and linguistic performance findings were reported for sixteen adult males who stutter and for ten adult nonstutterers. The groups were matched for age. The sixteen stuttering subjects represent a subgroup of the twenty described by Finitzo and co-workers (1991) and Pool and colleagues (1991), who had completed both SPECT and linguistic performance studies. The ten nonstuttering subjects reported no history of speech, language, hearing, or neurologic disorder. No subject reported taking psychoactive medications.

Details of linguistic performance testing are in Watson et al. (1994). Each subject's language skills were evaluated using tasks that assess relatively high-level production and comprehension processes. Discourse production was evaluated by an analysis of three stories told by the subjects using a discourse grammar that models the core information components essential to story structure (Labov & Waletsky, 1967). Components include setting, complicating action, and resolution.

Discourse comprehension was evaluated using two measures. One measure consisted of questions to probe comprehension of the complex story used in the production task. The second measure assessed subjects' ability to identify noun referents for pronouns within a different set of short stories read aloud by an examiner. Referents were major characters in the stories who were identifiable through the use of subtle linguistic cues within the text. A third task assessed subjects' ability to disambiguate grammatically or lexically ambiguous sentences (for example, "The duck is ready to eat."). Each subject's number of errors across all linguistic assessments was transformed into a z score relative

to the error mean and standard deviation of the ten nonstutterers. Subjects whose z score was greater than 3.0 were classified as linguistically impaired.

All nonstuttering subjects were classified as linguistically normal; six stutterers were identified as linguistically normal; ten stutterers were identified as linguistically impaired. Mean age of the linguistically normal subgroup of stutterers (44 ± 8.6) was significantly greater than the linguistically impaired subgroup (35 ± 6.3) [$t(14) = 2.35$, $p< 0.05$]. Mean years of education for the linguistically normal subgroup (15 ± 2.7) and for the linguistically impaired subgroup (14.5 ± 2.9) was not significantly different. Stuttering severity did not differ between the two groups of stutterers.

Figure 7.7 summarizes the distribution of errors across linguistic assessments by group. Nonstutterers showed the greatest percentage of errors on the ambiguous pronoun (7 of 19, 37%) and complex story expression (6 of 19, 32%) tasks. Linguistically normal stutterers showed the greatest percentage of errors on the sentence disambiguation (5 of 13, 38%) and ambiguous pronoun (4 of 13, 31%) tasks. Linguistically impaired stutterers showed greatest percentage of errors on the complex comprehension (37 of 111, 33%) and complex expression (32 of 111, 29%) tasks.

Between-group comparisons of rCBF data were performed for the four cortical regions identified by Pool et al. (1991) as showing asymmetric blood flow and that are classically associated with speech and language production (i.e., superior temporal, medial temporal, inferior frontal, and anterior cingulate).

Three comparisons were conducted: nonstutterers versus linguistically normal stutterers; nonstutterers versus linguistically impaired stutterers; and linguistically normal versus linguistically impaired stutterers. Scores for each subject were classified as above or below the median value for the combined data of the two groups being compared. This required calculation of a new median value for each between-group comparison.

Comparisons of the ten nonstutterers and six linguistically normal stutterers revealed no signifi-

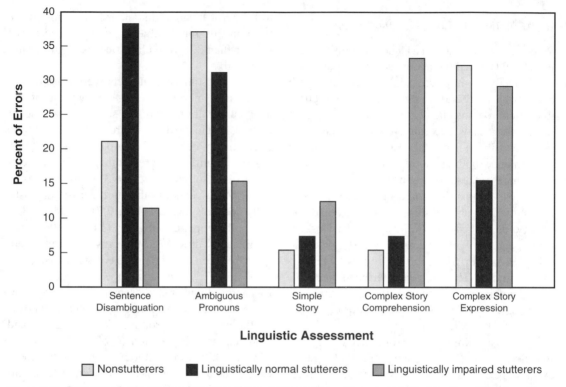

Figure 7.7   Percent of errors as a function of linguistic performance assessment for linguistically normal nonstutterers, linguistically normal stutterers, and linguistically impaired stutterers. (Adapted from Watson, B.C., Freeman, F.J., Devous, M.D., Sr., Chapman, S.B., Finitzo, T., & Pool, K.D. (1994). Linguistic performance and regional cerebral blood flow in persons who stutter. *Journal of Speech and Hearing Research*, *37*, 1221–1228. Reprinted by permission of the American Speech-Language-Hearing Association.)

cant differences in relative blood flow asymmetry for any of the four ROIs ($p > 0.05$). Comparisons of the ten nonstutterers and ten linguistically impaired stutterers revealed significant differences in relative blood flow asymmetry (L < R) for the middle temporal ($p < 0.025$) and inferior frontal ($p < 0.025$) ROIs. The linguistically impaired stutterers showed, on average, 11 percent lower rCBF in the left middle temporal ROI and 7 percent lower rCBF in the left inferior frontal ROI compared to the respective contralateral ROIs than did nonstutterers. Comparisons between linguistically normal and linguistically impaired stutterers revealed a significant difference in relative blood flow asymmetry (L < R) for the middle temporal ROI only ($p < 0.025$). The linguistically impaired stutterers

showed, on average, 11 percent lower rCBF in the left middle temporal ROI compared to the contralateral ROI than did linguistically normal stutterers.

The patterns of rCBF asymmetry observed in association with linguistic performance deficits are consistent with brain imaging findings that suggest a temporal lobe abnormality in a subgroup of stutterers (Finitzo et al., 1991; Pool et al., 1991; Rosenfield & Jerger, 1984). The finding that linguistic performance deficits in these stutterers are associated with asymmetric flows to the temporal region indicates that theories that attempt to explain fluency failures in stutterers must extend beyond speech motor processing to include language processing.

A CAVEAT: THERE IS STRENGTH IN NUMBERS

The brain imaging studies reviewed here are preliminary. Several have generated controversy (Fox, Lancaster, & Ingham, 1993; Pool, Finitzo, Devous, Freeman, & Watson, 1992; Pool, Finitzo, Devous, Watson, & Freeman, 1993; Viswanath, Rosenfield, & Nudelman, 1992). By far, the greatest limitation with respect to the theoretical significance of their findings is the small number of subjects studied. This limitation is particularly important in light of the subgroups of stutterers suggested by the findings. The validity of these subgroupings and of any conclusions based on comparisons among subgroups rests upon replication of these studies with larger samples.

With this caution in mind, it is worth noting that the design of the functional imaging studies reported by Finitzo et al. (1991) and Pool et al. (1991) strengthens the internal validity of their findings. First, subjects were studied using two different brain imaging technologies: one electrophysiologic and the other metabolic. The congruence of findings for the QEEG and SPECT studies (e.g., reduced Beta amplitudes on QEEG associated with hypoperfusion on SPECT) suggests that the observed phenomena are real. Second, imaging studies were combined with behavioral studies. The association between SPECT rCBF findings and behavioral findings with respect to speech and language performance for subgroups of stutterers is consistent with classic anatomoclinical principles of the cortical organization of speech and language.

TENTATIVE CONCLUSIONS AND IMPLICATIONS

These structural and functional brain imaging findings and their relation to speech and language performance in adult developmental stutterers permit several tentative conclusions. First, the majority of adult developmental stutterers examined have either no or relatively subtle cortical or subcortical structural anomalies. There are no obvious lesions or signs of degenerative disease. Second, most of these adult stutterers show some degree of anomalous brain function on electrophysiologic and/or metabolic imaging procedures. Third, anomalous brain functions are multifocal and involve cortical regions classically associated with speech motor (anterior cingulate and inferior frontal) and language (temporal) processing. Fourth, anomalies identified during resting brain imaging studies are consistent with deficits in speech motor and language performance.

According to D.R. Hofstadter (1980), theories must be subjected to a simple test: A meaningless interpretation is one that fails to posit any isomorphic connection between theorems of the system and reality. Under a meaningful interpretation, theorems and truths correspond; that is, an isomorphism exists between theorems and some portion of reality. Our next task is to see whether findings reviewed here permit us to propose a theory from which we can draw meaningful interpretations.

The findings of significant QEEG changes at left hemisphere sites (Finitzo et al., 1991), regional blood flow asymmetries, with left hemisphere flows relatively lower than right (Pool et al., 1991), and PET abnormalities in Broca's and Wernicke's areas (Wu et al., 1995) could lead to a reconsideration of older theories, such as those proposed by Orton and Travis, or of Kussmaul's nineteenth century aphasia/stuttering hypothesis. We believe that recent evidence provides a rationale for combining neurogenic (acquired) stuttering and developmental stuttering under one theoretical umbrella. These findings also support the integration of several contemporary theories of stuttering. To illustrate this point, we can refer to the table of contents of the first edition of this text. The following chapters appeared in the section entitled Theoretical Perspectives of Stuttering: "Stuttering as a Genetic Disorder" (Kidd, 1984)—the neurophysiologic abnormalities identified in these studies could have a basis in genetic inheritance; "Stuttering as a Cognitive-Linguistic Disorder" (Hamre, 1984)—these data support the existence of, at least, a linguistic component in stuttering; "Stuttering as a

Sequencing and Timing Disorder" (MacKay & MacDonald, 1984)—cortical abnormalities in temporal and cingulate regions are consistent with this perspective; "Stuttering as a Temporal Programming Disorder" (Kent, 1984)—again, findings support this perspective.

When brain imaging findings are examined in the broader context of speech motor and linguistic performance, the perspectives represented by the chapters cited above merge into a coherent picture of a neurophysiologic system that integrates cognitive, linguistic, and speech motor processes for the production of fluency. Wingate (1988, p. 267) implied the existence of such a system when he stated, "Stuttering is not simply a problem of words per se, but of words as the pivotal elements in a system that can transduce ideas and thoughts into an audible code—speech." Nudelman, Herbrich, Hoyt, and Rosenfield (1991) presented a model of stuttering that includes motor control and linguistic processing systems, and Wu et al. (1995) offered a neuroanatomic map of such a system.

In keeping with a systems perspective, stuttering can be considered as one symptom of a defect in a fluent speech generating system; a system that is diffusely represented in the central nervous system and includes motoric, linguistic, and cognitive processing. This perspective motivates development of theories and models that go beyond stuttering/disfluency and seek a more global understanding of the processes and neural bases of fluency. A simple example of such a model is illustrated schematically in Figure 7.8. In its most basic form, this system has three component processes: cognitive, linguistic, and speech motor.

At the Cognitive level, the communicative intent or motivation for an utterance exists. Thoughts, ideas, and feelings that underlie the drive to communicate are processed and, to varying degrees, are formulated and organized into conscious experience. Important influences at this level are the speaker's perceptions of himself, his message, his listener(s), and the communicative situation. A variety of cognitive processes subserved by perception, memory, experience, and affect (Miller, 1993) are involved. At the Linguistic level, the "message"

is encoded through both segmental and supra-segmental processing. Semantic selection and lexical retrieval occur. Syntactic and grammatical formulations are active. Semantic and syntactic sequences are encoded as phonologic and prosodic sequences. The Speech Motor level consists of both a preprogramming/programming stage and an execution stage. In the preprogramming/programming stage, the linguistic message (including both segmental and supra-segmental aspects) is encoded as phonetic and neuro-motor patterns. In the execution stage, these neuromotor patterns are realized as a sequence of muscle contractions and articulatory gestures. Experimental findings reviewed above point to an association between impairments in shaded component processes and abnormalities at shaded neuroanatomic sites in Figure 7.8.

All of these component processes must be efficient, synchronized, and fully integrated to generate optimal fluency. Some degradation in fluency will result if a component process is delayed or if integration or synchrony among components is disrupted. Fluency can thus be viewed as a reflection of the functional integrity and coordination of the components of the system. Impaired fluency reflects inefficiency or dysfunction in some component process, disruption in the integration of components, or both. Disorders of fluency could arise from differing forms of disruption at one or more sites within the neurological system (shown as the neuroanatomic sites in Figure 7.8) subserving these processes (see also McClean, 1990 for a discussion of potential neurophysiologic systems underlying fluency and stuttering). The shaded sites in Figure 7.8 are supported by brain imaging findings reviewed here.

Patterns of fluency failure offer insight into the neurophysiologic system and the nature of different fluency disorders. For example, while stuttering and cluttering are generally considered the primary disorders of fluency, aphasias are defined clinically by the binary categories of "fluent" and "nonfluent." Comparisons among these clinical populations may reveal important neurophysiologic similarities (for example, see Finitzo et al., 1991). Of course, impairments of fluency are not

Conceptual Model of Fluency

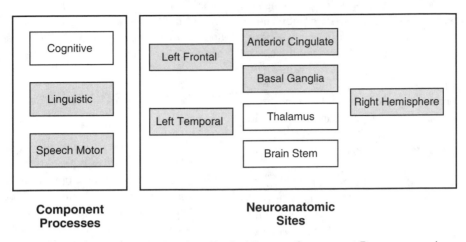

Figure 7.8   A schematic model of oral/verbal fluency. Component Processes and Neuroanatomic Systems are indicated. See text for details.

limited to the specific disorders of fluency. Application of a broader definition of fluency can lead to characterization of different degrees and types of fluency impairment in many disorders of communication. For example, the spoken (and in some cases, the written) language disabilities of dementia, psychosis, deafness, head trauma, developmental disorders of language or intelligence, neuroses of public speaking or "stage-fright," Parkinson's disease, dysarthria, laryngectomy, or right hemisphere stroke may demonstrate impaired or significantly degraded fluency.

Intra- and intersubject variations in fluency are well recognized both for disordered populations and "normal" speakers; however, the ability to quantify or otherwise reliably measure degree of fluency is virtually nonexistent. Standard measurement tools and behavioral definitions of the characteristics of fluency are lacking. The search for perception and production variables that comprise the construct of fluency can be guided by a general model of fluency, such as that shown in Figure 7.8. With that in mind, it may be useful to discuss fluency with reference to current models of the normal speech and language production process.

Starkweather (1987, 1993) has offered a par-

tial approach. He proposes a model of speech fluency that includes the dimensions of continuity, rate, effort, duration of segments, and coarticulation. Starkweather (1987) explicitly excludes linguistic processes from his model, stating, "Language fluency does not seem to be a part of the problem of stuttering. Adult speakers who stutter have not been shown to lack syntactic, semantic, pragmatic, or phonologic knowledge or skill, although few tests of these propositions have ever been made" (pp. 11–12). Findings reviewed here suggest that Starkweather's (1987) model of fluency should not have neglected the role of linguistic processes.

Other models (Borden & Harris, 1990; Levelt, 1989; Perkins, Kent, & Curlee, 1991) explicitly recognize that efficient integration of cognitive, linguistic, and motoric processes is critical to successful oral/verbal expression. For example, Levelt's (1989) model of the generation of fluent speech includes several "processing components" that are activated in the evolution from a speaker's communicative intent at the cognitive level to neuromuscular commands at the articulatory level. Levelt's model also includes error detection and correction components. Normal fluency occurs when operations within each processing component are accomplished successfully and efficiently. By implication, each processing component in Levelt's model is susceptible to disruption and is, therefore, a potential source of fluency failure. This implication is presented formally as the covert repair hypothesis (Postma & Kolk, 1993, Kolk & Postma, Chapter 9) which maps overt (stuttered or nonstuttered) disfluency types to errors at specific points in the utterance-formulation process and to the speaker's repair strategy.

Our understanding of fluency can be expanded by empirical tests of the models presented by Levelt (1989) and Perkins et al. (1991). The discussion by Postma and Kolk (1993) lays the foundation for such tests, and a study by Wolk, Edwards, and Conture (1993) illustrates one approach. Wolk et al. (1993) described two subgroups of children who stutter: a phonologically normal subgroup and a phonologically impaired subgroup. They speculated that their findings provide "partial support to the notion of two forms of stuttering—one that co-occurs with (and perhaps is dependent upon) disordered phonology and one that is independent of disordered phonology" (Wolk et al., 1993, p. 915). These forms of stuttering would be differentiated by the locus and type of disruption in the process of fluency generation.

Our understanding of the fluency failures identified as stuttering should benefit from investigating stuttering in the context of other disorders of fluency and from advances in the technology of brain imaging. Comparison of different clinical populations (for example, stuttering, aphasia, and cognitive impairment) on the same measures of motoric, linguistic, and cognitive performance and of CNS structure and function may elucidate the processes underlying production of fluency and consequences of their failure. We recall, once again, Wingate (1988) who concludes, "There are many parallels between stuttering and aphasia, ordinarily not clearly evident, that become discernible once the parameters of comparison are brought into focus" (p. 266). Present findings suggest that relevant "parameters of comparison" on which to focus include cognitive and linguistic processes. Additional insights are likely to accrue through application of new analytic approaches to brain imaging data and new imaging techniques.

AN IMAGE OF THE FUTURE

MRI

Traditional MRI offers excellent spatial resolution of brain structure, but no information on brain function. Recent development of functional MRI (fMRI) provides noninvasive measures of brain function by imaging fluid (blood or cerebrospinal fluid) displacement (Moonen, van Zijl, Frank, Le Bihan, & Becker, 1990). FMRI techniques yield high resolution images of coherent (vascular blood flow or circulation of cerebrospinal fluid) and incoherent (diffusion) fluid displacement. Finally, certain fMRI applications use contrast agents to change the magnetic properties of water hydrogen atoms, which permits assessment of cerebral perfusion, an indicator of increased neuronal activity.

FMRI has several advantages as a tool for stuttering research. Foremost of these is that fMRI is the only metabolic brain imaging technique that does not require ionizing radiation. Thus, repeat fMRI scans can be can obtained safely to monitor functional changes over time; for example, changes associated with experimental drug treatment of stuttering (Ludlow & Braun, 1993). FMRI and conventional MRI scans can be obtained in a single imaging session to allow direct comparison of structural and functional information. Two major limitations of current technology for speech research are the noise produced by this instrumentation and movement artifacts resulting from speech production.

QEEG

Conventional analyses of EEG signals, whether through visual inspection or topographic and quantitative techniques, are guided by the assumption that "the EEG is a very complex signal, hence it must be produced by a very complex system that can only be described in stochastic terms" (Pradhan & Dutt, 1993, p. 427). However, this assumption is being challenged by a new approach arising from nonlinear dynamics and chaos theory. The nonlinear approach to EEG analysis assumes that, "The EEG is a very complex signal, hence it may be produced by a simple, *but nonlinear* (emphasis added) system" (Pradhan & Dutt, 1993, p. 427). The output of a nonlinear system is determined completely by a set of system properties and initial conditions, but accurate prediction of this output is limited. The possibility that a relatively simple nonlinear system may account for complex features seen in EEG signals for normal and pathological subjects has implications for new methods of quantifying EEG as well as for models of the neurophysiologic basis of EEG.

The application of chaos theory and of fractal analysis (Goldberger & West, 1987) to EEG signals is relatively recent, and critical methodological issues are not resolved (Rapp, Bashore, Zimmerman, Martinerie, Albano, & Mees, 1990). The potential value of this approach lies in the focus that nonlinear dynamics places on the system that generates the signal, rather than on the signal itself (Rapp et al., 1990). This focus may reveal patterns of brain function that are unique to stuttering or that are shared among disorders of fluency.

SPECT

Advances in technology and the introduction of new techniques in dynamic SPECT brain imaging hold the promise for improved spatial and temporal resolution in identifying loci of CNS abnormality, particularly in subcortical regions, and for well-controlled studies of brain function at rest and during speech and language performance. The new generation SPECT scanners combine improved spatial resolution with full-volume imaging (Devous, 1992). Scans are no longer limited to discrete transverse sections and can include the entire brain volume. Consequently, the brain can be represented in sagittal or coronal as well as transverse orientations, and abnormalities may be identified on sagittal or coronal sections that were not discernible on transverse sections. Full volume brain scans also permit construction of three-dimensional SPECT images.

A second important advance in SPECT imaging is the ability to combine SPECT images of brain function with MRI or CT images of brain structure. Image coregistration permits the construction of a structure/function map of a particular brain region for each individual subject. This technique also facilitates comparison of an individual subject's scan to those of a normal group and comparisons among subject subgroups. This latter capability may yield important insights into neurophysiologic bases of heterogeneity within the stuttering population by allowing comparisons among subgroups of stutterers who differ on clinical indices of severity and typology of dysfluency.

A third important advance in SPECT imaging is the development of dual isotope imaging (Devous, Payne, & Lowe, 1992). This technique permits acquisition of two image sets during a single scan. The two scans are directly comparable since subject placement artifacts are eliminated. The full potential of the dual isotope technique is realized by the fact that radiopharmaceuticals used for SPECT scans represent brain function at the time of their administration rather than the time of the scan (Devous, 1992). The significance of this technique for stuttering research can be appreciated by considering the relation between resting rCBF and acoustic LRT described earlier. Recall that the subgroup of stutterers who showed relative rCBF asymmetry to left temporal regions at rest also showed normal LRT for vowel responses and prolonged LRT for sentence responses. With the dual isotope scan technique, one radiopharmaceutical can be administered during the vowel condition and a second radiopharmaceutical during the sentence condition. A subsequent analysis of the SPECT scan might reveal differential patterns of blood flow associated with response complexity and provide insights into neurophysiologic processes underlying stutterers' speech motor control.

Magnetoencephalography

Magnetoencephalography (MEG) is the study of the brain's magnetic field. The device used to obtain images is the superconducting quantum interference device (SQUID). A SQUID detects very small changes in magnetic fields and has been described as "the most sensitive detector of any kind available to scientists" (Clarke, 1994, p. 46). The application of a SQUID to brain imaging is based on the fact that electric currents, such as those resulting from nerve conduction, produce time-varying magnetic signals. Thus, an array of SQUID sensors can map spatial variations in magnetic fields produced by neural activity. This information can be used to reconstruct the region that produced the signals. For example, SQUID imaging can locate, very accurately, sources of electrical discharge associated with seizures. Coregistration of SQUID and MRI images permits anatomic localization of abnormality. SQUID imaging can also be applied to the study of CNS responses to stimulation in a manner analogous to evoked potential studies. The sensitivity of SQUID is such that a temporal resolution of 79 ms and a spatial resolution of 9 mm are reported for an auditory EP condition (Gallen & Bloom, 1993). Theoretical and analytical models of SQUID are being developed and refined. As this technology matures, SQUID may offer a sensitive, noninvasive (and nonionizing) alternative for functional brain imaging studies in stuttering.

SUMMARY

Recent evidence from brain imaging studies provides a coherent, albeit preliminary, view that stuttering occurs when a neurophysiologic system that integrates motoric, linguistic, and cognitive processes fails. This view is not fundamentally different from that voiced by Hartley, Combe, and Kussmal in the eighteenth and nineteenth centuries.

Investigation of the nature of this system should be the goal of stuttering research into the next century. Replication studies are needed to establish the validity of current findings and to elucidate neural mechanisms of failure of the proposed fluency-generating system. These studies must include larger sample sizes and complementary combinations of imaging techniques. Creative paradigms will be necessary and should include resting and performance tasks. Each brain imaging technology described above has specific strengths and weaknesses. For example, QEEG provides good temporal resolution for the study of electrophysiologic events recorded at the scalp, but poor spatial resolution regarding the cortical or subcortical origins of these events. SPECT and PET provide good spatial resolution of blood flow and metabolic activity throughout the cortex and subcortex, but poor temporal resolution. Future studies that combine the strengths of QEEG and SPECT or PET will overcome the limitations of each technology. FMRI is a potentially valuable research tool because there is no exposure to ionizing radiation. The ability to conduct repeated studies using fMRI has application for documenting neurophysiologic changes associated with the development or remediation of stuttering. Furthermore, the ability to obtain fMRI and conventional MRI scans in a single imaging session facilitates assessment of brain function and structure. Good spatial and temporal resolution and a lack of exposure to ionizing radiation make MEG a valuable tool for stuttering research.

Insights gained from future brain imaging studies may permit specification of a comprehensive neurophysiologic model of both fluent and dysfluent spoken language. Such a model may stimulate development of new strategies for the prevention and treatment of a variety of speech and language disorders whose shared characteristic is abnormal fluency.

REFERENCES

Bloodstein, O. (1983). *Handbook on stuttering* (Third edition). Chicago: The National Easter Seal Society.

Borden, G., & Harris, K. (1990). *Speech science primer: Physiology, acoustics, and perception of speech*. Baltimore: Williams & Wilkins.

Caruso, A.J., Abbs, J., & Gracco, V. (1988). Kinematic analysis of multiple movement coordination during speech in stutterers. *Brain, 111*, 439–455.

Chandra, R. (1987). *Introductory physics of nuclear medicine*. Philadelphia: Lea & Febiger.

Clarke, J. (1994). SQUIDs. *Scientific American*, August, 46–53.

Dembowski, J., & Watson, B.C. (1991). Acoustic reaction time related to models of central nervous system function. In H.F.M. Peters, W. Hulstijn, & C.W. Starkweather (Eds.) *Speech motor control and stuttering* (pp. 263–268). Amsterdam: Elsevier.

Devous, M.D., Sr. (1992). Comparison of SPECT applications in neurology and psychiatry. *Journal of Clinical Psychiatry, 53* (suppl 11), 13–19.

Devous, M.D., Sr. (1995). SPECT functional brain imaging. In F.I. Kramer & J. Sanger (Eds.), *Clinical applications of SPECT*. New York: Raven Press.

Devous, M.D., Sr., Payne, J.K., & Lowe, J.L. (1992). Dual-isotope brain SPECT imaging with Technetium-99m and iodine-123: Clinical validation using Xenon-123 SPECT. *The Journal of Nuclear Medicine, 33*, 1919–1924.

Devous, M.D., Sr., Stokely, E.M., Chehabi, H.H., & Bonte, F.J. (1986). Normal distribution of regional cerebral blood flow measured by dynamic single-photon emission tomography. *Journal of Cerebral Blood Flow and Metabolism, 6*, 95–104.

Finitzo, T., Pool, K.D., Freeman, F.J., Devous, M.D., Sr., & Watson, B.C. (1991). Cortical dysfunction in developmental stutterers. In H.F.M. Peters, W. Hulstijn, & C.W. Starkweather (Eds.), *Speech motor control and stuttering* (pp. 251–262) Amsterdam: Elsevier.

Fox, P.T., Lancaster, J.L., & Ingham, R.J. (1993). On stuttering and global ischemia—letter to the Editor, *Archives of Neurology, 50*, 1287–1288.

Gallen, C.C., & Bloom, F.E. (1993). Mapping the brain with MRI. *Current Biology, 3*, 522–524.

Goldberg, G. (1985). Supplementary motor area structure and function: Review and hypotheses. *The Behavioral and Brain Sciences, 8*, 567–616.

Goldberger, A.L., & West, B.J. (1987). Fractals in physiology and medicine. *Yale Journal of Biology and Medicine, 60*, 421–435.

Hamre, C.E. (1984). Stuttering as a cognitive-linguistic disorder. In R.F. Curlee & W.H. Perkins (Eds.), *Nature and treatment of stuttering: New directions*. (pp. 237–260). San Diego: College Hill Press, Inc.

Hari, R. (1983). Auditory evoked magnetic fields of the human brain. *Revue Laryngology Otology Rhinology, 104*, 143–148.

Hofstadter, D.R. (1980). *Gödel, Escher, Bach: An eternal golden braid*. New York: Vintage Books.

Ingham, R.J., Fox, P.T., & Ingham, J.C. (1994). Brain image investigation of the speech of stutterers and nonstutterers. *Asha, 36*, 188.

Kent, R.D. (1984). Stuttering as a temporal programming disorder. In R.F. Curlee & W.H. Perkins (Eds.), *Nature and treatment of stuttering: New directions* (pp. 283–302). San Diego: College Hill Press, Inc.

Kidd, K.K. (1984). Stuttering as a genetic disorder. In R.F. Curlee & W.H. Perkins (Eds.), *Nature and treatment of stuttering: New directions* (pp. 149–170). San Diego: College Hill Press, Inc.

Kussmaul, A. (1887). Die Storungen der Sprache. In H. Ziemssen (Ed.), *Cyclopaedia Medica*. Reported in Van Riper, C. (1982). *The nature of stuttering* (Second edition). Englewood Cliffs, NJ: Prentice Hall.

Labov, W. & Waletsky, J. (1967). Narrative analysis: Oral version of personal experience. In J. Helm (Ed.), *Essays on the verbal and visual arts* (pp. 12–44). Seattle: University of Washington Press.

Lehmann, D. (1989). Functional states of the brain and brain electrical fields. In K. Maurer (Ed.), *Topographic brain mapping of EEG and evoked potentials* (pp. 53–75). Berlin: Springer Verlag.

Lennox, W.G., Gibbs, F.A., & Gibbs, E.L. (1938). The relationship in man of cerebral activity to blood flow and to blood constituents. *Journal of Neurology and Psychiatry, 1*, 211–225.

Levelt, W.J.M. (1989). *Speaking: From intention to articulation*. Cambridge: MIT Press.

Ludlow, C.L., & Braun, A. (1993). Research evaluating the use of neuropharmacological agents for treating stuttering: Possibilities and problems. *Journal of Fluency Disorders, 18*, 169–182.

MacKay, D.G., & MacDonald, M.C. (1984). Stuttering as a sequencing and timing disorder. In R.F. Curlee & W.H. Perkins (Eds.), *Nature and treatment of stuttering: New directions* (pp. 261–282). San Diego: College Hill Press, Inc.

McClean, M. (1990). Neuromotor aspects of stuttering: Levels of impairment and disability. In J.A. Cooper (Ed.), *Research needs in stuttering: Roadblocks and future directions* (pp. 64–71). Rockville, MD: ASHA.

Miller, S. (1993). *Multiple measures of anxiety and psychophysiologic arousal in stutterers and nonstutterers during nonspeech and speech tasks of increasing complexity.* Unpublished doctoral dissertation, The University of Texas at Dallas, Dallas.

Moonen, C.T., van Zijl, P.C.M., Frank, J.A., Le Bihan, D., & Becker, E.D. (1990). Functional magnetic resonance imaging in medicine and physiology. *Science, 250*, 53–60.

Moore, W.H., Jr. (1984). Central nervous system characteristics of stutterers. In R.F. Curlee & W.H. Perkins (Eds.), *Nature and treatment of stuttering: New directions* (pp. 49–72). San Diego: College Hill Press, Inc.

Moore, W.H., Jr. (1990). Pathophysiology of stuttering: Cerebral activation differences in stutterers vs. nonstutterers. In J.A. Cooper (Ed.), *Research needs in stuttering: Roadblocks and future directions* (pp. 72–80). Rockville, MD: ASHA.

Newhouse, J., & Wiener, J. (1991). *Understanding MRI.* Boston: Little, Brown & Co.

Nudelman, H.B., Herbrich, K.E., Hoyt, B.D., & Rosenfield, D.B. (1991). A neuroscience approach to stuttering. In H.F.M. Peters, W. Hulstijn, & C.W. Starkweather (Eds.), *Speech motor control and stuttering* (pp. 157–162). Amsterdam: Elsevier.

Office of Technology Assessment (1978). *Policy implications of the computed tomography (CT) scanner.* Washington, DC: U.S. Government Printing Office.

Orton, S.T. (1927). Studies in stuttering. *Archives of Neurology and Psychiatry, 18*, 671–672.

Perkins, W., Kent, R.D., & Curlee, R.F. (1991). A theory of neurolinguistic function in stuttering. *Journal of Speech and Hearing Research, 34*, 734–752.

Physicians' Desk Reference (1991). Oradell: Medical Economics Data.

Pinsky, S.D., & McAdam, D.W. (1980). Electroencephalographic and dichotic indices of cerebral laterality in stutterers. *Brain and Language, 11*, 374–397.

Pool, K.D., Devous, M.D., Sr., Freeman, F.J., Watson, B.C., & Finitzo, T. (1991). Regional cerebral blood flow in developmental stutterers. *Archives of Neurology, 48*, 509–512.

Pool, K., Freeman, F.J., & Finitzo, T. (1985). Brain electrical activity mapping: Applications to vocal motor control disorders. In H.F.M. Peters & W. Hulstijn (Eds.), *Speech motor dynamics in stuttering* (pp. 151–160). Wien: Springer-Verlag.

Pool, K.D., & Finitzo, T. (1989). Three-dimensional dipole localization of auditory evoked potentials: A videotape presentation. San Francisco: American Association for the Advancement of Science, January.

Pool, K.D., Finitzo, T., Devous, M.D., Sr., Freeman, F.J., & Watson, B.C. (1992). Stutterers and cerebral blood flow—in reply. *Archives of Neurology, 49*, 347–348.

Pool, K.D., Finitzo, T., Devous, M.D., Sr., Watson, B.C., & Freeman, F.J. (1993). On stuttering and global ischemia—in reply. *Archives of Neurology, 50*, 1289–1290.

Postma, A., & Kolk, H. (1993). The covert repair hypothesis: Prearticulatory repair processes in normal and stutterers disfluencies. *Journal of Speech and Hearing Research, 36*, 472–487.

Pradhan, N., & Dutt, D.N. (1993). A nonlinear perspective in understanding the neurodynamics of EEG. *Computers in Biology and Medicine, 23*, 425–442.

Prescott, J. (1988). Event-related potential indices of speech motor programming in stutterers and nonstutterers. *Biological Psychology, 27*, 259–273.

Prescott, J., & Andrews, G. (1984). Early and late components of the contingent negative variation prior to manual and speech responses in stutterers and non-stutterers. *International Journal of Psychophysiology, 2*, 121–130.

Rapp, P.E., Bashore, T.R., Zimmerman, I.D., Martinerie, J.M., Albano, A.M., & Mees, A.I. (1990). Dynamical characterization of brain electrical activity. In S. Krasner (Ed.), *The ubiquity of chaos* (pp. 10–22). Washington, DC: AAAS.

Reiber, R.W., & Wollock, J. (1977). The historical roots of the theory and therapy of stuttering. In R.W. Reiber (Ed.), *The problem of stuttering: Theory and therapy* (pp. 3–24). New York: Elsevier.

Rosenbeck, J.C. (1984). Stuttering secondary to nervous system damage. In R.F. Curlee & W.H. Perkins (Eds.), *Nature and treatment of stuttering: New directions* (pp. 31–48). San Diego: College Hill Press, Inc.

Riley, G. (1980). *Stuttering severity instrument for children and adults: Revised edition.* Tigerd, OR: C.C. Publications, Inc.

Rosenfield, D., & Jerger, J. (1984). Stuttering and auditory function. In R.F. Curlee & W.H. Perkins (Eds.), *Nature and treatment of stuttering: New directions.* (pp. 73–87). San Diego: College Hill.

Ryan, B. (1974). *Programmed therapy for stuttering in children and adults.* Springfield, IL: Charles C. Thomas.

Scherg, M., & Von Cramon, D. (1985). Two bilateral sources of the late AEP as identified by a spatiotemporal dipole model. *EEG Clinical Neurophysiology, 32–44.*

Starkweather, C.W. (1987). *Fluency and stuttering.* Englewood Cliffs: Prentice Hall.

Starkweather, C.W. (1993). Issues in the efficacy of treatment for fluency disorders. *Journal of Fluency Disorders, 2&3,* 151–168.

Strub, R.L., Black, F.W., & Naeser, M.A. (1987). Anomalous dominance in sibling stutterers. Evidence from CT scan asymmetries, dichotic listening, neurophysiological testing, and handedness. *Brain and Language, 30,* 338–350.

Sugar, O., & Gerard, O.W. (1938). Anoxia and brain potentials. *Stroke, 1,* 558–572.

Travis, L.E. (1931). *Speech pathology.* New York: Appleton-Century-Crofts.

Van Riper, C. (1982). *The nature of stuttering* (Second edition). Englewood Cliffs: Prentice-Hall, Inc.

Viswanath, N.S., Rosenfield, D.B., & Nudelman, H.B. (1992). Stuttering and cerebral blood flow—letter to the Editor. *Archives of Neurology, 49,* 346–347.

Watson, B.C., Freeman, F.J., & Dembowski, J. (1991).

Respiratory/laryngeal coupling and complexity effects on acoustic LRT in normal speakers. *Journal of Voice, 5,* 18–28.

Watson, B.C., Pool, K.D., Devous, M.D., Sr., Freeman, F.J., & Finitzo, T. (1992). Brain blood flow related to acoustic laryngeal reaction time in adult developmental stutterers. *Journal of Speech and Hearing Research, 35,* 555–561.

Watson, B.C., Freeman, F.J., Devous, M.D., Sr., Chapman, S.B., Finitzo, T., & Pool, K.D. (1994). Linguistic performance and regional cerebral blood flow in persons who stutter. *Journal of Speech and Hearing Research, 37,* 1221–1228.

Webster, W.G. (1988). Neural mechanisms underlying stuttering: Evidence from bimanual handwriting performance. *Brain and Language, 33,* 226–244.

Wingate, M.E. (1988). *The structure of stuttering: A psycholinguistic analysis.* New York: Springer-Verlag.

Wolk, L., Edwards, M.L., & Conture, E.G. (1993). Coexistence of stuttering and disordered ohonology in young children. *Journal of Speech and Hearing Research, 36,* 906–917.

Wood, F., Stump, D., McKeehan, A., Sheldon, S., & Proctor, J. (1980). Patterns of regional cerebral blood flow during attempted reading aloud by stutterers both on and off haloperidol medication: Evidence for inadequate left frontal activation during stuttering. *Brain and Language, 9,* 141–144.

Wu, J.C., Maguire, G., Riley, G., Fallon, J., LaCasse, L., Chin, S., Klein, E., Tang, C., Cadwell, S., & Lottenberg, S. (1995). A positron emission tomography [¹⁸F]deoxyglucose study of developmental stuttering. *NeuroReport, 6,* 501–505.

Zimmerman, G., & Knott, J.R. (1974). Slow potentials of the brain related to speech processing in normal speakers and stutterers. *Electroencephalography and Clinical Neurophysiology, 37,* 599–607.

RECOMMENDED READINGS

Goldberg, G. (1985). Supplementary motor area structure and function: Review and hypotheses. *The Behavioral and Brain Sciences, 8,* 567–616. Goldberg presents a comprehensive review and integration of information regarding the role of the supplementary motor control area. Goldberg's model is cited often in the stuttering motor control literature.

Levelt, W.J.M. (1989). *Speaking: From intention to articulation.* Cambridge: MIT Press. Levelt presents a systematic exploration of the process of oral language generation. Multiple stages in the process can be conceptualized at possible functional sites of fluency failure.

Moore, W.H., Jr. (1990). Pathophysiology of stuttering:

Cerebral activation differences in stutterers vs. nonstutterers. In J.A. Cooper (Ed.), *Research needs in stuttering: Roadblocks and future directions* (pp. 72–80). Rockville, MD: ASHA. Moore has made significant contributions to the study of hemispheric function in stutterers. This chapter reviews his work and that of others in this area.

Pool, K.D., Devous, M.D., Freeman, F.J., Watson, B.C., & Finitzo, T. (1991). Regional cerebral blood flow in developmental stutterers. *Archives of Neurology, 48*, 509–512. This is the original report of SPECT rCBF findings for a large group of adult developmental stutterers.

PART THREE

ETIOLOGICAL VIEWS OF STUTTERING

As was noted in the Preface and in several chapters in this book, there are diverse descriptions of stuttering, its treatment and cause, extending from those in some of the earliest records of human civilization to those in this text. Contemporary researchers and theoreticians continue to ponder and to disagree about the origins of stuttering, leaving unresolved such basic issues as whether stuttering is a syndrome consisting of a collection of loosely related signs and symptoms that result from a number of different etiologies or from a common etiology; whether stuttering is best understood as an impairment in normal biological and psychological functions, as the result of early learning experiences, or as the interplay of biology and environment; whether stuttering arises from anomalous reactions to essentially normal speech disfluencies or whether, rather, these disfluencies are the expression of some anomalous cognitive, linguistic, or motor functions. Such divisions in theorizing reflect not only differences in beliefs about the nature of stuttering, but also differences concerning which level of description will provide more useful explanations of the disorder.

Current theories differ in their scope and objectives. As will be seen in this section, some theories focus on the variables that elicit stuttering events during ongoing speech but attend little to the original development of the disorder. Others are more concerned with original cause but offer little to explain immediate stuttering events. There have been few attempts to describe the variables that determine the duration or termination of individual stuttering events or of the conditions that lead to remission of stuttering or its persistence. Clearly, much work in this area remains to be done.

The etiological views that follow reflect different beliefs about the nature of stuttering and, implicitly, about the preferred level of explanation for the origins of stuttering. Oliver Bloodstein's anticipatory-struggle account is a cognitive theory that focuses on how a child's beliefs about the hazards of speaking can result in stuttered speech. It is an environmental theory to the extent that the child's maladaptive belief system emerges from encounters with the world.

Kolk and Postma present a psycholinguistic account of the sort that has attracted increasing attention in recent years. They describe stuttering as by-products of attempts to repair phonemic errors prior to articulation, but do not explain why some children, those who stutter, are susceptible to these kinds of phonemic problems but others are not.

Smith and Kelly introduce a dynamic, multifactorial approach that conceptualizes stuttering as emerging from the interplay of cognitive, linguistic, motoric, and emotional variables. Their approach integrates information from these various levels of observation using analytical techniques that are applicable to the functioning of nonlinear systems, but seems ultimately grounded in careful empirical studies of motor and physiological functioning in stutterers.

This section concludes with Perkins's essay arguing that explanations of stuttering and research that are not motivated at the outset by a well-articulated theory of both the origins and the maintenance of this disorder are destined to fail. Indeed, he believes that the lack of such a theory has led to a proliferation of etiological views and research that is too diffuse ever to lead to a coherent understanding of stuttering.

It remains to be seen whether the theory outlined by Perkins or any of the others represented in this book will rally researchers and clinicians in the way that those of Travis and Johnson did in the years of their pervasive influence on stuttering. For now, there is indeed a proliferation of theories and models, dealing, often, with different aspects of the stuttering problem so that they are not even competing explanations for the same phenomena. One test of their utility that is unique to fields such as communication disorders is the extent to which the various theories influence current approaches to therapy, as represented in the clinical management sections of this book and in the practices of clinicians working in the field.

CHAPTER 8

STUTTERING AS AN ANTICIPATORY STRUGGLE REACTION

OLIVER BLOODSTEIN

INTRODUCTION: STATEMENT OF THE THEORY

The anticipatory struggle hypothesis is first and foremost a cognitive theory of stuttering. It holds that stuttering stems largely from early speech experiences that infect a child's system of belief with the conviction that speech is difficult. A theory in all probability as old as stuttering itself, it has been advanced in crude form by every stutterer who ever observed that he could say any word in the language except when it was important to say it fluently, or when thinking of it as a difficult word or when expecting to stutter. What is missing from such casual statements of the theory is any attempt to explain why a stutterer's belief that a word is difficult should make it so. If this lack is not obvious at first glance, it is perhaps only because most of us have experienced similar effects on a small scale in such activities as typing, writing, or the playing of musical instruments, to say nothing of speech itself. Nevertheless, such an explanation is required.

Wendell Johnson's writings gave wide currency to the explanation that stuttering is nothing but the effort to avoid stuttering and originates as the effort to avoid normal childhood disfluency (see Johnson, 1967). This certainly explains how a belief in the difficulty of producing speech fluently might lead to stuttering, but it is suitable only for Johnson's own distinctive form of anticipatory struggle theory, which asserts that the problem results from parents' misdiagnoses of their children's normal speech hesitancies as stuttering.

An alternative model, which permits a much wider array of etiological possibilities, is the view that stuttering is the reflection of tension and fragmentation in speech. Whenever we are overwhelmed by the difficulty of a complex, automatic, serially ordered motor activity, we are likely, first, to initiate the activity with excessive tension, and second, to fragment the activity—that is, to break it up into manageable segments, and especially to repeat the first part of the activity until we gain the conviction to execute it as a whole. All of the surface features of stuttering, whether repetition, prolongation, hard attack on sound, or stoppage, may be viewed as manifestations of underlying tension and fragmentation in the initiation of speech units. On this assumption, it is clear that virtually any imaginable kind of speech pressure or chronic speech failure in childhood might lead to stuttering.

THE ROLE OF ENVIRONMENT

At the present time we are witnessing the revival of interest in constitutional and genetic influences on stuttering, an area of research that had been neglected for many years. Now the anticipatory struggle hypothesis clearly rests on the premise that stuttering is learned behavior, so it would be well to address the general question of environmental influences on stuttering before going on to specific evidence in support of the hypothesis.

Several independent sources of evidence can

be adduced to show that environmental influences play a decisive role in stuttering. To begin with, there are the findings from anthropological studies by Lemert (1953) and Morgenstern (reported by Johnson, 1967) suggesting that stuttering tends to flourish in cultures that impose heavy competitive pressures for achievement and conformity. Perhaps more telling is the very marked decline in the prevalence of stuttering that has taken place in the United States during recent decades (Van Riper, 1982, p. 49). This observation, revealing how stuttering may vary from era to era, is not well documented, but the agreement on it among clinicians of long experience is difficult to ignore. Even more conclusive evidence of the influence of environment comes from studies of stuttering in identical twins. Although the concordance of monozygotic twins for stuttering is quite high, cases in which only one member of the pair stutters are quite common (Howie, 1981; Luchsinger, 1959). The discordant cases, of course, can only be due to differences in environment.

Equally conclusive are the findings of Kidd and his colleagues. These workers applied a genetic model that made it possible for them to predict with considerable accuracy the proportion of stutterers' mothers, fathers, sisters, and brothers who would prove to be stutterers (Kidd, Heimbuch, & Records, 1981). These findings have lent strong support to the view that heredity often contributes in some way to the etiology of stuttering. But the genetic model that Kidd and his co-workers applied assumed that stuttering is the product of an interaction between genes and environmental factors. The same findings that speak for the influence of heredity, then, also underscore the power of environment.

Since the days when speech pathology was young, there has often been a tacit assumption that we will one day discover whether stuttering is an organic or functional disorder. Perhaps what we have been learning above all from recent genetic studies of stuttering is that we have been asking a nonsensical question. The effects of heredity, environment, physical makeup, and learning are probably inextricably interwoven in most cases of stuttering, as they are in so many other human traits.

Perhaps the most striking evidence of the part that environment plays in stuttering has come from a study by Farber (1981) of identical twins who had been separated at birth or soon afterward and reared apart. Farber reported data on ninety-five such cases gleaned from a review of the literature from 1923 to 1973. Remarkable similarities emerged in a variety of physical and behavioral traits. The similarity extended to speech characteristics: "The pitch, tone, and overall characteristics of the twins' voices were so stunningly alike that almost all investigators made mention of the similarity." The only exception among speech traits was stuttering. Among the ninety-five sets of twins, stuttering was noted in five cases. In all five, only one member of the pair was reported to stutter.

THE INFLUENCE OF BELIEFS

Both as children and adults, persistent stutterers are victimized by a proliferation of morbid beliefs. The incipient belief in the difficulty of speech that stutterers first verbalize in early childhood by saying "I can't talk" or "I can't say it" soon develops into a specific self-concept as a stutterer. This in turn gives rise eventually to the assumptions that certain words, sounds, or "letters" are difficult to say, that some listeners and situations are threatening, that stutterers are helpless to talk in any other way, and that stuttering is something to be hidden or avoided at all costs. Such beliefs are familiar to virtually all who have worked clinically with stutterers. What we are considering here is the theory that these beliefs not only result from, but also cause and serve to perpetuate and maintain, stuttering.

It is self-evident that if a stutterer could forget that he was a stutterer, this whole system of beliefs would vanish. For all practical purposes, then, we can reduce the anticipatory struggle hypothesis to the prediction that if a stutterer were to forget that he was a stutterer, he would have no further difficulty with his speech. On this prediction the theory stands or fails. Evidence that this is true would seem to constitute the most direct support for the theory.

Under ordinary conditions, to forget that one is a stutterer is a very difficult thing to do. Yet such forgetting does appear to take place in varying degrees, and the stuttering does seem to disappear as a result. The most striking examples are those rare "born-again" experiences in which stutterers either emerge from a religious reawakening convinced that they will never stutter again, or so narrowly escape from a life-threatening situation that their self-concepts as stutterers recede into comparative insignificance. A student of the writer's stopped stuttering when she became a Christian Scientist on the advice of one of her professors. A patient of Tawadros (1957) stopped stuttering when he battered several fingers in a machine shop accident that almost claimed his life. Other examples have been reported informally, but such cases are unfortunately not well documented.

More adequately documented is the observation that stuttering can be made to disappear for short periods of time by suggestion. The hypnotist who helps stutterers to speak fluently for days at a time simply by telling them that they will no longer stutter when they wake up from their trance is inducing them to forget that they are stutterers in the most straightforward way. This effect has been reliably reported by Moore (1946), who conducted a clinical study of hypnosis with forty stutterers, and by many others in observations of a more general sort going back to the nineteenth century. The effect of powerful suggestion in nonhypnotic forms is illustrated by a multitude of reports of at least temporary recovery from stuttering due to such therapies as breathing exercises, articulatory drills, diets, and periods of enforced silence, whose efficacy could only have been derived from the stutterer's faith in the outcome. A sensational example is the use of tongue surgery in 1841 when surgeons, buoyed by what at first seemed remarkable success, performed operations on scores of stutterers (Burdin, 1940).

Also well attested are the brief intervals of fluency stutterers experience when they forget for the moment that they are stutterers because they are carried away by excitement, enthusiasm, or anger, or because they are distracted by surprise or by fear of bodily harm. Subjects cited numerous examples in a questionnaire and interview study of conditions under which stuttering is reduced or absent (Bloodstein, 1950). In the same category are such situations as acting a part in a play, assuming an unaccustomed role, impersonating someone else, or speaking in a dialect, all of which are likely to result in fluency (Bloodstein, 1950). The well-known fact that virtually any change that stutterers make in their usual speech patterns results in immediate fluency appears to be due in large measure to the same "masquerade" effect. It is possible to speculate about other factors that may contribute in the case of certain artificial speech patterns, but the masquerade effect operates in all of them.

Finally, there are those revealing instances in which the vagaries of English spelling induce stutterers to "forget" that words beginning with certain sounds are difficult for them to say. Stutterers who are unable to say words beginning with *f* may have little difficulty with *photo*. They may be able to say *psychology* even if they ordinarily stutter on words beginning with s.

We have been discussing conditions under which stutterers appear to speak fluently because they forget their self-concepts as stutterers and their belief in the difficulty of speech. Conversely, stuttering seems to increase when stutterers are made more conscious of their speech difficulty or their role as speakers. For example, they often have great difficulty when speaking on the telephone, which reduces them to a voice. They almost always stutter when asked to repeat something the listener has failed to hear. Outside the speech clinic their stuttering has often been observed to increase noticeably when they discover that the person they are speaking to is a speech pathologist.

THE RELATION TO ANTICIPATORY EVENTS

The hypothesis that stuttering results from a belief in the difficulty of speech would seem to call for the occurrence of some kind of anticipatory reaction prior to stuttering, but the question of how to identify this reaction has been a source of confusion. For Johnson, the anticipation of stuttering was defined by the ability of stutterers to indicate accurately by a signal the word on which they are about to stutter. Most of the stutterers who served as subjects in early studies of anticipation by Johnson and his colleagues were able to predict the occurrence of their stutterings with considerable accuracy (Knott, Johnson, & Webster, 1937; Milisen, 1938; Van Riper, 1936). The accuracy was not perfect, but Johnson theorized that the anticipation of stuttering could sometimes occur at a low level of consciousness. The subjects of these studies were adults. Much later, Silverman and Williams (1972) found that children were far more variable in their ability to predict the occurrence of their stutterings; about half were able to predict less than 50 percent. So this method of investigation did not serve to confirm the anticipatory struggle hypothesis.

In another type of research, measures of autonomic arousal just prior to the stuttering block have suggested the presence of anticipation. It has been found that blocks are often preceded by a rise in pulse rate, vasoconstriction, disturbed breathing, increased electrical skin conductance, and motor disturbances (Brutten, 1963; Ickes & Pierce, 1973; Kurshev, 1968, 1969; Tanberg, 1955; Van Riper, 1936). Again, these are evidently not universal findings. However, they appear to be indications of anxiety rather than anticipation of difficulty. In subjects with high levels of anxiety about stuttering, we would naturally expect anticipation of stuttering to be accompanied by physiological arousal. But the anticipatory struggle hypothesis does not require the presence of anxiety. It is sufficient that the stutterer possess a certain eccentric system of assumptions about the imagined difficulty of speech and the unusual things that must be done to overcome that difficulty.

Of more consequence for the anticipatory struggle theory is the presence of some type of preparatory activity of the speech musculature prior to stuttering. Such activity has been reported in electromyographic studies by Shrum (1967) and Guitar (1975). In addition, Peters, Love, Otto, Wood, and Benignus (1976) found changes in brain waves preceding subjects' attempts on their difficult words, whether or not the words were stuttered. In a spectrographic study, Knox (1975) observed decreased rate, rise in pitch, and eccentric formant transitions on syllables spoken just prior to stuttering. Viswanath (1989) found that words preceding stuttered words were lengthened in duration.

It is evident that many kinds of anticipatory events are observable in advance of stuttering. Whether any of them can be found in association with all stutterings, and whether they are to be observed in young children as well as adults, are questions to which we do not have the answers.

The fact that some form of anticipation is seen to precede the stuttering block is no proof that it causes the block. It was perhaps for this reason that Goss (1952) took an entirely different approach to the study of stuttering in relation to anticipation. He systematically varied the time interval between the exposure of a word and a signal to the stutterer to say it. He found that for intervals between 2 and 10 seconds, the longer the interval the greater the probability of stuttering. (As the interval decreased below 2 seconds there was also a rise in stuttering, as a different kind of pressure apparently asserted itself.) Forte and Schlesinger (1972) observed the same effect in children. The importance of these findings is that they show stuttering to be not merely associated with but functionally dependent on anticipation. The more time there is to expect stuttering, the more likely it becomes.

THE ROLE OF STIMULI REPRESENTATIVE OF PAST STUTTERING

Although the anticipatory struggle hypothesis lends itself most readily to formulation in terms of attitudes and beliefs, it can also be framed in terms of observable behavior. In these terms, the theory states that stuttering in its developed form is a response to stimuli representative of past stuttering. To take a concrete example, suppose a stutterer, introducing a friend at a social gathering, blocks severely on the name "Gabriella." If stuttering is an anticipatory struggle reaction, will he be less likely, equally likely, or more likely to stutter on the name if he has to introduce the friend again a few moments later? The answer is more likely, of course, other things being equal. Coming back to attitudes and beliefs for a moment, he will remember his recent difficulty and will be even more certain than he was before that "Gabriella" is a difficult name for him to say.

So the theory says he will be more likely to block again. What are the facts? Among stutterers and their clinicians, the prevailing impression appears to be that the prediction is correct. It was, in fact, from such experiences as the one with Gabriella that the theory probably arose in the first place. Many stutterers, as is well known, tend to have personal lists of words that cause unusual difficulty. Clinical impression points to memorable past experiences of severe stuttering or severe social penalties for stuttering on these words as the source of the difficulty. Van Riper (1972, pp. 269–270) has presented a series of examples from his clinical experiences, such as the case of a young woman who could no longer say the word "well" after she had been harshly ridiculed when repeating it as a starting device. Incidents of this kind epitomize stuttering as an anticipatory struggle reaction.

An experimental paradigm of the tendency of stuttering to occur in response to stimuli associated with past stutterings was discovered by Johnson and Millsapps (1937). On subjects' copies of a reading passage they blotted out the words on which the subjects stuttered in successive readings. In subsequent readings the subjects were found to have stuttered to a significant degree on words adjacent to the blots. Johnson and Millsapps inferred that the blots had served as cues representative of past stutterings. This "adjacency" effect was confirmed in later studies by Brutten and Gray (1961) and Rappaport and Bloodstein (1971). The effect was also found in children (Avari & Bloodstein, 1974). These demonstrations of the adjacency effect perhaps offer as much evidence of a strictly experimental kind as has yet been possible to obtain in support of the anticipatory struggle hypothesis.

It might be argued that words blotted out in a reading passage might produce adjacent stutterings for reasons that had nothing to do with past stutterings. To check this, the writer in collaboration with one of his students tested the hypothesis that words blotted out at random would produce an adjacency effect (Rappaport & Bloodstein, 1971). The results were a striking confirmation of Johnson and Millsapps's interpretation. When a reading with randomly placed blots preceded an ordinary adjacency trial, the random blots produced no adjacent stutterings. But for subjects for whom the order of the two conditions was reversed, the random blots resulted in a marked adjacency effect for every subject. In other words, random blottings in and of themselves did nothing, but once subjects had been exposed to blottings of previously stuttered words, even new blots placed at random in a new passage continued to provoke stutterings.

EXPLANATORY POTENTIAL OF THE HYPOTHESIS

Since no theory of stuttering has yet been conclusively proved by a crucial laboratory experiment, and very possibly never will, the validity of a theory may ultimately have to rest on how well it explains the known phenomena of the disorder and perhaps on how well it enables us to predict phenomena yet unknown. In the preceding sections of this chapter we have already touched on certain aspects of stuttering that are explained particularly well by the anticipatory struggle hypothesis. Here we would like to show that the hypothesis is consistent with all of the many conditions and factors that are known to influence the occurrence of stuttering.

If we begin with the manner in which stuttering is distributed in the speech sequence, a fundamental fact about it is the consistency effect—the tendency of the stutterer to block on the same words from reading to reading of a passage. This shows that the stuttering is in part a response to stimuli in the reading passage, and is probably the best evidence we have of the role that learning plays in the distribution of stutterings.

Next in importance is the fact that the blocks tend to be distributed on different words from stutterer to stutterer (Hendel & Bloodstein, 1973). That is, factors that differ from case to case are far more powerful in determining what words are stuttered than are factors that operate for stutterers as a group. The studies do not indicate what the factors are, but clinical experience strongly suggests that the assumptions stutterers acquire about the difficulty of certain words are of major importance in determining the loci of blocks.

Lastly, there are the factors that affect the distribution of blocks for stutterers as a group. These have been investigated extensively (Brown, 1937, 1938, 1945; Brown & Moren, 1942; Danzger & Halpern, 1973; Griggs & Still, 1979; Hahn, 1942a, b; Johnson & Brown, 1935; Lanyon, 1968; Lanyon & Duprez, 1970; Quarrington, 1965; Quarrington, Conway, & Siegel, 1962; Schlesinger, Forte, Fried, & Melkman, 1965; Schlesinger, Melkman, & Levy, 1966; Soderberg, 1962, 1966, 1967, 1971; Taylor, 1966a, b; Wingate, 1967, 1979). As a result of these studies, we know that most stutterers tend to have more difficulty on words beginning with consonants than vowels; on longer words; on content words as opposed to function words and pronouns; on words at the beginning of the sentence; on words of low frequency of occurrence in the language; on words that have high "information value" in the sense that they are difficult to guess from the preceding context; and on words that receive the most stress. All this is consistent with the anticipatory struggle hypothesis. Such attributes of words tend to make them seem difficult or conspicuous. They are, consequently, the words on which stuttering is most likely to be anticipated.

The myriad conditions under which stuttering increases and decreases in frequency are also readily explained in terms of variations in anticipatory struggle. Most of them involve changes in the amount of communicative pressure of various kinds—the pressure of communicative responsibility, of time for motor planning of speech, of listener reactions, of concern about social approval, and of audience size. Other conditions involve suggestion, the factor of stutterers' attention to

their speech and their role as speakers to which we have already alluded, states of generalized tension, and the role of cues that evoke anticipation of stuttering. The writer has discussed these conditions at length in relation to the anticipatory struggle hypothesis elsewhere (Bloodstein, 1987, pp. 262–287). In general, the conditions under which stuttering is most frequent appear to be those that are most likely to evoke anticipation of stuttering, or in which the social penalties for stuttering are most severe.

We have saved for last one additional observation that must be included in any discussion of the variables to which stuttering is related, and that is the locus of stuttering within the word. Blocks occur on the first sound or syllable in over 90 percent of cases. Occasionally they are to be heard on accented syllables within words, but virtually never on final sounds or syllables. The absence of stuttering from the ends of words enjoys an unusual position among the phenomena of stuttering; it is one of the very few that have the status of a rule. A generalization to which there are only rare, if any, exceptions would appear to harbor some information of basic importance about stuttering. In the writer's view, it is the information that the stutterer's belief in the difficulty of speech revolves mainly around the execution of words rather than other units of speech. The stutterer who repeats or prolongs the first sound of a word is hardly having difficulty with the sound, as a moment's thought will show. What the stutterer appears to be doing is fragmenting the word—that is, uttering only the first part of it and repeating or prolonging that until gaining the conviction that is necessary to say the word as a whole. The stutterer seems to be acting out of a belief that the word is too difficult to articulate all at once in its entirety.

Note that this characterization of stuttering as mainly difficulty with words is supported by two independent observations. One is the failure of stuttering to occur at the ends of words. The other is evident in the factors that affect the distribution of stutterings in the speech sequence. These are all attributes of words—their length, grammatical function, initial sound, information value, and above all, the extent to which they are part of the stutterer's private glossary of difficult words. It is important to keep in mind, however, that if stuttering has to do in large part with the execution of words, this is true of the disorder in its developed form. When we deal with stuttering in very young children, the picture changes considerably, as we will see.

EARLY STUTTERING

We have attempted to show that the essential facts that we know about stuttering in its fully developed form are in accord with the anticipatory struggle hypothesis. The question now is whether the theory also fits what we know about the conditions surrounding the development of the problem in early childhood. Are they such as to instill a belief in the difficulty of speech? The evidence on this point takes a number of different forms.

In the first place, a large proportion of young stutterers appear to have experiences of speech or language failure before they are observed to stutter. Many have a history of delayed language development (Andrews & Harris, 1964; Berry, 1938; Blood & Seider, 1981; Milisen & Johnson, 1936; Morley, 1957). As a group, they tend to score lower than nonstuttering children on tests of language skill (Byrd & Cooper, 1989; Kline & Starkweather, 1979; Murray & Reed, 1977; Wall, 1980; Westby, 1979). From 15 to 50 percent of stuttering children have been reported to have articulatory or other speech defects (Andrews & Harris, 1964; Blood & Seider, 1981; Darley, 1955; Johnson & Associates, 1959; Kent & Williams, 1963; Louko, Edwards, & Conture, 1990; Morley, 1957; Schindler, 1955; St. Louis & Hinzman, 1988; Williams & Silverman, 1968).

Moreover, clinical interviews with parents of young stutterers reveal a considerable number of cases in which language difficulties, articulatory defects, and other chronic failures in communication appeared to act as provocations to stuttering, particularly in an environment of speech or language pressures. Elsewhere the writer has presented a series of accounts of such cases (Bloodstein, 1975). A clinical observation of some significance is that some children experience episodes of stuttering during periods of therapy for language disorders. Instances have been reported from widely scattered speech clinics, and two such cases were the subject of an article by Hall (1977).

In this connection the results of a study by Merits-Patterson and Reed (1981) are well worth pondering. They studied the ordinary disfluencies of nine young children who were receiving therapy for delayed language development, nine children with delayed language who were not receiving therapy, and nine children with normal language development. The children undergoing therapy were found to have more word and part-word repetitions than the others. There was no difference between the no-therapy language-delayed subjects and those with normal language.

Of course, many children who stutter have perfectly normal language and articulation, but the clinical examination in these cases often reveals evidence of pressures that undermine the child's faith in his or her ability to communicate acceptably. These pressures may take such varied forms as overabundant praise for precocious speech, parental perfectionism about speech, or speech models that set excessively high standards (Johnson & Associates, 1959, Chapter 4; Bloodstein, 1975).

In sum, there are various indications that the self-concept as a stutterer usually has its source in a more general self-concept as a poor speaker; and that the anticipation of stuttering on specific words originally develops from a more vague and general belief in the difficulty of speech. Without question, much of this evidence can be interpreted in other ways. And there are cases in which the simplest way to account for the stuttering is solely on the basis of a strong predisposition to stutter that seems to be hereditary in some families. But the evidence seems to indicate that, in the main, genes are not enough.

The role of communicative pressures in the etiology of stuttering seems to be reflected in the form that early stuttering takes. When we examine the stuttering of preschool children, we find that it usually differs in certain respects from that of older children and adults. One of the outstanding differences is the presence of a large amount of word repetition. To be sure, word repetition is a very prominent feature of normal childhood disfluency, too, and so there has long been some confusion over the question of whether it should be defined as stuttering. The best normative data we have, however, show it to be about four times as prevalent in stutterers' as in nonstutterers' speech (Johnson & Associates, 1959, p. 210). These normative data indicate further that word and part-word repetitions form the bulk of the stuttering in 2- to 8-year-old children. In clinical experience with 2- to 4-year-old stutterers, extended repetitions of words are often the essence of the problem. To exclude them as stutterings would therefore only seem to create the need to invent another word for abnormal disfluency. To this writer it seems a far simpler solution to say that stuttering and certain types of normal disfluency in early childhood belong on a single continuum, an assumption for which there is considerable evidence (Bloodstein, 1975, pp. 48–56).

Now the large number of word repetitions in the speech of young stutterers may be telling us something of significance about the relation of stuttering to language development. In the preceding section we alluded to the fact that repetitions of sounds or syllables obey a rule: They do not occur at the ends of words. There is a parallel rule that applies to word repetitions: They do not occur at the ends of syntactic units. With the rarest exceptions, the repeated word is the first word of a sentence, clause, or phrase (Bloodstein, 1974; Bloodstein & Grossman, 1981). For example, we may hear "'cause 'cause 'cause 'cause I'll get sick," but not "'cause I'll get sick sick." The child may repeat the first word of a verb phrase, as in "You won't feel feel feel good," but not the last word "good" and not the last word of a noun phrase as in "and his name name was Ira." What is the meaning of this rule? By the same reasoning that we applied to sound repetitions, we would have to infer that word repetitions represent a hesitancy in the initiation of syntactic units. Whereas developed stuttering is primarily a difficulty with words, the distribution of early stuttering would seem to reflect a more general difficulty that centers on whole utterances or their constituent phrases.

The hypothesis that early stuttering, or much of it, is difficulty with syntactic units points directly to the burden of language acquisition that children bear during the years when most cases of stuttering develop. Interestingly, it is a hypothesis that can be verified by a prediction that flows from it. If early stuttering does not represent difficulty with words, its distribution in the speech sequence should not be influenced by the various attributes of words that influence developed stuttering. The writer (Bloodstein, 1974) once made that prediction, on the strength of the discovery that the distribution of early stutterings was not influenced by the grammatical functions of words (Bloodstein & Gantwerk, 1967). Additional findings have been slow in coming, but such as they are, they are in accord with the prediction. Wall, Starkweather, and Harris (1981) reported that preschool subjects failed to reveal the usual tendency of stutterers to have more trouble with words beginning with consonants than words beginning with vowels. And in a small number of subjects, Bloodstein and Grossman (1981) found no evidence that the grammatical factor, the consonant versus vowel factor, or word length had any effect. Only word position made a difference; words at the beginnings of utterances were stuttered with unusual frequency, as we would expect if the subjects formulated their expectations of difficulty in terms of whole utterances.

In conclusion, we infer that stuttering gives several different indications of being an anticipatory struggle reaction even in its earliest manifestations. By the end of the preschool years, however, a significant change takes place in the form of that reaction. By that time persistent stutterers have begun to acquire self-concepts as stutterers. By about age 5, children also have some awareness of language; they know about words as isolatable constituents of speech (Prutting, 1979). The stage is thus set for a process of development of the problem through which it eventually comes to be dominated by the anticipation of stuttering fostered and maintained by a belief in the difficulty of words.

THE INTERACTION WITH HEREDITY

Since it is almost certain that both environment and heredity have something to do with the development of stuttering, a final question is how genes might interact with communicative pressures to produce the disorder. To this we can at present give no satisfactory answer, but it may at least be possible to refine the question.

One good place to start is with a simple but revealing fact: No matter how badly stutterers are blocked in their attempt on a word, they can almost invariably stop and immediately say some other word with perfect fluency. So the stuttering block is not simply an organically caused phenomenon like a paralysis, tetanal muscular spasm, or athetotic movement. How is this fact to be reconciled with what we know about the role of heredity? We can perhaps progress a bit toward some clarity if we recognize that the question of what causes stuttering is really two distinct questions. One is about the conditions under which the difficulty first arises. The other is why a person stutters on a given word at a given time, once the problem has developed.

The answer to the second question is that the reason stutterers block on a given occasion appears to be little more than their anticipation of stuttering, from all that we can tell from all of the conditions that seem to precipitate blocks and all of the factors that seem to be related to them. In other words, little or nothing that stutterers have inherited seems to play an important part. The hypothetical organic predisposition to stutter either has disappeared or exists in such minimal amount that it can be ignored. Essentially everything we observe about the conditions under which fully developed stuttering comes and goes is compatible with the assumption that it is primarily if not wholly an anticipatory struggle reaction. If this is true, it has the important practical implication that in the treatment of all but the youngest children, we should be able to proceed without fear of being hampered to a marked degree by any hereditary predisposition. The same can be said of any subtle anomalies that may appear to emerge from research on aspects of stutterers'

brain functioning. Whenever we are tempted to view such things in the light of their direct effect on the outcome of treatment, we need to call to mind the familiar image of the stutterer who tries again and again to say "Schenectady" and finally blurts out fluently, "I can never say Schenectady!"

It is only in connection with the first question—the etiology of stuttering—that the influence of heredity looms large. There is apparently something that some young children inherit in such measure that it makes them prone to outbreaks of extreme disfluency, especially in the presence of constant or recurring communicative pressures. Exactly what part genes play in this interaction is a total mystery. The role of communicative pressures is easier to speculate about. We have done so in this chapter in terms of tension and fragmentation in the utterance of syntactic units. But it may be worth noting that there are a number of different ways in which this factor might function in its interaction with heredity. To illustrate, let us return once again to the work of Farber (1981), that brought to light such strong evidence of the role of environment in stuttering. Farber reported on a series of identical twins who had been reared apart. In five cases in which stuttering was noted, only one member of the pair stuttered in each case. We might take this to mean that the environmental factor may be so powerful in many cases as to be a sufficient condition for the development of stuttering. And it is a fact that many stutterers report no history of stuttering in their families. But note that, for all we know to the contrary, all five of Farber's twin pairs may have inherited a predisposition to stuttering that manifested itself in only one member because the other was not exposed to the environmental conditions that are conducive to stuttering. Finally, it is even possible that the normal speaking twin in each case had experienced an early childhood episode of stuttering so brief or mild that it had been long forgotten when the twins were studied many years later. So perhaps the environmental factor usually contributes not so much to the etiology of stuttering as to the persistence of the disorder. These are some of the ramifications we must consider when we raise the question of how heredity and environment interact with each other in the causation of stuttering.

CLINICAL IMPLICATIONS

From a therapeutic point of view, the main lesson of the anticipatory struggle hypothesis is that the way to overcome stuttering completely and permanently is to forget that one is a stutterer. If there were a drug that could make us forget selectively some of what we know, how quickly we might eradicate stuttering, to say nothing of superstition, prejudice, delusions, irrational fears, guilt, and grief. Since we have no such remedy, the lesson of our hypothesis may not appear to have any immediate practical consequences. Yet it does serve to illuminate some fundamental facts we have learned as a clinical and scientific discipline about the phenomenon of recovery from stuttering. It explains why some stutterers recover after life-threatening or religious experiences that give them a totally new outlook on life. It goes far to explain the familiar case of the young man who stutters severely, earns college degrees, becomes established in a profession, acquires a family, gradually becomes possessed of a new concept of himself in which "stutterer" occupies a progressively diminishing place, and by imperceptible degrees seems to forget to stutter.

The anticipatory struggle hypothesis also helps us to account for the fact that children are far more likely to recover, both with and without formal treatment, than adults. It is difficult to suppose that a child's inborn predisposition to be abnormally disfluent increases with age, but it is credible that the beliefs that stuttering thrives on tend to become more and more firmly established.

Finally, the anticipatory struggle hypothesis helps to explain one of the broadest generalizations we can make about recoveries that result from treatment in adulthood: Essentially any method, no matter how unusual or bizarre, has a potential for eradicating stuttering for some person, somewhere, at some time. Speaking on inhalation, speaking with gestures, and the use of a foam rubber vibrator are among the long list of expedients for which success has been claimed in reports on single cases. (See *De Therapia Vocis et Loquelae*, the proceedings of the XIII Congress of the International Association for Logopedics and Phoniatrics, 1965.) It is true that very many of these apparent recoveries are probably temporary, but some seem to be lasting. For many years I have occasionally received mail from former stutterers who have cured themselves of the problem by some techniques of their own devising and, out of a sincere impulse to help others, want their discoveries to become known. Unfortunately, these therapeutic devices are unlikely to aid many other stutterers. But I believe this potential of stuttering to yield to almost any form of treatment contains an important message. In the comparatively rare cases in which therapy totally eliminates stuttering in adults, it appears to be because stutterers have become convinced that they will not stutter and no longer need to be concerned about their speech. Any therapy has the power to bring this about. The key to such conviction is commitment. The stutterer must eat, sleep, and breathe therapy with monklike devotion. Few stutterers are prepared to pay so high a price for total recovery. Most prefer to settle for improvement, and it is not the business of a speech clinician to disparage such a choice. Only the stutterer is competent to weigh the benefit against the cost.

REFERENCES

Andrews, G., & Harris, M. (1964). *The syndrome of stuttering*. London: Spastics Society Medical Education and Information Unit in association with Heinemann.

Avari, D.N., & Bloodstein, O. (1974). Adjacency and prediction in school-age stutterers. *Journal of Speech and Hearing Research, 17*, 33–40.

Berry, M.F. (1938). Developmental history of stuttering children. *Journal of Pediatrics, 12*, 209–217.

Blood, G.W., & Seider, R. (1981). The concomitant

problems of young stutterers. *Journal of Speech and Hearing Disorders, 46*, 31–33.

Bloodstein, O. (1950). A rating scale study of conditions under which stuttering is reduced or absent. *Journal of Speech and Hearing Disorders, 15*, 29–36.

Bloodstein, O. (1974). The rules of early stuttering. *Journal of Speech and Hearing Disorders, 39*, 379–394.

Bloodstein, O. (1975). Stuttering as tension and fragmentation. In J. Eisenson (Ed.), *Stuttering: A second symposium*. New York: Harper & Row.

Bloodstein, O. (1987). *A handbook on stuttering* (4th ed.). Chicago: National Easter Seal Society.

Bloodstein, O., & Gantwerk, B.F. (1967). Grammatical function in relation to stuttering in young children. *Journal of Speech and Hearing Research, 10*, 786–789.

Bloodstein, O., & Grossman, M. (1981). Early stutterings: Some aspects of their form and distribution. *Journal of Speech and Hearing Research, 24*, 298–302.

Brown, S.F. (1937). The influence of grammatical function on the incidence of stuttering. *Journal of Speech Disorders, 2*, 207–215.

Brown, S.F. (1938). Stuttering in relation to word accent and word position. *Journal of Abnormal and Social Psychology, 33*, 112–120.

Brown, S.F. (1945). The loci of stutterings in the speech sequence. *Journal of Speech Disorders, 10*, 181–192.

Brown, S.F., & Moren, A. (1942). The frequency of stuttering in relation to word length during oral reading. *Journal of Speech Disorders, 7*, 153–159.

Brutten, E.J. (1963). Palmar sweat investigation of disfluency and expectancy adaptation. *Journal of Speech and Hearing Research, 6*, 40–48.

Brutten, E.J., & Gray, B.B. (1961). Effect of word cue removal on adaptation and adjacency: A clinical paradigm. *Journal of Speech and Hearing Disorders, 26*, 385–389.

Burdin, G. (1940). The surgical treatment of stammering 1840–1842. *Journal of Speech Disorders, 5*, 43–64.

Byrd, K., & Cooper, E.B. (1989). Expressive and receptive language skills in stuttering children. *Journal of Fluency Disorders, 14*, 121–126.

Danzger, M., & Halpern, H. (1973). Relation of stuttering to word abstraction, part of speech, word length, and word frequency. *Perceptual and Motor Skills, 37*, 959–962.

Darley, F.L. (1955). The relationship of parental attitudes and adjustments to the development of stuttering. In W. Johnson (Ed.), *Stuttering in children and adults*. Minneapolis: University of Minnesota Press.

De Therapia Vocis et Loquelae. (1965). XIII Congress of the International Society for Logopedics and Phoniatrica.

Farber, S. (1981). *Identical twins reared apart: A reanalysis*. New York: Basic Books.

Forte, M., & Schlesinger, I.M. (1972). Stuttering as a function of time of expectation. *Journal of Communication Disorders, 5*, 347–358.

Goss, A.E. (1952). Stuttering behavior and anxiety theory. I. Stuttering behavior and anxiety as a function of the duration of stimulus words. *Journal of Abnormal and Social Psychology, 47*, 38–50.

Griggs, S., & Still, A.W. (1979). An analysis of individual differences in words stuttered. *Journal of Speech and Hearing Research, 22*, 572–580.

Guitar, B. (1975). Reduction of stuttering frequency using analog electromyographic feedback. *Journal of Speech and Hearing Research, 18*, 672–685.

Hahn, E.F. (1942a). A study of the relationship between stuttering occurrence and grammatical factors in oral reading. *Journal of Speech Disorders, 7*, 329–335.

Hahn, E.F. (1942b). A study of the relationship between stuttering occurrence and phonetic factors in oral reading. *Journal of Speech Disorders, 7*, 143–151.

Hall, P.K. (1977). The occurrence of disfluencies in language-disordered school-age children. *Journal of Speech and Hearing Disorders, 42*, 364–369.

Hendel, D., & Bloodstein, O. (1973). Consistency in relation to inter-subject congruity in the loci of stutterings. *Journal of Communication Disorders, 6*, 37–43.

Howie, P.M. (1981). Concordance for stuttering in monozygotic and dizygotic twin pairs. *Journal of Speech and Hearing Research, 24*, 317–321.

Ickes, W.K., & Pierce, S. (1973). The stuttering moment: A plethysmographic study. *Journal of Communication Disorders, 6*, 155–164.

Johnson, W. (1967). Stuttering. In W. Johnson, S.F. Brown, J.F. Curtis, C.W. Edney, & J. Keaster (Eds.), *Speech handicapped school children* (Third edition). New York: Harper & Row.

Johnson, W., & Associates. (1959). *The onset of stuttering*. Minneapolis: University of Minnesota Press.

Johnson, W., & Brown, S.F. (1935). Stuttering in relation to various speech sounds. *Quarterly Journal of Speech, 21,* 481–496.

Johnson, W., & Millsapps, L.S. (1937). Studies in the psychology of stuttering: VI. The role of cues representative of stuttering moments during oral reading. *Journal of Speech Disorders, 2,* 101–104.

Kent, L.R., & Williams, D.E. (1963). Alleged former stutterers in grade two. *Asha, 5,* 772.

Kidd, K.K., Heimbuch, R.C., & Records, M.A. (1981). Vertical transmission of susceptibility to stuttering with sex-modified expression. *Proceedings of the National Academy of Sciences, 78,* 606–610.

Kline, M.L., & Starkweather, C.W. (1979). Receptive and expressive language performance in young stutterers. *Asha, 21,* 797.

Knott, J.R., Johnson, W., & Webster, M.J. (1937). Studies in the psychology of stuttering, II. A quantitative evaluation of expectation of stuttering in relation to occurrence of stuttering. *Journal of Speech Disorders, 2,* 20–22.

Knox, J.A. (1975). Acoustic analysis of stuttering behavior within the context of fluent speech. Unpublished Ph.D. dissertation, University of Iowa, 1975.

Kurshev, V.A. (1968). Study of nonspeech respiration in stutterers. *Zhurnal Nevropatologii i Psikhiatrii, 68,* 1840–1841.

Kurshev, V.A. (1969). Unconscious reactions in stutterers. *Zhurnal Nevropatologii i Psikhiatrii, 69,* 1075–1077.

Lanyon, R.I. (1968). Some characteristics of nonfluency in normal speakers and stutterers. *Journal of Abnormal Psychology, 73,* 550–555.

Lanyon, R.I., & Duprez, D.A. (1970). Nonfluency, information, and word length. *Journal of Abnormal Psychology, 76,* 93–97.

Lemert, E.M. (1953). Some Indians who stutter. *Journal of Speech and Hearing Disorders, 18,* 168–174.

Louko, L.J., Edwards, M.L., & Conture, E.G. (1990). Phonological characteristics of young stutterers and their normally fluent peers: Preliminary observations. *Journal of Fluency Disorders, 15,* 191–210.

Luchsinger, R. (1959). Die Vererbung von Sprach und Stimmstoerungen. *Folia Phoniatrica, 11,* 7–64.

Merits-Patterson, R., & Reed, C.G. (1981). Disfluencies in the speech of language-delayed children. *Journal of Speech and Hearing Research, 24,* 55–58.

Milisen, R. (1938). Frequency of stuttering with anticipation of stuttering controlled. *Journal of Speech Disorders, 3,* 207–214.

Milisen, R., & Johnson, W. (1936). A comparative study of stutterers, former stutterers and normal speakers whose handedness has been changed. *Archives of Speech, 1,* 61–86.

Moore, W.E. (1946). Hypnosis in a system of therapy for stutterers. *Journal of Speech Disorders, 11,* 117–122.

Morley, M.E. (1957). *The development and disorders of speech in childhood.* Edinburgh: Livingstone.

Murray, H.L., & Reed, C.G. (1977). Language abilities of preschool stuttering children. *Journal of Fluency Disorders, 2,* 171–176.

Peters, R.W., Love, L., Otto, D., Wood, T., & Benignus, V. (1976). Cerebral processing of speech and nonspeech signals by stutterers. In Proceedings of the XVI International Congress of Logopedics and Phoniatrics. Basel: Karger.

Prutting, C.A. (1979). Process/prál, ses/n: The action of moving forward progressively from one point to another on the way to completion. *Journal of Speech and Hearing Disorders, 44,* 3–30.

Quarrington, B. (1965). Stuttering as a function of the information value and sentence position of words. *Journal of Abnormal Psychology, 70,* 221–224.

Quarrington, B., Conway, J., & Siegel, N. (1962). An experimental study of some properties of stuttered words. *Journal of Speech and Hearing Research, 5,* 387–394.

Rappaport, B., & Bloodstein, O. (1971). The role of random blackout cues in the distribution of moments of stuttering. *Journal of Speech and Hearing Research, 14,* 874–879.

Schindler, M.D. (1955). A study of educational adjustments of stuttering and nonstuttering children. In W. Johnson (Ed.), *Stuttering in children and adults.* Minneapolis: University of Minnesota Press.

Schlesinger, I.M., Forte, M., Fried, B., & Melkman, R. (1965). Stuttering, information load, and response strength. *Journal of Speech and Hearing Disorders, 30,* 32–36.

Schlesinger, I.M., Melkman, R., & Levy, R. (1966). Word length and frequency as determinants of stuttering. *Psychonomic Science, 6,* 255–256.

Shrum, W.A. (1967). *A study of speaking behavior of stutterers and nonstutterers by means of multichannel electromyography.* Unpublished Ph.D. dissertation, University of Iowa.

Silverman, F.H., & Williams, D.E. (1972). Prediction of stuttering by school-age stutterers. *Journal of Speech and Hearing Research, 15,* 189–193.

Soderberg, G.A. (1962). Phonetic influences upon stuttering. *Journal of Speech and Hearing Research, 5,* 315–320.

Soderberg, G.A. (1966). The relations of stuttering to word length and word frequency. *Journal of Speech and Hearing Research, 9,* 584–589.

Soderberg, G.A. (1967). Linguistic factors in stuttering. *Journal of Speech and Hearing Research, 10,* 801–810.

Soderberg, D.A. (1971). Relations of word information and word length to stuttering disfluencies. *Journal of Communication Disorders, 4,* 9–14.

St. Louis, K.O., & Hinzman, A.R. (1988). A descriptive study of speech, language, and hearing characteristics of school-aged stutterers. *Journal of Fluency Disorders, 13,* 331–355.

Tanberg, M.C. (1955). A study of the role of inhibition in the moment of stuttering. In W. Johnson (Ed.), *Stuttering in children and adults.* Minneapolis: University of Minnesota Press.

Tawadros, S.M. (1957). An experiment in the group psychotherapy of stutterers. *International Journal of Sociometry and Sociatry, 1,* 181–189.

Taylor, I.K. (1966a). The properties of stuttered words. *Journal of Verbal Learning and Verbal Behavior, 5,* 112–118.

Taylor, I.K. (1966b). What words are stuttered? *Psychological Bulletin, 65,* 233–242.

Van Riper, C. (1936). Study of the thoracic breathing of stutterers during expectancy and occurrence of stuttering spasm. *Journal of Speech Disorders, 1,* 61–72.

Van Riper, C. (1972). *Speech correction: Principles and methods* (5th ed.). Englewood Cliffs, N.J.: Prentice-Hall.

Van Riper, C. (1982). *The nature of stuttering* (2nd ed.). Englewood Cliffs, NJ: Prentice-Hall.

Viswanath, N.S. (1989). Global- and local-temporal effects of a stuttering event in the context of a clausal utterance. *Journal of Fluency Disorders, 14,* 245–269.

Wall, M.J. (1980). A comparison of syntax in young stutterers and nonstutterers. *Journal of Fluency Disorders, 5,* 345–352.

Wall, M.J., Starkweather, C.W., & Harris, K.S. (1981). The influence of voicing adjustments on the location of stuttering in the spontaneous speech of young child stutterers. *Journal of Fluency Disorders, 6,* 299–310.

Westby, C.E. (1972). Language performance of stuttering and nonstuttering children. *Journal of Communication Disorders, 12,* 133–145.

Williams, D.E., & Silverman, F.H. (1968). Note concerning articulation of school-age stutterers. *Perceptual and Motor Skills, 27,* 713–714.

Wingate, M.E. (1967). Stuttering and word length. *Journal of Speech and Hearing Research, 10,* 146–152.

Wingate, M.E. (1979). The first three words. *Journal of Speech and Hearing Research, 22,* 604–612.

SUGGESTED READINGS

Bloodstein, O. (1975). Stuttering as tension and fragmentation. In J. Eisenson (Ed.), *Stuttering: A second symposium.* New York: Harper & Row. Offers clinical evidence of the role of communicative pressures and failures in the etiology of stuttering.

Bloodstein, O. (1995, 1987). Stuttering as a response. In *A handbook on stuttering* (5th ed., Chapter 7). San Diego: Singular; Easter Seal Society. Reviews the research findings on the frequency and distribution of stutterings in the speech sequence and relates them to the anticipatory struggle hypothesis.

Bloodstein, O. (1993). The inception of stuttering. In *Stuttering: The search for a cause and cure* (Chapter 15). Boston: Allyn & Bacon. The most complete account of the author's views on the nature and etiology of stuttering.

Bloodstein, O. (1974). The rules of early stuttering. *Journal of Speech and Hearing Disorders, 39,* 379–394. Contains evidence that early stuttering consists of the fragmentation of whole utterances and their constituent phrases.

CHAPTER 9

STUTTERING AS A COVERT REPAIR PHENOMENON

HERMAN KOLK
ALBERT POSTMA

INTRODUCTION

In 1985, Kolk and van Grunsven proposed a theory of agrammatic aphasia that they called *adaptation theory* (for a recent review of this theory, see Kolk, 1995). The theory contained two basic elements. First, the *impairment* was assumed to be due to a temporal disruption of grammatical processing. On the one hand, there could be a delay in the activation of grammatical units (e.g., phrasal categories); on the other hand, such units could decay from memory too rapidly after being activated (see Haarmann & Kolk, 1991, for a computer simulation of these two hypotheses). A second major assumption was that the speech of agrammatic patients was the result of the way in which they *adapted* themselves to this impairment. Thus, agrammatic symptoms are caused by the use of adaptive strategies, rather then being the immediate outflow of the impairment itself.

Within the theory, the effect of the temporal disruption is that the "temporal window" for grammatical processing reduces in size. Adaptation to this reduction occurs in two ways. First, patients can simplify the form of their utterances such that the syntactic planning of these utterances fits into the reduced window. This form of adaptation accounts for the reduced variety of grammatical form and the telegraphic speech that

ACKNOWLEDGMENT: We thank Ed Conture for his detailed and helpful comments.

is typical for these patients (e.g., "two weeks in the hospital, very ill") (cf. Goodglass & Kaplan, 1972). It was labeled *preventive adaptation* to indicate that it is a strategy that prevents the syntactic process from being disrupted because of taking too much time.

A second form of adaptation was called *corrective adaptation*. If syntactic processing is disrupted as a consequence of the temporal problem, the syntactic representation that underlies the sentence to be uttered is bound to contain errors. Normal speakers are able to "monitor" their "inner speech" and detect errors in their speech plan (cf. Levelt, 1983), a topic that will be discussed in further detail below. We assume that aphasics are able to monitor inner speech as well. If they detect errors, they will try to repair these errors by going back to the beginning of the phrase or sentence and restarting the process. If such a repair strategy is frequently used, it causes speech to become slow and effortful. In this way, the corrective adaptation hypothesis accounts for the pattern of nonfluent speech that is typical for agrammatic aphasia (Goodglass & Kaplan, 1972).

This theoretical framework has obvious applications to stuttering (cf. Kolk, 1985, 1990, 1991). The speech of stutterers can also be slow and effortful at times, and what we observe as stuttering events could be the effect of repair strategies. On the other hand, nonfluent aphasic speech is not the same as stuttered speech. An explanation of what "errors" the stutterer is trying to repair and how such repairs take place was specified in the covert repair hypothesis (CRH) of stuttering (cf. Postma & Kolk, 1993).

This chapter provides an up-to-date overview of CRH and its empirical support, its strong points as well as its shortcomings, and its clinical implications. We begin with a brief review of psycholinguistic theory and research that is fundamental to an appreciation of CRH.

PSYCHOLINGUISTIC BACKGROUND

Speech Repairs

Whenever speakers say something they did not intend to say, or say it in a less appropriate way, there is a good chance that they will stop and attempt to repair the utterance. Levelt (1989), in his authoritative handbook on language production, distinguishes between two categories of repairs. *Appropriateness repairs* have the character of further specifications, of saying the same thing in a more felicitous way (e.g., "I want a glass of wine—white wine"). *Error repairs*, on the other hand, are triggered by the occurrence of a linguistic deviancy. A speaker could, for instance, choose the wrong word and then repair it (e.g., "I want a cup of—uh—a glass of wine"). Besides lexical errors, a host of other errors can be repaired, including syntactic errors (e.g., ungrammatical word order, wrong inflections), phonological errors, and prosodic errors (wrong lexical stress). A study of repairs occurring in spontaneous speech by Nooteboom (1980), found that 57 percent of lexical and 75 percent of phonological errors were repaired. The rest of our discussion will focus on error repairs.

An important feature of repairs is speech *interruption* (e.g., "I want a cup of—"), and Levelt has argued that speech is interrupted as soon as an error is detected (the so-called Main Interrupt Rule, to be discussed in more detail below). After the interruption, there is a pause of varying duration, which is often filled with such *editing terms* as "uh" and "um" (e.g., "I want a cup of—uh—"). Error repairs include editing terms in 62 percent of Levelt's

(1983) error corpus. Following this pause, the repair proper begins (e.g., "I want a cup of—uh—a glass of wine"). Most error repairs, more than 90 percent, according to Levelt (1983), involve some kind of *retracing*, either to the beginning of the word containing the error (e.g., "I want a cup of—glass of wine") or to a word prior to the troublesome item (e.g., "I want a cup of—a glass of wine").

Most discussions of self-repairs in speech distinguish between *overt* and *covert* self-repairs (e.g., Berg, 1986; Blackmer and Mitton, 1991; Hockett, 1967; Laver, 1973, Levelt, 1983, 1989; Postma & Kolk, 1992a, 1993). Overt repairs are those repairs in which an error was actually present in overt speech. With covert repairs, this is not the case. However, this type of speech event manifests other features of overt repairs: interruption, editing terms, and retracing. It is therefore assumed that we are dealing with a repair that is triggered by a planning error. Levelt (1983) defines covert repairs as those speech events that are characterized by either (1) an interruption plus an editing term (e.g., "I want a—uh—glass of wine"), or (2) an interruption followed by a retracing of one or more words (e.g., "I want a—a glass of wine"). In his error corpus, 25 percent of all error repairs were classified as covert.

If there are such things as covert repairs, then speakers must detect planning errors and intercept them before they are uttered. This is called *prearticulatory editing*. An important argument in support of such editing is the evidence of all sorts of output biases in speech errors. First, there is a strong lexical bias (Dell & Reich, 1981). Sound errors are more likely to result in words than in nonwords. For example, an error like "hold card cash" when "cold hard cash" was intended is much more likely to occur than is "I should be sheeing him soon" when "I should be seeing him soon" was intended. Nonwords are assumed to be easier for the editor to detect and, therefore, less likely to appear in slips of the tongue. Levelt (1989) discusses data indicating there are semantic and syntactic biases as well, and that speakers are able to suppress socially less acceptable speech errors. In an ingenious experiment, Motley, Camden, and

Baars (1982) had subjects say two-word phrases that would create taboo words if their initial consonants were exchanged (e.g., hit shed, tool kit). Two findings were reported. First, there was a tendency to avoid taboo words so that subjects made errors like "hit head" and "cool kit," but rarely said "shit head" or "cool tit." A second result was that speech errors that could easily have been a taboo word (like "cool kit") were accompanied by larger galvanic skin responses, which are known to reflect emotional arousal, than were neutral speech errors that had no taboo counterparts. The latter result suggests that the taboo word was present during processing at some level, although it was never articulated.

A second important argument for prearticulatory editing concerns the speed with which overt repairs can be made. Speakers are able to interrupt a wrong word during the initial consonant or consonant cluster. An example by Levelt (1983) is: ". . . is a v—a horizontal line." If this error were detected through auditory feedback, one would expect at least the vowel, and probably the consonant, to be articulated before speech could have been interrupted. This argument is particularly relevant for the analysis of stuttering, since stuttered speech is characterized by interrupted words and syllables.

Direct evidence for the existence of prearticulatory monitoring comes from experiments in which subjects are asked to monitor inner speech. One way in which this has been done is to have them internally recite tongue twisters and to report errors. Although there is no overt speech, people do report "inner" speech errors, although fewer than occur in overt speech. Moreover, the distributions of various error types are similar for both inner and overt speech (Dell & Repka, 1992). In a recent study (Wheeldon & Levelt, 1995), subjects were instructed to translate an English word internally into Dutch and to press a button as soon as they realized the translation contained a specified sound (e.g., "react now to the sound /l/ as in: ladder, follow, barrel"). The study demonstrated, among other things, that subjects could do this reliably and that target sounds occurring at the beginning of first syllables were detected faster than were sounds occurring at the beginning of second syllable. We will return to this finding later in discussing how CRH accounts for different disfluency types.

The Perceptual Loop Theory of Self-Monitoring

How is prearticulatory editing carried out? The most influential theory is Levelt's perceptual loop theory of self-monitoring (Levelt, 1983, 1989). Figure 9.1, from Levelt (1989), presents the basics of this theory. Suppose a speaker wishes to express a particular idea. This idea is first encoded by the conceptualizer as a nonlinguistic proposition, or *preverbal message*. This message is input to the formulator, which gives it a linguistic form. Formulating takes place in two steps. First, a grammatical encoding process provides a *syntactic surface structure*. Second, this syntactic structure triggers a phonological encoding process, which results in a *phonetic plan* for the utterance. The phonetic plan is an internal representation of how the utterance should be articulated, and is also called the *articulatory plan*. It is assumed that the articulator accepts this plan as input and realizes it as overt speech.

This covers the production part of the model. What about monitoring? Levelt assumes that monitoring involves two perceptual loops, one internal and the other external. The external loop starts with overt speech. Overt speech is picked up by the audition component, which transforms it into a *phonetic string*. The speech comprehension system "parses" this string, that is, analyzes it phonologically, lexically, and syntactically, and the end result of this parsing process—*parsed speech*—is fed to the conceptualizer again, which created the original message. Included within the conceptualizer is the monitor, which checks overt speech for inappropriate meanings or linguistic deviances, sends out interrupt signals, and starts the repair process when an error is detected.

In addition to the external loop, Levelt's model contains an internal loop. The internal loop is much like the external loop, except that the articulator and audition components are bypassed. The speech comprehension system accepts both the acoustically derived phonetic string and a phonetic plan as input. The phonetic plan constitutes

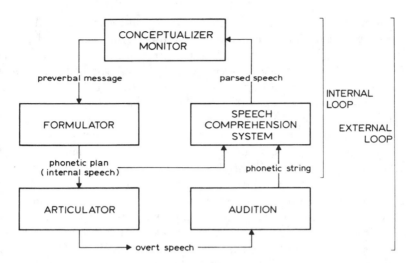

Figure 9.1 Levelt's perceptual loop theory of self-monitoring. (From Levelt, 1989. Copyright 1989 by MIT Press. Reprinted by permission.)

a representation of internal speech, which is processed by the same parsing routines as overt speech. Parsed inner speech is scrutinized by the monitor, which checks it for inappropriateness and linguistic errors. It should be noted that Levelt's model also includes a short internal loop within the conceptualizer that evaluates preverbal messages before formulation begins and makes any needed covert appropriateness repairs.

Levelt's model assumes that monitoring is carried out via the speech comprehension system. His main argument rests on parsimony. If the speech comprehension system can detect linguistic errors in the speech of others, shouldn't it be able to detect a speaker's own errors as well? This appears to be a valid argument for the monitoring of overt speech. However, covert monitoring requires an important extra assumption. Given that the speech comprehension system processes the acoustically derived phonetic structures of overt speech, Levelt has to assume also that a phonetic plan is so similar to acoustically derived phonetic structures that it can be handled by the speech comprehension system. That such a thing can occur is not self-evident and this aspect of the model still needs to be tested.

The perceptual loop theory has two major ri-

vals. First, it has been proposed that monitoring is a much more pervasive process that extends throughout the conceptual, syntactic, lexical, and phonological levels of processing within the production system. This type of monitor is called a "production system monitor," because the whole production system is open to inspection, at least in principle (Laver, 1973, 1980; van Wijk & Kempen, 1987). The proposal clearly is less parsimonious than Levelt's perceptual loop hypothesis. In particular, it entails a "reduplication assumption": The knowledge of how language should look would be contained not only in the production system itself, but also in the monitor.

A second alternative of self-monitoring has been advanced by Mackay (1982, 1987, 1992). Mackay has taken a connectionist approach to language perception and production. His "node structure theory" posits that language processing is carried out by the spread of activation among a large number of inter-connected nodes. Different layers in this network of nodes represent different linguistic processing levels. So there are, among others, conceptual nodes, lexical nodes, phonological nodes, and feature nodes. The network also has input (sensory analysis nodes) and output (muscle movement nodes) layers that serve both comprehension (from sensory to conceptual nodes) and production (from conceptual to movement nodes).

As in other connectionist theories (e.g., Dell, 1986), activation spreads from one node to every other node it is connected to. This means that activation spreads in both forward and backward directions. To give a simplified example, a lexical node for the word ROOF activates its constituent phonemes (/r/ /u/ /f/), and each of these segments, being connected to the lexical node, ROOF, sends activation back to this node. This is called *activation feedback* in connectionist theory. Now, suppose one of the segments has been activated in error, say /l/ is activated instead of /f/. The segments /r/ and /u/ would still feed back activation to ROOF, but /l/ would not. So the lexical node receives less return activation, which would signal the selection of a wrong phoneme. The lexical node can do this because nodes have both a production and a perception function in Mackay's model. In this way, errors can be detected before they result in overt speech through activated movement nodes.

An important property of Mackay's theory is its lack of a central monitor of the type postulated in Levelt's model. It assumes that nodes at a given layer in the network "monitor" layers lower in the hierarchy. Error detection can occur much quicker than in the Levelt model, which requires that production errors result in deviations in the phonetic plan before such deviations can be detected.

The connectionist account of monitoring is parsimonious because a mechanism for error detection is part of the overall structure of the theory, and no special device has to be postulated. So the connectionist account and the perceptual loop hypothesis account equally well for prearticulatory monitoring, and there are no compelling empirical data to choose one over the other at present. The most relevant data are probably measures of the speed at which error detection and repair take place (cf. Blackmer & Mitton, 1991).

Phonological Encoding

Phonological encoding is the process that uses a syntactic representation to derive a phonetic plan that is specific enough to serve as a set of instructions for the articulators. It is assumed that words are represented as abstract grammatical units, called *lemmas*. The first step of phonological encoding is retrieving the phonological counterpart of the lemma, the *lexeme*, from the mental lexicon. The lexeme represents all of a word's form information, both segmental—the set of phonemes that the word contains—and metrical. Metrical word form corresponds to what was labelled the *frame* by Shattuck-Hufnagel (1979). The frame is a series of slots that will be filled with individual phonemes; it is thought to contain various kinds of supra-segmental information. Such information includes the number of syllables, stress levels of syllables, and their structure, like the division between onset (prevocalic segments) and rhyme (remaining segments), and the subdivision of rhyme into a nucleus (vowel) and coda (postvocalic segments) (cf. Levelt, 1989).

Segmental and metrical information are integrated by a process called *segment-to-frame-association* (Levelt, 1992), which produces a phonological representation. An important property of this phonological representation, according to Levelt, is its division into syllables. Such *syllabification* does not respect word boundaries, so in utterances such as "I demand it," syllabic structure is "I-de-man-dit" instead of "I-de-mand-it."

Syllabified phonological representations give rise to the final prearticulatory stage. According to Levelt and Wheeldon (1994), individual syllables activate relevant entries in a mental syllabary. These entries correspond to "gestural scores" that specify the tasks to be performed to pronounce a syllable. So, a gestural score might specify that the lips have to be closed. The specific ways in which this task is carried out are the domain of the articulatory motor system.

Dell (Dell, 1986, Dell & O'Seaghdha, 1991) has proposed a connectionist model of phonological encoding that is of particular importance to this chapter because it has been applied to the analysis of disorders of phonological encoding, in particular aphasic disorders (Martin, Dell, Saffran, & Schwartz, 1994). We will follow the description of this model, as it is presented in Dell and O'Seaghdha (1991). Figure 9.2 is borrowed from their paper and provides an overview.

A distinction is made between semantic nodes, lexical nodes, and phonological (segment) nodes. The syntactic level is left out, for the sake of simplicity. Semantic nodes correspond to semantic features and to concepts in Levelt's model. Lexical nodes are comparable to lemmas. Between each of these three layers, there is bidirectional spreading of activation. Lexical access involves the following six steps:

1. *Input to semantic nodes.* A number of semantic units receive input from external or internal sources and become active. Suppose, for example, that the intended word is CAT and that the three semantic nodes connected to CAT receive input.
2. *Activation spreading from the semantic to the lexical nodes.* Activation spreads from semantic to all connected lexical nodes. In this example, CAT receives activation, but so do DOG and RAT, because they are also connected to two of the activated semantic nodes.
3. *Selection of the most active lexical node.* Of the three activated lexical nodes, CAT receives the most activation, because it has the highest number of links to the activated semantic nodes. Therefore, CAT is selected.
4. *Extra activation given to the selected lexical node.* The selected lexical node is given a triggering jolt of activation, so CAT will receive this extra jolt.
5. *Activation spreading from the lexical to the phonological nodes.* Activation continues to spread as before, but because of the extra activation of selected lexical nodes, appropriate phonological nodes become significantly activated. So, both DOG and RAT transmit activation to the phonological nodes they are connected to, but CAT transmits more activation to its segment nodes.
6. *Selection of the most active phonological nodes.* The most active phonological nodes (segments) are selected and associated with a phonological frame, which would happen to /k/,/æ/ and /t/ in our example.

Dell developed this model to account for speech errors, so how would such errors occur? Without extra assumptions, the intended lexical and phonological nodes will always be selected, because they have the best connections to the activated semantic nodes. To account for errors, it is assumed that the system is subject to *noise*. That is, activation

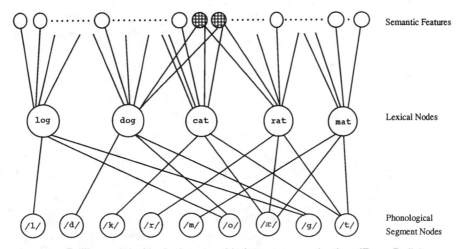

Figure 9.2   Dell's model of lexical retrieval in language production. (From Dell & O'Seaghdha, 1991. Copyright 1991 by The American Psychological Association. Reprinted by permission.)

levels go up and down, according to a particular stochastic (probabilistic) function. Such noise is assumed to result from ongoing information processing that is not specified in the model. As a consequence, a lexical or phonological node corresponding to a nonintended word (e.g., /r/ and RAT), can receive higher activation than the intended counterpart (e.g., /k/ and CAT). Understandably, this will happen more often if the two nodes are closely related in meaning to begin with, such as DOG and CAT, and, therefore, share many semantic features.

Two properties of Dell's model are of particular importance in the explanation of speech errors. The first is activation feedback. We discussed this principle in dealing with Mackay's monitoring theory, but the feedback principle is also important for other reasons. For instance, it is essential in explaining "malapropisms," speech errors in which a word is replaced by a phonologically related word (e.g., MAT for CAT). Figure 9.2 shows that RAT and DOG are connected to the same semantic nodes as CAT, so semantic errors are understandable. However, there are no such common connections of CAT and MAT at the semantic level. How then do such errors occur? The explanation is that CAT and MAT have common connections at the phonological level; they share a connection with the segments, /æ/ and /t/. And if activation spreads in a backward direction, from the phonological to the lexical level, not only is CAT reactivated, but MAT receives activation as well. In a number of cases, activation levels of CAT and MAT may become similar enough to lead to a substitution error, with MAT selected instead of CAT.

A second property pertains to speaking rate. Steps 3 and 6 state that the most active unit is chosen; however, it takes time for a node to reach its activation peak or asymptote (see Figure 9.3). Before reaching an asymptote, an intended unit must compete with other coactivated units. The chance of making a substitution error early in this period is high. Therefore, the model predicts that faster speaking rates lead to more errors. When speaking rate is high, the point at which selection is made moves from S to S- and the competition among units increases. Dell (1986) provides the relevant

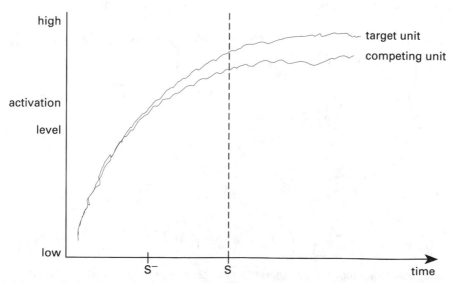

Figure 9.3 Activation and selection. Normal activation rate. Two points of selection: normal (S) and early (S–).

model description as well as empirical confirmation of this prediction. It is in effect a demonstration of the well-known speed-accuracy tradeoff. Interestingly enough, as speech rate increases, not only does error rate increase, there is also a change in error pattern. When selection is made so fast that there is not enough time for feedback from the phonological back to the lexical level, the model predicts a decrease in lexical bias effects, so that the number of non-word errors (e.g., TAT) increases, relative to word errors (RAT). It also predicts a decrease in the number of perseveration errors (reselection of CAT when it is no longer the target), because these errors also depend upon activation feedback (from /k/-/æ/-/t/ back to CAT). Both predictions were confirmed by Dell (1986) under conditions of fast speech.

This account of speech rate effects leads to unexpected consequences. Suppose we do not speed up selection, which leads to higher speech rates, but slow down activation, keeping S where it is (see Figure 9.4). The model predicts the same effects as when selection is speeded up: (1) more

errors overall, (2) more perseverations, (3) more nonword errors. But how can activation rate be manipulated to test this prediction? Dell and Repka (1992) had subjects produce tongue twisters after varied amounts of *practice*. Those who received little practice, and presumably had relatively slow activation rates, should show the same error pattern that is exhibited with high speech rates. This prediction was confirmed. A second way to study variations in speed of activation is to analyze the errors of children. Because children have received relatively little "practice" in phonological encoding, they should show more errors, more perseverations, and more nonword errors. Stemberger's (1989) analysis of children's speech errors confirms this prediction.

This framework has tremendous potential for the explanation of language and speech disorders. In fact, it has been used to account for aphasic naming errors (Schwartz, Saffran, Bloch, & Dell, 1994) and errors of repetition as well (Martin et al., 1994). Next, we will describe how we use this framework to account for stuttering.

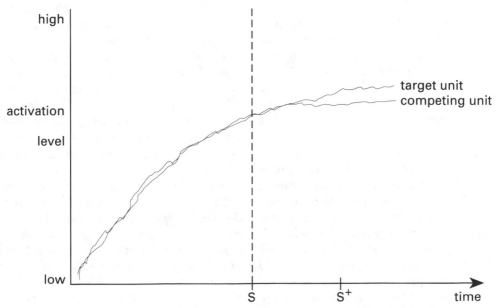

Figure 9.4 Activation and selection. Low activation rate. Two points of selection: normal (S) and late (S+)

THE COVERT REPAIR HYPOTHESIS

Stuttering: A Slowing of Phonological Encoding

The basic assumption underlying the covert repair hypothesis (CRH) is that stuttering constitutes a covert repair reaction to some flaw in the speech plan. Just as the covert self-repairs among normal speakers that have been reported by Levelt (1983) and other researchers frequently include speech interruptions, retracings, and editing terms (e.g., "interjections"), so do stutterings. There is good reason, therefore, to consider the possibility that stuttering is a covert repair phenomenon.

Before detailing the covert repair process in stutterers, we will discuss what we believe they are repairing. In other words, what is the underlying impairment to which a stutterer adapts by means of covert repair? To answer this question, it is important to remember that the speech disfluencies of normal speakers and stutterers are distributed differently. Adult stutterers evidence many more sound and syllable repetitions than do nonstutterers but similar numbers of word and phrase repetitions (cf. Wingate, 1988). And these findings are keys to the answer.

Sound and syllable repetitions require a speaker to interrupt speech within a word. Levelt (1983, 1989) has formulated an important constraint on such within-word interruptions. To understand this constraint, a bit more detail is needed with respect to the repair process. Following Nooteboom (1980), Levelt argued that speech is interrupted as soon as the "trouble" is detected. Levelt calls this the Main Interruption Rule. It implies that sentences, phrases, and words can all be interrupted (e.g., "I want a cu—a glass of wine"). However, Levelt noted one important exception that involves appropriateness repairs. In appropriateness repairs, an inappropriate lexical item tends to be interrupted only *after* the word has been completed (e.g., "I want a glass of wine, red wine"). In error repairs involving a linguistic deviance, on the other hand, there is no such exception. In these repairs, the erroneous word tends to be interrupted immediately. As Levelt pointed out,

"The bulk of within-word interruptions are cases where the broken-up word is an error itself" (Levelt, 1989, p. 481).

If we generalize to the population of stutterers, it follows that the sound and syllable repetitions that characterize adult stuttering must be viewed as *error* repairs. What kind of errors could be involved? What is the underlying difficulty that triggers a repair reaction? To address these questions, we begin with Levelt's (1989) distinction of the four kinds of overt error repairs:

1. Lexical repairs (e.g., "I want a cu- glass of wine").
2. Syntactic repairs (e.g., "Why he did - why did he leave?")
3. Morphological repairs (e.g., "My mother call me - calls me every day")
4. Phonological repairs (e.g., "I want a ga- a glass of wine")

Turning now to the question of what sort of difficulty might trigger a covert repair reaction in stutterers, are their sound and syllable repetitions covert repairs of a *lexical* error? It appears not. If a speaker says "I want a cu- cu- cu- cup of coffee," there appears to be a problem with "cup," but not in the sense that the speaker had intended to say a different word. If so, he would have revised his speech plan to include a different lexical item and would have made an overt rather than a covert speech repair (e.g., "I want a cu- cu- cu- glass of wine"). The same argument holds for *syntactic* errors that require the speaker to revise what he has already uttered and would, therefore, resemble an overt rather than a covert repair (e.g., "Why he d- d- did he leave?").

A third possibility is that the covert repairs of stutterers are triggered by errors in selecting *inflectional morphology*, such as plural inflection of nouns and agreement of verbs. If a speaker detected an incorrect verb inflection, she would interrupt and repair the error, without changing the word's beginning. For example, "My mother ca- ca- calls me every day" might be uttered if a speaker had forgotten to plan an inflection and was planning to say—inappropriately—"My mother call me every day." A covert repair of inflectional errors would not require a revision of the part of a word that is already uttered, so this is certainly a logical possibility. However, we think it is unlikely that stutterers' underlying difficulty is related to the production of inflectional morphology. If that were the case, stuttering would be limited primarily to inflectable words. In English, these are usually nouns and verbs. Stuttering by adult speakers of English, however, is definitely not limited to nouns and verbs. St. Louis (1979) reported, using data collected by Brown from oral readings of adult stutterers, that adjectives, which are only occasionally inflected (in comparative and superlative constructions), were stuttered more than nouns. Similarly, adverbs were stuttered more often than verbs. For preschool children who stutter, it has been reported that disfluencies occur particularly often on pronouns and conjunctions, both of which are uninflectable in English (Bloodstein & Gantwerk, 1967).

This leaves possibility number four, a difficulty with *phonological* encoding, which we will elaborate further below. But first, a fifth possibility, not mentioned by Levelt but discussed by Postma and Kolk (1993), has to be considered: The event that triggers stutterers' repair reactions could be an error at the motor level. There are two ways in which motor impairments may play a role. First, *motor programming* could be implicated. If programming errors arose and were detected by the monitor, that might trigger corrective reactions. Recent research findings, which we noted earlier, permit us to consider this hypothesis in more detail. In the development of a phonetic plan, we distinguished between the syllabified phonological representations and the syllabic gestural scores retrieved from the mental syllabary. These gestural scores are viewed as motoric representations, because they specify what basic motor movements should be made, such as closing the lips. Such gestural scores could be scrutinized for errors by the monitor and when such errors are detected, trigger a covert-repair.

The recent study by Wheeldon and Levelt (1995) seems to exclude this possibility. They asked subjects to indicate whether a specific sound occurred in a word that they were about to produce but had not yet uttered. As indicated above, it turned out that it took longer to detect a particular phoneme in the second syllable than in the first one. Wheeldon and Levelt computed the average difference per subject between monitoring latencies for word-initial segments and second-syllable initial segments. They then measured the average time lapse from the onset of the first syllable to the onset of the second syllable when the subjects actually pronounced these words. Now, if the subjects are monitoring a phonetic representation —consisting of a sequence of gestural scores— the difference in monitoring latencies should be a function of the spoken duration of the intervening syllable. This is because the phonetic representation should mirror precisely the real-time characteristics of the spoken word. It turned out, however, that there was no such relation (a zero correlation was observed). It was even the case that the difference in monitoring latencies did not correlate with the number of intervening phonemes. Wheeldon and Levelt conclude that the structures that are subject to monitoring are the syllabified phonological representations and not the phonetic ones, consisting of syllable gestures. It appears then that there is no prearticulatory monitoring of the motor plan in normal speakers. From this, it would follow that the errors stutterers are trying to repair are not errors in motor planning.

A second possibility is that *motor movements*, not plans, are monitored, and when incipient movements are detected as wrong, through proprioceptive and tactile feedback, speech is interrupted *before* any perceptually identifiable distortion of speech has occurred (cf. Postma & Kolk, 1993). Postma and Noordanus (in preparation) recently completed a study in which they asked normal speakers to recite tongue twisters rapidly and to indicate if they made an error by pressing a button. The conditions included: silent recitation (no articulatory movements, no voice), lipped speech (only movements, no voice), speaking aloud with and without noise. If kinesthetic and tactile feedback play a role, one would expect more errors to be detected in the lipped than in the silent condition. This was not the case; there was only a small difference in the opposite direction. On the other hand, if there are only two feedback loops available to a speaker, one internal and the other external (see Figure 9.1), a different prediction would be made. In the silent recitation and lipped conditions, only the inner loop can be used, so these conditions should produce similar numbers of error detections. The aloud-without-noise condition, in contrast, should produce more errors, because now both loops are available. The aloud-with-noise condition should be somewhere in between, because the inner loop is available plus some of the outer loop, given that auditory masking may not be complete and bone conduction is still present. This was indeed the pattern that was found. If these results are replicated, they constitute important evidence that prearticulatory speech monitoring relies solely on an internal and an external loop, just as Levelt claims. We can say, therefore, that if stutterers are repairing, they probably are not repairing errors at the motor execution level.

It seems reasonable to conclude that covert repair notions of stuttering are most compatible with describing the underlying impairment as one that is phonological in nature. Can such an impairment be characterized further? One characteristic of stuttering is that it is affected by speaking rate; it is reduced when speech rate is decreased (Adams, Lewis, & Besozzi, 1973; Andrews, Howie, Dosza, & Guitar, 1982; Perkins, Bell, Johnson, & Stocks, 1979; Postma & Kolk, 1990). Accordingly, a number authors (e.g., Mackay & MacDonald, 1984; Van Riper, 1982) have suggested that stuttering is a time-related disorder. In Dell's connectionist model of phonological encoding described above, time is an important control structure; this model seems particularly well suited, therefore, to characterize stutterers' phonological problems.

We have hypothesized that phonological encoding of stutterers is slower than that of normal speakers (Kolk, 1991; Postma & Kolk, 1993). If so, Dell's model would indicate that reliable segment selection requires more time in stutterers than in normal speakers. In fact, stutterers' segment selection was depicted in Figure 9.4. If there is an activation delay, there is a greater chance that incorrect phonemes are selected and integrated into the speaker's phonetic plan. This delay does not lead to an increase in overt speech errors because such errors are covertly repaired.

Given this framework, two familiar facts about stuttering fall into place. First, if stutterers speak more slowly, so that segment selection moves from S to S+, fewer encoding errors will be made and stuttering will be reduced. Secondly, if the same passage is read over and over again (i.e., adaptation effect), there is also a decrease in the frequency of stuttering (cf. Brenner, Perkins, & Soderberg, 1972). As we noted above, a similar reduction in the number of speech errors in normal speakers is called a practice effect. Dell's model accounts for these effects by increasing activation rate as a function of practice.

Our framework also suggests a connection with the *onset of stuttering*. As was mentioned earlier, children appear to be relatively slow in phonological encoding; they show the same pattern of speech errors as adults who are reciting tongue twisters without having practiced the task. Stuttering, of course, typically emerges during preschool years, and in most children it disappears sometime before puberty. Speech error data suggest that phonological encoding is slower for all children to begin with, and normal children apparently develop their phonological skills fast enough to accommodate their growing communicative needs. Stuttering children, on the other hand, may develop these skills later. Those who do would be the children who recover; those who do not, would become adult stutterers.

The picture of slow phonological development as giving rise to stuttering is consistent with the findings in a longitudinal study by Wijnen (1991). Wijnen compared the disfluency patterns of two 2-year-old children. In both children, disfluencies increased and then declined before age 3. This appears to be typical of that age period (Yairi, 1982). It has often been claimed that such temporary disfluencies are the byproduct of grammatical development, which starts around that age. However, Wijnen demonstrated that this was a reasonable hypothesis for only one of the children, T. The disfluencies of the other child, H, seemed more related to phonological difficulties. Wijnen presented the following list of findings. These findings, except for those on the language development test, were obtained when disfluencies for both children were at their peak, between age 2:7 and 2:8. At that time, H was a severe stutterer, while T's stuttering was mild, the ratio between H's and T's frequency of disfluency was 10:1.

1. Language development test. On this test, H, the severe stutterer, was advanced for his age, whereas T's performance lagged behind.
2. Percent grammatically incomplete sentences. H had a significantly smaller percentage of grammatically incomplete sentences than did T.
3. Syntactic repairs. H made fewer syntactic repairs than did T, the ratio being almost 1:9.

These observations support the hypothesis that H, in contrast to T, showed no signs of a delay in grammatical development. Two other observations indicate that H had a phonological problem.

1. H made twice as many phonemic error repairs as T.
2. The majority of H's repetitions (76%) were part-word repetitions; the others were whole word or phrase repetitions. Conversely, part-word repetitions were a minority of T's repetitions.

Taken together, these findings clearly suggest that H evidenced a temporary delay in the development of his phonological skills and that this delay coincided with the sudden decrease in speech fluency.

Stuttering Events: Covert Repairs of Errors of Phonological Encoding

In our theory, we connect stuttering and the phenomenon of covert repair that is observed in normal speakers. We are not suggesting, however, that the covert-repair process is somehow disrupted in stutterers. Rather, we have demonstrated that speech monitoring skills in stutterers are normal (Postma & Kolk, 1992b). What we do believe is abnormal in stutterers is that their phonetic plans contain many more flaws and therefore more occasions for error correction. We see stuttering as a "normal" repair reaction to an abnormal phonetic plan. That is, *stuttering is not the error.* It is, in terms of Kolk (1991), a symptom of adaptation, not a symptom of impairment.

How does a stutterer eliminate phonological encoding errors? The simplest possibility is that, upon detection of an error, the encoding process for the word or the syllable in which the error occurred is *restarted.* Why would a restart strategy be effective? In Dell's timing model, the noise component makes activation levels of individual nodes vary stochastically. This means that by simply repeating the attempt, the chance to make an additional encoding error reduces rapidly. If we estimate the chance of making such an error on the first attempt is .10, the chance that two attempts would both be unsuccessful reduces to .01, while the chance to make three errors in a row would only be .001. If the chance of an error is higher initially, more restarts may be necessary. For instance, if it were as high as .80, twenty restarts are needed before error probability is reduced to less than .01.

One important accomplishment of CRH is that it accounts for the *types of disfluencies* exhibited most often by people who stutter. The account is based upon Levelt's Main Interrupt Rule, discussed above. This rule asserts that speech is interrupted immediately upon error detection. We have noted that the main exception to this rule is speakers' tendency to finish the word they are articulating. However, if a word contains an error, speakers may interrupt immediately. Because most stutterings involve within-word interruptions, stutterers apparently do not wait until the end of the word, let alone until the end of the phrase, but interrupt immediately upon detecting an error. There is, therefore, good reason to assume that the point of interruption is closely related to the point of *detection* in stuttering, which is the first step in our account of disfluency types.

The second step is to tie the point of detection to the point of *occurrence* of an error in the word plan. We previously noted Wheeldon and Levelt's (1995) finding that it took subjects longer to detect a particular phoneme when it occurred in the second rather than the first syllable of a word to be produced. This implies that monitoring takes place from left to right and that errors occurring later in a preplanned string will be detected later. Accordingly, we formulated the following hypothesis: Variation in the position of an error in the word plan leads to variation in when speech is interrupted and, consequently, to different manifestations of the word's repair. If we assume there is a constant short detection latency, we can distinguish three situations that differ with respect to how early or late in the word that encoding errors occur. The meaning of "early" depends on the structure of the word; our description will be based on words or syllables having a C(C)VC(C) structure (e.g., "crab"). We will not consider whole-word repetitions, since these are not typical among adults who stutter.

1. Early occurrence. The error occurs at the beginning of word onset, for instance, on the first consonant of "cup." At the moment it is detected, no audible sound has been produced, nor has there been any prearticulatory positioning. If, right after detection, the word or syllable encoding program is restarted, we will observe a *silent pause*. If the error occurs slightly later, prearticulatory positioning has taken place, and restarts will result in repeating this positioning. No sound will be produced by continuous repositioning, but there will be a build-up of muscle tension and we will observe *tense pausing* or *blocking*.

2. Intermediate occurrence. The error is located in a noninitial but still early segment of the word or syllable. It could occur later in word onset, for example, in the second consonant of "place," or it could be located in the vocalic nucleus, as in the vowel of "lips." Restarts

will now result in either a *sound repetition* (e.g., "p- p- p- place"), or, in the case of a continuant sound, in a prolongation (e.g., "ll-lllllips"). A *prolongation* is conceived, therefore, as a smooth consecutive repetition of the same phoneme.

3. Late occurrence. If the error occurs in the syllable coda, for instance in the final consonant of "cup" or in the final consonant cluster of "lips," restarts will result in *part-word repetitions* (e.g., "cu- cu- cu- cup").

Two less frequently occurring types of disfluency do not immediately follow from the restart hypothesis, because they do not involve the beginning of syllables. These are prolongation of noninitial sounds (e.g., "cuuuup") and broken words (e.g., "cu- p"). One could assume that there is a restart from the beginning of the word, but part of the word's onset ("c" and "cu," respectively, in the above examples) would not be articulated. On the other hand, these disfluencies could result from a second type of strategy that Kolk (1991) described as a *postponement strategy*. This strategy consists of delaying articulation of part of the word, which allows the stutterer's activation process more time to be completed and increases the chance of selecting the intended unit (in Figure 9.4, the point of selection is moved from S to S+). Postponement could be responsible for the occurrence of both noninitial sound prolongations and broken words.

It is clear then that a direct relationship between the position of an error and disfluency type can be derived from principles of normal repair behavior. However, a vexing question remains: What determines the initial occurrence of the error? We have hypothesized that stutterers suffer from a slowing of phonological encoding. As should be clear from comparing Figures 9.3 and 9.4, this theory views phonological encoding of stutterers as differing only quantitatively, not qualitatively, from that of nonstutterers. This means that encoding errors of stutterers are subject to the same factors as those of normal speakers. If this is correct, we would expect the same determinants to affect stutterings and normal speech errors. The still limited evidence available seems to support this prediction. The following factors, known to affect disfluencies in adult stutterers (cf. St. Louis, 1979), have also been reported to influence normal speech errors.

1. Word-initial position (Mackay, 1970a; Shattuck-Hufnagel, 1987)
2. Sentence-initial position (Mackay, 1970b)
3. Syllable stress (Boomer & Laver, 1968)
4. Consonant-vowel contrast (Mackay, 1970a)
5. Content-function word contrast (Garrett, 1975; Stemberger, 1984; Nooteboom, 1973)

These similarities suggest that speech errors and stuttered disfluencies may result from the same underlying mechanisms. This does not mean that we know what these mechanisms are. It is unknown, for example, why stressed syllables elicit more speech errors than do unstressed ones or why consonants are more error prone than vowels. The search for causal determinants remains a topic for future research.

EMPIRICAL SUPPORT

In addition to the data already discussed, there are a number of empirical findings that support the various assumptions we have presented so far. We will divide the discussion into two parts. First, there are findings related to the hypothesis that there is a slowing of phonological encoding. Second, there are experimental data supporting the notion that stuttering events are manifestations of covert repair behavior.

Slow Phonological Encoding

There are a variety of empirical indications that stuttering is intimately related to processing speed. We have mentioned the adaptation (practice) effect, as well as the finding that stuttering is reduced when stutterers are asked to slow their speech rate. Slowing speech is one of a list of so-called fluency-enhancing conditions (cf. Andrews et al., 1983). Andrews et al. (1982) reported that speech rate also decreased in six other conditions

that enhanced fluency, such as speech under delayed auditory feedback, singing, and speaking in synchrony with a metronome. In a number of conditions, however, no changes in speech rate were observed. Let us take a closer look at two of these conditions, to see how CRH would account for such apparently contradictory findings: chorus reading (reading from a newspaper in unison with two fluent speakers) and shadowing.

When a word or a phoneme is presented to a speaker, the activation level of the internal representation of that item is increased. This is called *priming*. Priming facilitates subsequent processing of that item. Within spreading activation theories, it is assumed that priming causes an item to reach threshold faster, because activation begins at a higher initial activation level. If stutterers suffer from a slowing of phonological encoding, priming should help them, because it speeds their phonological encoding processes. Now, in shadowing, the words to be spoken are presented auditorily, just before they are produced. In chorus reading, not only are the spoken words potential sources of priming, there is also the written text. Both auditory and visual presentation of the word can serve to preactivate the phonological representations that stutterers need for their speech plan.

At present, two experiments have studied the effects of priming with stuttering subjects. The first is a reaction time study by Wijnen and Broers (1994) with adults who stutter, which employed a paradigm developed by Meyer (1990, 1991). In this paradigm, subjects learn short lists of word pairs. After learning, they are presented with the first word and told to produce the second one as quickly as possible. Response words can be either phonologically similar or dissimilar to one another. It was found that list homogeneity has a positive effect on speech initiation time. For instance, when all words begin with the same consonant, reaction times are shorter than when they begin with different consonants, as if the consonant of the first word primes the consonant of the following word. Wijnen and Broers repeated this experiment with stutterers and normal controls using two types of homogeneity: one in which only the first consonant was the same (e.g., "tailor," "tennis"), and one in which both the first consonant and the subsequent vowel were shared (e.g., "burglar," "burden"). Nonstutterers showed a priming effect in the consonant-only condition and a still larger effect in the consonant vowel condition. For stutterers, a negligible effect was observed in the consonant-only condition, while the consonant-vowel condition evidenced a substantial priming effect.

What does this result mean for our slowing-down hypothesis? Priming preactivates one or more segments of the phonetic plan, so that they get ahead of their competitors more quickly. With stutterers, however, these units are assumed to have slower rise times, which means they need more preactivation to show the priming effects found in normal speakers. This is exactly what was found. When only the first consonant was preactivated, this apparently was not enough for stutterers, and only when both the consonant and vowel were preactivated was the gain large enough for them to evidence a priming effect.

A second priming study was reported by LaSalle and Carpenter (1994) and involved 3- to 6-year-old normally fluent boys. The purpose of this study was to see if a phonological priming effect could be found, not on reaction time, but on speech output. The children had to retell two stories. The experimental manipulation involved the word's final consonant, the coda. One story was loaded with words carrying the same coda, /ŋ/, as in "king," "young," and "wrong." The repeated production of this coda should work as a prime. The control story was of similar length and syntactic structure but had words with normally varying endings. As predicted, subjects produced significantly more within-word disfluencies in the experimental than in the control condition.

We hypothesized that the origin of stuttering lies in a temporary or permanent delay in the development of phonological encoding skills. We discussed Wijnen's (1991) longitudinal study of two children in which phonological difficulty co-occurred with stuttering in one of the children. This relation has been brought to the fore in recent years by Conture and his co-workers (Louko, Edwards,

& Conture, 1990; Wolk, Conture, & Edwards, 1990; Wolk, Edwards, & Conture, 1993). Wolk and colleagues (1990) observed that 30 to 40 percent of the children who stutter also exhibit disordered phonology. Louko and colleagues (1990) found that, compared to nonstuttering children, children who stutter exhibit a greater number and a greater variety of phonological processes. These processes refer to systematic sound changes that affect sequences or classes of sounds, such as deletion of one consonant from a consonant cluster. Finally, it has been reported that children receiving speech therapy for articulation or phonological problems may exhibit increases in the frequency of their disfluencies during treatment (cf. Bernstein Ratner, 1995). Although the nature of the relationship between stuttering and the number and type of phonological difficulties such children exhibit is still unclear, the fact that there is an association between the two problems is consistent with the CRH view on the development of stuttering.

Stuttering and Self-Repair

In a number of studies, we have sought evidence relating to the repair part of CRH by studying the effects of accuracy demands on three types of speech events: speech errors, self repairs, and disfluencies. CRH predicts a particular kind of patterning: Disfluencies should behave like self-repairs rather than speech errors. In a study with normal speakers (Postma, Kolk, & Povel, 1990), we asked subjects to rapidly repeat tongue twisters. There were two conditions. In the first condition, subjects were instructed that, besides speed, accuracy was also very important, and they received feedback after each block of trials on how well they did in terms of both accuracy and speed. In the second condition only speed was emphasized. As expected, error rate went down under accuracy instruction, but overt self-repairs were unaffected.

At first, this contrast between errors and self-repairs may seem paradoxical. If error rate goes down, there are fewer occasions for the repair mechanism to come into action. So repair rate should decrease with error rate. In fact, this is what we find when we compare the data for tongue twisters with the data obtained with normal control sentences. Control sentences elicit many fewer errors than do tongue twisters, the ratio being about 1:5. Accordingly, there are also fewer self-repairs, with a ratio of about 1:4. But when accuracy is manipulated, error rate and repair rate diverge. To account for this repair-error dissociation, we argued that accuracy instruction had two effects. First, it focused speakers' attention on the process of speech programming, causing the number of programming errors to decrease. This should result in a decrease in the number of errors in the phonetic plan and bring about a subsequent decrease in the number of overt errors. Second, it would lead speakers to monitor their speech plan and their output more thoroughly to optimize their performance. This would increase the chance that an error would be detected and repaired. Apparently, these two effects are similarly strong, so that the net effect is nil.

Given this empirical contrast between speech errors and self-repairs, what happens to speech disfluencies? On the one hand, if disfluencies, like speech errors, result from trouble in speech programming, we would expect them to decrease in number when special attention is given to the programming task.

Conversely, CRH assumes that disfluencies are the result of a repair process and should, therefore, behave like self-repairs and show no effects from accuracy instruction. The latter finding was obtained with normal speakers by Postma, Kolk, and Povel (1990) and was later replicated by Postma and Kolk (1992a). Postma and Kolk (1990) did the same experiment with stutterers and found their disfluencies behaved like self-repairs, also, which supports the hypothesis that both normal and stuttered disfluencies are caused by covert repair processes.

Another type of evidence that disfluencies result from covert repairs comes from a dual task experiment by Arends, Povel, and Kolk (1988). Levelt's perceptual loop hypothesis of speech monitoring posits that monitoring is a *controlled* process that requires attention (for a discussion of the distinction between automatic and controlled

processes, see Schneider and Shiffrin, 1977). If the covert repairs that cause stuttering are also based on controlled processing, giving stutterers a secondary task that requires their attention should make them less able to monitor their speech and stuttering should decrease. Arends et al. (1988) had eleven adult stutterers perform a continuous tracking task in which a dot was tracked as it moved over a computer screen during three speech conditions: counting forward, counting backward by threes, and storytelling. Disfluency measures were percentages of disfluent syllables. There was very little stuttering observed during counting forward. Counting backward elicited more stuttering, and here the authors observed a dual-task effect: Stuttering decreased in frequency as the result of performing the tracking task, although the effect did not reach statistical significance. During storytelling, there was still more stuttering: Again, stuttering was reduced in frequency in the dual-task condition and this time the effect was significant. The authors also divided the stuttering subjects into two subgroups. Four subjects whose percentage of disfluent syllables exceeded 15 percent were classified as severe. The remaining seven subjects were classified as mild stutterers. Analysis of variance demonstrated a significant subgroup x task interaction. The dual-task effect during storytelling was highly significant for the severe subgroup, but not for the for the mild subgroup of stutterers. Another measure of these subjects' stuttering, the duration of disfluencies, was expressed as a percentage of total speaking time. This measure was also sensitive to the dual-task manipulation during storytelling and showed a task x subgroup interaction. Now the task effect was significant for both the severe and the mild stutterers. It is important to note that introduction of a dual task did not lead the stutterers to slow their speech. So the reduction in disfluencies was not caused by a change in speaking rate.

We described this last study extensively because its results are controversial. The notion that stuttering is reduced if a stutterer attends to something other than speech has long been advocated, especially by Bloodstein (cf. Bloodstein, 1987, pp. 275–278); however, clear experimental support for this distraction hypothesis has not been forthcoming, and most studies show no effect (see Thompson, 1985, for a discussion). Furthermore, so far, there has not been a convincing theoretical rationale for why stuttering should be reduced when a speaker is "distracted." Indeed, some assume that there are reasons to expect just the opposite, that stuttering should increase as a consequence of a second task (cf. Andrews et al., 1983, p. 240). The Arends study suggests that distraction effects do occur, at least if the secondary task is sufficiently attention demanding and if severe stutterers are studied. CRH provides a rationale for this effect.

CRITICAL APPRAISAL

CRH is a new hypothesis and in need of further elaboration and testing. Although it accounts for the origin of stuttering (slow development of phonological encoding skills), it does not explain why such slowness occurs in some children only, or why it disappears in most individuals but persists in some. Neither does it provide an explicit description of how stuttering changes from childhood to adult forms. In particular, a theory of how the accessory behaviors and associated features develop is not yet available (cf. Conture & Kelly, 1991). In both respects, however, we think that the general background from which CRH was developed does suggest tentative answers to these questions. First, work in aphasia could lead to an identification of neurological factors that underlie the dynamic changes in processing of language and speech. Such factors could then be connected to what is known about the development of the brain and, in this way, a more complete scientific picture of stuttering as a developmental disorder could emerge that could, in turn, suggest reasons for individual differences in the development of phonological skills. Second, theories of adaptive processes in aphasia may also help us to understand the development of accessory behaviors, which are no doubt related to the ways in which stutterers learn to cope with their impairment.

POSSIBLE EXTENSIONS OF THE CRH

At present, we see two major areas of development of CRH in the near future. The first has to do with *word prosody*. Current psycholinguistic theory describes the process of word production as an integration of a prosodic word frame with segmental content (Dell, 1986; Levelt & Wheeldon, 1994; Shattuck-Hufnagel, 1987). The prosodic part of the theory, however, is relatively underdeveloped. Although there is at least one fairly well developed proposal (Levelt & Wheeldon, 1994), there is not yet a computer model with a sufficiently specified prosodic component, and there is little experimental work. We will probably see a rapid growth of the latter in the coming years. In a recent dissertation, Meyer (1994) demonstrated that the priming paradigm, probably the must powerful paradigm in current use in psycholinguistics, is applicable to prosody production. One of Meyer's findings showed that one can facilitate the production of a particular word by presenting in advance another word with different segmental content but the same metrical structure (e.g., "bar" primed "tip" but not "silk"). Thus, a prosodic priming paradigm makes it possible to study the dynamic properties of the frame construction process and of frame-to-segment association in normal speakers and stutterers. In this way, one may be able to determine if the slowing we have postulated relates only to segment production or if it extends to the production of word prosody and its integration with segmental content. This will be of primary importance for CRH, but is of equal relevance for other hypotheses that have located the stutterer's deficit, or at least an important part of it, in the prosodic component of speech (e.g., Perkins, Kent, & Curlee, 1991; Wingate, 1988).

A second area of future development concerns *syntax*. There is an empirical relation between stuttering and syntax for which CRH has, as yet, no explanation. Two types of findings have consistently been reported. First, in both adults (e.g., Koopmans, Slis, & Rietveld, 1991; Prins, Hubbard, & Krause, 1991) and children (e.g.,

Wall, Starkweather, & Cairns, 1981; Yairi & Lewis, 1984), stuttering is more likely to occur at the beginning of sentences. Secondly, sentence length and complexity are positively related to the amount of disfluency, not only in children (e.g., Kadi-Hanifi & Howell, 1992); Logan & Conture, 1995), but in adults as well (e.g., Gordon & Luper, 1989; Wells, 1979).

One way to explain these two findings is to hypothesize that stutterers have a sentence-planning deficit and that this deficit is somehow responsible for the occurrence of stuttering. If we assume that sentence planning occurs primarily in the beginning of clauses, we can account for the concentration of disfluencies at that position. Furthermore, since long and complex sentences require more planning, they should also elicit more stuttering.

The hypothesis predicts that stutterers' sentences are grammatically different from sentences of normal speakers. In support of this hypothesis, it has been reported that children who stutter tend to use simpler linguistic structures (Wall, 1980). However, a recent study by Kadi-Hanifi and Howell (1992) found that stuttering children in different age groups had normal usage of various syntactic constructions (e.g., simple, embedded, doubly embedded, and the like). This same group, however, demonstrated clear effects of syntactic complexity on stuttering frequency. So it seems that, among children with normal grammatical skills, stuttering is still affected by syntactic factors. This dissociation is counter-evidence to the hypothesis that stuttering is caused by sentence planning problems.

If we now return to the hypothesis that it is only the phonological impairment that is causally related to stuttering, how can these syntactic effects be explained? We could follow Mackay's account for the sentence-beginning effect in speech errors and maintain that later parts of sentences are primed by the syntactically and semantically related words occurring earlier, making the earlier parts harder to activate (Mackay, 1987, p. 159). For the length/complexity effect, we could argue that more errors in phonological encoding occur

because longer sentences are spoken faster (cf. Malecot, Johnston, and Kizziar, 1972).

Another line of attack is to assume that syntactic effects are related to the degree of monitoring. Berg (1992) found that speech errors occurring at the beginning of words have a higher chance to be repaired by normal speakers than do errors at later positions. He also reported that the chance for an error to be repaired is higher in stressed than in unstressed syllables. Apparently, people monitor different parts of an utterance with different levels of scrutiny. Perhaps, the beginning of sentences are more intensely monitored than are later parts, because they carry the most important or the least redundant information. Similarly, speakers could monitor long/complex sentences more heavily, because these sentences present a higher risk of making various kinds of errors: pragmatic, lexical, and syntactic. As a byproduct of more intensive monitoring, there would also be a higher chance of detecting errors of phonological encoding. Such accounts must remain speculation for the time being; however, it is clear what empirical data are needed to test these possibilities.

SUMMARY

We can conclude that CRH offers a fruitful framework for the study of stuttering. Not only can it account for a large number of empirical phenomena, it also suggests how to proceed from here. For the further development of the CRH, it is important that its nesting within modern psycholinguistic theory is maintained. Current research in phonological encoding and self-monitoring should be tremendously helpful, both theoretically and methodologically. Besides, it is important to learn from the study of pathology of other behaviors, like aphasia.

Clinical work may profit from some of the insights offered by CRH. The hypothesis can help to disentangle the clinical relationship between stuttering and disorders of phonology in children (cf. Louko et al., 1990). Furthermore, it has implications for treatment procedures that involve changes in utterance rate and complexity. Clinicians often try to bring about slower speech in these children by (1) asking them directly to slow down; (2) asking them to wait a little longer before taking turns in a conversation; (3) asking parents to speak more slowly when talking to their children. CRH provides a theoretical rationale for these treatment procedures.

REFERENCES

Adams, M.R., Lewis, J.L., & Besozzi, T.E. (1973). The effect of reduced reading rate on stuttering frequency. *Journal of Speech and Hearing Research, 16,* 671–675.

Andrews, G., Craig, A., Feyer, A., Hoddinott, S., Howie, P., & Neilson, M. (1983). Stuttering: A review of research findings and theories circa 1982. *Journal of Speech and Hearing Disorders, 48,* 226–246.

Andrews, G., Howie, P.M., Dosza, M., & Guitar, B.E. (1982). Stuttering: Speech pattern characteristics under fluency inducing conditions. *Journal of Speech and Hearing Research, 25,* 208–216.

Arends, N., Povel, D.J., & Kolk, H. (1988). Stuttering as an attentional phenomenon. *Journal of Fluency Disorders, 13,* 141–151.

Berg, T. (1986). The problems of language control: Editing, monitoring and feedback. *Psychological Research, 48,* 133–144.

Berg, T. (1992). Productive and perceptual constraints on speech-error correction. *Psychological Research, 54,* 114–126.

Bernstein Ratner, N. (1995). Treating the child who stutters with concomitant grammatical and phonological impairment. *Language, Speech, and Hearing Services in Schools, 26,* 180–186.

Blackmer, E.R., & Mitton, J.L. (1991). Theories of monitoring and the timing of repairs in spontaneous speech. *Cognition, 39,* 173–194.

Bloodstein, O. (1987). *A handbook on stuttering.* Chicago: National Easter Seal Society.

Bloodstein, O., & Gantwerk, B.F. (1967). Grammatical function in relation to stuttering in young children. *Journal of Speech and Hearing Research, 10,* 786–789.

Boomer, D.S., & Laver, J.D.M. (1968). Slips of the tongue. *Journal of Disorders of Communication, 3,* 2–12. Reprinted in V. Fromkin (Ed.) (1973). Speech errors as linguistic evidence. The Hague: Mouton.

Brenner, N.C., Perkins, W.H., & Soderberg, G.A. (1972). The effect of rehearsal on frequency of stuttering. *Journal of Speech and Hearing Research, 15,* 285–294.

Conture, E.G., & Kelly, E.M. (1991). Young stutterers' nonspeech behavior during stuttering. *Journal of Speech and Hearing Research, 34,* 1041–1056.

Dell, G. (1986). A spreading activation theory of retrieval in sentence production. *Psychological Review, 93,* 283–321.

Dell, G.S., & O'Seaghdha, P. (1991). Mediated and convergent lexical priming in language production; A comment to Levelt et al. (1991). *Psychological Review, 98,* 604–614.

Dell, G.S., & Reich, P.A. (1981). Stages in sentence production: An analysis of speech error data. *Journal of Verbal Learning and Verbal Behavior, 20,* 611–629.

Dell, G.S., & Repka, R.J. (1992). Errors in inner speech. In B.J. Baars (Ed.), *Experimental slips and human error: Exploring the architecture of cognition.* New York: Plenum Press.

Garrett, M.F. (1975). The analysis of sentence production. In G. Bower (Ed.), *The psychology of learning and motivation: Vol. 9.* New York: Academic Press.

Goodglass, H., & Kaplan, E. (1972). *The assessment of aphasia and related disorders.* Philadelphia: Lea and Febiger.

Gordon, P.A., & Luper, H.L. (1989). Speech disfluencies in nonstutterers: Syntactic complexity and production task effects. *Journal of Fluency Disorders, 14,* 429–445.

Haarmann, H.J., & Kolk, H.H.J. (1991). A computer model of the temporal course of agrammatic comprehension: The effects of severity and sentence complexity. *Cognitive Science, 15,* 49–87.

Hockett, C.F. (1967). Where the tongue slips there slip I. To honor Roman Jakobson: Vol. 2. (*Janua Linguarum, 32,* 910–936) The Hague: Mouton.

Kadi-Hanifi, K., & Howell, P. (1992). Syntactic analyses of the spontaneous speech of normally fluent and stuttering children. *Journal of Fluency Disorders, 17,* 151–170.

Kolk, H.H.J. (1985). Stoornis en aanpassing bij afasie en stotteren [Deficit and adaptation in aphasia and stuttering]. In: P.H. Damste and P. Janssen (Eds.),

Foniatrie: Aandacht voor de mens of aandacht voor de stoornis? [Phoniatrics: Attention to the person or to the deficit?] Lisse: Swets & Zeitlinger.

Kolk, H.H.J. (1990). Stuttering as corrective adaptation. NICI Technical Report 90-06.

Kolk, H.H.J. (1991). Is stuttering a symptom of adaptation or of impairment? In H.F.M. Peters, W. Hulstijn, & C. W. Starkweather (Eds.), *Speech motor control and stuttering.* Amsterdam: Elsevier Science Publishers.

Kolk, H.H.J. (1995). A timing approach to agrammatic production. *Brain and Language, 50,* 282–303.

Kolk, H.H.J., & van Grunsven, M.F. (1985). Agrammatism as a variable phenomenon. *Cognitive Neuropsychology, 2,* 347–384.

Koopmans, M., Slis, I., & Rietveld, T. (1991). The influence of word positions and word type on the incidence of stuttering. In H.F.M. Peters, W. Hulstijn, & W. Starkweather (Eds.), *Speech motor control and stuttering.* Amsterdam: Elsevier Science Publishers.

LaSalle, L.R., & Carpenter, L.J. (1994). The effect of phonological simplification on children's speech fluency. Paper presented at the Annual Conference of the American Speech Hearing and Language Association, New Orleans, LA, November.

Laver, J.D.M. (1973). The detection and correction of slips of the tongue. In V.A. Fromkin (Ed.), *Speech errors as linguistic evidence.* The Hague: Mouton.

Laver, J.D.M. (1980). Monitoring systems in the neurolinguistic control of speech production. In V.A. Fromkin (Ed.), *Errors in linguistic performance: Slips of the tongue, ear, pen, and hand.* New York: Academic Press.

Levelt, W.J.M. (1983). Monitoring and self-repair in speech. *Cognition, 14,* 41–104.

Levelt, W.J.M. (1989). *Speaking: From intention to articulation.* Cambridge, MA: MIT Press.

Levelt, W.J.M. (1992). Accessing words in speech production: Stages, processes and representations. *Cognition, 14,* 41–104.

Levelt, W.J.M., & Wheeldon, L.R. (1994). Do speakers have access to a mental syllabary? *Cognition, 50,* 239–269.

Logan, K.J., & Conture, E.G. (1995). Length, grammatical complexity, and rate differences in stuttered and fluent conversational utterances of children who stutter. *Journal of Fluency Disorders, 20,* 35–61

Louko, L.J., Edwards, M.L., & Conture, E.G. (1990).

Phonological characteristics of young stutterers and their normally fluent peers: Preliminary observations. *Journal of Fluency Disorders, 15,* 191–210.

Mackay, D.G. (1970a). Spoonerisms: The structure of errors in the serial order of speech. *Neuropsychologia, 8,* 323–350.

Mackay, D.G. (1970b). Context-dependent stuttering. *Kybernetik, 7,* 1–9.

Mackay, D.G. (1982). The problems of flexibility, fluency, and speed-accuracy trade-off in skilled behavior. *Psychological Review, 89,* 483–506.

Mackay, D.G. (1987). *The organization of perception and action: A theory for language and other cognitive skills.* New York: Springer.

Mackay, D.G. (1992). Errors, ambiguity, and awareness in language perception and production. In B.J. Baars (Ed.), *Experimental slips and human error: Exploring the architecture of cognition.* New York: Plenum Press.

Mackay, D.G., & MacDonald, M. (1984). Stuttering as a sequencing and timing disorder. In W.H. Perkins & R. Curlee (Eds.), *Nature and treatment of stuttering: New directions.* San Diego: College-Hill.

Malecot, A., Johnston, R., & Kizziar, P.-A. (1972). Syllabic rate and utterance length in French. *Phonetica, 26,* 235–251.

Martin, N., Dell, G.S., Saffran, E.M., & Schwartz, M.F. (1994). Origins of paraphasia in deep dysphasia. Testing the consequences of a decay impairment to an interactive spreading activation model of lexical retrieval. *Brain and Language, 47,* 609–660.

Meyer, A. (1990). The time course of phonological encoding in language production: The encoding of successive syllables in a word. *Journal of Memory and Language, 29,* 524–545.

Meyer, A. (1991). The time course of phonological encoding in language production: Phonological encoding inside a syllable. *Journal of Memory and Language, 30,* 69–89.

Meyer, P.J.A. (1994). Phonological encoding: The role of suprasegmental structures. Unpublished doctoral dissertation, University of Nijmegen.

Motley, M.T., Camden, C.T., & Baars, B.J. (1982). Syntactic criteria in prearticulatory editing: Evidence from laboratory induced slips. *Journal of Psycholinguistic Research, 10,* 503–522.

Nooteboom, S. (1973). The tongue slips into patterns. In V. Fromkin (Ed.), *Speech errors as linguistic evidence.* The Hague: Mouton.

Nooteboom, S. (1980). Speaking and unspeaking: Detection and correction of phonological and lexical errors in spontaneous speech. In V. Fromkin (Ed.), *Errors in linguistic performance: Slips of the tongue, ear, pen and hand.* New York: Academic Press.

Perkins, W.H., Bell, J., Johnson, L., & Stocks, J. (1979). Phone rate and the effective planning time hypothesis of stuttering. *Journal of Speech and Hearing Research, 22,* 747–755.

Perkins, W.H., Kent, R.D., & Curlee, R.F. (1991). A theory of neuropsycholinguistic function in stuttering. *Journal of Speech and Hearing Research, 34,* 734–752.

Postma, A., & Kolk, H.H.J. (1990). Speech errors, disfluencies and self-repairs in stutterers under two accuracy conditions. *Journal of Fluency Disorders, 15,* 291–303.

Postma, A., & Kolk, H.H.J. (1992a). The effects of noise masking and required accuracy on speech errors, disfluencies and self-repairs. *Journal of Speech and Hearing Research, 35,* 537–544.

Postma, A., & Kolk, H.H.J. (1992b). Error monitoring in people who stutter. Evidence against auditory feedback defect theories. *Journal of Speech and Hearing Research, 35,* 1024–1032.

Postma, A., & Kolk, H.H.J. (1993). The covert repair hypothesis: Prearticulatory repair processes in normal and stuttered disfluencies. *Journal of Speech and Hearing Research, 36,* 472–487.

Postma, A., Kolk, H.H.J., & Povel, D.J. (1990). On the relation among speech errors, disfluencies and self-repairs. *Language and Speech, 33,* 19–29.

Postma, A., & Noordanus, C. (in preparation). Speech monitoring under different feedback conditions.

Prins, D., Hubbard, C.P., & Krause, M. (1991). Syllable stress and the occurrence of stuttering. *Journal of Speech and Hearing Research, 34,* 1011–1016.

Schneider, W., & Shiffrin, R.M. (1977). Controlled and automatic human information processing: I. Detection, search and attention. *Psychological Review, 84,* 1–66.

Schwartz, M.L., Saffran, E.M., Bloch, D., & Dell, G.S. (1994). Disordered speech production in aphasics and normal speakers. *Brain and Language, 47,* 52–88.

Shattuck-Hufnagel, S. (1979). Speech errors as evidence for a serial order mechanism in sentence production. In W.E. Cooper & E.C.T. Walker (Eds.), *Sentence processing: Psycholinguistic*

studies presented to Merrill Garrett. Hillsdale, NJ.: Lawrence Erlbaum.

Shattuck-Hufnagel, S. (1987). The role of word-onset consonants in speech production planning: New evidence from speech error patterns. In E. Keller & M. Gopnik (Eds.), *Sensory processes in language.* Hillsdale, NJ: Lawrence Erlbaum.

Stemberger, J.P. (1984). Structural errors in normal and agrammatic speech. *Cognitive Neuropsychology, 1,* 281–313.

Stemberger, J.P. (1989). Speech errors in early childhood language production. *Journal of Memory and Language, 28,* 164–188.

St. Louis, K.O. (1979). Linguistic and motor aspects of stuttering. *Speech and Language, 1,* 89–210.

Thompson, A.H. (1985). A test of the distraction explanation of disfluency modification in stuttering. *Journal of Fluency Disorders, 10,* 35–50.

Van Riper, C. (1982). *The nature of stuttering* (2nd Ed.). Englewood Cliffs, NJ: Prentice-Hall.

van Wijk, C., & Kempen, G. (1987). A dual system for producing self-repairs in spontaneous speech: Evidence from experimentally elicited corrections. *Cognitive Psychology, 19,* 403–440.

Wall, M.J. (1980). A comparison of the syntax of young stutterers and nonstutterers. *Journal of Fluency Disorders, 5,* 345–352.

Wall, M.J., Starkweather, C.W., & Cairns, H.S. (1981). Syntactic influences on stuttering in young child stutterers. *Journal of Fluency Disorders, 6,* 283–298.

Wells, G.B. (1979). Effect of sentence structure on stuttering. *Journal of Fluency Disorders, 4,* 123–129.

Wheeldon, L.R., & Levelt, W.J.M. (1995). Monitoring the time course of phonological encoding. *Journal of Memory and Language, 33,* 311–334.

Wijnen, F.N.K. (1991). The role of language formulation in developmental disfluency. Proceedings of the XIIth International Congress of Phonetic Sciences. Aix-en-Provence: Universite de Provence.

Wijnen, F.N.K., & Broers, I. (1992). Phonological priming effects in stutterers. *Journal of Fluency Disorders, 19,* 1–20.

Wingate, M. (1988). *The structure of stuttering: A psycholinguistic perspective.* New York: Springer-Verlag.

Wolk, L. Conture, E.G., & Edwards, M.L. (1990). Coexistence of stuttering and disordered phonology in young children. *The South African Journal of Communication Disorders, 37,* 15–20.

Wolk, L. Edwards, M.L., & Conture, E.G. (1993). Co-existence of stuttering and disordered phonology in young children. *Journal of Speech and Hearing Research, 36,* 906–917.

Yairi, E. (1982). Longitudinal studies of disfluencies in two-year old children. *Journal of Speech and Hearing Research, 24,* 490–495.

Yairi, E., & Lewis, B. (1984). Disfluencies near the onset of stuttering. *Journal of Speech and Hearing Research, 27,* 154–159.

SUGGESTED READINGS

Berg, T. (1986). The problems of language control: Editing, monitoring and feedback. *Psychological Research, 48,* 133–144. This article provides a general overview of the issues in the control of language production.

Dell, G. (1986). A spreading activation theory of retrieval in sentence production. *Psychological Review, 93,* 283–381. This influential paper presented the first spreading activation model of phonological encoding.

Kolk, H.H.J. (1991). Is stuttering a symptom of adaptation or of impairment? In H.F.M. Peters, W. Hulstijn, & W. Starkweather (Eds.), *Speech motor control and stuttering.* Amsterdam: Elsevier Science Publishers. This publication contains the first exposition of the covert repair hypothesis and describes its relation to other theories.

Levelt, W.J.M. (1983). *Speaking: From intention to articulation.* Cambridge, MA: MIT Press. This standard book on language production has especially relevant chapters on phonological encoding [9 and 10] and self-repair [12].

Levelt, W.J.M., & Wheeldon, L.R. (1994). Do speakers have access to a mental syllabary? *Cognition, 50,* 239–269. This reference provides the most up-to-date version of the theory of phonological encoding.

Postma, A., & Kolk, H.H.J. (1993). The covert repair hypothesis: Prearticulatory repair processes in normal and stuttered disfluencies. *Journal of Speech and Hearing Research, 36,* 472–487. This article presents the most extensive description of the covert repair hypothesis and its relationship to theories of monitoring.

CHAPTER 10

STUTTERING: A DYNAMIC, MULTIFACTORIAL MODEL

ANNE SMITH
ELLEN KELLY

INTRODUCTION

We recently had the pleasure of a visit from a colleague, Maria McCarthy, who works in Melbourne, Australia. Her view of stuttering arises from her extensive experience in family counseling programs for children with fluency disorders. In one of our discussions, Maria McCarthy suddenly said, "You know, the problem with theories of stuttering is that they try to give linear accounts of something that is fundamentally a nonlinear phenomenon." We were excited to hear this pronouncement, because this is precisely the conclusion that we have reached in our work, which has focused on several different aspects of the disorder (i.e., physiological correlates and parent-child interactions). The question we address in this chapter is how researchers and clinicians working from disparate perspectives can arrive at a common theoretical framework, one that is multileveled, nonlinear, and dynamic. To do so, we briefly survey the theoretical landscape on stuttering as it appears in the late twentieth century. Following this, we revisit and update our theoretical framework, which has its foundation in the work of Zimmermann (Zimmermann, 1980; Zimmermann, Smith, & Hanley, 1981).

ACKNOWLEDGMENT: Preparation of this chapter was supported in part by grants to A. Smith (DC00559) and E. Kelly (DC00073) from the National Institutes of Health, Institute on Deafness and Other Communicative Disorders.

A LOOK AT THE THEORETICAL LANDSCAPE

Three new theories of stuttering that have appeared in the past five years suggest that the fundamental causal elements for disfluency in stuttering lie in higher level linguistic processes, in planning of linguistic elements and/or adjustment of plans via internal monitoring loops (Karniol, 1995; Perkins, Kent, & Curlee, 1991; Postma & Kolk, 1993). Perkins, Kent, and Curlee (1991) suggest that disfluencies arise when there is dyssynchrony between paralinguistic and linguistic systems that is coincident with time pressure imposed on execution processes. Postma and Kolk (1993) propose a theory of stuttering based on the speech production model of Levelt (1989). Their covert-repair hypothesis emphasizes the role of monitoring loops that are used to detect and correct phonological errors in speech planning and production. It is proposed that those who stutter place the wrong elements into an articulatory buffer and that the detection and correction of these frequent errors leads to disfluency. Misalignment of planning elements is posited at a different level by Karniol (1995), who speculates that disfluencies occur when revised sentence alignment plans are not appropriately integrated with plans generated prior to initiation of the utterance.

We would argue that, although these new models pinpoint factors that may be related to stuttering, they do not provide a comprehensive theoretical framework for experimental and clinical work in the area. These models have in common three problems: (1) They attempt to account for stuttering as an event (e.g., a part-word repetition), rather than as a dynamic disorder; (2) they are linear, positing a core problem from which all stuttering-related phenomena are thought to flow; and (3) they are narrowly focused on putative linguistic processes and thus fail to capture the complex integration of systems at multiple levels involved in fluency breakdown. This is not to say that these models are not relevant to stuttering. Their authors suggest that planning processes may be problematic in stuttering. While we agree that the processes targeted in each model may play a role in stuttering, we do not believe they constitute a holistic framework from which an understanding of stuttering can emerge.

We believe that workers in the area of stuttering should adopt a multifactorial, nonlinear, and dynamic framework. Furthermore, from our own work and conversations with experimentalists investigating stuttering, it appears that many of us are already working with a multifactorial model. In many cases, however, the model is not explicitly formulated. One reason may be that multileveled, dynamic models are not tidy, and they are, therefore, difficult to articulate. The tidiness of static, compartmentalized, and single-level approaches has been noted by Fentress (1986), but as he states, "Tidiness and relevance are not synonymous," and "Complexity and rigor are not necessary antonyms" (p. 101). His comments were directed to models of the development of coordinated movement, but they are equally relevant here. Tidy, static models are intellectually attractive, but stuttering is not a tidy disorder. Equally important is the recognition that complex models can be subjected to rigorous experimental tests. Although experimental work may focus on a single level at a time, the results must be interpreted within a comprehensive framework. Important insights about stuttering may arise from observations at a single level, but it is also likely that insights will arise from examining the relationships between seemingly disparate levels of analysis (e.g., Peters & Starkweather, 1990; Riley & Riley, 1980; Watson, Freeman, Devous, Chapman, Finitzo, & Pool, 1994).

In this chapter we update our theoretical view of stuttering, which has been strongly influenced by nonlinear dynamics (Bassingthwaighte, Liebovitch, & West, 1994; Deering & West, 1992; Fentress, 1986; Glass & Mackey, 1988; Thelen, 1986). Our view has much in common with other multifactorial models of stuttering, including the demands and capacities model of Starkweather (1987), the three factor model of Wall and Myers (1995), and other multidimensional accounts (e.g., Conture, 1990; Peters & Guitar, 1991; Riley & Riley, 1984; Van Riper, 1982).

A MULTIFACTORIAL, NONLINEAR, DYNAMIC FRAMEWORK FOR STUTTERING

The Problem with Defining Stuttering

A major roadblock for stuttering research and treatment has been defining stuttering. In our earlier work (Zimmermann et al., 1981), we suggested that classical definitions of stuttering (e.g., Wingate, 1964) rely too heavily on perceptual/linguistic evaluation of the speech acoustic signal. This remains a significant problem. To conceptualize this problem, we ask: Where is stuttering? Some of the levels at which phenomena associated with stuttering can be observed are:

1. The perceptual system of the listener
2. Instability in linguistic processes
3. The repetition of a syllable seen in an acoustic record
4. A series of eye blinks or foot taps
5. Tremor in muscle activity during speech
6. An aberrant configuration of the chest wall for respiration
7. An increase in skin conductance prior to speech
8. An alteration in metabolic activity of the brain
9. A DNA sequence
10. Avoidance of situations in which speaking to an audience is required

Stuttering "is" all of these phenomena and exists at all of these levels. Stuttering looks quite different when examined as social avoidance behavior, respiratory patterning, or as a repeated event in an acoustic record; however, these are simply different images of a complex disorder, one that operates at many levels and over a broad range of time frames, from milliseconds to years.

Although the disorder of stuttering can be observed at multiple levels, one level of analysis has been elevated above all others: the perceptual evaluation of the speech acoustic signal. In the attempt to objectify the definition, diagnosis, and treatment of stuttering, we have been seduced by units. Part-word repetitions, audible prolongations, silent blocks, and so on. have become the units of stuttering. The acceptance of these units has had a broad impact on theory, experimentation, and treatment.

Theoretically, stuttering is conceptualized as an event that may be categorized in linguistic terms, for example, repetition of a syllable. Models therefore attempt to account for repetition and prolongation of linguistic elements. Arguing for their view of stuttering as a phonological encoding problem, Postma and Kolk (1993) emphasize that "stuttering occurs more frequently on consonants than on vowels, on syllable and word initial positions " (p. 481). Karniol (1995) makes a similar case, noting that "stuttering is more likely on the same words in sentence contexts than in isolation" (p. 111). Stuttering may only be described as "occurring on a consonant" or "on a word" if it is thought of as a compartmentalized event, but the units of stuttering are a convenient fiction that have no biological reality. They are fictive in time and space.

As an illustration of this point, suppose that a child says "it's my buh-buh-ball." We would count this as a single disfluency in the traditional stuttering measurement system (i.e., a syllable repetition with two iterations). When physiological events surrounding this "stuttering moment" are examined, we might find that 2 seconds prior to the syllable repetition there was an inspiration characterized by excessively large air flow; that 5 seconds prior and 3 seconds following the "event," there were significant increases in autonomic arousal. Examining the interpersonal context of the "event," we might observe that the child's older brother had challenged him over possession of the ball 15 seconds earlier. The dynamic processes that contribute to fluency failure occur

at multiple levels and over varying time frames. We suggest that stuttering units are a fiction that has been created as a shorthand to describe the behavior of complex biological systems operating within a dynamic environmental context. Furthermore, "events" that are classified as distinct units in the traditional classification system (e.g., silent block versus sound prolongation) may be shown to reflect the operation of similar processes when considered at a different level of analysis.

The practice of defining stuttering in perceptual/linguistic terms presents a major roadblock, because the units are accepted as real. Stuttering theories, therefore, invoke linguistic models to explain how to produce "a stuttering event," that is, a sound or syllable repetition. Auditory feedback and other "loop" models experience frequent revivals (e.g., Harrington, 1988; Postma & Kolk, 1993), because feedback loops can produce reiterations. We suggest that accounting for prolongations or repetitions should not be the goal of stuttering theory. Rather, a comprehensive theory of stuttering, as shown in Figure 10.1, should account for fluency failures in a multidimensional space that includes family history, social context, linguistic processes, emotional/autonomic factors, speech motor organization, and other factors. We do not intend to imply that the traditional units of stuttering measurement should be abandoned; rather, we suggest that the inherent limitations of these units be fully appreciated. These units are merely a tool that has been used as a window on the disorder. Unfortunately, to paraphrase Maslow (1966): If the only tool you have is a hammer, you treat everything as if it were a nail.

It is apparent that measuring stuttering as unitary events has also had a major impact on diagnosis and treatment. The problems with reliability of judgments of "stuttering events" have been outlined in detail in a series of papers by Ingham, Cordes, Gow, and Finn (e.g., Cordes, 1994; and see review in Cordes & Ingham, 1994). We suggest that the reason for lack of success in the reliable identification and classification of stuttering events according to the traditional Johnsonian categories, or any others, is the use of a primitive and

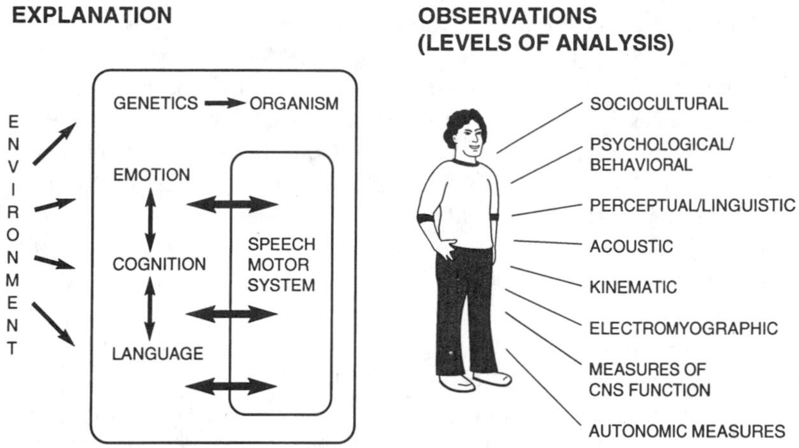

EXPLANATION

**OBSERVATIONS
(LEVELS OF ANALYSIS)**

Figure 10.1   The model we propose distinguishes between the type of explanation that we seek for stuttering and the many levels of analysis that will be needed to contribute to that explanation (adapted from Zimmermann, 1984).

impoverished measurement system. This approach is analogous to taking a car to a mechanic who diagnoses and fixes problems solely by listening to the engine. Certainly an experienced master mechanic can tell a great deal by listening to sounds of the engine, but reliability among mechanics is likely to be low, as the cues used to judge problems are not objectively definable and cannot easily be shared across garages. Cordes and Ingham (1994) suggest that, instead of asking the mechanic to specify what the problem is, we should ask him or her to simply say if "something" is wrong. With this procedure, as they have demonstrated for interval judgments of stuttering (Is this interval "stuttered" or "not stuttered?"), interobserver reliability is somewhat improved.

While it may be possible to improve interobserver and interclinic reliability for counting stuttering by using the interval judgment method or any other unit-level analysis, we question the goal of this enterprise. If the goal is simply to improve reliability for counting stuttering, Cordes and colleagues' (Cordes, Ingham, Frank, & Ingham, 1992) intervals, Yairi's stuttering-like disfluencies (Yairi & Ambrose, 1992a), or Conture's (1990) within-word disfluencies would all be viable units. If, however, the goal is to improve the diagnosis and treatment of stuttering, these may not be the

best approaches. To return to our analogy of the auto mechanic, we suggest that, rather than simplifying the task of judging the acoustic signal, one must look under the hood.

In other words, developing reliable ways of counting "stuttering events" is not the best means to improve the diagnosis and treatment of stuttering. We have argued in the past on theoretical grounds that any event-related definition of stuttering must fail (Smith, 1990). We also believe that event-oriented diagnosis and treatment is not optimal. One of the assumptions underlying the "stuttering-as-event" reliability pursuit is that perceptual judgments of the acoustic output of the client will remain the primary means available to diagnose stuttering and to assess the effects of therapy. Certainly, clinicians employing stuttering modification techniques and self-help groups would object to that assumption.

There are multiple levels of observation and many new tools open to us. Clinical research is needed to determine what combination of variables has the best predictive value in answering the question of whether a given child will develop a chronic stuttering problem. There are many studies that provide evidence of the types of measures that may be useful in predicting chronic stuttering: family history, tests of language and phonological development, indices of speech rate (including percent of speaking time in fluency failure), detailed topography of early disfluencies, and so on (Ambrose, Yairi, & Cox, 1993; Conture & Kelly, 1991; Kelly, 1994; Kelly & Conture, 1992; Meyers & Freeman, 1985a,b; Wolk, Edwards, & Conture, 1993; Yairi & Ambrose, 1992b; Zebrowski, 1991, 1994). Studies are in progress to identify physiological measures that may be useful in the early detection of stuttering (e.g., Kelly, Smith, & Goffman, 1995). The advent of noninvasive, functional brain imaging techniques with enhanced temporal and spatial resolution also should aid us in studying central nervous system correlates of fluency and fluency failure. Diagnosis will be improved by a multi-leveled approach; similarly, better assessment of treatment efficacy will depend on developing multidimensional scales for assessing improvements in fluency. The clinician of the twenty-first century will most likely have a battery of diagnostic tests that will include examination of linguistic, phonological, familial, and motor variables.

In summary, traditional, event-related definitions of stuttering have limited our ability to understand, diagnose, and to treat the disorder. Fluency occupies a multidimensional space that is poorly characterized by disfluency counts. We cannot assume that clinicians of the twenty-first century will diagnose and treat stuttering primarily on the basis of perceptual judgments of disfluencies.

Stuttering as a Nonlinear, Emergent Phenomenon

We propose that stuttering be viewed as an emergent, dynamical disorder (Mackey & Milton, 1987). This implies that stuttering refers to processes that change in time, rather than to compartmentalized, static events. As we have suggested above and as Fentress (1986) has noted, "While for many purposes derived concepts such as 'units,' 'modules,' and 'stages' serve well to highlight important categories of events, they can obscure rather than reveal the operation of underlying dynamic processes" (p. 78). A signature characteristic of dynamic systems is nonlinearity. Thus, a very small change in one pa-

rameter may produce very large changes, even qualitative shifts, in the output behavior of the system (for an excellent introduction to nonlinear dynamics, see Glass & Mackey, 1988).

Concepts from nonlinear dynamics, fractal physiology (e.g., Bassingthwaighte et al., 1994) and chaos theory (Gleick, 1987) recently have been applied to almost every branch of the physical, biological, and social sciences. The "dynamic, emergent intelligence" of the starship's computer system recently was a focus of an episode of a popular television series (Star Trek). It is reasonable to question whether we are simply being caught up in the current, nonlinear fashion and whether these theoretical concepts really have any specific, useful application to understanding stuttering. We would argue that nonlinear dynamic theories have become widely popular because they afford new insights into a broad range of phenomena, from fluid mechanics to the emergence of personality disorders. To demonstrate the implications of nonlinear dynamics for stuttering, we will consider applications to stuttering theory and experimentation.

Implications of Nonlinear Dynamics for Stuttering Theory.   Perhaps the most significant impact that nonlinear dynamics will have for stuttering theory is on understanding the etiology of the disorder. As in an earlier paper (Zimmermann et al., 1981), we defined stuttering as a diagnostic category. The important question then becomes: What factors contribute to the emergence of this diagnosis? A major insight that arises from nonlinear dynamics is that sudden, dramatic shifts in the behavior of systems may occur. Traditional models of stuttering (e.g., Bluemel, 1932; Bloodstein, 1960a,b; Froeschels, 1921; Johnson, 1942) were linear, in the sense that early stuttering behaviors were thought to be simple events (sound or syllable repetitions) that grew into more complex and severe stuttering behaviors with accompanying "secondary characteristics." In linear models of the development of stuttering, some simpler, kernel component (this could be a sound, syllable repetition, placing the wrong phoneme into an articulatory buffer, an inappropriate lag in a feedback loop, etc.) leads ultimately to the complex behaviors of chronic stuttering in adults.

It is now clear from the work of Yairi, Van Riper, and others (e.g., Van Riper, 1982; Yairi & Ambrose, 1992a,b; Yairi, Ambrose, & Niermann, 1993) that at the time stuttering is first diagnosed in young children, stuttering behaviors are often complex and severe, involving "secondary characteristics." Just as the onset of stuttering may be sudden and severe, its disappearance can be remarkably swift. Figure 10.2 suggests some of the aspects of a nonlinear view of the emergence of stuttering. The size of the symbols represents the relative strengths of factors A through E, which play a role in the emergence of stuttering. Each collection of symbols represents an individual. Important characteristics of this type of model are: (1) The factors are dynamic, changing over time, (2) the factors are present to widely varying degrees in the various individuals diagnosed as stuttering, and (3) a small change in one of these factors, or a change in the interaction between factors, may produce the sudden appearance of highly aberrant speech (and non-

speech) behaviors associated with stuttering. Note, however, that a sudden onset of complex or severe symptoms is not necessary for this model. A nonlinear, multifactorial, dynamic account incorporates the heterogeneity well known to be characteristic of the individuals who fall into the diagnostic category of stuttering. The paths of different individuals into (and out of) the stuttering diagnostic space may be quite distinctive. Another significant aspect of this model is that an individual may have many of the underlying dynamics and observable behaviors characteristic of stuttering, yet not be diagnosed as stuttering (e.g., the individual represented by the collection of factors that lies outside the stuttering diagnostic space of Figure 10.2).

Dynamic theories emphasize the strong impact of behavioral context (Fentress, 1986; Thelen & Smith, 1994). The factors that contribute to stuttering may be present in an individual, but not be judged by the individual or his or her culture as presenting a problem in communication. Considerable overlap exists for many of these factors between individuals diagnosed as stuttering and those catego-

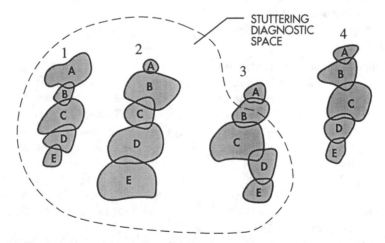

Figure 10.2 The stuttering diagnostic space is indicated by the broken lines. Each collection of shaded areas represents an individual. Individuals 1 and 2 are both diagnosed as stuttering; however, each of these individuals has a different weight on the factors that underpin the disorder. Individual 3 has many of the contributing factors, but moves in and out of the stuttering diagnostic space, while individual 4 has many of the contributing factors but is not diagnosed as stuttering. The essence of our model, then, is that stuttering emerges from the complex, nonlinear interaction of many factors. No single factor can be identified as "the cause" of stuttering.

rized as normally fluent. In this regard, the model makes clear that stutterer/nonstutterer differences do not equal "the cause" of stuttering. In other words, it is a misconception that the "cause of stuttering" will be found by identifying the one experimental variable present in all individuals who stutter and absent in all who do not stutter. Stuttering emerges in individuals when complex, multileveled, and dynamic processes interact to produce failures in fluency that the individuals and their culture judge to be aberrant. There is no core factor—a brain lesion, a DNA sequence, a type of disfluency, a feedback loop—that generates all the phenomena associated with stuttering. In summary, the model we propose, as suggested in Figures 10.1 and 10.2, is multileveled and dynamic. We emphasize that multiple levels of observation and analysis will be necessary to understand this complex disorder. Further, this multiplex of observations must be combined to create a comprehensive explanation of the emergence and development of stuttering within the large array of individuals who are affected by it.

Implications of a Nonlinear, Dynamic Theory for Experimentation in Stuttering.   Some of the implications of this theory for experimental work have already been alluded to:

1. Upon completion of an experiment on one or several factors related to this complex, dynamic disorder, the results must be interpreted within a comprehensive framework. It is our hope that in the future, the elephant and the blind men analogy so often invoked in relation to stuttering research (Culler & Freeman, 1984; Johnson, 1958; Zimmermann, 1984) will no longer be relevant.

2. Experiments focusing on stutterer/nonstutterer differences will not reveal the single key factor or "true cause" of stuttering. This point provides insight into the variable results of studies of many phenomena in the stuttering literature. For example, suppose that Factor E of Figure 10.2 is an emotional factor (the individual has high levels of autonomic arousal when fluency problems occur). We do an experiment to determine how those diagnosed as stuttering differ from those not diagnosed as stuttering on Factor E. By chance,

our first sample of stuttering subjects includes a majority who resemble individual 2, who has a strong emotional component underlying his or her fluency problems. In our first study looking at the means of the stuttering and nonstuttering groups, we find significant stutterer/nonstutter differences. By chance, in our follow-up study of Factor E, we draw a new sample of stuttering subjects, the majority of whom do not have a strong emotional component. In the second study, we do not find differences in the stuttering/nonstuttering means. This example points to the reason for the confusing experimental literature in stuttering.

If we understand that we are looking for multiple factors related to stuttering, rather than a "key factor" that explains all stuttering phenomena, we recognize that to play a role in stuttering, a factor need not be significant in all individuals diagnosed as stuttering. Just as all individuals at risk for cardiovascular disease are not overweight or smokers, all individuals at risk for developing stuttering do not exhibit significant deviations from the nonstuttering population on measures of motor, linguistic, phonological, emotional, familial, or other factors.

3. Stuttering is not an event with real boundaries in time or space. Experimentally we often find it convenient to use static, compartmentalized representations, such as the traditional units of stuttering (part-word repetition, etc.), to identify intervals of time for data analysis. This allows us to provide a "landmark" or index, so that others may know approximately where in the perceptual/linguistic stream we chose to capture our images of the disorder. We must avoid, however, being fooled by a collective belief in the reality of these units. Fentress (1986) makes this point by citing the theoretical physicist David Bohm:

> *The image of vortices in a stream, noted by Bohm (1980), conveys a good initial sense of the problem; i.e., a vortice is a recognizable category of dynamic movements of fluids. These movements can reflect a stream's more stable structural characteristics (cf. anatomy) that are often far removed from the locus of the vortice itself, as well as changes in water level (cf. "drive"!) etc. Stabilities in biological systems are always relative (p. 79).*

Recently there has been a great deal of experimental effort and discussion on the question of how the boundaries of the "stuttering event" can be delineated (e.g., Armson & Kalinowski, 1994; Ingham, Cordes, Ingham, & Gow, 1995). If stuttering is viewed from the perspective we have encouraged, trying to find the boundaries of "stuttering events" is analogous to trying to find the boundaries of a vortice in a stream. The relevant questions are not whether a particular cubic centimeter of water at one moment in time is really part of the vortice or the surround, or whether some millisecond of an acoustic record is part of a stuttering disfluency or the fluent surround. The critical question is: What are the underlying dynamics of these perceptually salient features of the speech production process? In other words, what are the dynamic processes that lead to the apparent fluency failures suffered by those who stutter?

New Methods of Analysis Generated from Nonlinear Dynamics. A multileveled, dynamic framework not only aids us in generating the critical experimental questions concerning the disorder of stuttering, but leads us to new methods of analysis and new explanatory principles. It becomes apparent that we need to examine phenomena using multiple levels of analysis and sampling across a range of time frames (in both real and developmental time scales, e.g., Peters & Starkweather, 1989). Principles then used to explain these phenomena must transcend levels of analysis (Fentress, 1986). For example, one principle often invoked in dynamical accounts of the behavior of complex systems is the continuum of stability and instability. This is a principle that cuts across linguistic, cognitive, emotional, and motor levels of analysis.

The stability/instability continuum can be examined experimentally. Traditionally, we examine a time series of measurements, using analysis techniques that most often concentrate on linear properties, such as the mean and variance. In the past twenty years, there has been increasing recognition that such linear tools of analysis are inadequate to describe highly nonlinear systems with powerfully interacting components (see Bassingthwaighte et al., 1994, Chapter 7 for an excellent discussion of the tools for analysis of nonlinear systems). Some of the new techniques, such as the power spectral density function, are familiar. However, the dynamic perspective provides new ways of interpreting these functions.

One feature of nonlinear dynamic systems is that they may show bifurcations—sudden, qualitative changes in the form of the output. A bifurcation may be suggested by observing changes in the periodicity of the output (e.g., the sudden appearance of a new periodicity). Our work examining the spectra of EMG amplitude envelopes of adults and children who stutter (Denny & Smith, 1992; Kelly et al., 1995; Smith, Denny, & Wood, 1991; Smith, 1989; Smith, Luschei, Denny, Wood, Hirano, & Badylak, 1993) suggests that the motor system bifurcates during periods of extreme instability, that is, those periods in which we easily perceive disfluencies in the acoustic signal.

Mackey and Milton (1987) have defined a dynamical disorder as one "that occurs in an intact physiological control system operating in a range of control parameters that leads to abnormal dynamics" (p. 16). One sign of a dynamical disorder is the "appearance of a regular oscillation in a physiological control system not normally characterized by rhythmic processes" (p. 17). The rhythmic synchronization of motor unit firing that produces these peaks in the EMG power spectra in the 5–15 Hz range is not a feature of the normal operation of speech motor systems. Thus, under this view, neuromuscular oscillations in stuttering represent bifurcations into a qualitatively different state. Because these oscillations tend to occur more frequently during longer disfluencies (Denny & Smith, 1992), we speculate that such bifurcations represent the extreme, unstable end of the continuum. The critical question becomes: What are the control parameters that lead to this bifurcation? Some candidate parameters that we are considering are autonomic arousal (which may be related, in turn, to variables such as pressure in conversational turn taking, status of the listener, etc.), speech rate, and respiratory drive.

Another new approach of nonlinear dynamics is to consider the complexity of the system. Indices of complexity may reveal features of the underlying dynamics, for example, whether variations in the output are truly random (noise) or deterministic (chaotic). Some of the methods of analysis include spectral analysis of rate/time functions and plots in "pseudo-phase space" (Bassingthwaighte et al., 1994). To illustrate these concepts, consider breathing rate during quiet, resting breathing and during conversational speech. We can measure the duration of each breathing cycle over, for example, 50 cycles of each behavior. These data comprise an event series in which sampling is not uniform in the time domain; the data must be interpolated to produce uniform sampling intervals (DeBoer, Karemaker, & Strackee, 1984). The reciprocal of the interpolated function represents a uniformly sampled rate function (breathing rate in breaths/min as a function of time).

With the breathing rate functions for each task, we can create phase delay plots as shown in Figure 10.3. Breathing rate at time t is plotted against breathing rate for the same task at time t+d (d is a delay; in this case we used 4 sec). From these plots, we can see that the variation in breathing rate is, as we would expect, much greater in conversational speech than in quiet breathing. It is interesting to note that pseudo-phase plots for the adult who stutters appear to be more complex, both for quiet breathing and for conversational speech. In addition to being used for the phase plots, the rate functions may be subjected to standard methods of power spectral estimation. Shown in the far right panel of Figure 10.3 are the spectra for the rate functions for each task. These plots may reveal unusual periodicities in the variation of the output (Bassingthwaighte et al., 1994). The slope of such spectra has been interpreted as an index of complexity (Goldberger, 1992; Goldberger, Rigney, Mietus, Antman, & Greenwald, 1988; Kaplan, Furman, Pincus, Ryan, Lipsitz, & Goldberg, 1991). These are only preliminary data from two subjects; however, we note that the adult diagnosed as stuttering has a relatively larger distribution of energy in the higher frequency region and thus a different spectral slope.

As an addendum to this discussion of complexity, it is important to note that increased complexity may not always be a sign of reduced or abnormal function. Using the methods described above to study heart rate variability, Goldberger and colleagues (Goldberger et al., 1988; Kaplan et al., 1991) have found that young, healthy subjects have greater complexity in heart rate variability than do older subjects and patients with cardiovascular disease. Thus, aging or disordered states may be associated with a loss in the normal complexity of biological systems.

As we have noted in earlier sections of this chapter, the dynamic perspective leads us to think about the phenomena of interest with many different time scales (with intervals ranging from very short to very long). Problems of scaling and recognition of repeating patterns are central to the new methods for the analysis of dynamic systems (e.g., Bassingthwaighte et al., 1994). In traditional analyses of time series data, we often pick single points in time from which to take certain measurements (e.g., vowel steady state for formant estimation; onset of a movement and its peak velocity). In dynamic analyses we are encouraged to "throw time out" to create a different window on the potential form of the underlying dynamics.

For example, instead of measuring a series of single points from a displacement waveform representing a sequence of lip movements for a sentence, we (Smith, Goffman, Zelaznik, McGillem, & Ying, 1995) rescaled the data in time and space to look at the stability of the entire movement sequence. We have preliminary data from adults who stutter and matched nonstuttering subjects. Shown in Figure 10.4 are (left panel) the original waveforms of lip motion for ten repetitions of the sentence, "Pop took his socks off." The middle panel shows the waveform after time and amplitude rescaling (normalization). It is clear that the ten productions of the nonstuttering subject were highly repeatable; that is, the waveforms tend to converge on a single pattern. In contrast, for the subject who stutters, the ten rescaled waveforms tend to remain highly variable (all ten utterances were judged to be fluent). To capture this range of

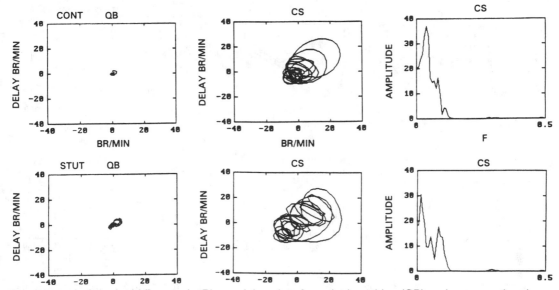

Figure 10.3   Left and middle panels: Phase delay plots for quiet breathing (QB) and conversational speech (CS) for breathing rate data from a normal speaker (top row) and an adult who stutters (bottom row). The mean rate has been subtracted (zero represents the mean rate for each plot), and the delay used was 4 seconds. Much larger variation in rate occurs in CS compared to QB. The subject who stutters shows evidence of less stable breathing rate for both tasks. Far right panels: Spectra of breathing rate data for CS for each subject. The subject who stutters appears to have a relatively higher distribution of energy in the higher frequency region, but no unusual periodicity in rate is apparent.

spatiotemporal variability, we then computed an index (the spatiotemporal index, or STI), which is the cumulative sum of the 50 standard deviations computed at 2 percent intervals across normalized time. For the normally fluent subject, the STI is 12.46. For the stuttering subject, the STI was approximately double this value, or 25.69. Thus, time and amplitude rescaling allows us to capture aspects of variability by considering the entire waveform rather than selecting isolated points in time for measurement. These data provide further evidence that, even when we cannot perceive disfluency, the underlying dynamics of the speech production process for those who stutter may be different from those of speakers who do not have fluency problems (e.g., Peters & Boves, 1988)

The above examples of methods from nonlinear dynamics have been drawn from physiological studies. Much of our work examines the physiological aspects of stuttering; therefore, these examples and data are convenient for us. The application of

these principles and methods, however, is not limited to physiological signals. We have noted that an important principle in dynamic models is the behavioral context. Fentress (1986) and others (e.g., Thelen & Smith, 1994) have stressed the importance of "contextual affordances" in the emergence of behaviors. There are obviously many factors external to the organism that play a significant role in the emergence of stuttering.

Clearly, the principles outlined above could be incorporated into many levels of analysis. For example, in the development of stuttering, interactions between conversational partners, such as caregivers and the child, at the onset of stuttering and over time, may be significant. In traditional, linear analyses, overall frequencies and means of specific behaviors (e.g., speech rate, interspeaker pauses, and interruptions) have been compared. Results of these studies have been equivocal (cf. Kelly, 1994; Kelly & Conture, 1992; Meyers & Freeman, 1985a,b; Schulze, 1991). With the

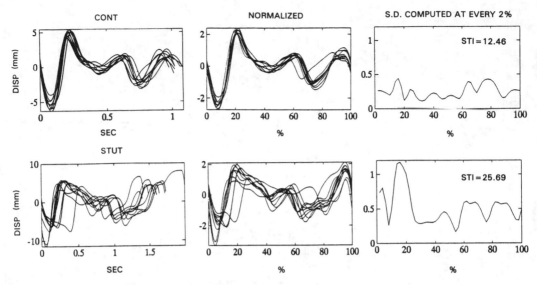

Figure 10.4 Left panel: Unprocessed displacement waveforms for a normal speaker (top) and an adult who stutters (bottom). Overlaid traces are displacement waveforms of the lower lip for ten fluent productions of "Pop took his socks off." Alignment points are the peak velocities of the first and last opening movements. Middle panel: Data after rescaling by normalization. The normal speaker shows a more regular pattern. Right panel: Standard deviations computed at 2 percent intervals from the rescaled data. The spatiotemporal index (STI) is the sum of the 50 standard deviations. The much higher STI of the subject who stutters suggests much greater variability in the patterning of speech movements over repetition of this utterance.

development of techniques such as computer-automated sequential analyses, we are beginning to examine the relations between and among parents' and children's speech behaviors (including stuttering) at specific points in time, as well as over the course of longer intervals (e.g., hours, days, weeks, months), and in varying contexts (e.g., home, school, clinic). In this way, dynamic fluctuations in children's stuttering and parents' and children's conversational behaviors may be examined in conjunction with other factors related to the development of stuttering. Long-term analyses may reveal nonlinear fluctuations in a wide range of variables related to fluency failure.

SUMMARY

The nonlinear dynamic framework provides a rich world of analysis techniques as well as new ways of thinking about familiar analyses. These methods encourage us to conceptualize and to characterize

experimentally the dynamics of the underlying processes. In the case of stuttering, we are rooted in arguments about what is "really" a "stuttered" disfluency and whether we can reliably count "stuttered events." The field must move beyond attempts to identify isolated fluent, disfluent, or stuttered moments reliably. Parents and clinicians are able to agree when a fluency problem exists, despite potential interclinic differences (e.g., Ingham & Cordes, 1992) in disfluency counts. Instead, it is our task to explain the complex, dynamic interplay of the factors that leads to the diagnosis of stuttering. With the new methods and theories available to us, the armamentarium of the clinician of the twenty-first century should be considerably different than it is today. We predict that multileveled indices of stability, complexity, and nonlinearity, together with the more traditional measures of familial, linguistic, phonological, and motor factors, will be critical to improved success in the early diagnosis and treatment of stuttering.

REFERENCES

Ambrose, N.G., Yairi, E., & Cox, N. (1993). Genetic aspects of early childhood stuttering. *Journal of Speech and Hearing Research, 36*, 701–706.

Armson, J., & Kalinowski, J. (1994). Interpreting results of the fluent speech paradigm in stuttering research: Difficulties in separating cause from effect. *Journal of Speech and Hearing Research, 37*, 69–82.

Bassingthwaighte, J.B., Liebovitch, L.S., & West, B.J. (1994). *Fractal physiology*. New York: Oxford University Press.

Bloodstein, O. (1960a). The development of stuttering: I. Changes in nine basic features. *Journal of Speech and Hearing Disorders, 25*, 219–237.

Bloodstein, O. (1960b). The development of stuttering: II. Developmental phases. *Journal of Speech and Hearing Disorders, 25*, 366–376.

Bluemel, C.S. (1932). Primary and secondary stammering. *Quarterly Journal of Speech, 18*, 187–200.

Bohm, D. (1980). *Wholeness and the implicate order*. London: Routledge & Kegan Paul.

Conture, E.G. (1990). *Stuttering* (2nd Ed.). Englewood Cliffs, N.J.: Prentice Hall.

Conture, E.G., & Kelly, E.M. (1991). Young stutterers' nonspeech behavior during stuttering. *Journal of Speech and Hearing Research, 34*, 1041–1056.

Cordes, A.K. (1994). The reliability of observational data: I. Theories and methods for speech-language pathology. *Journal of Speech and Hearing Research, 37*, 264–278.

Cordes, A.K., & Ingham, R.J. (1994). The reliability of observational data: II. Issues in the identification and measurement of stuttering event judgements. *Journal of Speech and Hearing Research, 37*, 279–294.

Cordes, A.K., Ingham, R.J., Frank, P., & Ingham, J.C. (1992). Time-interval analysis of interjudge and intrajudge agreement for stuttering event judgements. *Journal of Speech and Hearing Research, 35*, 483–494.

Culler, M., & Freeman, F. (1984). Stuttering: The six blind men revisited. *Journal of Fluency Disorders, 19*.

DeBoer, R.W., Karemaker, J.M., & Strackee, J. (1984). Comparing spectra of a series of point events particularly for heart rate variability data. *IEEE Trans Biomed Eng, 31*, 384–387.

Deering, W., & West, B.J. (1992). Fractal physiology. *IEEE Eng Med Bio*, 40–46.

Denny, M., & Smith, A. (1992). Gradations in a pattern of neuromuscular activity associated with stuttering. *Journal of Speech and Hearing Research, 35*, 1216–1229.

Fentress, J.C. (1986). Development of coordinated movement: Dynamic, relational, and multileveled perspectives. In M.G. Wade & H.T.A. Whiting (Eds.), *Motor development in children: Aspects of coordination and control* (pp. 77–105). Dordrecht: Martinus Nijhoff Publishers.

Froeschels, E. (1921). Beitrage zur symptomatologie des stotterns. *Monatsschr. Ohrenheilk, 55*, 1109–1112.

Glass, L., & Mackey, M.C. (1988). *From clocks to chaos*. Princeton, N.J.: Princeton University Press.

Gleick, J. (1987). *Chaos: Making a new science*. New York: Viking Penguin.

Goldberger, A.L. (1992). Fractal mechanisms in the electrophysiology of the heart. *IEEE Eng Med Bio*, 47–52.

Goldberger, A.L., Rigney, D.R., Mietus, J., Antman, E.M., & Greenwald, S. (1988). Nonlinear dynamics in sudden cardiac death syndrome: Heartrate oscillations and bifurcations. *Experientia, 44*, 983–987.

Harrington, J. (1988). Stuttering, delayed auditory feedback, and linguistic rhythm. *Journal of Speech and Hearing Research, 31*, 36–47.

Ingham, R.J., & Cordes, A.K. (1992). Interclinic differences in stuttering event counts. *Journal of Speech and Hearing Disorders, 17*, 171–176.

Ingham, R.J., Cordes, A.K., Ingham, J.C., & Gow, M.L. (1995). Identifying the onset and offset of stuttering events. *Journal of Speech and Hearing Research, 38*, 315–326.

Johnson, W. (1942). A study of the onset and development of stuttering. *Journal of Speech Disorders, 7*, 251–257.

Johnson, W. (1958). The six men and the stuttering. In J. Eisenson (Ed.), *Stuttering* (pp. xi–xxiv). New York: Harper & Brothers.

Kaplan, D.T., Furman, M.I., Pincus, S.M., Ryan, S.M., Lipsitz, L.A., & Goldberg, A.L. (1991). Aging and the complexity of cardiovascular dynamics. *Biophysics Journal, 59*, 945–949.

Karniol, R. (1995). Stuttering, language, and cognition: A review and a model of stuttering as suprasegmental sentence plan alignment (SPA). *Psychological Bulletin, 117*, 104–124.

Kelly, E.M. (1994). Speech rates and turn-taking behaviors of children who stutter and their fathers. *Journal of Speech and Hearing Research, 37,* 1284–1294.

Kelly, E.M., & Conture, E.G. (1992). Speaking rates, response time latencies, and interrupting behaviors of young stutterers, nonstutterers, and their mothers. *Journal of Speech and Hearing Research, 35,* 1256–1257.

Kelly, E.M., Smith, A., & Goffman, L. (1995). Orofacial muscle activity of children who stutter: A preliminary study. *Journal of Speech and Hearing Research, 38,* 1025–1036.

Levelt, W.J.M. (1989). *Speaking: From intention to articulation.* Cambridge, Mass.: MIT Press.

Mackey, M.C., & Milton, J.G. (1987). Dynamical diseases. In S.H. Koslow, A.J. Mandell, & M.F. Shlesinger (Eds.), *Perspectives in biological dynamics and theoretical medicine* (pp. 16–32). New York: The New York Academy of Sciences.

Maslow, A.H. (1966). *The psychology of science.* New York: Harper & Row.

Meyers, S.C., & Freeman, F.J. (1985a). Interruptions as a variable in stuttering and disfluency. *Journal of Speech and Hearing Research, 28,* 428–435.

Meyers, S.C. & Freeman, F.J. (1985b). Mother and child speech rates as a variable in stuttering and disfluency. *Journal of Speech and Hearing Research, 28,* 436–444.

Perkins, W.H., Kent, R.D., & Curlee, R.F. (1991). A theory of neuropsycholinguistic function in stuttering. *Journal of Speech and Hearing Research, 34,* 734–752.

Peters, H.F.M., & Boves, L. (1988). Coordination of aerodynamic and phonatory processes in fluent speech utterances of stutterers. *Journal of Speech and Hearing Research, 31,* 352–361.

Peters, H.F.M., & Starkweather, C.W. (1989). Development of stuttering throughout life. *Journal of Fluency Disorders, 14,* 303–321.

Peters, H.F.M., & Starkweather, C.W. (1990). The interaction between speech motor coordination and language processes in the development of stuttering. *Journal of Fluency Disorders, 15,* 115–125.

Peters, T.J., & Guitar, B. (1991). *Stuttering: An integrated approach to its nature and treatment.* Baltimore, MD: Williams & Wilkins.

Postma, A., & Kolk, H. (1993). The covert repair hypothesis: Prearticulatory repair processes in normal and stuttered disfluencies. *Journal of Speech and Hearing Research, 36,* 472–487.

Riley, G.D., & Riley, J. (1980). Motoric and linguistic variables among children who stutter. *Journal of Speech and Hearing Disorders, 37,* 314–320.

Riley, G.D., & Riley, J. (1984). A component model for treating stuttering in children. In M. Peins (Ed.), *Contemporary approaches in stuttering therapy.* Boston: Little, Brown.

Schulze, H. (1991). Time pressure variables in the verbal parent-child interaction patterns of fathers and mothers of stuttering, phonologically disordered and normal preschool children. In H.F.M. Peters, W. Hulstijn, & C.W. Starkweather (Eds.), *Speech motor control and stuttering* (pp. 441–452). Amsterdam: Elsevier Science Publishers.

Smith, A. (1989). Neural drive to muscles in stuttering. *Journal of Speech and Hearing Research, 32,* 252–264.

Smith, A. (1990). Toward a comprehensive theory of stuttering: A commentary. *Journal of Speech and Hearing Disorders, 55,* 398–401.

Smith, A. (1990). Factors in the etiology of stuttering. *American Speech-Language-Hearing Association Reports, Research Needs in Stuttering: Roadblocks and Future Directions, 18,* 39–47.

Smith, A., Denny, M., & Wood, J. (1991). Instability in speech motor systems in stuttering. In H.F.M. Peters, W. Hulstijn, & W. Starkweather (Eds.), *Speech motor control and stuttering* (pp. 231–242). Amsterdam: Elsevier.

Smith, A., Goffman, L., Zelaznik, H.N., Ying, G., & McGillem, C. (1995). Spatiotemporal stability and patterning of speech movement sequences. *Experimental Brain Research, 104,* 493–501.

Smith, A., Luschei, E., Denny, M., Wood, J., Hirano, M., & Badylak, S. (1993). Spectral analysis of activity of laryngeal and orofacial muscles in stutterers. *Journal of Neurology, Neurosurgery, and Psychiatry, 56,* 1303–1311.

Starkweather, C.W. (1987). *Fluency and stuttering.* Englewood Cliffs, N.J.: Prentice-Hall, Inc.

Starkweather, C.W., Gottwald, R.S., & Halfond, M. (1990). *Stuttering prevention: A clinical method.* Englewood Cliffs, N.J.: Prentice-Hall.

Thelen, E. (1986). Development of coordinated movement: Implications for early human development. In M.G. Wade & H.T.A. Whiting (Eds.), *Motor development in children: Aspects of coordination and control* (pp. 107–124). Dordrecht: Martinus Nijhoff Publishers.

Thelen, E., & Smith, L.B. (1994). *A dynamic systems approach to the development of cognition and action*. Cambridge, Mass.: MIT Press.

Van Riper, C. (1982). *The nature of stuttering* (2nd ed.). Englewood Cliffs, N.J.: Prentice-Hall.

Wall, M.J., & Myers, F.L. (1995). Theories of stuttering and therapeutic implications. In *Clinical management of childhood stuttering* (2nd ed.). Austin, Tex.: Pro-ed.

Watson, B.C., Freeman, F.J., Devous, Sr., M.D., Chapman, S.B., Finitzo, T., & Pool, K.R. (1994). Linguistic performance and regional cerebral blood flow in persons who stutter. *Journal of Speech and Hearing Research, 37,* 1221–1228.

West, B.J. (1990). Fractal forms in physiology. *International Journal of Modern Physics, 4,* 1629–1669.

Wingate, M.E. (1964). A standard definition of stuttering. *Journal of Speech and Hearing Disorders, 29,* 484–489.

Wolk, L., Edwards, M.L., & Conture, E. (1993). Coexistence of stuttering and disordered phonology in young children. *Journal of Speech and Hearing Research, 36,* 906–917.

Yairi, E., & Ambrose, N.G. (1992a). A longitudinal study of stuttering in children: A preliminary report. *Journal of Speech and Hearing Research, 35,* 755–760.

Yairi, E., & Ambrose, N.G. (1992b). Onset of stuttering in preschool children: Selected factors. *Journal of Speech and Hearing Research, 37,* 782–788.

Yairi, E., Ambrose, N.G., & Niermann, R. (1993). The early months of stuttering: A developmental study. *Journal of Speech and Hearing Research, 36,* 521–528.

Zebrowski, P.M. (1991). Duration of the speech disfluencies of beginning stutterers. *Journal of Speech and Hearing Research, 34,* 483–491.

Zebrowski, P.M. (1994). Duration of sound prolongation and sound/syllable repetition in children who stutter: Preliminary observations. *Journal of Speech and Hearing Research, 37,* 254–263.

Zimmermann, G.N. (1980). Stuttering: A disorder of movement. *Journal of Speech and Hearing Research, 23,* 122–136.

Zimmermann, G.N. (1984). Articulatory dynamics of stutterers. In R.F. Curlee & W.H. Perkins (Eds.), *Nature and treatment of stuttering: New directions* (pp. 131–147). San Diego, Calif.: College-Hill.

Zimmermann, G.N., Smith, A., & Hanley, J.M. (1981). Stuttering: In need of a unifying conceptual framework. *Journal of Speech and Hearing Research, 24,* 25–31.

SUGGESTED READINGS

Bassingthwaighte, J.B., Liebovitch, L.S., & West, B.J. (1994). *Fractal physiology*. New York: Oxford University Press.

Fentress, J.C. (1986). Development of coordinated movement: Dynamic, relational, and multileveled perspectives. In M.G. Wade & H.T.A. Whiting (Eds.), *Motor development in children: Aspects of coordination and control* (pp. 77–105). Dordrecht: Martinus Nijhoff Publishers.

Glass, L., & Mackey, M.C. (1988). *From clocks to chaos*. Princeton, N.J.: Princeton University Press.

Mackey, M.C., & Milton, J.G. (1987). Dynamical diseases. In S.H. Koslow, A.J. Mandell, & M.F. Shlesinger (Eds.), *Perspectives in biological dynamics and theoretical medicine* (pp. 16–32). New York: The New York Academy of Sciences.

Smith, A. (1990). Factors in the etiology of stuttering. *American Speech-Language-Hearing Association Reports, Research Needs in Stuttering: Roadblocks and Future Directions, 18,* 39–47.

Thelen, E. (1986). Development of coordinated movement: Implications for early human development. In M.G. Wade & H.T.A. Whiting (Eds.), *Motor development in children: Aspects of coordination and control* (pp. 107–124). Dordrecht: Martinus Nijhoff Publishers.

Zimmermann, G.N. (1980). Stuttering: A disorder of movement. *Journal of Speech and Hearing Research, 23,* 122–136.

CHAPTER 11

HISTORICAL ANALYSIS OF WHY SCIENCE HAS NOT SOLVED STUTTERING

WILLIAM H. PERKINS

The science of stuttering, or of anything else, is two-thirds architecture, one-third sports. Starting with architecture, the architect's first task is to define the project in order to, second, design a structure that meets all of the client's needs within the context of a specific site with as elegantly simple a solution as possible. For science, this is comparable to designing an explanation of stuttering that fits all of the defining characteristics of the problem within the context of the individual who stutters with as parsimoniously simple a theory as possible.

Implications of this analogy are instructive. Consider simplicity. The simpler the theory that explains the greatest complexity, the greater its beauty. For example, Einstein's $E=MC^2$ explains all aspects of mass and energy. When asked what would have happened to his theory if early experiments had not confirmed it, he replied, "The experiments would have been wrong." His reason— the theory was too elegantly simple to be wrong. In fact, beauty is of such importance that it is considered by a Nobel physicist to be a stronger test of a final theory of the physical world than empirical evidence (Weinberg, 1992).

Think of the consequences of designing and constructing the bedroom of a house without concern for where, at minimum, the living room, kitchen, and bathroom would be, how they would fit together, how the house would look. If all the rooms were designed independently by different architects in different styles, a hodgepodge would be inevitable.

For stuttering, the equivalent would be to have a theory of onset, a different theory of normal disfluency, then several theories of how normal disfluency becomes abnormal stuttering, a theory of primary stuttering, a theory of secondary stuttering, a theory of neurogenic stuttering, a theory of developmental stuttering, a theory of linguistic stuttering, a theory of articulatory stuttering, a theory of severity, a theory of genetic stuttering, a theory of cluttering stuttering, and the list goes on. Unfortunately, of course, as this text bears witness, this is essentially what we do have.

The one common element running through these theories would be that they are attempts to explain some aspect of what most everyone thinks they can recognize when they hear it. If stuttering were a house and each of these theories a separately designed and constructed room, the architectural hodgepodge we started with would seem beautifully simple by comparison.

Just as an elegant architectural design must take into account everything about the building— room requirements and relationships, plumbing, heating, interior and exterior appearance in relationship to the setting—so must an elegant theory explain all aspects of stuttering. At minimum, a bare bones theory must account for the universal defining feature, that is, the characteristic that is necessary and sufficient to identify stuttering, whether by speakers or listeners. Obviously, this objective, for either architecture or theory construction, cannot be met by assembling bits and pieces of different solutions by different people at different times. If stuttering is ever to be solved, a unified conception of the entire problem will be required as the foundation.

Thus far, we have considered two of the three fundamental requirements for a scientific solution of stuttering, which can be stated as follows (Perkins, 1996):

1. "The invariant characteristic that defines the categorical difference between stuttered and nonstuttered disfluency must be established as a valid and reliable constraint on any theoretical explanation."

2. "A logically constructed, comprehensive, noncontradictory, necessary and sufficient, testable explanation of cause and effects of stuttering must be formulated."

Now for sports, the basis of the third requirement. All sporting events, from their ancient beginnings, have had a common objective—to determine a winner. Competitive sports without winners are not competitive sports. Rules, regulations, and referees have been used to insure that the winner is, indeed, the strongest.

By the same token, science was devised to accomplish exactly the same objective in the arena of knowledge. Science is designed to reveal the nature of reality with all its messy empirical inconsistencies and contradictions. Unlike mathematics, which is concerned with abstract proof and truth, science proceeds in incremental steps toward this revelation by disproof. The luxury of proof is beyond its scope for the same reason it is beyond the scope of sports. The winner of the Super Bowl is best only in comparison with the teams it beats. This is not proof that it is and will forever be the best. The possibility always threatens that eventually it can, and will, be beaten. A team remains as winner only as long as it avoids defeat.

So it must be with theories if they are to serve a purpose. A theory that cannot be defeated is as useless as a team that cannot be beaten. To *insure* winning, that team's games would have to be unjustly rigged to prevent the possibility that a stronger opponent might win. To insure fair tests of theories, methodological procedures for unbiased observation and analysis have been devised. The objective of scientific methodology is to test the strength of a theory by trying to disprove it, which means that it must be constructed so as to be vulnerable to disproof. Its strength is only as great as the strength of efforts to defeat it.

Here, then, is the third leg for the basis of scientific progress:

3. "Theoretical inferences must be rigorously tested under replicable conditions before they can be accepted as definitive statements" (Perkins, 1996).

The order in which these legs are constructed and applied is not optional. Until the essence of stuttering that differentiates it from nonstuttered disfluency (which includes transient disfluency that only sounds like stuttering) is unambiguously identified, no basis exists for constructing a theory. After all, how could we have a theory of something that does not exist? And without a theory, how can powerful methodology designed to test it be put to proper use?

Within this framework of requirements for scientific progress, let us briefly review the history of systematic investigation of stuttering. It began with the Orton-Travis theory of cerebral-dominance proposed in 1929. Travis described it in the first text in the field (1931, p. 96).

My point of view is that in most cases the act of stuttering is a neuromuscular derangement secondary to general reduction in cortical lead control. The latter is conceived to be due to transient and mutually inhibitative activities of the right and the left cerebral hemispheres. In the stutterer, instead of nervous energy being mobilized by one center of greatest potential, it is mobilized by two centers of comparable potential. Because both of these centers when operating singly function in reaction patterns of opposite motor orientation and configuration, there is produced in the peripheral speech organ an undesirable competition in the resulting muscular movements. The symptoms of stuttering are then mainly the peripheral signs of the rivalry between the two sides of the brain. They are of two kinds: those, such as clonic and tonic blocks, which show evidences of the simultaneous lead of the two centers of opposite sign; and, those such as prolonged inspiration and the interruption of expiration, which indicate the alternate lead of two centers of opposite sign.

As a scientific theory it was notable in several respects. Although the essence of stuttering was not explicitly defined, it was implied by the nature of the theory, to wit: "Symptoms of stuttering are then mainly the peripheral signs of the rivalry between the two sides of the brain." Implied is a rivalry over which the speaker has no control.

This theory, moreover, was explicit enough to be tested, which it was. It provided the basis for three major predictions: that stutterers are either left-handed or ambidextrous, that changing handedness against natural dominance would cause stuttering, and that strengthening natural dominance would reduce stuttering (Bloodstein, 1987, p. 58). It failed the test of all three predictions and was buried for several decades, only to be dug up recently in the hope of resuscitating it as evidence that the cause of stuttering is neurogenic. Its major shortcoming was that Travis's primary interest was not in stuttering. He pioneered EEG and EMG, so his was an EEG/EMG theory of stuttering. His chief concern was to determine how much of stuttering could be explained electrophysiologically. After testing it, the answer turned out to be not much.

For personal reasons, Travis left Iowa for the University of Southern California in 1939. His research at Iowa had been handsomely supported. At USC, the only support available from a university with virtually no endowment was for a football team. Thus ended a brilliant career as an experimental scientist. He turned from research to psychoanalytic therapy of stuttering, an approach requiring privacy and confidentiality, so he became insulated from the very rigors of science he had practiced at Iowa.

Succeeding him at Iowa was Wendell Johnson, who along with Charles Van Riper, were considered by Travis (Personal communication, 1955) to be among his most brilliant students. Both Van Riper and Johnson had gone to Iowa because they stuttered. The only therapy available there was in the form of a test of Travis's cerebral-dominance theory. Both had their nondominant arms immobilized in plaster casts, presumably to strengthen the dominant hemisphere, far longer than needed for them to be thoroughly convinced that this treatment was not effective.

They, therefore, set out to devise their own therapy. Van Riper (1992) wrote that they agreed on the core of stuttering being a brief loss of control of the speech mechanism; that all else was a reaction to that core. He had found how to stutter easily, so he built his therapy around techniques for managing stuttering. Recently, he told me that Johnson emphasized advertising stuttering because he didn't stutter enough to want to be bothered with Van Riper's (Personal communication, 1993) approach.

Out of this background, and at least equally important, out of Johnson's expertise in general semantics (for which he was famous outside the new field of speech pathology) came his diagnosogenic theory of stuttering. It was an explicit rejection of everything about Travis's cerebral-dominance theory, arm cast and all.

Johnson argued, in speeches I heard as well as in his writing, that stuttering was not a symptom of anything, not of brain conflicts nor of psychoneurotic conflicts. Stuttering was no more than what he defined it as being—an anticipatory, apprehensive, hypertonic, avoidance reaction (Johnson, Brown, Curtis, Edney, & Keaster, 1948). It was not a consequence of organic breakdown or repressed needs, it was a learned response to a semantically erroneous label.

Thus was born the diagnosogenic theory of stuttering, also known in its early years as the semantogenic theory to emphasize its semantic origin. This was a theory of stuttering acquisition in young children that explained its development arising out of the misdiagnosis of what he called "normal nonfluency," until Robert West pointed out that nonfluency meant no fluency, at which time it became "normal disfluency," which it still is. Usually it was parents who mislabeled these fluency breaks as stuttering, considered a pejorative label, to which the child was hypothesized to react strongly enough to try to avoid it by struggling not to be normally disfluent. As mislabeling and struggles to avoid disfluency persisted, the child eventually learned the anticipatory, apprehensive, hypertonic avoidance reactions that characterized stuttering as Johnson defined it.

Johnson's theory did not lend itself to reliably measurable predictions, so it was not readily available to disprove. Its two major premises—that parents were hypersensitive to stuttering and that children were normally disfluent at time of onset of stuttering—were tested as best they could be. Insufficient attitude differences among parents and big differences in stuttering in children's syllable/sound disfluency—which, ironically, became the operational definition of stuttering—weakened the theory, but not enough to defeat it.

Johnson revised it to the interaction hypothesis. Diagnosis of stuttering was then an interaction between the child's disfluencies and the parents' evaluation of those disfluencies. This revision, however, never did begin to attract the attention of its diagnosogenic predecessor. Furthermore, this revision made the theory even more untestable. If the child began stuttering, then it was a function of either the child's disfluencies or the parent's evaluation. With these two options, no condition existed that could not be explained as to why the child either did or did not stutter.

Viewed in terms of our three scientific requirements for a good theory, the diagnosogenic explanation had problems from the beginning. The definition Johnson used excluded the core disruption of stuttering that Van Riper (1992) reported they agreed as students was the essence of the problem. Every term in Johnson's definition nonetheless describes a reaction to that core—anticipatory/apprehensive/hypertonic/avoidance/reaction. He argued, though, that this reaction was what the child learned in response to having normal disfluencies mislabeled as stuttering.

Aside from the incongruity of how stuttering could be a learned response and still be involuntary (in the sense that it cannot be prevented—this is what all definitions mean, dictionary and scientific alike), the failure of the theory to survive Johnson's death should have discredited his definition; what his theory provided was an alternative to primary stuttering to account for what would otherwise have to be considered secondary reactions to involuntary core disruptions. But his definition did not die. With it, he claimed that because there is no observable difference between normal disfluency and primary stuttering (which can, but need not, be true), the concept of secondary stuttering is useless. At least as far as Johnson's public statements were concerned, stuttering had no primary core disruption. It consisted entirely of what Van Riper, and others who stutter, considered to be secondary reactions to a primary core. For them, these disruptions might not have sounded different from normal disfluency, but they felt different to speakers.

Far from Johnson's definition being mortally wounded by disproof, irony of ironies, it is Johnson's major surviving relic. But what a relic. As we will see, it has been the dominant influence on stuttering research for a half century. Along with this influence, we encounter another paradox. Both his definition (which rejects existence of a primary core of stuttering) and his theory (which legitimated listener judgments of stuttering) are preserved as a basis of anticipatory stuttering by the very explanation that rejects these effects of his definition and theory. The argument for this statement is presented elsewhere (Perkins, 1996). It is beyond the scope of this chapter, except to say that the explanation provides a mechanism by which Johnson's anticipatory-reaction definition (which describes a potentially voluntary coping response) can turn stutter-like normal disfluency into primary core uncontrollable stuttering.

As for Johnson's theory, it was ingenious to say the least. It was flawed, though, in two major ways. It was not comprehensive for the same reason Travis's theory was not comprehensive. Neither was primarily a theory of stuttering in all of its complexity. Both were applications of other theories to stuttering. Travis investigated what could be learned about stuttering electrophysiologically, and later, psychoanalytically. Johnson investigated what could be learned about stuttering from application of his expertise in general semantics. Their inquiries did not extend beyond these bounds.

The other major difficulty with the diagnosogenic theory, and certainly with its successor, the interaction hypothesis, was its resistance to testing and disproof. Neither of its two basic premises lent themselves to unambiguous measurement. Theoretically, misidentifying normal disfluency as stuttering was so punishing that a child responded negatively enough to acquire all the characteristics of Johnson's anticipatory definition. The problem was what to measure as a basis for such a strong reaction. Surely the word "stuttering" to a child who has never heard it before is not inherently punishing. So what must be measured—tone-of-voice, angry looks, spanking, rejection, general attitude?

Finally, how rigorously was methodology used to test the theory? Although attempts were made to determine whether parent attitudes could be responsible for a child's reactions to disfluency, they were largely inconclusive (Bloodstein, 1987; Johnson & Associates, 1959).

Similarly, children's disfluency patterns were studied for evidence that they differed from normal disfluency. What was revealed was a much higher proportion of syllable/sound disfluencies in children judged to be stuttering, but this difference was minimized by stressing that these were only parts of total normal disfluencies. By the total count, stutterers and nonstutterers did not differ much (Johnson & Associates, 1959). Nonetheless, syllable/sound disfluency was eventually adopted as the operational definition of stuttering (Wingate, 1964).

Admittedly, the diagnosogenic theory was difficult to test. One approach that could have been taken, but never was, would have been to determine if any amount of "normal-disfluency stuttering" would produce the predicted punishing effects required for the various anticipatory reactions. As an even stronger test, I know from personal experience of enough cases of severe initial onset stuttering to have raised serious doubts about the theory. Those doubts have recently been confirmed (Yairi, Ambrose, & Niermann, 1993).

Instead, the primary effort seemed more toward finding support for Johnson's explanation than toward disproving it. To this end, the observational and analytic statistical methodologies still in vogue were used. Not until Wingate (1962) reanalyzed Iowa data from earlier research were these results and the theory critically analyzed.

The survival of Johnson's influence was not just from the power of his ideas, which were intriguing. The entire situation was an example of why Kuhn's (1970) paradigm shifts in science occur or do not occur. Johnson, along with Travis, West, and Van Riper were the brilliant charismatic leaders who founded our profession. They were great teachers who attracted bright students. Their magnetism was so strong that many of those students identified with them and became disciples. For them, belief displaced scientific doubt.

Be that as it may, when Johnson replaced Travis at Iowa, he not only inherited a strong research program in stuttering, along with a full complement of talented graduate students to pursue his ideas, he also inherited leadership of the entire field, including publication policies and standards. Until his death in 1965, Wendell Johnson was *the* dominant figure in establishing speech pathology as a profession and the paradigm for investigating the profession's dominant topic, which at that time was stuttering.

Without this backdrop, the course of stuttering theory and research is difficult to understand. Although other programs provided strong directions for therapy, especially Van Riper's, none approached the influence on investigations of stuttering as did those of Johnson and his students.

The diagnosogenic theory placed onset of stuttering in the ear of the listener. This was the origin of important implications. If normal disfluency was semantically misjudged by listeners as being stuttering, then it was listeners who defined the nature of stuttering. It was their judgments, therefore, that had to be studied. In theory, those judgments were the cause of stuttering, which was the child's reaction to disfluency, as Johnson defined it. Beyond them, no other notable cause was needed.

Effects of judgments were studied by investigating groups of parents and children, so, following the prevailing pattern of psychological methodology, statistical analysis of group data became a mandated characteristic of publishable research. A precept of science is that observations be replicable. Since listener judgments are made in response to objective acoustic stimuli, they were not only replicable but were easily tested for inter- and intrasubject reliability. Not surprisingly, observable, objective, replicable listener judgments of stuttering also became publication requirements. These mandatory characteristics constituted the mainstream pattern for investigating stuttering. They are still applied long after the demise of Johnson's theory for which they were most appropriate.

The diagnosogenic theory did not die heroically by outright disproof, it sank slowly as support leaked away. Still, it lives on in the spirit of the continuity hypothesis. Oliver Bloodstein (see his chapter in this volume), an outstanding student of Johnson's, hypothesized an alternative mechanism for onset of stuttering. Recognizing that stuttered and nonstuttered early childhood disfluencies apparently could not be categorically distinguished, Bloodstein (1961, 1970, 1975) proposed that stuttering develops from the tensions and fragmentations of struggling to acquire speech. This idea has survived for over three decades, especially the premise that stuttering lies along a continuum with, and develops out of, normal disfluency. The only hitch in this explanation is that the tensions and fragmentations he calls stuttering do not necessarily constitute involuntary loss of control of the speech mechanism. They are the consequences of the volitional struggle with speech acquisition frustrations, so they are only nonstuttered disfluency that sounds like stuttering. The mechanism alluded to earlier that turns Johnson's anticipatory reactions into involuntary stuttering would do the same for Bloodstein's tensions and fragmentations (Perkins, 1996).

Bloodstein is also responsible for the term "anticipatory-struggle" as a category for theories and therapies stemming from Johnson's definition of stuttering. Included under this rubric are therapies descendant from the approach of Van Riper as well as Johnson, and the attempts to explain how stuttering develops by learning along a continuum out of normal disfluency. Perhaps not surprisingly, virtually all of these attempts have followed in the footsteps of Travis and Johnson in that nothing about stuttering was explained beyond the limits of the theory being applied. Wischner (1950) offered a learning theory explanation; Sheehan (1953), an approach-avoidance-conflict theory explanation; Shames and Sherrick (1963), an operant theory explanation; and Brutten and Shoemaker (1967) a comprehensive learning theory account of how both classical and instrumental conditioning are involved in the acquisition and development of stuttering. Theirs was the last attempt at theorizing before the behavioral revolution brought formal theory construction to a halt.

Goldiamond, in 1965, tested Johnson's prediction that the effect of punishment of stuttering is to increase it. If true, this would violate learning principles. He used delayed-auditory-feedback (DAF) disruption as punishment. His subject, in the course of the experiment, discovered that very slow droning speech not only freed him from DAF disruption but also from any feeling of stuttering. This led to the development of fluency skills, such as rate control (Curlee & Perkins, 1969; Perkins, 1973), and to operant procedures, such as time out and gradually increased length of utterance, which made establishment of fluency an easily achievable objective (Costello, 1975; Ryan, 1971).

This objective turned the traditional point of therapy upside down. Van Riper's therapy stressed achievement of easy stuttering, Johnson's even advocated advertising it with faked stuttering. Both urged avoiding avoidances until there was no stuttering to hide—stutter openly. With the behavioral objective of fluency, launched by Goldiamond, the prospect loomed of promoting avoidance and hiding as a clinically sanctioned tactic for achieving fluency. Unfortunately, this is not an infrequent prospect. It is the primary reason I abandoned fluency as an objective. Nonetheless, the ease with which fluency could literally be established overnight, at least within the clinic, was too strong a lure to resist.

Not only was there an explosion in behavioral treatment, but also in behavioral treatment research (Ingham, 1984). With a fluency objective, contingent reinforcement could be applied to both stuttering and fluency. Scientific measurement of treatment effects was now a reality. Another irony, the anticipatory-struggle requirement of listener identification of stuttering eased the way for operant therapists to establish their diametrically opposite objective by clinician identification of fluency and stuttering for contingent reinforcement purposes. Establishment of fluency, formerly the province of quacks, was now, with treatment measurement accountability, scientifically respectable. The behavioral bandwagon was in high gear.

The premise for such therapy is that stuttering is a form of behavior that can be modified by operant principles. This premise has been demonstrated to apply regardless of the cause of stuttering. Operant principles constitute a theory of learning that does not lend itself in any special way to explaining what causes stuttering. Although maintenance of fluency in adults has proven to be a universally thorny problem, the ease with which an operant approach makes fluency available in the clinic has gained it overwhelming popularity.

With an effective therapy for fluency available for which no understanding of causation was necessary, the stage was set to nail down the lid on the theory-construction coffin. Demise of the cerebral-dominance theory, after three dozen studies, was assured when Johnson ascended to Travis's throne at Iowa. Johnson took control of the research machinery, turned it around, and headed in the opposite direction. It chugged along in pursuit of Johnson's ideas and their derivations, with dozens of studies, for over two decades. But by the 1960s it had just about run out of steam. All it took was the behavioral revolution, which made theory construction seem irrelevant, to bury any interest in theories.

With formal theories out of the way, investigators trained in research methodology were now free to pursue their hunches and assumptions wherever they led. The signposts they followed were marked by statistical significance, which in itself is a warning. Statistics imply that the roads indicated by significant differences are filled with variability potholes, and are narrowed by small mean differences. The more sophisticated the statistic, the smaller the difference and the greater the variability that can yield a significant difference.

Unable to find a big enough environmental lead during the Johnson years to constitute a thoroughfare to an understanding of stuttering, research traffic has turned back toward neurological assumptions, which picked up where the Travis era left off. In fact, at least twice as many hemispheric studies have been done since that era as during it. Research has headed in any direction in which conceivable differences between stutterers and nonstutterers might be found. Two in particular—auditory and reaction-time abilities—have been pursued (Bloodstein, 1987; Perkins, 1996). Over the years, these fishing expeditions have cycled back and forth between constitutional and environmental assumptions because, despite some significant differences, neither direction has revealed a strong enough lead to generate incisive questions, let alone explain stuttering.

The basic problem has been in failure to follow the principles of science as they were designed to be used. Ayala and Black (1993), in a guiding statement for courts as to what is science and what is not, provide a succinct description of these principles. Science involves:

> *two intertwined kinds of intellectual effort: invention or discovery [the architectural part] and validation or corroboration [the sports part]. Most new scientific ideas begin with imagination and conjecture . . . Newton is said to have been inspired by a falling apple . . . Once a new idea or discovery has been articulated, its validation requires that it go through empirical testing capable of proving it false. (p. 234)*

In explaining the origins of his own theories, which have withstood all attempts to disprove them, Einstein said, "Bernstein's book limited itself almost throughout to qualitative aspects . . . a work which I read with breathless attention." By thinking qualitatively rather than quantitatively, Einstein is said to have "gained early a broad conceptual overview of physics on which to build and add more technical details" (Holton, 1994, p. 48).

By abandoning theory construction, the need to clarify what is and is not stuttering has been moved to the back burner, where the only thing keeping it simmering is the operant need to identify stuttering for administration of contingent reinforcement. For this purpose, Ingham and his associates (Ingham, Cordes, & Finn, 1993) have demonstrated a reasonably adequate, partial clinical solution. In no way, though, does it solve the failure of a half century of effort to establish a definitive categorical difference for listeners between stuttered and nonstuttered disfluency (Perkins, 1990).

Efforts have been made to define this difference physiologically (Zimmerman, 1980; Zimmerman, Smith, & Hanley, 1981). This is an exercise in reductionism, which adds nothing because the differences described can be no more or better than the listener-defined stuttering behavior with which they are correlated. The results are so ambiguous that they are interpreted as only *possibly* having causal implications. The expectation is that when sufficient data are gathered, they might possibly be the basis for a theory of stuttering (Smith, 1992). The illogic of this remarkable position is discussed elsewhere (Perkins, 1992, 1996). By reporting results of descriptive research only associated with stuttering, they escape the rigors of experimental tests of cause and effect.

What has happened is that the precision tools of methodology designed for tests of explicit theoretical predictions are being used to troll in any direction for a statistically significant lead. This is a fundamental misconception of science. It is an attempt to substitute the hard-nosed empirical methods of corroboration for the imaginative conjectural thinking that often characterizes clinical decision making. Only after speculative ideas as to what might cause stuttering have been formulated can the power of experimental methodology be marshalled to test an idea by trying to falsify it. Misapplication of empirical research methods has resulted inevitably in an array of Catch-22 situations.

Because the accepted paradigm for doing science only permits experimental evidence, clinical evidence in general and case histories in particular (deemed to be mere "story telling"), are excluded as untrustworthy. By this standard, Newton's inspiration from a falling apple, about as nonexperimental as evidence could get, would have disqualified his conception of gravity as unscientific. What is excluded are observations of clinicians whose professional obligation is to understand cause and effect relationships within the individuals for whom they are responsible for tailoring treatment to their specific needs. Their observations are excluded as leads because they are considered to be nonexperimental, so they cannot be investigated to qualify them for empirical research. How, then, is science served by invalidating the observations of clinicians who are dealing with cause and effect in every clinical encounter in favor of investigators who admittedly may never have even talked with a person who stutters outside an experimental situation (Smith, 1992; Perkins, 1992)?

This leads to the next Catch-22.

Since the paradigm is to do group research using appropriate statistical analysis, with individual results rarely reported, whatever significant results are found apply only to the group. They do not apply to those who vary from the group. But cause and effect operate only within the individual. How can we understand why an individual stutters when the research paradigm allows only statistically analyzed group results?

Finally, definitional Catch-22s. The starting point in trying to understand any phenomenon, stuttering in particular, is to be able to identify it categorically and unambiguously. How can we have a theory of something we cannot identify? Obviously, a definition that distinguishes what we are trying to understand is a fundamental requirement. Such a definition will have to be necessary and sufficient for making that distinction if it is to be adequate. This means it will have to be invariant. It cannot operate some times and not others. To detect such a difference would exclude any need for statistics.

Yet, the listener definition mandated by the research paradigm has never come close to providing such a distinction, despite a half century of serious effort to establish even reliability, to say nothing of validity. So we are caught in a Catch-22 by persisting in requiring listener judgments to define stuttering, and we are caught in another Catch-22 by the paradigm requirement of group research and statistical significance. If the paradigm requires following statistically significant leads from listener judgments, how can the invariant difference needed for an adequate definition of stuttering ever be found if the paradigm biases against following anything but variable differences for which statistics are needed?

The most insidious consequence of this paradigm for "doing science" is that it is self-perpetuating. It does not provide for self-correction. It has prevailed for a half century with no inherent limit on how much longer it could continue. The reason is threefold. First, the prevailing assumption is that any statement not based on experimental evidence is not good science. Smith (1992) provides an excellent example of this assumption in her critique of a theory of neuropsycholinguistic function in stuttering: "Perkins, Kent, and Curlee do not offer compelling experimental evidence to force our attention to the particular dyssynchrony hypotheses they favor (p. 807)." Obviously, the inventive "architectural" component of science that provides the basis for empirical testing does not exist in Smith's conception of science. Without architecture, a comprehensive internally consistent theory is virtually impossible.

What does exist for Smith is pursuit of statistically significant leads from empirical research. Consider this statement of hers: "Many workers in the area have recently adopted multifactorial models of stuttering. . . . We have much to do before the role of many of the factors is understood well enough to allow the specification of a formal, integrated, multifactorial model of stuttering" (Smith, 1992; pp. 807–808). Implicit in this call for research are the assumptions that make this approach to science both barren and self-perpetuating. Because Smith's critique excludes pursuing anything but experimental leads, her call for much work is a call for further group research on statis-

tically significant leads. This assumption is barren because it perpetuates weak leads. Statistics are unnecessary when differences are so regular as to be obvious, which is why discovery of such differences is an integral part of the architectural component. These differences are more likely to be observed by alert clinicians who detect patterns of individual behavior. After all, causes of stuttering operate only within individuals. To expect to find consistent causal differences in groups who stutter is to assume all stuttering occurs for the same reasons—hardly likely if stuttering is the multifactorial problem Smith describes. Thus, by investigating empirical leads from groups of stutterers, the causal leads can hardly be anything but weak. This assumption also contributes to self-perpetuation because without a theory to test, virtually all research now derives from significant results of varieties of prior studies, of which there is an endless supply.

Smith's prediction, that when the multitude of factors suspected of causing stuttering are understood then a multifactorial model of stuttering will be possible, embodies another assumption that guarantees perpetuity for this approach. She says, "the writers generally suggest that many different factors, including linguistic, cognitive, motoric, and sociocultural factors play a role in the development and maintenance of stuttering" (pp. 807–808). Indeed, I suspect that these factors probably are *associated* with stuttering, but stated as broad categories, they are meaningless in so far as how they could be *causally* related to stuttering. As matters stand, empirical evidence merely *suggests* that they may even be associated with stuttering. Further, such evidence as exists is from groups of stutterers, so it only applies to some, not all, who stutter. For these factors to be of value to a comprehensive theory, they must be shown experimentally to be necessary and sufficient, at minimum, for the common characteristic that defines stuttering, whatever that may be.

But, again, the categorical qualitative distinction between stuttered and nonstuttered disfluency as judged by listeners has been sought vigorously by mainstream investigators for over a half century—

with no success. It is the central problem. Without that distinction, how can those in the mainstream have a theory of something they cannot even identify except collectively by frequency of occurrence?

This scientific situation fits Tuchman's (1984) description of political folly: "If pursuing disadvantage after disadvantage has become obvious[ly] irrational, then rejection of reason is the prime characteristic of folly" (p. 380). How could the mainstream not have concluded long ago that continued pursuit of disadvantageous research is folly? The answer is in the assumption implicit in Smith's call for more research. It is that when they have gathered all of the necessary data, then, and only then will the answer become apparent. But since the course they are pursuing is without scientific merit, how are they ever to discover when enough is enough?

The reason this course is without merit is because it has abandoned the basic strategy of science that makes it akin to sports, which produces winners and losers. Formal theories are designed to be vulnerable to disproof by testing logically deduced hypotheses. Without an internally consistent theory, only assumptions are available to guide research. But they are untestable because they are too vague to generate specific predictions that could be defeated. Thus, mainstream hypothesis testing proceeds in a vacuum. It can continue endlessly because no assumption is ever defeated. One lead from a significant difference is just as good as any other lead.

Unfortunately, assumptions are typically unrecognized, hence uncorrectable. Two such assumptions have literally prevented a scientific solution of stuttering. One is that "doing science" consists exclusively of using only empirical methodology, which precludes inventive theory construction. The other is that listeners are better qualified to define stuttering than are stutterers themselves. If concern were about the effect of stuttering on audiences, then a listener definition would be necessary, as it was for Johnson's diagnosogenic theory. But listeners hear only the top of the stuttering iceberg; the difference for them between stuttered and nonstuttered disfluency is indistinguishable (Moore & Perkins, 1990). This is not a fatal flaw for therapy, but it is if solving stuttering is the goal. Since stuttered and nonstuttered disfluency sound alike, the difference is assumed to be quantitative, not qualitative. For the speaker, who is privy to what is below the surface, the difference is categorically *qualitative*.

The net effect of this situation, unfortunately, has been to widen the gap between research and therapy. At least anticipatory-struggle theories provided a semblance of relevance to avoidance-reduction therapies. As matters stand, with behavior therapy divorced from cause and effect theories and with research directed by methodological requirements, connections among research, theory, and therapy have all but vanished. Clinicians are left with no scientific guidance as to what problems have to be solved for treatment to be optimally effective.

By correcting the methodological and definitional assumptions, and by working primarily from four decades of clinical observation (a source of evidence that Smith, in her critique we discussed, branded as unscientific), plus what little experimental causal evidence is available, a comprehensive solution of stuttering becomes possible (Perkins, 1996). That a basic understanding with fundamental relevance can be achieved by proper application of principles of science has, moreover, been demonstrated. The scope of this chapter permits only a synopsis of the solution and what it can accomplish.

The approach to an explanation was guided by a series of questions. Answers could be generated in any fashion. They could come from anything from dreams to rational speculations. They could also, of course, come from empirical observations, but only those that qualified. Essential longitudinal evidence, for example, described developmental characteristics from onset to adulthood such as gender differences, recovery differences, objective and subjective nature of stuttering.

On the other hand, empirical differences between stutterers and nonstutterers or about conditions under which frequency or severity of stuttering varied, for instance, were only acceptable if they were close to invariant. Variable differences implied that they did not apply to all who stutter, so they could provide neither a necessary nor sufficient contribution to a solution of stuttering.

In brief, a credible explanation of stuttering could not violate causal evidence about stuttering, or neurolinguistic, psycholinguistic, cognitive, nor evolutionary evidence related to it.

The first question was fundamental. Does stuttering exist as an unambiguously identifiable phenomenon? If it cannot be qualitatively and categorically identified, then it cannot be the basis for a coherent logical explanation with specific predictions. A theory of something that does not exist has little merit or future. There are two answers to this fundamental question.

The answer that has prevailed since the beginning of systematic research has to be *no*. For this, listeners have defined stuttering by what they can hear and see. They can be trained to high levels of agreement with themselves and each other when asked to count frequency of stuttering. But when asked to identify words on which stuttering occurs, they have never come close to acceptable agreement, despite a half century of continuous trying. Accordingly, Siegel (Personal communication, 1995) thinks "of 'stuttering' as a 'construct' rather than a thing."

If people who do the stuttering provide the answer at time of occurrence of stuttering, then the result is entirely different. It is an unqualified *yes*. This answer is based on a decade of asking clients in my clinic how they know when they stutter, on systematic descriptive research (Sue-O'Brien, 1993), and on experimental research in which the subject who produced samples of faked and real stuttering accurately distinguished between them without error in over five dozen trials at time of productions. But when the subject and eighteen listeners tried to discriminate faked from real an hour after production, the subject was no more accurate than were the listeners. All of them were merely guessing (Moore & Perkins, 1990).

This result only confirmed the consistent client answers to my question. Not one person who stuttered had any doubt about knowing when they stutter. I must add that what they said was stuttering at time of occurrence, I sometimes did not detect as much of a disfluency. Conversely, what I thought was obvious stuttering on some occasions they disagreed with as not being stuttering at all. Clearly, they were detecting stuttering by some other means than what I could hear, which leads to the question of what that alternative basis could be.

What condition is necessary and sufficient categorically and qualitatively to differentiate chronic clinical stuttering from transient stuttering and normal disfluency? The most obvious answer is historical. For background, a dictionary distinction is needed between *stuttering*, "usually refers to spasmodic repetition or exaggeration of sounds or syllables," and *stammering*, "generally refers to involuntary pauses or breaks in speech" (Morris, 1970). Although this dictionary distinction is still recognized elsewhere in the world, in the United States it disappeared sometime before 1931 when it did not appear in Travis's *Speech Pathology*. Listeners, who were then being used to judge stuttering, could not determine by listening whether a disfluency was involuntary or not, so as Johnson et al. (1948) wrote, the two terms were considered to be synonymous.

Unfortunately, what was eliminated was the only qualitative difference between stuttered and nonstuttered disfluency—chronic clinical stuttering is involuntary. Acoustically, this difference is observable in fluency fractures within the syllable, not between syllables (Stromsta, 1986). Subjectively, such fractures leave speakers helpless to prevent, correct, or terminate loss of control of the speech mechanism. This is the one universal description in answer to my question, "How do you know when you stutter?" This is how Moore and Perkins's (1990) subject experimentally distinguished faked from real stuttering accurately more than five dozen times without exception. And it is what Van Riper (Personal communication, 1993) described when I asked him my question. "I would agree that . . . the feeling of helplessness and inability to control the speech mechanism is a common experience. When fluency inexplicably turns to gluency, when you can't squeak out a sound, when tremors infest your jaw and lips, when you find yourself repeating or blatting syllables or sounds uncontrollably, you lose the integrity of the self. You feel controlled by mysterious forces outside your skin sack. Always there is that sense of mystery once the stuttering is over. Wot happened?"

Many added such characteristics as tight chest, tight throat, tight stomach, and tremors. But the other most frequent additional characteristic was disproportional terror of helplessness invariably described in life-threatening analogies, such as helplessly falling, helplessly submerged, helplessly trapped in a burning building.

Why is a speaker definition of stuttering, which seems to be more subjective, preferable to a listener definition? It would not be if listener reaction were being studied, nor if, as Johnson theorized, stuttering developed out of negative listener reactions.

If clinical stuttering as experienced by speakers is the concern, however, then the difference in definitions is critical to understanding the nature of stuttering. (Parenthetically, the distinction is not important for therapy since no harm is done by reducing nonstuttered as well as stuttered disfluency.) The reasons for preference are these:

First, each listener's judgment of stuttering is every bit as subjective as a speaker's. Worse, the listener is not privy at all to the subjective experience of stuttering. For the speaker at time of occurrence, helpless loss of control of the speech mechanism is every bit as real, if not more so, than the experience of hearing speech disruptions.

Second, the most critical scientific difference is that a listener definition provides virtually no constraint on what a viable solution could be, whereas a speaker definition tightly constrains any acceptable answer. All that listeners hear as stuttering is syllable-sound disfluency, so it has become the operational definition of stuttering for research, as well as for operant therapy. But transient stuttering, for which three out of four children will recover without help, usually within a year (Yairi et al., 1993), and many forms of normal disfluency also include syllable-sound disfluency.

The research literature is replete with reports of a wide array of conditions, such as those Smith (1992) identified, that affect syllable-sound disfluency. Understandably, no one has figured out how any of these conditions could cause stuttering, and for good reason. How can causal connections for such a wide array of conditions affecting frequency of disfluency be determined when effects of these conditions could just as well be attributed to normal disfluency or transient stuttering as to chronic stuttering? Because no such distinction is possible, no listener-definition constraint exists on potentially causal conditions of clinical stuttering. No causal connection can be tested, let alone disproved, so research is free to wander off in virtually any direction, which, indeed, it has.

By contrast, a speaker definition is so constraining that it all but requires a specific solution to stuttering. Whether starting off from the subjective experience or from the overt act of stuttering, both of these constraints lead to the same solution. The experience is helpless loss of control of the speech mechanism. The implied constraint is that the speaker is unaware of the cause of disrupted fluency. Thus, two questions must be answered. The broader one is, What causes speech disruption? The most constraining one is, What aspect of speech is so far beyond awareness that the speaker is unable to prevent disruption?

The broad answer first. Two major components comprise speech—syllables, which provide breath stream energy, and symbolic sounds, which are articulatory modulations of the breath stream. The syllable does not contain only prosodic vocal components of speech. Indeed, it need not contain any verbal components at all, it can consist solely of nonverbal screams or laughs, for instance. Research has shown that when syllables do contain speech, the phonological articulatory operations and the prosodic vocal operations are processed separately in the brain (Shattuck-Hufnagel, 1983). So when speaking, articulatory movements must be coordinated with the syllabic breath stream. The answer to the broad question, then, is that any condition disturbing syllable-sound coordination will produce stutter-sounding disfluency. This leaves the remaining much narrower subjective question, What aspect of speech can account for chronic stuttering being experienced as involuntary?

Constraints imposed by the act of stuttering also lead to this same narrow question. The most definitive experimental evidence about stuttering is that when children suspected of stuttering recover without help, their initial disfluency near onset will have been intersyllabic, they are disfluent in whole syllables. This implies that the cause of disruption is linguistic uncertainty. The syllable, being the unit of spoken language, is the physiological structure for speech. Linguistic utterances are organized exclusively around whole syllables. For those children, however, who become chronic, their initial disfluency is intrasyllabic, fractures occur within the syllable. First is disruption of coarticulation that initiates the syllable, followed within 300 msec by termination of what started out to be normal voice onset (Stromsta, 1986). The remaining question this time is what can account for this peculiar sequence of intrasyllabic disintegration?

For this latter question, the implied answer has to be that coordination of breath stream and articulation occur at the production level of voice and articulation. That coarticulation disintegrates at onset of the syllable whereas voice terminates a fraction of a second later is clear indication that speech sounds are not integrated into their syllables within the brain, as MacNeilage and colleagues (MacNeilage, Studdert-Kennedy, & Lindblom, 1985) concluded from Shattuck-Hufnagle's (1983) research. If they were, then voice and articulation would fracture at the same time.

What must happen, instead, is dyssynchronous timing of breath stream requirements for articulatory production. Each sound has pressure, duration, pitch, and voicing specifications that have to be met at precisely the proper instant for high-speed coarticulation of normal speech to occur. Meanwhile, normal voice onset initiates the syllable, indicating that the speaker is prepared to produce the syllable to be uttered. Thus, linguistic uncertainty is excluded as cause of disintegrated coarticulation. But as Stromsta (1986) asserts, it is the disruption of laryngeal pressure differentials (that drive cord vibration) by chaotic articulatory movements, which terminate voice after the syllable has been initiated.

This leads to the key question, What aspect of speech is there, if linguistic components are excluded, that could discoordinate the syllabic breath stream from the articulatory movements for the sounds intended for that syllable? The required answer turns out to be the same as for the experiential question, Why is stuttering involuntary? Because stuttering is so obviously an articulatory breakdown, a linguistic cause seems self-evident. But this cause is excluded for three major reasons. One we have just discussed—speech production is organized around whole syllables, but chronic stuttering occurs within the syllable.

The second reason is experimental evidence. Using frequency of stuttering in normal speech as a baseline, whispering reduces stuttering 90 percent, and articulatory speech with no voice eliminates it invariably (Perkins, Rudas, Johnson, & Bell, 1976). Since the only speech operation common to all conditions is articulation, cause of stuttering can hardly be attributed to segmental production disorders.

Of special interest are the puzzling effects of pitch and vocal quality, which are the only components of a syllable eliminated by whispering, the condition accounting for 90 percent reduction of stuttering. Intuitively, the other two syllable components, loudness and duration, which are still active elements in whispering, would seem to have more likely effects on stuttering, but eliminating them in voiceless speech only reduced stuttering an additional 10 percent. The most plausible explanation is that this is evidence supporting an assertiveness conflict as a cause of stuttering, which we will soon consider.

The third reason is that everything about symbolic aspects of speech is learned and must be readily subject to voluntary correction, so nothing about linguistic aspects of spoken language are relatively unavailable to awareness. This includes all aspects of prosody—syllable stress (effecting meaning) involves control of pitch, loudness, and duration; inflection (distinguishing questions from statements) involves control of pitch; and intonation (emphasizing ideas) involves pitch, loudness, and duration. Thus, all distinctive aspects of spoken language must be readily available to voluntary correction, so no linguistic operation can account for stuttering being involuntary.

What other component of speech remains if all linguistic components are eliminated? Obviously, constraints on an answer to why stuttering is involuntary are narrow indeed. Only two possible leads are available, one involving articulatory modulation of breath stream energy, the other involving production of that breath stream.

Considering how extensively loudness, duration, and especially pitch are required for prosody, hardly any breath stream component seemingly remains that is not under linguistic control. But such a component does exist—tone of voice. It is sometimes mistakenly included in prosody, when in reality it is entirely independent of linguistic symbolic functions. Tone of voice is exclusively a signal system of how we feel about ourselves, what we are saying, and to whom we are saying it.

Ironically, tone of voice is the only communication system we have inherited from our ancient mammalian ancestors, yet it has rarely been recognized for what it is, let alone investigated scientifically. It is most evident as the infant's communication system prior to acquisition of speech. The symbol system as it develops is overlaid on it, so whether an utterance includes a linguistic component is optional. What is not optional is tone of voice as the foundation of a syllable.

Elements of tone of voice include vocal quality and speech rate, both of which are entirely independent of linguistic control. Additionally included are pitch, loudness, and syllable duration not commandeered by prosodic requirements.

Evidence of the primacy of tone of voice in phonetic processing can be seen in the necessary sequence of the operations involved. Once phonological determination of segments for syllables to be uttered is completed, including proportional durations of segments, tone of voice for the utterance must be established before segmental phonetic speech-motor specifications can be processed. The reason is because segmental durations will depend on syllable durations, which will depend on speech rate, which is dependent on the affect to be expressed by tone of voice. One speaks faster, for instance, when excited than when tired, regardless of the message to be uttered.

The foremost consideration that typically makes tone of voice unavailable to awareness is that its evolutionary roots are so deeply embedded that there are no tone-of-voice rules to be learned, it is reflexively self-expressive when speaking spontaneously. Only when controlled for acting, singing, or certain fluency therapies is it managed voluntarily. Note, these are conditions under which stuttering is usually eliminated. Thus, tone of voice under typical circumstances is invariably automatic, hence beyond awareness.

The question remains, however, how tone of voice could have any effect on stuttering, regardless of how involuntary it is when speaking spontaneously. The short answer is that if a mechanism exists by which tone of voice could delay normal timing of the breath stream, this would dyssynchronize breath stream requirements for nomally timed articulatory movements, thereby disrupting coarticulation as Stromsta's (1986) research described.

Since tone of voice is the vehicle for spontaneous self-expressive speech, any self-expressive conflict would be sufficient to involuntarily delay syllabic (breath stream) processing. The delay would be caused by the demonstrated effect of competition for neural resources—it retards task performance (Kinsbourne, 1982).

The suspected conflict is about being openly assertive. The evidence for this is robust, extensive, and complex, so here is only a brief sample (Perkins, 1996). Because the alternative to overt stuttering is silence, severity of stuttering is a direct measure of assertiveness. Another equally self-evident example is freedom from stuttering when speaking alone where assertiveness is not an issue.

Unlike this assertiveness conflict, which may seem so far off the beaten path as to be unbelievable, articulatory processing, the other potential cause of involuntary stuttering, is closer to familiar territory. Johnson's traditional definition, that stuttering is an anticipatory, apprehensive, hypertonic avoidance reaction is accurate for my purpose, as far as it goes. But being anticipatory of difficulty, it describes a coping response potentially available to voluntary control.

Similarly, Bloodstein's (1995) description of early childhood stuttering as fragmentation of syntactic structures is a consequence of struggles to cope with language acquisition complexities. Not only does this imply potential for voluntary control, it also specifies fragmentations as being linguistic in origin, hence involving whole syllables, which implies spontaneous recovery. This then is a credible account of transient, but not chronic, stuttering.

To understand why both Johnson and Bloodstein have described causal conditions for involuntary stuttering requires a brief detour into recent research that differentiates independent voluntary and involuntary control systems. The voluntary system involves the cortex and limbic system in cognitive learning; it is used for tasks requiring voluntary attention, so it operates at slow speeds. The involuntary system involves the extrapyramidal-cerebellar system for high-speed control of automatic operations (Petri & Mishkin, 1994).

With this background, consider the effect of expecting to stutter on a particular word or sound. For the same reason that walking across a narrow beam over a gorge would convert my automatic stride into a one-movement-at-a-time crawl, expectancy to stutter converts automatic coarticulation to voluntary preparation to guide articulators through the predicted disruption. This prophecy is self-fulfilling because the typical attempt is to rush to push through the block. The inevitable consequence is discoordination of an automatic high-speed syllabic breath stream with carefully controlled low-speed articulatory movements to produce observable involuntary stuttering.

For voluntary control of articulation to be a viable explanation of chronic stuttering onset requires a period of learning. Children must have long enough exposure to syllable-sound-disfluency-producing conditions to begin to expect difficulty with certain situations, words, and sounds with which they begin preparing to struggle. This can, but need not, result from the speech acquisition difficulties Bloodstein (1995) describes. On the other hand, a

self-expressive conflict, probably over assertiveness, would operate from onset of connected speech, so it would produce a version of involuntary stuttering that would predictably become exacerbated by anticipatory stuttering. Thus, early onset of full blown stuttering could not be from anticipation of speaking difficulty. Instead, it would have to develop gradually as voluntary struggles to acquire spoken language turn increasingly into involuntary disruptions caused by anticipatory attempts to deal with difficult situations, words, and sounds.

Note that this cause of involuntary stuttering has nothing to do with a defective articulatory nor syllabic system. When articulatory control is shifted to the low-speed monitoring system while syllabic control remains under the high-speed feedback system, both of which function independently, the inadvertent consequence is discoordination of articulatory movements with breath stream requirements for those movements.

For stuttering to be observable, however, requires more than just involuntary syllable-sound dyssynchronization. It requires a critical element already discussed in connection with self-expressive conflict—assertive pressure to continue an involuntarily disrupted utterance. Otherwise, speakers could stop and wait for synchrony to be re-established before proceeding, with no one the wiser. Only the speakers would know they had stuttered.

What we have presented in overview is a demonstration that by applying the problem-solving strategies of science, a comprehensive, coherent, testable explanation of stuttering can be formulated. This is not to argue that this theory is correct in all respects. Far from it. Although the original premise of stuttering being a consequence of dyssynchronized syllable-sound processing remains intact, it has already been altered from its original form as new evidence has appeared (Perkins, 1996; Perkins, Kent, & Curlee, 1991).

Let me reiterate that the ultimate test of a theory is not how well it conforms to acceptable ideas, acceptable evidence, acceptable methodology, or acceptable anything else. It can be, and often is, done in the ways I have criticized. Many scientists in many disciplines practice trial and error research. There is no law against it; occasionally it is productive, but not often. Its probability of success is very low. By contrast, all of the great advances in science have emanated from theories: of gravity, evolution, relativity, quantum mechanics, molecular biology, cosmology, psycho- and neurolinguistics. These theories have prospered because they have successfully met endless efforts to defeat them.

In the final analysis the origin of a theory is of no consequence. It could arise from mold on muck under a toadstool and survive as a brilliant solution if it makes predictions undefeated by empirical testing. The theory, from which this digest excerpt comes, arose out of a dream a dozen years ago (almost on a par with mold under a toadstool). It at least has the distinction of being the first comprehensive theory of stuttering, unlike the partial theories that have preceded it. Also, it explains all of the situations under which stuttering is typically eliminated. Moreover, it has survived several intentional and unintentional tests. The first was performed, using the method of strong inference (Platt, 1964), to test the foundation premise on which the entire theory was constructed (Moore & Perkins, 1990). It would not have been published if results of that test had not been without exception.

Another test, unbeknownst to me until recently, was performed near mid century. It was the only long-term full-scale longitudinal experiment to determine acoustic predictions of which children would recover and which would become chronic. It was 90 percent accurate (Stromsta, 1986). It was a test of this theory because the physiological and acoustic characteristics of those who became chronic were predictable from the theory's cause of stuttering.

Still another critical, although unintentional, experimental test was performed recently, which experimentally falsified the Neilsons' neural resource premise, on which the capacity-demands theory is built. Their premise posits "inadequate resources for sensory-motor information processing" as the basis of stuttering (Neilson & Neilson, 1987, p. 325). What the Dalhousie group demonstrated, by altering auditory feedback, which increased demand, and by increasing rate, which reduced capacity, was a decrease, not an increase in stuttering, a result congruent with this neuropsycholinguistic theory. Delayed auditory feedback results were also explained in the Dalhousie research as equivalent to known "shadow speech" effects, whereas half-octave alternations of vocal feedback were compared to elimination of stuttering with choral speech (Kalinowski, Aronson, Roland-Mieszkowski, & Stuart, 1993). The comparisons were apt, but not explanatory. Again, though, the comprehensive demonstration theory's cause of stuttering could have predicted and does explain these effects.

This theory also contains a multitude of other predictions awaiting experimental testing. These are a brief sampling (Perkins, 1996):

- Severity of stuttering is a function of assertive pressure to continue an involuntarily disrupted utterance.
- Preponderance of stuttering in males, waning of severity with age, and changes in severity from day to day or over long periods, is a function of level of testosterone.
- Disproportional fear of stuttering is a function of terror of helplessness which originates from unattended crying in infancy.

Finally, on a clinical note, the principles of science, in conjunction with the new theory, have been used to demonstrate how strong leads can be generated for answers to such critical questions as:

- What is the essence of stuttering?
- What causes transient stuttering?
- What causes core primary chronic stuttering?
- What causes severe reactions to core stuttering and secondary coping reactions?
- Can chronic stuttering be prevented?
- Can chronic stuttering be cured?
- If all who stutter are different, how can causation in individuals be determined?
- How can stuttering and its causes be measured?

Despite this endorsement, I hold no brief for the life expectancy of these ideas. Theories are born to be buried. They are only as good as the last attempt to defeat them has failed. This is merely a stepping stone en route to more accurate approximations of the reality of stuttering.

Science provides powerful tools for determining the nature of stuttering. But as with all tools, they must be used for the purpose for which they were designed if they are to be maximally effective. The history of stuttering research provides strong evidence of our mastery of empirical methodology for testing conceptions of stuttering. When imaginative creative theories of equal strength, based on questions derived from valid assumptions, become available for testing, then science will, indeed, become capable of solving stuttering.

REFERENCES

Ayala, F., & Black, B. (1993). Science and the courts. *American Scientist, 81*, 230–239.

Bloodstein, O. (1961). The development of stuttering: III. Theoretical and clinical implications. *Journal of Speech and Hearing Disorders, 26*, 67–82.

Bloodstein, O. (1970). Stuttering and normal nonfluency: A continuity hypothesis. *British Journal of Disorders of Communications, 5*, 30–39.

Bloodstein, O. (1975). Stuttering as tension and fragmentation. In J. Eisenson (Ed.), *Stuttering: A second symposium*. New York: Harper & Row.

Bloodstein, O. (1987). A handbook on stuttering. Chicago: National Easter Seal Society.

Bloodstein, O. (1995). *A handbook on stuttering*. San Diego: Singular Publishing Group, Inc.

Brutten, G., & Shoemaker, D. (1967). *The modification of stuttering*. Englewood Cliffs, N.J.: Prentice-Hall.

Costello, J. (1975). The establishment of fluency with time-out procedures. *Journal of Speech and Hearing Disorders, 40*, 216–231.

Curlee, R., & Perkins, W. (1969). Conversational rate control therapy for stuttering. *Journal of Speech and Hearing Disorders, 34*, 245–250.

Goldiamond, I. (1965). Stuttering and fluency as manipulable operant response classes. In L. Crasner & L. Ullman (Eds.), *Research in behavior modification*. New York: Holt, Rinehart, & Winston.

Holton, G. (1994, September). Of love, physics and other passions: The letters of Albert and Mileva, Part 2. *Physics Today*, 37–43.

Ingham, R. (1984). *Stuttering and behavior therapy*. San Diego: College-Hill Press.

Ingham, R., Cordes, A., & Finn, P. (1993). Time-interval measurement of stuttering. *Journal of Speech and Hearing Research, 38*, 1168–1176.

Johnson, W., & Associates (1959). *The onset of stuttering*. Minneapolis: University of Minnesota Press.

Johnson, W., Brown, S., Curtis, J., Edney, C., & Keaster, J. (1948). *Speech handicapped school children*. New York: Harper & Row Publishers.

Kalinowski, J., Aronson, J., Roland-Mieszkowski, M., & Stuart, A. (1993). Effects of alterations in auditory feedback and speech rate on stuttering frequency. *Language and Speech, 36*, 1–16.

Kinsbourne, M. (1982). Hemispheric specialization and the growth of human understanding. *American Psychologist, 37*, 411–420.

Kuhn, T. (1970). *The structure of scientific revolution, 2nd ed.* Chicago: University of Chicago Press.

MacNeilage, P., Studdert-Kennedy, M., & Lindblom, B. (1985). Planning and production of speech in normal and hearing-impaired individuals. *Asha Reports, 15*, 15–21.

Moore, S., & Perkins, W. (1990). Validity and reliability of judgments of authentic and simulated stuttering. *Journal of Speech and Hearing Disorders, 55*, 383–391.

Morris, W. (Ed.). (1970). *The American heritage dictionary*. Boston: American Heritage Publishing Co.

Neilson, M., & Neilson, P. (1987). Speech motor control and stuttering. *Speech Communication, 6*, 325–333.

Perkins, W. (1973). Replacement of stuttering with normal speech: II. Clinical procedures. *Journal of Speech and Hearing Disorders, 38*, 295–303.

Perkins, W. (1990). What is stuttering? *Journal of Speech and Hearing Disorders, 55*, 370–382.

Perkins, W. (1992). Marching to different drummers: A reply to Smith. *Journal of Speech and Hearing Research, 35*, 1033–1040.

Perkins, W. (1996). *Stuttering and science*. San Diego: Singular Publishing Group.

Perkins, W., Kent, R., & Curlee, R. (1991). A theory of neuropsycholinguistic function in stuttering. *Journal of Speech and Hearing Research, 34*, 734–752.

Perkins, W., Rudas, J., Johnson, L., & Bell, J. (1976). Stuttering: Discoordination of phonation with articulation and respiration. *Journal of Speech and Hearing Research, 19*, 509–522.

Petri, H., & Mishkin, M. (1994). Behaviorism, cognitism, and the neuropsychology of memory. *American Scientist, 82*, 30–37.

Platt, J. (1964). Strong inference. *Science, 146*, 347–353.

Ryan, B. (1971). Operant procedures applied to stuttering therapy for children. *Journal of Speech and Hearing Disorders, 36*, 264–280.

Shames, G., & Sherrick, C. (1963). A discussion of nonfluency and stuttering as operant behavior. *Journal of Speech and Hearing Disorders, 28*, 3–18.

Shattuck-Hufnagel, S. (1983). Sublexical units and suprasegmental structure in speech production and planning. In P. MacNeilage (Ed.), *The production of speech*. New York: Springer-Verlag.

Sheehan, J. (1953). Theory and treatment of stuttering as an approach-avoidance conflict. *Journal of Psychology, 36*, 27–49.

Smith, A. (1992). Commentary on "A theory of neuropsycholinguistic function in stuttering." *Journal of Speech and Hearing Research, 35*, 805–809.

Stromsta, C. (1986). *Elements of stuttering*. Oshtemo, Mich.: Atsmorts Publishing.

Sue-O'Brien, D. (1993). *Stuttering: Dimensions of an unfolding experience*. Unpublished dissertation, University of Southern California.

Travis, L. (1931). *Speech pathology*. New York: Appleton.

Tuchman, B. (1984). *The march of folly*. New York: Ballentine Books.

Van Riper, C. (1992). Stuttering. *Journal of Fluency Disorders, 17*, 81–84.

Weinberg, S. (1992). *Dreams of a final theory*. New York: Pantheon.

Wingate, M. (1962). Evaluation and stuttering. Part I: Speech characteristics of young children. *Journal of Speech and Hearing Disorders, 27*, 106–115.

Wingate, M. (1964). A standard definition of stuttering. *Journal of Speech and Hearing Disorders, 29*, 484–489.

Wischner, G. (1950). Stuttering behavior and learning. *Journal of Speech and Hearing Disorders, 15*, 324–335.

Yairi, E., Ambrose, N., & Niermann, R. (1993). The early months of stuttering: A developmental study. *Journal of Speech and Hearing Research, 36*, 521–528.

Zimmerman, G. (1980). Articulatory behaviors associated with stuttering. *Journal of Speech and Hearing Research, 23*, 108–121.

Zimmerman, G., Smith, A., & Hanley, J. (1981). Stuttering: In need of a unifying conceptual framework. *Journal of Speech and Hearing Research, 24*, 25–31.

PART FOUR

CLINICAL MANAGEMENT OF CHILDREN

The chapters in this section cover a broad range of clinical perspectives about the evaluation and management of childhood disorders of fluency. Although approaches to assessment and therapy for young stutterers differ, there is general agreement that treatment outcomes for children are usually better and more enduring than those for adults, but this very success raises the vexing questions of how soon children should receive therapy and what the form of that therapy should be. On these questions there is far less agreement. Based on the pattern of signs and symptoms obtained from parent interviews and observations and analyses of speech assessments, clinicians have to decide whether a child is beginning to stutter or is just at the high end of a normal disfluency continuum, and whether it is better to err by overselecting normally disfluent children or overlooking potential stutterers.

Furthermore, many of the assumptions that guided therapy in the past are being challenged by new data concerning the conditions under which stuttering initially develops. Yairi has shown that parents of young children who begin to stutter are not fundamentally different, even in respect to their concern and tolerance for childhood disfluency, from other parents, and that the onset of stuttering is not always gradual or protracted. As a consequence, it no longer seems responsible to respond to the earliest stages of stuttering by routinely admonishing parents not to call attention to their child's speech on the assumption that the less done with the child, the better. Intervention has become more aggressive, involving the child as well as the environment. On the other hand, few of the intervention methods used with young stutterers derive directly from theories about the cause of the disorder, or have been adequately tested through research. As will be readily apparent in this section, the methods used to assess and treat the early emergence of stuttering are guided more by intuition and clinical experience than by solid research, not because the authors have ignored such research, but rather because the difficult studies that need to be done have not yet been carried out.

Closing this section is a chapter by St. Louis and Myers concerning the puzzling, complex nature of cluttering and its possible relationship with stuttering and other disorders of speech and language. It is just possible that, in our eagerness to distinguish between stuttering and cluttering, we may have overlooked underlying similarities that may elucidate both disorders.

As is always the case with stuttering, much work remains to be done, including when is the right time to begin treating it. Like all other issues concerning the origins of behavior, it is rarely clear where the boundaries between normal and abnormal should be drawn, and so there will be disagreement about how to decide when stuttering has emerged to stay, and how aggressively to intervene in the lives of children when such is suspected. These and other issues are explored in the following chapters.

CHAPTER 12

EVALUATING CHILDHOOD STUTTERING

EDWARD G. CONTURE

This chapter discusses current approaches to the assessment of stuttering in children between 2 and 7 years of age, and I need to acknowledge, with appreciation, the work of others in this area (e.g., Adams, 1977, 1980, 1991; Conture & Caruso, 1987; Conture & Yaruss, 1993; Costello & Ingham, 1984; Culatta & Goldberg, 1995; Fosnot, 1992; Gordon & Luper, 1992; Gregory & Hill, 1992; Hayhow, 1983; Ingham, 1985; Johnson, Darley, & Spriestersbach, 1963; Peters & Guitar, 1991; Pindzola, 1986; Pindzola & White, 1986; Wall & Myers, 1984, 1995; Williams, 1974; Zebrowski, 1994). Relatively recent advances in procedures (Bahill & Curlee, 1993) and information (e.g., Conture & Kelly, 1991; Yairi & Ambrose, 1992a; Yairi, Ambrose, & Niermann, 1993) that appear particularly relevant to assessing stuttering in 2- to 7-year-old children, the age range within which most children begin to stutter, are also discussed.

Given the amount of literature that could be cited, I will need to employ a selective, less than exhaustive coverage of relevant literature. And while coverage will be somewhat selective, every attempt will be made to insure that it is as non-doctinaire and factual as possible. My discussion of past approaches to the assessment of childhood stuttering as well as recent advances in relevant knowledge will be followed by a description of clinical practice, that is, the procedures most clinicians use when assessing a child known or suspected to be stuttering.

Both quantitative (e.g., number of stutterings per 100 words spoken) and qualitative (e.g., listener judgments of a speaker's physical tension) assessments are covered. In an ideal world, assessment of childhood stuttering would involve a set of clearly specified criteria that are based on readily measurable events. By applying these criteria, trained professionals could readily classify children as either a person who stutters or one who does not (see Conture, 1990b; Young, 1984 for more general discussion of the identification/classification of stuttering and stutterers). And once this classification decision was made (i.e., the child is or is not a stutterer), it would be ideal if the same clinician had available a related set of criteria to help decide where along a continuum of no, low, moderate, or high risk for continuing to stutter to place the child.

At present, less than ideal means are available for making these two, interrelated decisions. And, as I try to make clear, any decision made as a result of assessment is significantly influenced by the nature and number of observations, information, and measurements.

OBJECTIVES

The first objective of this chapter is to discuss how to make these two interrelated decisions: (1) Does the child stutter, and if the answer is yes, (2) Does

Acknowledgment of Grant Support: Preparation of this paper was supported in part by an NIH research grant (DC000523) to Syracuse University.

the child have no, low, moderate, or high risk for continuing to stutter? Related to these two decisions, but somewhat different from both, is an assessment of the severity of the child's problem as well as his or her need for and the type of treatment needed. In order to make these two decisions, of course, we must collect information from a variety of sources.

A second objective is to describe the procedures needed to obtain this information: (1) direct interview of child's primary caregivers, which in most cases will be the child's mother and/or father; (2) direct observation of the child, including formal as well as informal testing; and (3) written reports, documents from other professionals about the child, including forms or questionnaires about the child that caregivers have filled out in advance of direct observation of the child. Of course, other sources of information, such as the child's teacher, may be available, but as much as possible, I like to base decisions on information gathered from the three sources mentioned. Given the enormous variety in types as well as forms of reported information derived from source (3), I will concentrate on sources (1) and (2).

It is not my objective (Conture & Caruso, 1987; Conture, 1990a, pp. 35–84; Conture & Yaruss, 1993), to provide a cookbook, how-to, or recipe orientation to the assessment of childhood stuttering. Rather, I will present a problem-solving, maneuver-according-to-circumstances approach. Such an approach permits a clinician to maneuver according to the circumstances that are actually, not theoretically, presented by children and their environment. As trite as it may sound, it is nonetheless true that one of the few constants to expect when assessing childhood stuttering is change. Indeed, any assessment procedure that cannot adequately deal with changes or variations in people and their behavior will be unable to deal adequately with the realities of assessing childhood stuttering. While absolute criteria and cut-off scores for this or that behavior may make us feel more secure, the reality is that people and their behavior vary within and among themselves. Thus, clinical strategies must be structured, from beginning to end, to describe

and take account of the variations in children, their parents, and their respective behaviors.

My discussion will be framed in a relatively "ideal" clinical situation in which can be obtained the greatest amount and variety of observations as well as information. I fully realize that many clinical situations, places where I have worked, do not match the "ideal." Thus, I will note, when appropriate, some of the "real" problems, concerns, and issues that may preclude obtaining an ideal amount and variety of information. The approach to be discussed, while applicable to evaluations of stuttering in children through early junior high school age, is most applicable to preschool (3- to 6-year-old) and early elementary school (7- to 9-year-old) children.

TACTICS AND PROCEDURES

Publications

I will focus on two forms of publications: (1) general reviews of assessment procedures and (2) reviews of more specific assessment approaches.

General Reviews.   Beginning clinicians and/or students who are interested in learning about the assessment of childhood stuttering should start by reading several general reviews or descriptions of approaches to the assessment of childhood stuttering (e.g., Conture & Yaruss, 1993; Gordon & Luper, 1992; Hayhow, 1983; Pindzola, 1986). Some of these publications (e.g., Gordon & Luper, 1992; Pindzola, 1986) provide brief but informative descriptions and critiques of most available (in)formal testing procedures, whereas others provide overviews of most available diagnostic procedures (e.g., Conture & Yaruss, 1993; Hayhow, 1983). For example, Conture and Yaruss (1993) describe the use and development of case history forms, parent interviews, formal and informal tests, evaluations of findings, and so forth. Such reviews provide a foundation on which clinicians and students can, with further study and experience, erect their own conceptual and procedural superstructure. It should be noted, however, that most of the (in)formal tests discussed in these reviews document only the frequency, type, and severity of a child's stuttering (e.g., Iowa Scale for Rating the Severity of Stuttering [Johnson et al., 1963]). In contrast, the Stuttering Prediction Instrument (Riley, 1984), attempts to estimate the child's relative risk for continuing to stutter, that is, the chronicity of the child's stuttering.

Specific Reviews. The second type of publication, a review of one or more selected approaches, generally provides much more detail about a specific approach to the assessment of stuttering (Adams, 1980; Conture, 1990a; Conture & Caruso, 1987; Costello & Ingham, 1984; Culatta & Goldberg, 1995; Fosnot, 1992; Gregory & Hill, 1992; Johnson et al., 1963; Peters & Guitar, 1991; Pindzola & White, 1986; Wall & Myers, 1984, 1995; Williams, 1974; Zebrowski, 1994). Specific guidelines and criteria may be provided also (e.g., Adams, 1980), for example, criteria for: (1) defining instances of stuttering, (2) determining severity of stuttering, (3) deciding which children appear more or less at risk for continuing to stutter, and so forth. Some provide detailed descriptions of a specific assessment approach (e.g., Wall & Myers, 1995) that typically originate from the authors' basic assumptions about what stuttering is; what may cause, exacerbate, or maintain it; and how best to treat it. These discussions of a particular approach to evaluating childhood stuttering (e.g., Peters & Guitar, 1991) provide a more motivated or rationale-based approach than do general reviews. The importance of motivation to the assessment of childhood stuttering will be discussed later.

Whether general or specific, most approaches to assessing childhood stuttering involve, to a greater or lesser degree, three general components: (1) a case history form (filled out by the child's caregivers before or at the time of the evaluation), (2) an interview of the child's parents, and (3) a direct examination of the child. The extent to which a clinician employs (1), (2), and (3), as well as makes decisions on the information derived from each, probably depends, in large part, on the clinician's basic assumptions about stuttering in addition to such other variables as the clinician's experience, what is possible to do within the work setting, and so forth.

Variations Between and Within People. Behavioral variations within and between people are one part of the factual engine that drives much of an assessment vehicle. Unless we take variation into consideration, we really cannot adequately account for the child's behavior. We can never be certain that the child we are assessing is having a "good," "bad," or "in-between" day in terms of speech, language, and other related behavior. And our relative uncertainty about the representativeness of a child's behavior has tremendous implications for assessment.

To account for each child's behavioral variations, I try to make as many observations from as many sources and over as long a period of time as possible. In this way, I attempt to cast an observational net that is both wide and deep in terms of the quantity and quality of information it captures. Developing and using such an observational net repeatedly with the same child, if necessary, increases the chance that I will observe the child's "usual" as well as best and worst performances. Although I try to increase my chances of capturing the most salient aspects of the child's behavior, I can never be certain that I have done so. Remaining cognizant of such uncertainty should help temper any ideas clinicians may entertain about "completely" understanding the child as well as qualify any decisions to be made concerning the child.

Some deal with such uncertainty by recommending treatment for any child whom a parent or referring agency expresses concerns about. Perhaps they do this because they realize that they can never know everything there is to know about a child and because they cannot know for sure who does and does not need therapy. Consequently, they decide (actually, by not deciding) to recommend therapy for all children, and the sooner the better. Conversely, others may deal with uncertainty by slowly, deliberately, cautiously gathering information, which results in their becoming mired in an indecisive, wait-and-see mode. Perhaps they do this because they realize there are many different pieces of information they need to know. Thus, they try to collect the uncollectable or ALL needed information, which keeps them from ever making any decisions. Rather than selecting either of these two extremes, clinicians should try to deal with uncertainty by striking some sort of balance between those forces encouraging them to be overly reflective (i.e., "when in doubt, delay") and those that encourage them to be impulsive (i.e., "any-action-is-better-than-none").

That said, how should clinicians go about developing and using an observational net of sufficient breadth and depth to arrive at timely, reasonable, factually based decisions? Obviously, there are no clear-cut, easy answers, and what follows is just one way for assessing childhood stuttering. An ideal outline is presented with the full realization that realities of everyday clinical situations influence, modify and may even prevent us from carrying out an ideal approach.

An Outline for Assessment

I will discuss assessment in three interrelated sections. First, I will provide an overview of assessment procedures, in table form (Table 12.1) and then in the text. This overview presents an idealized sequence of observations, information synthesis, and decision-making strategies that I have found useful when assessing childhood stuttering. Second, I will cover the process of interviewing parents. Third, I will discuss the direct assessment of the child and his or her speech, language, and related behavior. To begin, I will present a conceptual framework for the sequence of events and procedures I use when assessing childhood stuttering.

Motivated Observations. Probably nothing is more important to effective and efficient assessment of childhood stuttering than developing an organized collection of motivated observations. Obtaining as many observations as we can, without a motivation or reason for doing so, is likely to scatter and obfuscate rather than focus and clarify our understanding of the child we are trying to assess. It is not unusual to find diagnostic formats

TABLE 12.1   An Outline of an Idealized Sequence of Observations, Information Synthesis and Decision-Making for the Assessment of Stuttering in Children

(1) **Motivated Observations:** Develop organized collection of motivated observations.

(2) **Many, different observations:** Make as many, different observations as possible.

(3) **Repeated observations:** Expect to make repeated observations of some children.

(4) **Organize/Synthesize information:** Attempt to organize/synthesize relevant information gathered from observations.

(5) **Evaluate information:** Determine meaning of and evaluate organized, synthesized observations.

(6) **Decide on classification and chronicity:** Decide if the child can be

    (a) meaningfully classified as a person who stutters, and

    (b) if so, what is the child's risk for continuing to stutter—no, low, medium, or high?

that make many different types of observations; however, it is not always readily apparent what motivates these observations. My own motivation comes from a belief (Conture, 1990a, pp. 35–84) that childhood stuttering involves a complex interaction between a child's environment and the skills and abilities a child brings to that environment. Thus, when assessing children who stutter, I am motivated to observe, as best I can, both the child's environment (e.g., parents' attitudes, behaviors, and beliefs) and the child's abilities/behaviors (e.g., expressive language skills, speech motor development, and frequency, type, duration, and severity of speech disfluencies). Thus, it should not come as a surprise that my diagnostic evaluations are organized to facilitate my ability to observe both the child and the child's environment, separately as well as together.

Many Different Observations. I want to make as many different, relevant observations as possible. Which observations are relevant? Those related to my fundamental belief about childhood stuttering, the child's behavior and environment. Again, observations should be related to beliefs and assumptions about what childhood stuttering is, and what may cause, exacerbate, and/or maintain it. By obtaining many different observations, using the widest and deepest observational net possible, I hope to capture the most complete picture of the child, relevant events, and their variations.

To do this, clinicians need to assemble and know how to administer and evaluate a large battery of formal tests as well as informal observations. A number of formal tests are now available, for example, *Stuttering Severity Instrument for Children and Adults* (SSI) (Riley, 1980), *Stuttering Prediction Instrument for Young Children* (SPI) (Riley, 1984), and *Stocker Probe Technique for the Diagnosis and Treatment of Stuttering in Young Children* (Stocker, 1976). In addition, there is also available a "computer-based decision support system to evaluate incipient stuttering" (i.e., Bahill & Curlee, 1993). Of course, collecting all of this objective and subjective information is only half the task; it still has to be organized and synthesized and then evaluated so that the meaning of these observations and information can be used to make a decision about the child's classification and chronicity.

Repeated Observations. Some children will require repeated (in)formal observations. After assessment, children fall into one of three categories: (1) No clear need for therapy, (2) clear need for therapy, and (3) unclear need for therapy. More than a few of the children diagnosed initially as stuttering recover without therapy (e.g., Yairi, 1993; Yairi, Ambrose, & Niermann, 1993; Yairi, Chapter 3, this text). However, the more important question, at least in my opinion, is not whether a particular percentage of children (e.g., 50%, 60%, or 75%) will eventually recover without therapy— a number of human problems spontaneously remit without treatment—but of those children initially classified as stuttering, which ones are likely to recover without therapy? A retrospective examination of the diagnostic records of 100 children who were known or suspected to be stuttering

(Yaruss, LaSalle, & Conture, 1996) suggests that, even after a thorough initial diagnostic evaluation, it was not clear for approximately 40 percent of these children whether therapy was needed. Thus, the first assessment of these children is often not the last. Repeating observations with these children should be expected, since only with the passage of time can a greater degree of certainty about the child's difficulties be established.

Synthesize Information Derived from Observations. Clinicians need to organize and synthesize the information that has been gathered and strive to bring this information together into a coherent, organized package, ideally on a 1- or 2-page summary sheet (such a "sheet" is presented in Conture, 1990a, p. 55; Conture & Yaruss, 1993, p. 62). It is not sufficient merely to collect large amounts of information and expect its meaning to emerge spontaneously. And, of course, organizing and synthesizing information requires clinicians to include relevant but exclude irrelevant information as well. Pindzola and White (1986) present a good example of an organizational structure for assessing childhood stuttering.

It is here, when trying to organize and synthesize observations and test findings, that the first issue, motivated observations, becomes crucial. Unless there is a motivational scaffold, some motivation or reason for obtaining all of the different information that was collected, such information would be like a dictionary having a complete but unalphabetized listing of words. Such a collection of words may be impressive in number and variety but of little practical use and meaning without some organizational structure. Clearly, clinicians need a means of synthesizing all of the collected observations and information, of bringing it together into an integrated whole. They need to see the forest, not merely the trees, so that they can provide an overview for the child's parents, referral sources, and other agencies. An excellent example of a well-motivated, organizational scaffold for assessing childhood stuttering is Wall and Myers's (1995, pp. 161–194) three-factor model (i.e., psycholinguistic, physiological, and psychosocial) for observing, synthesizing, and evaluating assessment information of childhood stuttering.

Evaluation of Information.   Clinicians need to evaluate the collected information and give meaning to all of the observations and information they have collected. For example, what does it mean that the child's expressive language skills exceed those of his or her peer group? Or, what does it mean that a child's speaking rate is above, but diadochokinetic rate is below, age expectation? Is it of significance that one child attends to one object, event, or person too long, while another seems unable to attend to any object, event, or person for any extended period? Likewise, what does it mean if a mother constantly interrupts, or nearly so, every time a child begins to talk? What do such observations mean in terms of whether a child should be classified as a stutterer, at risk for continuing to stutter, or in need of therapy?

Decisions Based on Information.   Finally, clinicians must make decisions based on the information that has been gathered. These decisions, of course, are what the child's parents and referring agencies want. Making such decisions is one of the major tasks clinicians are paid to do. Given the expenditures of time and money that any treatment regimen will entail, clinicians need to base decisions about therapy on the best, most up-to-date, and widest ranging information available.

ASSESSMENT CRITERIA

The Child's Environment: Interviewing the Parents

My rationale and method for interviewing parents is thoroughly discussed elsewhere (e.g., Conture, 1990a; Conture & Yaruss, 1993), and I will discuss only some essential elements here. To begin, let me be clear that most clinicians are uncertain about how parental beliefs, feelings, or behavior relate to childhood stuttering. Simply put, a great deal more needs to be known about how a variety of parental variables do or do not relate to the cause, exacer-

bation, or maintenance of childhood stuttering (see Conture & Zebrowski, 1992 for further discussion of the relationship between parental behaviors and childhood stuttering). I do believe that parents are often a child's most frequent and important listeners and conversational partners. As such, at the very least, they are in a position to make a number of observations that may help clinicians help their child. The objective is to find out what parents say in response to such questions as the following (see Conture & Yaruss, 1993, p. 9):

1. How can the clinician help the child/the parents? What, if anything, do the parents believe that the clinician can do to help them or their child?
2. What, in general, concerns the parents? What are the parents concerned about, if, in fact, they are concerned? Their concerns need not be limited to speech or language and may include, for example, concerns about the child's social development.
3. What specifically concerns the parents? What is the specific nature of their concern, in their words or through their demonstrations? Although some clinicians may believe that parents of children who stutter are more likely than parents of nonstuttering children to label or classify speech behaviors as stuttering, research [Zebrowski & Conture, 1989] suggests that the two groups of parents do not differ appreciably in what they do and do not classify as stuttering.
4. How long have parents been concerned? How long have they had such concerns? It is also relevant to find out if other adults who know the child have expressed similar or different concerns about the child.
5. What have the parents done, if anything, to help their child or to deal with their concerns (again, in their words or through their demonstrations)? If they have read something about stuttering, it may be helpful to know what they have read and what they have learned from having read it. Such written (e.g., Ainsworth & Fraser, 1988; Conture & Fraser, 1989; Cooper, 1979] and videotaped [e.g.,

Conture, 1994] material often serves, as it should, as the beginning rather than end of dialogue between clinicians and parents about the child and the parents' relation to the child.

6. What do parents believe caused or is maintaining the problem? What do the parents, explicitly or implicitly, say has caused their child's problems? What do they believe may exacerbate or maintain it?

7. What other concerns do the parents have? Are there other concerns (past, present or future) about the child? This relates to (2) and (4) above and may need to be asked in several ways to obtain a full and adequate understanding of parents' concerns.

8. Are there any other issues the parents want to discuss? What questions or concerns do the parents have that haven't been addressed, in whole or in part, or that haven't already been mentioned (i.e., "Is there anything I have not covered that you'd like to ask me or talk about with me?")?

A detailed listing of sample questions that explore these and other related issues is available elsewhere (Conture, 1990a, pp. 293–296; Conture & Yaruss, 1993, pp. 72–76), and Table 12.2 lists specific topic areas relating to child development, family life, descriptions of the child's problem, and so forth that should be explored.

Issues Pertaining to Questioning Parents

Follow-up Questioning.   In addition to knowing what questions to ask parents, it is equally important to know how to follow up parents' responses to questions. Indeed, some responses should lead to more questions, and sometimes these follow up questions will lead to important information about, or a key to, a child's problem.

Example of follow-up questioning: "Johnny is talking much better now." Let me briefly explore a common situation in which a mother seems to be reporting that her child's speech (dis)fluency is variable. This might start with the clinician asking, "How is Johnny's talking right now?" to

TABLE 12.2   Questions Asked of Parents of Children Known or Suspected to Be Stuttering Should Cover the Following Topics

General development

Family history

Speech-language development and history

Academic information

Social information

History/description of child's problem

Child's current speech, language, and voice abilities

Influence of listeners, type of speech, and speaking situations on child's speech

Parental reactions, theories, and attempts to help

Family interactions, including siblings

Child's psychosocial development in relation to peers, siblings, and any apparent reactions/awareness of speech problems or difficulties

Miscellaneous, for example, questions about previous evaluations or therapy, parental history of therapy, etc.

which the mother responds, "Oh, it is much better than it was before." This response should make the clinician want to know what the mother means. So, a follow-up might be, "What was it (her child's speech) like before?" And the mother again responds, "Oh, it was much worse earlier this year" At this point, the clinician has several options:

1. *Discontinue this line of questioning.* This would indicate that the clinician believes that the mother thinks the child is talking better now than in the past or that the mother thinks the child's speech problem is variable.

2. *Continue this line of questioning.* This would indicate that the clinician believes that the mother thinks that the quality or quantity of her child's speech is variable but is not sure exactly what she means. Is she referring to the usual developmental fits and spurts in a child's speech and language acquisition? Or is she describing significant changes in the nature or frequency of her child's speech prob-

lem? Or is she just relatively unreliable in recalling her child's past behavior?

3. *Discontinue for now but later continue this line of questioning and make note of mother's comment in your diagnostic report.* This would indicate that the clinician senses the mother is becoming concerned, or unnecessarily anxious about these questions. Perhaps she thinks that this is a serious issue or that the clinician sees the variability of her child's speech as a problem. While it's important to get a clear idea from the mother regarding the nature and amount of variability in the child's disfluency, it is also important not to worry the mother unduly about something that may, with further questioning, be revealed as normal variation or of marginal clinical significance.[1]

Regardless of which alternative is chosen—continue, discontinue, or delay continuing a line of questioning—the decision has to be made fairly quickly, and it will be based, in large part, on the clinician's judgments about whether further questioning is likely to elicit responses from the mother that can influence evaluation decisions about the child, treatment recommendations, or the child's therapy. Such judgments require the kind of knowledge that comes from experience, experience that has been guided by motivated questioning that is linked to evaluation objectives.

Unclear Parent Answers to Seemingly Clear, Straightforward, Clinician Questions. Clinicians need to be concerned about the reliability of parents' responses to questions as well as that of

their own judgments and measures. Do the parents provide different answers to the same question asked in different forms? Do they routinely offer unclear, vague answers to clear, straightforward questions? Do they seem unusually confused in responding to routine types of questions? Because parents' responses, like those of all people, vary in reliability and credibility, *Second Opinion* (Bahill & Curlee, 1993), a computer-based decision support system for evaluating incipient stuttering, includes a "certainty factor" (CF). Each item of information entered into the computer is given a CF, whether based on parents' responses, the clinician's observations, or data gathered from the child. In this way, if a clinician is uncertain of the reliability or credibility of some information, it can be assigned a "weight," from 0 to 100 percent, to reflect the clinician's estimate of the accuracy of the information provided.

Most parents, in my opinion, do not consciously or unconsciously lie about their child or the child's behavior. Most respond as best as they can based on imperfect, human, memories of what happened several years, months, or days ago. Basically, clinicians need to assess the reliability of parents' responses to questions. Some are simply not good observers of their children and can provide only vague, if not inaccurate, information. Others may be so concerned about saying the "right" thing about their child that they continually try to say what they think the clinician wants to hear. Still others may avoid answering directly, even when they know the answer, because they are afraid it may implicate them somehow as a "cause" of their child's problem. Lastly, some parents know the information needed, are willing to tell the truth, but are just not sufficiently articulate to clearly convey what they know, believe, or feel about their child.

Questions Are Complete but Just Not Appropriate. During some assessments, a clinician may have asked a complete set of questions, but not just the right ones about the child being evaluated. For example, a child's good grades in school might lead clinicians to skip asking about school. If they had,

---

[1]Any event, issue, observation, or behavior is clinically significant if it, in whole or part, somehow influences or helps determine decisions about diagnostic classification, likelihood for remaining in that classification, need for or type of therapy, as well as chances for recovery through therapy. Such events differ from those that represent a clinically thorough procedure. For example, attempting to document thoroughly the age at which a child was able to tie shoes will have little influence on a clinician's decisions about diagnostic classifications, a child's risk for continuing in a classification, or the need to begin treatment without delay.

they might have discovered that the child frequently complains of stomachaches or headaches before or after arriving at school and frequently visits the nurse's office, particularly before tests, complaining of such problems. For whatever reason (e.g., home or school pressures), the child appears to be trying so hard to excel in school, to get good grades (i.e., he believes he is either "all right" or "all wrong") that he is showing stress-related symptoms. Such perfectionism on his part may indicate that he is also intolerant of any mistakes in his speech or language (i.e., he feels he is either "all right" or "all wrong" when he talks), an attitude that has the potential for adversely affecting his ability to benefit from treatment.

The Child's Skills, Abilities, and Behaviors

Direct Observation of the Child's Speech, Language, and Related Behavior. Obviously, I cannot cover all areas of development that clinicians must consider when assessing children who stutter (e.g., speech, voice, language, audition, motor). I will not discuss such related behaviors as intelligence, for example, but will focus on specific aspects of speech that are related to speech (dis)fluency. One very important assumption to keep in mind is that effective assessment of childhood stuttering requires clinicians to search carefully for subtle harbingers that a child's stuttering may not be a temporary or transient difficulty. It is most important, I believe, before reading the following criteria and rationale for measuring specific aspects of stuttering in young children, to reflect on my basic assumption about the assessment of childhood stuttering: *The main objective is to identify subtle harbingers that incipient stuttering may not be a temporary or transient difficulty.* For most 2- to 7-year-olds, stuttering, at the time of the first diagnostic evaluation, typically will not be (1) very stable, (2) grossly apparent (i.e., easily perceptible to the casual listener), or (3) severe. Yes, it is possible that incipient stuttering, for as many as three in ten children, will be (1) highly consistent, (2) grossly apparent, (3) quite severe and (4) easily perceptible to even casual observers shortly

after onset. However, for the remaining seven out of ten, the problem is much less stable, apparent, and severe.

It should be kept in mind, also, that I am discussing the assessment of young children, those in the lower half of the 2- to 7-year-old age range, many of whom (1) cannot be easily nor meaningfully classified as stutterers, and (2) if they are, their risk for continuing to stuttering is unknown. It is not enough to classify a child as a stutterer, the more important task is trying to determine the degree to which a child is at risk for continuing to stutter. Thus, at the time of their first diagnostic evaluation, these children have yet to receive any treatment, and most will be displaying relatively subtle deviations from the speech of their peers and few, if any, signs that their stuttering is nontransitory.

For example, advanced training and experience are not needed to recognize that a 3-year, 6-month-old is stuttering or is at risk for continuing to do so if the child stutters on 25 percent of the words spoken, with a 2-second average duration, half of which consist of physically tense "blocks." Again, it is possible, but not probable that we will encounter, during an initial evaluation of incipient stuttering, a problem of this severity, frequency, duration, type, and overt manifestations. In fact, clinicians looking for "gross" signs of stuttering, at or near its onset, may waste a lot of time waiting for such problems to emerge. When such less-subtle signs do become apparent, clinicians may be dealing with a more entrenched problem that could evolve into one that is chronic. Table 12.3 lists some of the subtle harbingers that I and my colleagues' research has found to be indicators of childhood stuttering, its severity and chronicity. I believe that these criteria are additive (i.e., the more of them exhibited, the greater the risk) and noncontradictory (i.e., presence of one does not preclude the presence of others).

Stuttering Frequency

Basic Criterion. If a child exhibits three or more within-word (stuttered) speech disfluencies per 100 words of conversational speech, I believe that

TABLE 12.3 Indicators That a Child Can Be Meaningfully Classified as a Stutterer and/or at Risk for Continuing to Stutter

(1) **Stuttering (within-word disfluency) Frequency:** Average of three or more within-word (stuttering) disfluencies per 100 words of conversational speech in a sample of 300 words or more.

(2) **Sound Prolongation Index:** 25 percent or more of a child's total stutterings are sound prolongations that may be estimated by assessing the percentage of sound prolongations per ten nonsystematically selected within-word disfluencies.

(3) **Mother-Child Speaking Behaviors:** Average difference of two or more syllables per second in the speaking rates of mother and child during conversational speech, and increases in simul-talk duration or the duration of parent-child interrupting behaviors may be associated with increases in a child's stuttering severity.

(4) **Stuttering-Stuttering Clusters:** Presence of any stuttering-stuttering clusters in a child's two-element speech disfluency clusters.

5) **Selected Nonspeech Behavior:** Eyeball movements to the side and/or eyelid blinking during stuttering.

---

the child is at risk for continuing to stutter. However, the degree of risk depends on other factors, not only whether three or more stutterings per 100 words are exhibited by the child. There is no single criterion discussed in this section that would, by itself, be sufficient to permit me to classify a child as a stutterer or to determine the child's degree of risk for continuing to stutter.

Rationale.   While there is no way to avoid making errors when classifying children who stutter, seldom have I found children who exhibit fewer than three stutterings per 100 words to be at an appreciable risk for continuing to stutter. This clinical observation is supported by research findings of Johnson and associates (1959) and Yairi and

Lewis (1984). Several years ago, I discussed Johnson and associates' data and suggested that three within-word disfluencies per 100 word criterion would result in 100 percent "correct rejections" of the children who do not stutter and about 60 percent "hits" of those who do stutter (Conture, 1990a, Table 1-1, p. 11). The errors or "misses" comprise the nearly 40 percent of the study's children who stuttered but who produced fewer than three within-word disfluencies per 100 words.

Unfortunately, I know of no way to avoid making some "false positives" or "misses" (see Conture, 1990a, p. 12, Figure 1-1) when assessing childhood stuttering (see, Conture, 1990a, pp. 10–13). For example, lowering the criterion from three to two within-word disfluencies per 100 words would likely increase correct classification of stutterers to nearly 70 percent, but it would also decrease correct rejections of children who do not stutter to less than 90 percent. On rare occasions, which I estimate may happen during evaluations of one in thirty children who do not stutter, a child who otherwise appears to be a nonstutterer will exhibit three to five within-word disfluencies per 100 words. Typically, when re-evaluated three to six months later, the child will exhibit within-word or stuttered speech disfluencies below this criterion. Continued work is needed, perhaps along the lines of Ingham and colleagues (e.g., Cordes, Ingham, Frank, & Ingham, 1992), to develop more reliable means for judging the presence as well as frequency of instances of stuttering. Such judgments are essential to thorough assessments of childhood stuttering.

Procedure.   My experience indicates that a fairly representative impression of a child's speech fluency can be obtained by assessing about 300 words of conversational speech between the child and a parent. Obviously, a larger sample is better, because it is more likely to capture more of the variability in a child's speech fluency. Although samples can always be repeated, for example, one to six months later, depending on the needs of the child, a 300-word sample of parent-child conversation is a reasonable-sized sample with which to begin.

Stuttering Duration

Basic Criterion. There is no clearly discriminating duration for within-word speech disfluencies that reliably differentiates young children who stutter from their nonstuttering peers. I can say, however, that many children at various levels of risk for continuing to stutter produce within-word speech disfluencies that are shorter than 1 second. Zebrowski (1994, pp. 225–226), in reviewing her studies and those of others on the duration of childhood stuttering, states that the duration of sound/syllable repetitions and sound prolongations of young children averages about one-half second, and ranges from one-quarter of a second or less to about one-and-one-half seconds. In addition, research indicates that there is no significant difference in the duration of sound/syllable repetitions and sound prolongations of very young children who stutter and those who do not (Kelly & Conture, 1992; Zebrowski, 1991).

Rationale. The duration of stuttering is probably more useful for describing the quality (i.e., the severity) of stuttering, whereas the frequency of stuttering is more useful for describing its quantity (i.e., presence). Thus, I use measures of stuttering duration as a qualitative index of stuttering, in particular its severity. Many seem to make the reasonable assumption that the longer the duration of stuttering, the more severe the problem, as does, for example, the *Stuttering Severity Instrument* (Riley, 1980).

Procedure. There are no standardized procedural guidelines for the measurement of stuttering duration, but my experience has been that measuring the duration of ten nonsystematically selected stutterings in the conversational speech of children and averaging them gives a reasonable estimate of the duration of their typical stutterings. Of course, the more a child stutters, the more stutterings one can measure; therefore, to be consistent across children, I sample ten stutterings nonsystematically throughout a child's conversation, usually with a parent, which is a compromise between oversampling children who stutter infrequently and undersampling those who stutter frequently.

Sound Prolongation Index

Basic Criterion. If sound prolongations exceed 25 percent of a child's total stutterings, I believe that the child is at greater risk for continuing to stutter than one whose sound prolongations are less than 25 percent of all stutterings. For example, if a child produces, on average, twelve stutterings per 100 words, of which five are sound prolongations (42%), that child is at greater risk than if he or she had produced only one or two sound prolongations per twelve stutterings. Research (e.g., Johnson & Associates, 1959; Yairi & Lewis, 1984) has shown that children who do and who do not stutter exhibit the same types of speech disfluencies. Thus, every disfluency type produced by children who stutter is produced by some children who do not stutter; however, it is also the case that the absolute number of within-word disfluencies differs between the two groups (see Conture, 1990a, Table 1-1, p. 11).

Rationale. Schwartz and Conture (1988) showed that the percentage of stutterings that were sound prolongations (the sound prolongation index) was one of three variables that significantly differentiated among children who stutter. Sound prolongations reflect a cessation in the forward flow of speech production, which we believe indicates a more advanced stage of stuttering. In a sound/syllable repetition, forward movement of the speech production system has also stopped, but there is movement, albeit reiterative. In a sound prolongation, forward articulatory movement has apparently ceased, and the articulators maintain a "fixed" articulatory posture. In the next stage in the development of stuttering, a "block" or blockage, the cessation or stoppage of speech production involves a longer, generally more physically tense and perceptibly more noticeable cessation or stoppage of speech movement. Usually, long before "blocks" become a routine part of a child's disfluency repertoire, sound prolongations are consistently present, which suggests that the child's problem may not be transitory.

Procedure. Using the same 300-word sample from which frequency of stuttering was computed, one can estimate the percent of total stutterings that sound prolongations represent. For example, if thirty within-word disfluencies were produced by a child in the 300 words, of which fifteen were sound/syllable repetitions (50%), ten were sound prolongations (33%), and five were monosyllabic whole-word repetitions (17%), the child would have exceeded the 25 percent prolongation index, and I would consider this as an indication that stuttering might not be transitory.

Mother-Child Speaking Rate

Basic Criterion. If a preschool child habitually exhibits an average articulatory speaking rate (Costello, 1983) of 210 or more syllables per minute, the child is probably speaking too fast (Pindzola, Jenkins, & Lokken, 1989). However, even more instructive, I believe, is a comparison of the child's and parents' speaking rates. If the child's mother speaks two or more syllables per second faster than the child, on average, the chances increase that the child is stuttering more severely (Yaruss & Conture, 1995). Obviously, more work is needed to understand how differences in the speaking rates of children who stutter and their parents may be related to stuttering frequency, severity, or chronicity; however, we presently have some indication that stuttering severity is related to mothers' speaking rates that exceed those of their stuttering children by more than two syllables per second, a relation we should probably examine when assessing childhood stuttering.

Basic Rationale. I believe that it is difficult for a child to be fluent when speaking at a rate that exceeds the activation rate for phonological encoding. Anything that makes a child speed up his or her planning for speech (e.g., producing longer utterances) may cause the child to misselect speech units. And as the frequency of misselection increases, as suggested by Postma and Kolk (1993), the child is apt to make unintended phonological selection errors, errors that he or she may detect,

and in attempting to repair or modify them, exhibit disfluent speech.

Procedure. For both the child and parents, clinicians should calculate overall speaking rate (average number of syllables spoken per minute, including stuttered and nonstuttered syllables) as well as articulatory speaking rate (average number of syllables spoken per minute in segments of nonstuttered speech). Because articulatory speaking rate is less contaminated by longer pauses and stuttering, it has become the preferred speaking rate measure for assessing speaking rate in childhood stuttering. Unfortunately, it is still not clear how large a sample one has to collect from within the 300-word sample in order to arrive at a valid and reliable estimate of the child's speaking rate. Several colleagues and I (e.g., Kelly & Conture, 1992; Logan & Conture, 1995), concluded that ten utterances is a bare minimum and twenty-five to thirty utterances a reasonable compromise between under- and oversampling for estimating a child's speaking rate.

Disfluency Clusters

Basic Criterion. If a child produces any within-word disfluency clusters (i.e., two or more within-word disfluencies on adjacent sounds, syllables or words within an utterance; see Hubbard & Yairi, 1988), the child should be re-evaluated, unless, of course, stuttering is otherwise apparent, and treatment, not re-evaluation, has been recommended. Stuttering-stuttering clusters seem to occur rarely in the speech of children who do not stutter (LaSalle & Conture, 1995). Even among children who do stutter, such within-word disfluency clusters occur, on average, in only 25 to 40 percent of their total speech disfluency clusters.

Procedures. Clinical procedures for measuring speech disfluency clusters are not well developed. *Second Opinion* (Bahill & Curlee, 1993) asks whether 50 percent or more of the child's disfluencies are in clusters; however, LaSalle and Conture's (1995) study indicates that stuttering-stuttering, two-element disfluency clusters average about 32 percent of stuttering children's disfluency clusters (standard error of mean = about 4%), whereas children who do not stutter never produced a stuttering-stuttering, two-element disfluency cluster.

One prudent means of measuring speech disfluency clusters is to tabulate the total number of two-element, speech disfluency clusters in a child's conversational speech. Since children who do and do not stutter produce speech disfluency clusters (Hubbard & Yairi, 1988; LaSalle & Conture, 1995), the mere presence of these clusters does not distinguish the two groups. However, any stuttering-stuttering clusters in a child's corpus of two-element clusters may be a subtle sign that the child's stuttering problem is not transitory. And while it may seem reasonable to assume that the higher the percentage of total disfluency clusters that are stuttering-stuttering, the greater the chance that the child's stuttering problem is not transient, this assumption awaits further investigation.

Basic Rationale.   I do not know what causes stutterings to cluster together any more than anyone knows what causes stutterings to occur in isolation; however, a number of clinicians have observed that the presence of speech disfluency clusters (e.g., Bahill & Curlee, 1993) indicates a more advanced problem. Thus, the presence of stuttering-stuttering clusters is something clinicians will want to note.

Nonspeech Behaviors

Basic Criterion.   The absolute number of nonspeech behaviors associated with stutterings seems to significantly differentiate subgroups of children who stutter (Schwartz & Conture, 1998). However, I have come to believe that the types and the overall frequency of these behaviors provide clues about the presence and chronicity of stuttering in children. First, Conture and Kelly (1991) reported that even the fluent speech of children who do not stutter includes a wide variety and number of nonspeech behaviors. Thus, nonspeech behaviors, just like speech disfluencies, are produced by both stuttering and nonstuttering children. And, much like disfluency types, there is a great deal of

overlap in the type and frequency of nonspeech behaviors that occur during the conversational speech of both talker groups. Because nonspeech behaviors are exhibited by children who stutter at or near the onset of the problem (Schwartz, Zebrowski, & Conture, 1990; Yairi, Ambrose, & Niermann, 1993), the occurrence of such behavior does not necessarily indicate that the child's stuttering is a long-standing or firmly established problem. However, two nonspeech behaviors are produced significantly more often by children who stutter: eyeball movement to the side and eyelid blinking. For reasons that are still unclear, children who exhibit such behaviors during speech, particularly during within-word disfluencies, are more often classified as children who stutter.

Basic Rationale.   Although any nonspeech behavior during stuttering may be of interest, Conture and Kelly (1991) found that the above two types clearly differ between children who do and do not stutter. Other nonspeech behaviors, such as raising the upper lip (as in a sneer or sign of disgust or distaste), pressing the lips together (when producing a sound that does not require bilabial contact), or dropping the jaw (when producing a sound that does not require bilabial opening) are also observed more often among children who stutter. Obviously, further research is needed to understand their causes, but for now, they appear to be one more subtle harbinger of a stuttering problem that is not transitory. Likewise, more research is needed to study the bidirectional nature of such nonspeech behaviors as mother-child eye contact (e.g., LaSalle & Conture, 1991), and how these behaviors become associated with, and perhaps influence, childhood stuttering.

Support for Procedures

Much of what I have covered in this chapter has resulted from years of clinical trial and error by myself and other clinicians at many different sites. Typically, the diagnostic methods that clinical experience has indicated are helpful have been retained, while those that proved of little benefit have been discarded. However, given the recently increased emphasis on research into childhood stuttering (e.g., Yaruss & Conture, 1993; Yairi & Ambrose, 1992a, b; Yairi, Ambrose & Niermann, 1993), it is clear that diagnostic approaches are becoming increasingly blended with information that is derived from well-controlled research studies of childhood stuttering at or near onset.

If this were an ideal world, there would be standard procedures and common rationales for the diagnosis and assessment of childhood stuttering. But in the real world, no such standard exists. Nevertheless, a number of speech-language pathologists appear to be working relatively independently, but concurrently, towards a consensus (e.g., Conture, 1990a, pp. 34–85; Culatta & Goldberg, 1995, pp. 49–107; Peters & Guitar, 1991, pp. 129–187; Zebrowski, 1994, pp. 215–245). A consensus does not mean absolute, but relative, agreement. Indeed, different speech-language pathologists differ in their interpretation of findings or in the weight placed on particular observations and information. The following areas of consensus appear to support, in whole or in part, various aspects of the approach I have described for the assessment of childhood stuttering.

First, most clinicians attempt to interview the child's parents. From the relatively elaborate procedure for parent interviewing that I favor to a more modest set of questions asked by some (e.g., Culatta & Goldberg, 1995, p. 55), most clinicians who work in this area believe that interviewing the parents is an essential part of the assessment of childhood stuttering.

Second, most clinicians attempt to objectify the child's speech disfluencies and related behaviors. From the relatively elaborate, observer-dependent means of specifying speech disfluencies, as exemplified in the *Stuttering Severity Instrument* (Riley, 1980) to the less elaborate, speaker-dependent means of describing speech behavior (e.g., "Tell me about your problem," Culatta & Goldberg, 1995, p. 61), most clinicians quantify, to some degree, a child's speech, language, and other related behaviors. By and large, the time is long past when merely noting an opinion that this or that child stutters was all that was necessary to

recommend that a child begin treatment. Modern-day clinicians want and typically try to verify their opinions through many different types of (in)formal observations.

Third, most clinicians routinely use (in)formal tests. While related to objectification, the use of (in)formal tests to assess childhood stuttering is a bit different. In using available tests, such as the *Stuttering Prediction Instrument* (Riley, 1981), clinicians can corroborate and judiciously interpret their subjective impressions about a child with findings from tests designed to assess childhood stuttering. The routine use of such tests "standardizes" clinicians' assessments, from one child to the next, and helps clinicians organize and objectify the results of assessment procedures more consistently. This also leads to more consistent decision making about diagnostic classifications as well as chronicity judgments.

Fourth, most clinicians make multiple as well as repeated measures. Sometimes a process or a person has to be observed several times before a clear picture emerges, especially if the process or person is highly variable. To obtain such a picture, therefore, many clinicians currently collect a variety of data on speech, language, and related behavior (e.g., Conture, 1990a, p. 55) and document changes that occur in these data, especially in a child's speech disfluencies over time (e.g., Zebrowski, 1994, p. 233).

SUMMARY

Advances in clinical application typically lag advances in knowledge. Basic information is often slow to find its way into the clinic. There are many reasons for this, and one that is particularly important is that clinicians know that findings from one research study are not always replicated in subsequent studies. Likewise, they know that findings from research studies cannot always be replicated in the clinic. Thus, encouraging new findings from seemingly careful research studies are not always replicable in other research laboratories or in clinics.

Clinicians, in their daily practice, have their

own form of replication. They do this by using certain methods repeatedly and coming to rely on those that they find to be of benefit with most clients, at least some of the time. Unfortunately, some clinicians may use a procedure about which they have little understanding of why or how it works. In such cases, when a clinical procedure "doesn't work," it simply "doesn't work" because the clinician was essentially clueless about why the procedure worked in the first place. In all fairness, though, everyday realities of clinical practice do not always allow clinicians to develop rationales for an approach or a full understanding of why it may or may not be effective.

Effectiveness

Speech-language pathologists are probably most effective in describing the characteristics of a child's speech disfluency problem, its frequency, duration, and type. Although a bit less effective, clinicians have become increasingly able to distinguish children who stutter from those who do not and to distinguish among the relative severity levels that a stuttering child exhibits. Although everyone can and does make mistakes sometimes, on occasion deciding that a child is stuttering who, in fact, does not or that child is not stuttering who does (Conture, 1990a, p. 11–12), we seem to be increasing our ability, through research, as well as refinements in clinical practice, to minimize such errors.

Ineffectiveness

Speech-language pathologists are probably least effective in assessing a child's risk for continuing to stutter and in predicting a child's and family's ability to benefit from therapy. Knowing that a child is stuttering and also knowing that a child will continue to stutter are two different kinds of knowledge. Believing that a child needs therapy and predicting that a child will benefit from therapy are also based on different kinds of information. It would be nice if the current knowledge base permitted clinicians to engage in the primary prevention of childhood stuttering (i.e., preventing the onset of stuttering be-

havior), something that any clinician would welcome. However, the truth of the matter is that present treatment efforts directed at childhood stuttering, which are preceded, presumably, by careful assessment, are related to secondary prevention, which attempts to prevent a worsening of a problem or its evolution into a chronic disability.

Diagnostic Evaluation as Orientation to Treatment

One truism is that therapy begins with a diagnostic evaluation. Not only is the clinician trying to figure out whether a problem exists and its probable risk for continuation, but just as importantly, the clinician is also trying to orient the child and the child's parents to the problem, what it is, what it is not, and what may lie ahead in terms of its management. It is important for clinicians to note that initial assessment sessions are the optimal time for orienting a child and the child's family to stuttering and to how the clinician expects treatment to proceed. Indeed, such orientation may be the main benefit that the child and family receive from a diagnostic session. More often than is appropriate, speech-language pathologists do not take full advantage of this opportunity for orientation. Much too often a child and family begin treatment essentially clueless about the breadth and depth of the child's problem, what treatment will be about, and why.

Maneuver According to Circumstances

When reading some of the literature on stuttering, I sometimes get the impression that assessment of childhood stuttering is viewed as a puzzle within a riddle surrounded by an enigma. And while much about this problem is not well understood, much progress in understanding childhood stuttering has been made and in how to assess and treat it. While efforts to advance understanding of childhood stuttering must continue, this childhood communication disorder can be appropriately assessed and effectively treated, particularly if clinicians blend their empirically derived clinical procedures with findings from both basic and applied research studies of children who stutter.

Facts can be pesky things, and oftentimes cannot be scoured away, regardless of the strength of one's theoretical cleanser. Only if clinicians maneuver in response to the circumstances or the facts presented by a child, which may not be those that have been taught or that are expected, is it likely, in the long haul, that they will be able to assess and treat the child effectively. Paradoxically, only by adjusting assessment procedures to account for the "real circumstances" of children are speech-language pathologists likely to increase their chances of developing more ideal means for assessing childhood stuttering and its risks for continuation.

REFERENCES

Adams, M.R. (1977). A clinical strategy for differentiating the normally nonfluent child and the incipient stutterer. *Journal of Fluency Disorders, 2,* 141–148.

Adams, M.R. (1980). The young stutterer: Diagnosis, treatment and assessment of progress. *Seminars in Speech, Language, and Hearing, 1,* 289–299.

Adams, M.R. (1991). The assessment and treatment of the school-age stutterer. In W. Perkins (Ed.), *Seminars in Speech and Language, 12,* 279–290.

Ainsworth, S., & Fraser, J. (Eds.). (1988). *If your child stutters: A guide for parents* (3rd Ed.). Memphis, TN: Stuttering Foundation of America.

Bahill, A.T., & Curlee, R.F. (1993). *User's guide to childhood stuttering: A second opinion.* Tucson, AZ: Bahill Intelligent Computer Systems.

Conture, E.G. (1990a). *Stuttering* (2nd Ed.). Englewood Cliffs, N.J.: Prentice-Hall.

Conture, E.G. (1990b). Childhood stuttering: What is it and who does it? In J.A. Cooper (Ed.), *Research needs in stuttering: Roadblocks and future directions. ASHA Reports, 18,* 2–18.

Conture, E.G. (Producer) (1994). *Stuttering and your child: A videotape for parents* [30-min videotape]. Memphis, TN: Stuttering Foundation of America.

Conture, E.G., & Caruso, A.J. (1987). Assessment and diagnosis of childhood disfluency. In L. Rustin, D. Rowley, & H. Purser (Eds.), *Progress in the treatment of fluency disorders* (pp. 57–82). London: Taylor & Francis.

Conture, E.G. & Fraser, J. (Eds.). (1989). *Stuttering and your child: Questions and answers.* Memphis, TN: Stuttering Foundation of America.

Conture, E.G., & Kelly, E.M. (1991). Young stutterers' nonspeech behaviors during stuttering. *Journal of Speech and Hearing Research, 34,* 1041–1056.

Conture, E.G., & Yaruss, J.S. (1993). *A handbook for childhood stuttering: A second opinion.* Tucson, AZ: Bahill Intelligent Computer Systems.

Conture, E.G., & Zebrowski, P. (1992). Can childhood speech disfluencies be mutuable to the influences of speech-language pathologists, but immutable to the influences of parents? *Journal of Fluency Disorders, 17,* 121–130.

Cooper, E. (1979). *Understanding stuttering: Information for parents.* Chicago, Ill.: National Easter Seal Society for Crippled Children and Adults.

Cordes, A.K., Ingham, R.J., Frank, P., & Ingham, J.C. (1992). Time-interval analysis of interjudge and intra judge agreement of stuttering event judgments. *Journal of Speech and Hearing Research, 35,* 483–494.

Costello, J.M. (1983). Current behavioral treatments for children. In D. Prins & R.J. Ingham (Eds.), *Treatment of stuttering in early childhood: Methods and issues.* San Diego: College-Hill Press.

Costello, J.M., & Ingham, R.J. (1984). Assessment strategies for stuttering. In R.F. Curlee & W.H. Perkins (Eds.), *Nature and treatment of stuttering: New directions.* San Diego: College-Hill Press.

Culatta, R., & Goldberg, S. (1995). *Stuttering therapy: An integrated approach to theory and practice.* Boston: Allyn & Bacon.

Fosnot, S.M. (1992). *Fluency development for young stutterers: Differential diagnosis and treatment.* Buffalo, N.Y.: EDUCOM Associates.

Gordon, P.A., & Luper, H.L. (1992). The early identification of beginning stuttering I: Protocols. *American Journal of Speech-Language Pathology, 1,* 43–53.

Gregory, H.H., & Hill, D. (1992). Differential evaluation, differential therapy for stuttering children. In R.F. Curlee (Ed.), *Stuttering and related disorders of fluency* (pp. 23–44). New York: Thieme Medical Publishers.

Hayhow, R. (1983). The assessment of stuttering and the evaluation of treatment. In P. Dalton (Ed.), *Approaches to the treatment of stuttering*. London: Croom Helm.

Hubbard, C.P., & Yairi, E. (1988). Clustering of disfluencies in the speech of stuttering and nonstuttering preschool children. *Journal of Speech and Hearing Research, 31*, 228–233.

Ingham, R.J. (1985). Assessment of stuttering in children. In J. Gruss (Ed.), *Stuttering therapy: Prevention and early intervention*. Memphis, Tenn.: Speech Foundation of America.

Johnson, W., & Associates. (1959). The onset of stuttering. Minneapolis: University of Minnesota Press.

Johnson, W., Darley, F., & Spriestersbach, D. (1963). *Diagnostic methods in speech pathology*. New York: Harper & Row.

Kelly, E.M., & Conture, E.G. (1992). Speaking rates, response time latencies, and interrupting behaviors of young stutters, nonstutterers and their mothers. *Journal of Speech and Hearing Research, 35*, 1256–1267.

LaSalle, L.R., & Conture, E.G. (1991). Eye contact between young stutterers and their mothers during stuttering. *Journal of Fluency Disorders, 16*, 173–199.

LaSalle, L.R., & Conture, E. (1995). Disfluency clusters of children who stutter: Relation of stutterings to self-repairs. *Journal of Speech and Hearing Research, 38*, 965–977.

Logan, K., & Conture, E. (1995). Length, grammatical complexity, and rate differences in stuttered and fluent conversational utterances of children who stutter. *Journal of Fluency Disorders, 20*, 35–61.

Peters, T.J., & Guitar, B.G. (1991). *Stuttering: An integrated approach to its nature and treatment*. Baltimore, Md.: Williams & Wilkins.

Pindzola, R.H. (1986). A description of some selected stuttering instruments. *Journal of Childhood Communication Disorders, 9*, 183–200.

Pindzola, R., Jenkins, M., & Lokken, K. (1989). Speaking rates of young children. *Language, Speech and Hearing Services in the Schools, 20*, 133–138.

Pindzola, R.H., & White, D. (1986). A protocol for differentiating the incipient stutterer. *Language, Speech, and Hearing Services in School, 17*, 2–15.

Postma, H., & Kolk, H. (1993). The covert repair hypothesis: Prearticulatory repair processes in normal and stuttered disfluencies. *Journal of Speech and Hearing Research, 36*, 472–487.

Riley, G. (1980). *Stuttering severity instrument for children and adults* (rev. ed.). Austin, Tex.: Pro-Ed.

Riley, G. (1981). *Stuttering prediction instrument for young children*. Austin, Tex.: Pro-Ed.

Schwartz, H.D., & Conture, E. (1988). Subgrouping young stutterers: Preliminary behavioral observations. *Journal of Speech and Hearing Research, 31*, 62–71.

Schwartz, H.D., Zebrowski, P.M., & Conture, E.G. (1990). Behaviors at the onset of stuttering. *Journal of Fluency Disorders, 15*, 77–86.

Stocker, B. (1976). *Stocker probe technique for the diagnosis and treatment of stuttering in young children*. Tulsa, Okla.: Modern Education.

Wall, M., & Myers, F. (1984). *Clinical Management of Childhood Stuttering*. Baltimore, Md.: University Park Press.

Wall, M., & Myers, F. (1995). *Clinical management of childhood stuttering* (2nd Ed.). Baltimore, Md.: University Park Press.

Williams, D.E. (1974). Evaluation. In C.W. Starkweather (Ed.), *Therapy for stutterers* (pp. 9–19). Memphis, Tenn.: Speech Foundation of America.

Yairi, E. (1993). Epidemiology and other considerations in treatment efficacy research with preschool-age children who stutter. *Journal of Fluency Disorders, 18*, 197–220.

Yairi, E., & Ambrose, N. (1992a). A longitudinal study of stuttering in children: A preliminary report. *Journal of Speech and Hearing Research, 35*, 755–760.

Yairi, E., & Ambrose, N. (1992b). Onset of stuttering in preschool children: Selected factors. *Journal of Speech and Hearing Research, 35*, 782–788.

Yairi, E., Ambrose, N., & Niermann, R. (1993). The early months of stuttering: A developmental study. *Journal of Speech and Hearing Research, 36*, 521–528.

Yairi, E., and Lewis, B. (1984). Disfluencies at the onset of stuttering. *Journal of Speech and Hearing Research, 27*, 154–159.

Yaruss, S., & Conture, E. (1993). F2 transitions during sound/syllable repetitions of children who stutter and predictions of stuttering chronicity. *Journal of Speech and Hearing Research, 36*, 883–896.

Yaruss, S., & Conture, E. (1995). Mother and child speaking rates and utterance lengths in adjacent fluent utterances: Preliminary observations. *Journal of Fluency Disorders, 20*, 257–278.

Yaruss, S., LaSalle, L., & Conture, E. (1996). One hundred children who stutter: Their initial diagnostic report. Manuscript in preparation.

Young, M.A. (1984). Identification of stuttering and stutterers. In R.F. Curlee & W.H. Perkins (Eds.), *Nature and treatment of stuttering: New directions.* San Diego: College-Hill Press.

Zebrowski, P.M. (1991). Duration of the speech disfluencies of beginning stutterers. *Journal of Speech and Hearing Research, 34,* 483–491.

Zebrowski, P. (1994). Stuttering. In J. Tombline, H. Morris, & D. Spriestersbach (Eds.), *Diagnosis in speech-language pathology* (pp. 215–245). San Diego: Singular Publishing Group, Inc.

Zebrowski, P.M., & Conture, E.G. (1989). Judgments of disfluency by mothers of stuttering and normally fluent children. *Journal of Speech and Hearing Research, 32,* 307–317.

SUGGESTED READINGS

Conture, E., & Yaruss, S. (1993). *A handbook for childhood stuttering: A second opinion.* Tucson, AZ: Bahill Intelligent Computer System. Conture and Yaruss provide a thorough overview of assessment of childhood stuttering, from parent interviewing to evaluation of the child in conjunction with *Childhood stuttering: A second opinion* (Bahill & Curlee, 1993).

Gordon, P., & Luper, H. (1992). The early identification of beginning stuttering I: Protocols. *American Journal of Speech-Language Pathology, 1,* 43–53. Gordon and Luper provide a helpful resource for clinicians who want to know about material typically used for assessment of childhood stuttering.

Pindzola, R., & White, D. (1986). A protocol for differentiating the incipient stutterer. *Language, Speech and Hearing Services in the Schools, 17,* 2–15. Pindzola and White present clearly organized guidelines for assessment of childhood stuttering, which nicely integrates pertinent theory, research findings and clinical practice.

Wall, M., & Myers, F. (1995). *Clinical management of childhood stuttering* (2nd Ed.). Baltimore, MD: University Park Press. Wall and Myers provide a well-motivated approach for assessing childhood stuttering (pp. 161–194), which includes various psycholinguistic, physiological, and psychosocial variables and their interrelationships. While all such variables cannot be measured, presently, in the manner or to the degree desired, a strong case is presented for considering and measuring the variables discussed.

CHAPTER 13

THERAPY FOR YOUNGER CHILDREN

C. WOODRUFF STARKWEATHER

INTRODUCTION

The past ten years have seen a revolution in the treatment of young children who stutter or are at risk for stuttering. The prevailing attitude in previous years was to wait and see. The odds seemed to be that the child would outgrow the problem. That may or may not be true. Ingham's (1984) review of the "spontaneous recovery" literature suggested that the odds may not really favor spontaneous recovery and were, at best, even. Yairi, in this volume, has presented evidence supporting the other view.[1] In any event, a re-examination of the logic behind waiting (Starkweather, Gottwald, & Halfond, 1990) makes it evident that, although waiting might work well for those children who were going to recover anyway, waiting too long left those who would not recover spontaneously with the burden of chronic stuttering. Finally, a re-examination of the efficacy of fluency-shaping programs made it evident that adult stutterers have rather meager therapy choices—a substantial probability of relapse (Boberg & Kully, 1984), speech that could be free of stuttering only at the cost of extraordinary vigilance over a very long period of time (Peters & Guitar, 1991), and a decrease in both speech melody and speech rate (Franken, Peters, & Tettero, 1989). On the other hand, most young children who successfully completed early intervention or prevention programs have natural sounding speech, no need to be vigilant, and only a remote possibility of relapse (Gregory & Hill, 1984; Starkweather, Gottwald, & Halfond, 1990).

Through the increased use of early intervention strategies with very young children, clinicians also discovered that the young child was much easier to change than an adult (Starkweather & Gottwald, 1993).[2] Most children under 5 still spend most of their time with parents who are fully invested in, and able to exert substantial control over, their children's environment. The possibility of environmental manipulation is considerably reduced once the child enters school.

The treatments developed for preschool children are both efficient and effective, with essentially complete remission of symptoms, no side effects (e.g., slow rate, monotone voice), and little relapse in about 95 percent of cases. The duration of treatment is short compared to that for adults—8 weeks to a

---

[1] There is some question whether the recoveries described in this study were spontaneous, since the parents of the children were apparently counseled. In my experience, parent counseling alone can account for complete recovery in approximately 20 percent of cases.

[2] Although amply attested to with regard to stuttering by thousands of clinical trials, the tendency of infants and young children to be more strongly influenced than adults by a rich panorama of environmental events is confirmed by a number of important studies in epigenesis (Brauth, Hall, & Dooling, 1991; Kagan, 1991; Kagan & Moss, 1962; Rathburn, DiVirgilio, & Waldfogel, 1958; Waddington, 1960, 1962). These studies led Jerome Kagan to conclude "There is therefore a great deal of plasticity in development with respect to behavior" (Kagan, 1991, p. 13). Children are far more changeable than adults. Similarly, with regard to emotional factors "most of the longitudinal studies are in general agreement that until 5 or 6 years of age, it is very difficult to find preservation of individual differences in the child" (Kagan, 1991, p. 13).

year (Gregory & Hill, 1984; Starkweather & Gott-wald, 1993; Starkweather, Gottwald, & Halfond, 1990), depending on the intensity of treatment. With effective and efficient treatment available, the limited efficacy of adult treatment, and the proportion of spontaneous recovery smaller than previously believed, it seems foolish to wait and see.

NORMAL FLUENCY

It is useful to understand the nature of normal fluency, as a behavior, before undertaking to modify abnormal fluency. One needs to know what to aim for. In a general sense, the word "fluency" suggests easy and smooth movement, but with regard to stuttering, "fluency" has in the past been used to mean the absence of stuttering, but this seems wrong. Starkweather (1987) argued that fluency is more than the absence of stuttering; it is a set of speech production skills defined by specific variables. Both the continuity (smoothness) and the rate of speech contribute to a speaker's overall fluency.

When discussing stuttering, the word "fluency" is not used in its linguistic sense, where it refers to easy sentence formulation, word finding, word pronunciation, and pragmatic skill. People who stutter have the same knowledge and use of syntax, semantics, phonology, and pragmatics as people whose fluency is normal. Although there is evidence that stuttering children, as a group, are slightly delayed in their language development (Kline & Starkweather, 1979), individual case histories make it clear that some stuttering children are advanced in language development (Amster, 1989), so it seems unlikely that stuttering is related to language development in any universal way. There are, nevertheless, individual cases in which stuttering development seems clearly related to aspects of language development, such as awkward or hesitant sentence formulation, slow word finding, or phonological processes that are delayed or deviant (Louko, Edwards, & Conture, 1990). Furthermore, a subgroup of young stuttering children develop stuttering along with, and apparently because of, unusually precocious language development (Amster, 1989).

Speech fluency, as contrasted with language fluency, refers to the consistent ability to move the structures of the vocal tract easily, rapidly, smoothly, and with appropriate timing relative to other vocal tract activities. The words *easily* and *consistently* are key to this definition. People who stutter can, and on most occasions do, move the vocal tract quickly, smoothly, and with appropriate timing. But at certain times they can do so only with the use of extraordinary physical or mental effort. To distinguish stuttering behavior from normal nonfluency, we need to look at the amount of effort the person uses, as shown by (1) the frequency of breaks in the continuity of speech; (2) the relative frequency of extraneous behaviors, such as syllable repetitions, sound prolongations, hesitations, broken words, tense pauses; (3) the duration of these discontinuities; (4) the inability to achieve a normal rate of speech; and (5) the presence of extraneous compensatory, avoidance, or defensive behavior, not usually found in the speech of nonstutterers. When extraneous behaviors (including thoughts, feelings, beliefs, and perceptions) occur too frequently, last too long, or are abnormal in type, the presence of stuttering can be inferred.

Time plays a central role in these definitions. All behavior is bound by time, and for behavior to be considered "extraneous," there must be too much of it during a certain amount of time. And, when speech time is the issue, it can be measured in terms of words or syllables as well as seconds and milliseconds. The two sets of measures are closely related. This means that when people who stutter slow down their speech, they are not really engaging in extraneous behavior; they are, instead, stretching the time constraint so that whatever behaviors they are performing become less extraneous. In simpler terms, they are giving themselves the time they need to say what they want.

I see little virtue in making loss of control (or involuntariness) central to a definition of stuttering. Nonstutterers, when they lose speech continuity, are also out of control and usually produce behavior that is extraneous to their intention. Normal nonfluency is no more voluntary than stuttering disfluencies. The primary difference is in the duration of the behavior. So loss of control fails the crucial definitional test—it doesn't separate the normal from the abnormal. This is not to say that people who stutter don't feel out of control. Of course they do. And because this helpless state lasts longer for stutterers, they are more likely to find it uncomfortable, even excruciating, than nonstutterers do during normal nonfluency.

The Continuity of Speech

The continuity of speech refers to the smoothness and efficiency with which information is produced. It is important to recognize that the flow of information can be broken by the interposition of extraneous phrases even though speech is continuous. For example, a person who says, "I went to the, I mean the, I mean the, I want to say the, I mean I went to the, perhaps I want to say I went to the zoo" produces a smooth flow of words, but there is information only in the last five words. The rest is extraneous.

Another way to separate extraneous from nonextraneous production is to infer the intended utterance. Levelt (1989) has shown that native speakers are capable of reliably identifying the intended sentence from a speaker's production, in spite of errors, slips of the tongue, interposed extraneous elements, grammatical mistakes, and so on. This ability can be used to separate the parts of a speaker's sentence that are intended from those that are extraneous to intention. Such a separation enables the clinician to identify reliably the parts of an utterance that break the continuity of information flow, so that they can be categorized, counted, and measured.

Recent writings have stressed the difficulty of reliably identifying, categorizing, and measuring stuttering behaviors (Young, 1984; Cordes & Ingham, 1994), but these difficulties stem from two unnecessary practices. The first is the attempt to count stuttering behaviors on line, as they occur. It would be wonderfully useful if we could do this, but few clinicians try it. A tape recorded sample, which permits repeated listening, will remain the object of analysis for some time. The second is the attempt to

distinguish normal nonfluencies from stuttering. This, too, seems an unnecessary clinical practice. Stutterers may well have normal nonfluency in addition to their stuttering, but if the clinician simply tries to measure the level of fluency, instead of the level of stuttering, the differentiation of normal from abnormal discontinuity ceases to be a measurement problem. Since an improvement in the level of fluency is what treatment is designed to accomplish, the evaluation of therapy effectiveness can be reliably made. So, by (1) not trying to identify and count stuttering on line, and (2) measuring the occurrence of behaviors that are extraneous to the intended utterance, reliable and useful clinical measures are possible (Starkweather, 1993).

Types of Discontinuities

Normal speakers pause and hesitate, sometimes filling the pauses with "um," "uh," or other sounds to signal to listeners that they wish to retain their conversational turn. Normal adult speech is peppered with these pauses (Goldman-Eisler, 1961). Filled pauses appear in children's speech beginning around 4 to 5 years of age. Before that, children most often simply repeat the word they are in the process of saying until the next part of the utterance is ready to be produced. In most cases, this does not take long, so repetitions in normal preschool children are seldom longer than two units, like, like, like this. Consequently, whole-word and whole-syllable repetitions are a somewhat younger type of discontinuity. Prolongations also occur in the speech of normal children, although, like repetitions, they tend to be rather brief.

The Rate of Speech

The rate of speech is also an aspect of fluency. Speakers, both normal and abnormal, can speak with markedly reduced pauses and hesitations or other forms of discontinuity when they slow their rate of speech. Furthermore, the speaker who is able to produce long strings of syllables at a rapid rate, without showing an increase in the number of discontinuities, is recognized as an extraordinari-

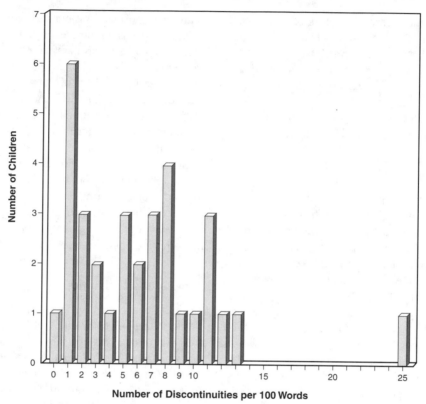

Figure 13.1   Speech continuity in 2-year-old children.

ly fluent speaker. So rate and continuity seem to be two sides of the same coin. There is a trading relation between them such that the faster the rate, the more likely it is that the speaker will be discontinuous, and vice versa.

In young children, rate of speech increases from the slow, overarticulated speech of the 2-year-old to the rapid, coarticulated speech of the 6-year-old (Amster, 1984). In assessing the fluency of children at risk for stuttering, both speech rate—with behaviors extraneous to the intended utterance included—and articulatory rate—where only the intended utterance is included—are collected.

STUTTERING DEVELOPMENT

Stuttering is a disorder that changes over time, both for the better and for the worse. These changes can be rapid or slow, and sometimes there are periods when it seems not to be changing. In addition, changes in stuttering take place against a

background of other dynamic events—the child's motoric, linguistic, emotional, and cognitive development, and changes in the family. Both the child's development and the family's development are influenced by the presence of stuttering (or any other problem), and in return, changes that occur in the child and family also influence the development of the disorder. With all these changes occurring simultaneously, it can be difficult to understand what is going on. Nevertheless, there is great potential for change in development, and the successful management of stuttering in a young child often depends on an accurate assessment of these forces and the implementation of strategies that make them work for improved fluency.

Precursors to Stuttering

Yairi (1981) examined the fluency of normally speaking 2-year-olds. Figure 13.1 shows these data. It is evident that a third of these children, those

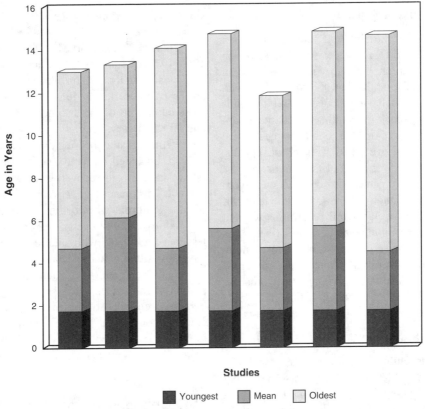

Figure 13.2 Seven studies of stuttering onset.

showing 0–3 disfluent words per 100 words, are speaking almost as fluently as adults. A middle third, showing 4–9 disfluencies per 100 words, are slightly more disfluent than adults. Only the upper third, showing more than 10 percent disfluent words, are clearly more disfluent than adults. It is this upper third that may be at risk for the development of stuttering. Levels above 3 percent are sufficient to worry parents (Starkweather, Gottwald, & Halfond, 1990), and parental concern is important for two reasons. Parents know their children well and have a keen appreciation for how they differ from their peers. Also, concern over fluency that parents feel may, in some cases, cause the parents to react and behave in ways that make it more difficult for the child to develop normal fluency. For example, many concerned parents react nonverbally when the child's speech is disfluent (Conture & Kelly, 1988), showing fear, anger, worry, humiliation, or disgust on their faces. Young children are at-

tentive to nonverbal behavior and consequently may learn that stuttering is something to be afraid of, angry about, ashamed of, and so on. Therefore, clinicians need to assess parental concern and reactions to see if the child may be learning that stuttering is frightening, awful, or shameful.

AGE AT ONSET

Figure 13.2 shows the results of seven studies of stuttering onset. It is evident that stuttering typically begins during the preschool (2–5) years, a finding confirmed by Andrews and Harris (1964). It is worth noting that the youngest child in each of the seven studies was under 2 years old; thus, fully developed stuttering can and does occur in very young children. Also, it should be noted that the oldest children in these studies were 10 to 12, and although onset at these ages is relatively rare (Andrews & Harris, 1964), it does happen.

Characteristics of Stuttering in Children

Variability. The variability of stuttering has been well documented (Wieneke & Janssen, 1987). In very young children, variability may be somewhat less than that for adults, but it is still substantial. When defensive behavior is present, and it often is in young children, it is childlike in character, appearing as reticence or occasionally as mechanical forcing of words, eye blinking, head movements, trying to pull the words out of the mouth with the fingers, or squeezing the cheek to push a stuck word out. It is also common for young children to exhibit many whole- or part-word repetitions without struggle. There is, in fact, a full range of behaviors shown by stuttering children, from the most benign, multiple, whole-word repetitions with little or no struggle to advanced stuttering with avoidance, struggle, and secondary characteristics.

Changes in Stuttering Behavior with Time

As stuttering children continue to cope with it, there is a general tendency for the disorder to become more severe with the addition of coping behaviors, avoidance behaviors, and struggle (defensive behavior). In addition, there is a tendency, by no means universal, for stuttering to become more frequent. When there is increased struggling, the time occupied by stuttering will increase relative to the total amount of time spent talking. The developmental course of the disorder seems almost independent of the child's age; there are very young children with advanced symptoms and a few 5- or 6-year-olds who still do not struggle at all. Figure 13.3 lists common tendencies for changes in stuttering that occur over time.

One of the striking features of early stuttering is its tendency to come and go (Bloodstein, 1960). This episodic nature of the disorder is quite frustrating for both parents and clinicians. It tends to create in parents periods of panic that alternate with periods of relief, and for clinicians, a welter of cancelled appointments. There are also changes in the distribution of stuttering. Younger children are more likely to stutter with equal severity in all situations, and as much on some words as on others (Bloodstein, 1960).

There are two studies (Sheehan & Martyn, 1966, 1970) that suggest a very high spontaneous recovery rate, but the data on which these conclusions are based are seriously flawed by poor sampling, loose definitions of the disorder, of "spontaneous," and of "recovery." Ingham (1984) carefully reviewed the literature bearing on spontaneous recovery and concluded, correctly I believe, that the actual rate of spontaneous recovery is between 30 and 50 percent. This means that between 50 and 70 percent of the children who begin stuttering in their preschool years will become chronic stutterers unless they are treated with an effective management program. Although these data seem a sufficient reason to intervene with very young children, it is important to remember that a significant minority— perhaps even half—of the children treated will recover without treatment, so it behooves the clinician to make the treatment of these children as efficient as possible.

1. Changes in type
   a. more fragmented
   b. faster repetitions
   c. more struggle/tension

2. Changes in severity
   a. more frequent
   b. longer durations

3. Changes in the distribution of stuttering
   a. becomes situation, word, and listener dependent
   b. becomes chronic

4. Spontaneous recovery in 50%

Figure 13.3 Changes in stuttering with time.

Finally, there is some evidence—not conclusive, but compelling—that there is a critical period for the persistence of stuttering. In the well-known longitudinal study of Andrews and Harris (1964), 93 percent of those children whose stuttering persisted beyond one year were stuttering during the 5 1/2 to 6 1/2 age range. Only 7 percent of those whose stuttering did not occur during this period were persistent.

A word needs to be said about pediatricians. Although there has been a noticeable increase in referrals to speech clinicians from pediatricians, perhaps as a result of the efforts of the Stuttering Foundation of American to educate this important group of health care providers, it is still common for pediatricians to advise the parents of very young stutterers to "wait and see." When such advice carries the authority of a pediatrician, it is often followed, at least for a while, until the parents realize that the pediatrician must have been wrong and seek the advice of a speech-language pathologist. The difficulty is that the child usually becomes more severe during this time and the disorder more complex, making recovery, although still possible to achieve, a longer project than it need have been (Starkweather & Gottwald, 1993).

The Speech of Adults to Stuttering Children

Figure 13.4 shows the speech characteristics of adults when speaking to children who stutter. Meyers & Freeman, 1985a,b) compared the speech of adults talking to children who stuttered (not their own) with that of adults talking to children who did not stutter. They found that (1) adults talk faster to stuttering children than to nonstuttering children of the same age and (2) adults are likely to interrupt children who stutter more often than they do children who don't. Hutt (1987) compared the speech of mothers talking to sons with that of mothers talking to daughters, all of whom were normal speakers. She found that these mothers talked faster to boys than to girls of exactly the same age. Together, these studies suggest that how parents

talk to their children may be influenced by the presence of stuttering and by the child's gender. The speech rate of parents is a variable that influences time pressure on the child, as are interruptions. Amster (1989) has shown that a highly verbal environment, where there is a low tolerance for silence, seems conducive to the development of stuttering. It seems evident that assessment of aspects of the child's communicative environment can increase a clinician's understanding of stuttering in a particular child.

THE DEMANDS AND CAPACITIES MODEL

The Demands and Capacities Model (DCM) is a useful tool for understanding and harnessing the dynamics of child and family development. The DCM is not a theory of stuttering. It says little or nothing about the cause of stuttering. What it does do is organize the research literature in a way that helps clinicians understand what forces influence the development of fluency in children, and with this knowledge, consider the development of stut-

---

Faster speech rate than to nonstuttering children

More interruptions than to nonstuttering children

Speech rate is faster to boys than to girls

Some parents talk excessively to their child

Some parents show negative nonverbal reactions

Figure 13.4 Parents' speech to their children who stutter.

tering in a particular child. In short, it helps clinicians plan therapy. There are at least four areas of development that seem related to fluency—speech motor control, language development, social and emotional functioning, and cognitive development. It is possible that future research will identify other areas, but at the moment, these are the areas in which research findings show a connection to fluency development.

Speech Motor Control

It seems evident that people who stutter cannot move the structures of the vocal tract as quickly, or time such movements as accurately, as do people who are normal speakers (Starkweather & Myers, 1979; Zimmermann, 1980). These data, however, were taken from adults, so it is possible that the differences observed are a result of stuttering, rather than a cause, or being related to the cause. Similarly, a rather robust finding in the literature is that stutterers do not react to an external stimulus as quickly as nonstutterers do (Adams & Hayden, 1976; Starkweather, Hirschman, & Tannenbaum, 1976), but here too most of the data have been gathered on adults. What evidence there is for children (Cross & Luper, 1979) suggests that the reaction-time differences in children are larger than those in adults, although this may reflect the presence of concomitant disorders. It is not clear, however, what role rapid reactions to external stimuli play in speech production, if any, nor is it clear how reaction time is related to speech production skill. Slowed movement is a natural consequence of having a speech mechanism that is stiffened by extraneous muscle activity, and it is uncertain whether the differences that have been observed between stutterers and nonstutterers in reaction time are related to a cause of the disorder or are themselves a result of the disorder.

It seems evident, too, that adult stutterers are not as able as adult nonstutterers to coordinate the movements of the larynx (Freeman & Ushijima, 1978), mouth (De Nil & Brutten, 1988; Shapiro, 1980) and respiratory apparatus (Peters & Boves, 1987). In addition, van Lieshout et al. (van Lieshout, Peters, Starkweather, & Hulstijn, 1993) found that stutterers had higher levels and longer durations of elevated muscle activity than did nonstutterers in a simple lip-rounding gesture used to initiate a sentence. Figure 13.5 shows the results of this study. Producing movements of speech with a vocal apparatus that is stiffened by extraneous muscle activity could result in movements that are slow and tremulous. One of the more interesting aspects of van Lieshout's results is that the elevated extraneous muscle activity among stutterers did not subside immediately after the gesture was made. This suggests that stutterers have not only elevated muscle activity, but that this extraneous activity is also slow to return to normal levels after the gesture is completed. This finding is consistent with those of another study in which muscles that are not part of the vocal tract were examined. Barrett and Stoeckel (1979) showed that stutterers were less able than were matched peers to inhibit movements of the contralateral eye during a winking task. The ability to move speech structures rapidly, smoothly, and without extraneous muscle activity appears to be a skill that underlies fluent speech, and one of the capacities for fluency is smooth, rapid movement of the speech mechanism.

Language Development

A number of studies have shown that, on the whole, children who stutter are somewhat slower in their language development than are children whose fluency is normal (Andrews, Craig, Feyer, Hoddinott, Howie, & Neilson, 1983; Kline & Starkweather, 1979). At the same time, there is compelling clinical evidence that some stuttering children have advanced language development, which may be attributable to overstimulation of language by the child's parents (Amster, 1989). These apparently contradictory characteristics can be reconciled when a child's motor performance is considered. Children who are slow developing language may be urged on by their parents to perform, and in some cases sent for therapy to stimulate their development. There is some evidence that language stimulation therapy may be respon-

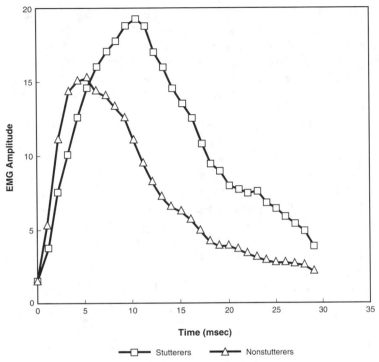

Figure 13.5 EMG level over time during a speech gesture.

sible for the development of stuttering in some children (Merits-Patterson & Reed, 1981), and it seems reasonable that parental efforts to accelerate slow language development could have the same effect. The advanced child, however, delights his or her parents with long, complex sentences, and seeks to recreate the delight. In both cases, the child may try to perform linguistically beyond his or her motor capacity, and difficulties with fluency may be the result. Language therapy that is based on under- rather than overstimulation does not seem to result in stuttering (Goorhuis-Brouwer, 1987; Personal communication, 1988).

Social and Emotional Functioning

Although the evidence seems clear that anxiety does not cause the disorder of stuttering (Peters & Hulstijn, 1984), it is equally evident that, given high levels of disfluency, the presence of anxiety or prolonged stress typically exacerbates the problem. As a result, children who are emotionally ma-

ture and socially comfortable in circumstances that tend to elicit anxiety in children (meeting strangers, separation from parents, performance situations, talking in front of a group) may have a capacity that makes it easier for them to talk more fluently. In contrast, the child who is easily frightened, has relatively more of the common fears of children, or is socially insecure, can be expected to have less fluency under the same anxiety-producing circumstances. Clinically, I have found it useful to ask parents to choose a word that best describes their child's personality. A high proportion respond that their child is nervous, high strung, anxious, fearful, clingy, or tense.

Cognitive Development

The relation of cognition to fluency is not clear. There is no evidence of a relationship between general intelligence and stuttering, except the weak one reported by Andrews, Craig, Feyer, Hoddinott, Howie, & Neilson (1983). This relation can be explained by the reliance of such testing on speech. This is true, although to a lesser extent, even for nonverbal tests, since subvocal speech plays a role in reasoning. It may also be partly explained by the increased prevalence of stuttering among the retarded (Gens, 1951; Gottesleben, 1955). In spite of the lack of evidence for some sort of relationship between general intelligence and stuttering, it seems likely that children whose cognitive development is further along have a better tool with which to deal with the problems that disfluency (normal or abnormal) presents. Those whose cognitive development includes the metalinguistic ability to think about speech as a process will probably find it easier than less cognitively mature children to consider the consequences of various reactions to disfluency and so may be able to avoid the trap of struggle and forcing.

Environmental Demands on Fluency

Many events in a child's communicative environment can challenge the fluent (easy) use of the speech mechanism. The various demands can be categorized most usefully in terms of the demands placed on a child's capacities for fluency.

Demands on Motor Skills. Possibly the most pervasively challenging environmental demand on speech is time pressure. Whenever circumstances suggest that there is less time in which to say something, there is a corresponding pressure to talk more rapidly, and this makes stuttering behaviors more likely and more severe. Time pressure can be gross or fine. Gross time pressure comes from such circumstances as a family getting ready to leave for school and work in the morning. There is a lot to do and a schedule to meet, and everyone feels the need to do things quickly, including talking. Other gross time pressure situations include ordering in a fast food restaurant when there are people waiting behind you, talking to people who talk rapidly, or when there is a specific time limit on talking or a charge for talking per unit of time, as on a long distance call.

Fine time pressure situations involve much smaller units of time but have more negative consequences. An example is introducing yourself. It takes very little hesitation to look as if you have forgotten your own name. A hesitation of less than half a second in saying one's name can be embarrassing. Answering the telephone is another fine time pressure situation. A half second delay in saying hello can lead to the caller repeating "Hello? Hello?" or wondering whether to hang up. Similar situations are saying other familiar items of information, such as your own phone number, address, or answering questions with obvious answers. Children seem to respond much more to gross time pressure than to fine time pressure.

It is possible, although hardly well established, that certain combinations of movements or certain conditions of speaking also increase demands on the motor system. Starkweather et al. (Starkweather, van Lieshout, Hulstijn, & Peters, 1989) and van Lieshout and colleagues (van Lieshout, Starkweather, Hulstijn, & Peters, 1995) found that words positioned early in a sentence, longer words, words in longer sentences, and words conveying higher loads of information required adjustments in the rate and timing of speech production in nonstuttering speakers. These additional demands on coordination—the momentary decreases or increases in the velocity of movement and the adjustments in relative timing of different parts of the speech mechanism—may play a role in the tendency for stuttering to occur at clause boundaries, on longer rather than shorter words, on longer sentences, and on words that carry more information. In addition, it has been known for some time that longer sentences are produced more rapidly than shorter ones (Amster, 1984; Malecot, Johnston, & Kizziar, 1972), which also increases motor demands.

There are also learned reactions as a consequence of stuttering on specific sounds and words, in certain situations, and when talking to certain listeners. Such experientially based reactions can trigger more stuttering. Children clearly have fewer of these reactions than adults, although it is not unusual for even very young children to stutter more in front of some listeners than others and on certain sounds.

Demands on Language Production (Performance) Skills.

As children develop from age 2 through 5 years, their linguistic knowledge increases dramatically, and with this increase in competence comes a corresponding increase in performance. Language development often occurs in spurts, and it is not unusual for the child at risk for stuttering to show dramatic reductions in fluency shortly after spurts of language development. Wexler and Mysak (1982) found that shortly after a new linguistic form was acquired, the probability that it would be produced disfluently increased. Whether additional complexity of sentences makes it harder for a child to formulate such sentences or whether there is an indirect demand on the motor system (i.e., complex sentences are almost always longer in this age group and, therefore, are produced more rapidly) is difficult to know. Possibly both linguistic and motoric demands are increased by spurts of language development.

Increases in vocabulary have a similar effect. As a child knows more words and uses them, a larger lexicon is created from which each word has to be chosen. In addition, recently learned words tend, on the whole, to be longer. This means that semantic development, like syntactic development, places increased demands, both on the language act of word-finding and on the motor acts required to produce new words.

In pragmatics, also, the child's increased awareness of when to use specific forms increases the number of decisions that have to be made when talking in any given situation, and this may create hesitancy or uncertainty, and consequently a greater probability of disfluency. In addition, as children become pragmatically more adept, their parents are more likely to allow them the freedom to enter more complex communication situations.

It is also plausible that increased phonological knowledge may increase demands on the speech production process. The child who is aware of phonological errors is more likely to hesitate before producing a combination that is new and less familiar, or perhaps more difficult. Similarly, the child with a history of difficulty in producing specific sounds or sound combinations is likely to approach them more tentatively perhaps even with some apprehension, which increases the challenge to produce those words fluently.

There are several ways in which children's home and (play)school environment may make it more difficult for them to produce fluent speech by increasing speech and language production demands. First, when children who are advanced in their speech development produce forms that are more adult than is expected for their age, parents typically react with considerable pleasure. Thoughts of Harvard begin to dance in their heads, and this delight in their child's performance is likely to be translated into parental reactions, both verbal and nonverbal, that reinforce the child for these more adult productions. Children at this age are quick to read nonverbal behavior—not so long ago they were nonverbal themselves—and they want to please their parents. So there is a natural tendency for parents' reactions like this to have the effect of increasing children's language performance. This is probably a pleasant circumstance and harmless in most families, but if the child is at risk for stuttering, whether by virtue of a slowly (perhaps even normally) developing motor system or by genetic predisposition, then advanced language production skills may challenge the child's more slowly developing motor skills in a way that results in increased disfluency.

Second, if a child's language or phonological development is delayed, attempts to stimulate the child or correct errors may result in the child's forcing or struggling to produce "correct" speech. Thus, attempts to improve the child's performance, whether in syntactic or phonological areas, may lead to struggle and forcing.

Demands on Social/Emotional Skills.

When children are thrust before an audience and asked to perform, most react with anxiety and perhaps anger. Similarly, if they are asked to act as go-betweens in marital disputes, to translate for non-English-speaking parents, to say specific politeness markers on demand from parents, or to talk in any emotionally charged situation, they find it more difficult, as do many adults, to speak fluently. The circumstances may differ for children, but the effects of talking in emotionally charged circumstances are similar.[3]

The fluency of children's speech is also powerfully influenced by high levels of positive feeling, such as excitement or happiness, which is strikingly illustrated by the following anecdote. A 4-year-old girl was left with a sitter for two weeks while her parents went on their first vacation without her. Although they called frequently while they were away and spoke with their daughter, and although she was fluent during these calls, she blocked severely the first time she re-encountered them on their return. She continued to block after this event for a number of weeks. It seemed as though the intensity of her happiness at seeing her parents, and perhaps the suddenness with which its intensity increased, was responsible for her sudden inability to move her speech apparatus easily.

The kinds of events that elicit high levels of anxiety and excitement in children are, of course, different than those for adults. Moving into a new house, going to a new school, playschool, or camp, visits by grandparents, birthday parties, holidays, illness of a relative, death of a relative, separation from a relative, and the return of a relative after separation are among the experiences that seem to disrupt a child's fluency.

Demands on Cognitive Skills.   All speaking places some demand on cognition, but some types of speaking are more demanding than others. Perhaps the most common cognitively demanding speech situation begins when parents say, "Tell me what you did in playschool today." This request calls for the child to remember a large number of

events, select from them the ones to recount, sequence them, adopt a narrative mode, and then produce enough detail to satisfy the parent. Another common circumstance arises when parents are teaching their children. Although teaching is a legitimate, important aspect of parenting, some parents seem to teach excessively. One parent I knew, an art teacher, conducted continuous lessons with his son about the color, texture, composition, and form of nearly everything that attracted their attention. The child was continuously on edge whenever they were together, trying to make sure that he could see and think correctly about all of these aspects. As soon as the father began to interact in a less instructional way with his son, the boy's disfluencies returned to normal. The real issue in this case was not that the parent was teaching the child, but that he did so at the expense of other types of interactions. As a result, the father became a stimulus that elicited the child's apprehension.

Using the Demands and Capacities Model in Assessment

The DCM provides useful guidelines for understanding what specific skills a child may lack for producing fluent speech and for understanding what aspects of the child's environment may be challenging those skills. Consequently, evaluations of preschool children with fluency difficulties should assess their motor, language, cognitive, and emotional development as well as the demands placed on them by their communicative environment. Environmental assessment is the key to successful management of preschool children.

At a minimum, environmental assessment should gather information about the differences between parent and child in speech rate, total talking time, speech continuity, grammatical complexity, and vocabulary. In addition, at least informal assessments should be made of the child's phonological, syntactic, pragmatic, emotional, and cognitive development. Of course, screening assessments of vocal function and hearing are also routinely made with this population.

---

[3]This topic is considerably more complex and requires a discussion beyond what current space permits. Bloodstein (1987) notes that many adults report being made more fluent by highly emotional circumstances, and it seems likely, if not clear, that many adults are not strongly affected by them, although many are. When one looks at children, the tendency for emotion (anxiety and excitement) to precipitate or exacerbate stuttering seems stronger. This is an area where more research would be very useful.

Testing Hypotheses.   Because a fair proportion, as many as half, of these children are likely to recover without intervention, the clinician is responsible for making treatment as efficient as possible. One way of doing this is to test the effectiveness of a procedure before implementing it. If a large difference between the parents' and child's speech rates suggests that a reduction in parental rate might increase fluency, this hypothesis can be tested in the first or second session by observing the effects of altering the clinician's (or if possible the parents') rate of speech. If the child becomes notably more fluent under these conditions, then speech rate reduction in the home environment over a longer period of time is justified.

Often, when a hypothesis about rate, questions, interruptions, or the like, is tested, immediate results may be negative. Clinicians need to be aware that the absence of a noticeable effect during hypothesis testing is not convincing evidence that such an effect will not occur in time. Positive effects (a reduction in the child's disfluency following a change in rate), are a clear go-ahead to use a method in treatment, but negative results (no change in the child's fluency level following a change in the clinician's or parent's rate in the clinic) are not sufficient evidence for abandoning it. Nevertheless, if its continued use does not produce the desired result, it should be abandoned in favor of methods that are found to be effective. In preschool children who have been stuttering for no longer than a year, environmental changes—if they are the right environmental changes—can be expected to produce results within a few days or weeks.

TYPES OF STUTTERING DEVELOPMENT

There are a number of ways in which stuttering can develop. After a review of some 100 cases, there appear to be certain specific "tracks of development," just as Van Riper (1973) suggested. Van Riper identified four tracks, but my clinical experience suggests that there may be more.

Garden Variety

The track that is most common is still the most puzzling. These are children who appear to be normal in every other respect and whose environments do not seem to be particularly stressful. Nevertheless, they often do not produce speech in a smooth way. Typically, these children begin showing speech that is excessively repetitious between ages 2 and 5 years, and this repetitious speech places them in an "at risk" category. Their repetitions are usually of whole words or whole syllables, as the child lets the word or syllable run its course, without attempting to shorten it. Clinicians can identify this type of repetition by listening carefully for the closing of the syllable. To be "excessive" the child must produce at least 3 percent of words with at least three units of repetition. Three units of whole-word repetition sound like, like, like, like this—that is, there are three additional words.

Another criterion is the parents' concern. If parents are worried about a child's fluency, then the family should be seen, at least for counseling, because (1) the parents are much more familiar with the child than a clinician can ever hope to be, and (2) the presence of parental concern may result in verbal or nonverbal reactions to the occurrence of disfluency that can convey to the child that there is something quite wrong with his or her speech. This, in turn, can lead to the child's beginning to struggle and force out words. Once a child is struggling to talk, it is clear that stuttering is no longer simply a risk, but is, in fact, present.

Slowly Developing Speech Motor Skills

A second track is characterized by speech motor skills that seem immature. Such children may drool, stick their tongues out when drawing or lettering, talk quite slowly, or articulate with immature precision. Sometimes, but not always, their gross motor abilities are also behind schedule. These children often present with a developmental phonological disorder, which raises a number of issues that clinicians will need to deal with, as Louko, Edwards, and Conture (1990) discussed.

Although these children have slowly developing speech motor skills, they have normal language skills. As a result, they formulate sentences that are of normal length and complexity for their age, but they cannot easily (i.e., fluently) say these sentences. Possibly also, such children, or their parents, have come to react to these slow labored speech productions as being too slow. In any event, children in this track try to talk more rapidly, which results in an infusion of muscular tension into the speech mechanism during speech attempts. Such surges of tension are likely to occur most commonly on longer sentences, which require a more formidable motor plan that is executed more quickly (Amster, 1984).

Rapidly Developing Language Skills

Another developmental track is needed for children whose language development is advanced. These children show remarkably advanced forms of language production at an early age and are motorically normal. As a result, these children appear to know how to produce sentences that are more complex and longer than their motor systems are capable of handling. Often these children are members of families in which speech and language are important and whose adult members talk a great deal. As a result, they have been called "language overstimulation" cases (Amster, 1989). Hearing so much speech, their language develops rapidly and seemingly outstrips their ability to coordinate the movements of the oral, vocal, and respiratory mechanisms. Like the child whose speech motor control development is slow, they have most difficulty on longer sentences, where complex motor planning needs to be executed at faster rates of speech.

Environmental Pressures

Most children in this track seem to be normal in both their motoric and linguistic development, but they have the misfortune to have been born into a difficult environment. There may be poverty, many siblings, marital discord, chaos in the home, a great deal of time pressure in the home, frequent relocations, a difficult or frequently changing playschool environment, or family illness. These conditions, and others, create stress in children. Most children seem to cope with stressors like this without stuttering, and the evidence suggests that anxiety is not so much a cause as an exacerbating influence on it. Nevertheless, such stressors in a child's life often seem to play a role in making stuttering develop more quickly into a more severe problem.

Although relatively rare, a few children who experience serious emotional trauma will begin stuttering shortly thereafter. As mentioned previously, a "traumatic" experience of intense happiness seems to be able to produce stuttering also. Our knowledge about psychogenic stuttering, in adults as well as in children, is largely anecdotal. There just aren't enough cases—and they seem quite different from each other—to be able to compile a general or average picture. In adults, psychogenic stuttering responds readily to treatment and is rarely a chronic problem. Since most preschool children respond readily to treatment, there is no apparent difference in outcome for this population.

Although it is highly unusual, some parents punish their children for stuttering. Perhaps they do this in desperation, led on by the memory of having used punishment with success for other problems. In my experience, they show relief when advised to stop, often having already seen that punishment makes stuttering worse rather than better. Punishment is known to suppress behavior in an indiscriminate way. The negative stimulation associated with it tends to produce a generalized inhibition against performing any behavior unless there is an alternative behavior readily available, and in the case of the child who stutters, parental punishment typically results in the child talking less, trying to hide the stuttering or hold it in so that it won't show. These reactions lead children to try talking without letting very much come out of their mouths, and to show generalized tension, often twitching of the whole body and small, tense movements that seem unrelated to speech, but are very abnormal in their appearance.

It should be noted that, in addition to punishment that is intentionally used by parents to try to control stuttering, punishment may also be inherent in some inadvertent nonverbal reactions to the child's disfluency. Parents who "can't stand to look at" a child who stutters, or who feel intensely ashamed when their child stutters in front of other people, or who are very afraid that the child will grow up with a serious speech handicap, are likely to show these feelings in their nonverbal behavior when the child stutters. These nonverbal reactions have a punitive effect on the child, who feels that he or she is causing the parents to be afraid, or ashamed, or pained. A common result is an increase in struggle and forcing behaviors, as well as a tendency to hide or suppress stuttering. But perhaps even more important, the child learns also to be afraid, hurt, or ashamed of stuttering. In real-life situations, stuttering is not an operant, in the nontautological sense[4]; it seems not to follow the law of effect in these circumstances, and, of course, it is obvious that it does not follow the law of least effort (see Chapter 4, this volume).

_____

[4]A behavior can be classified as an operant simply by demonstrating that it can be manipulated by its consequences, but this sense of the word is essentially tautological. When a variety of behaviors are examined, behaviors acquired by different learning processes and behaviors that are not learned at all but are physiologically based reflexive activity, it is clear that all behaviors are operants in this tautological sense (DiCara & Miller, 1968; Miller, 1969). So this sense of the word is relatively useless as a way to classify behavior, particularly for clinical purposes; it tells us nothing about the learning processes by which the behavior was acquired or the circumstances under which it is performed. The nontautological sense of the word has to do with the history of the behavior, the circumstances under which it is performed, and the consequences it generates. An operant can be defined nontautologically as a behavior that (1) has been acquired through operant processes, or (2) is reinforced when it is performed under ordinary circumstances. An operant in this sense of the word will follow the law of effect and the law of least effort, and it will be performed happily and willingly by the person. Stuttering can under certain laboratory conditions be shown to follow the law of effect, although in a number of studies this did not occur, but under typical circumstances, stutterers are resistant to performing stuttering behaviors voluntarily (Bloodstein & Shogan, 1972), so it seems appropriate to conclude that it does not follow the law of effect. That it does not follow the law of least effort is obvious. For a more elaborate, and excellent, discussion of this subject, the interested reader is referred to Bloodstein (1987, pp. 301–11).

Some children do not have to cope with a difficult or stressful environment, but they seem to be particularly susceptible to stress. Parents often describe them as nervous, sensitive, high strung, perfectionistic, or delicate. When stressors that would be minor to most children come along, these children can't seem to handle them. If they are disfluent, it doesn't take much of a change in the daily routine to elicit a major stuttering episode. A bad night's sleep can become a disaster that may take a day or two to recover from. For such children, parents should be advised about the importance of good rest, a regular daily routine, clearly stated and consistently maintained structure, and general health. An orderly time-structured environment often promotes parental serenity as well as the child's fluency. It is sometimes hard to know whether some parents are generally frazzled or whether the chaos in their lives originates with the child's fluency problem. In fact, it doesn't matter much. Clinicians can manage these cases with calm counsel about the utility of routine and structure, and usually the child's fluency improves quite quickly.

Child with Low Self-Esteem

It is also difficult to separate cause from effect in children with low self-esteem. Although low self-esteem is seen more often in older children, it does occur in the preschool age group. Many such children show early signs of attention deficit disorder (ADD) or hyperactivity—signs such as difficulty in complying with directions, diminished awareness of the needs of others, or poor impulse control. These signs, of course, are commonly observed in most normally developing younger preschool children, so clinicians need to balance the child's age against such behavioral signs. One clue to stuttering-related low self-esteem in these young children is frequent difficulty in initiating topics or asking questions without stuttering. In initiating a topic or in asking a question, children put themselves on the line a little. The new topic may be ignored, and questions, too, reveal a need. When such utterances are related to disfluency, a relation to the child's self-esteem can be suspected.

Low self-esteem can also be produced as a consequence of a disorder. Certainly this happens in older children as a result of peer reactions to stuttering behavior, but it may also happen in very young children because of difficulty in communicating or the reactions of parents or others. Some parental reactions may result in a child feeling ashamed, and shame can be a powerfully negative force in the development of both stuttering (Bennett, 1994) and low self-esteem. Children manifest low self-esteem in a number of different ways. Some children who feel that they are not worth much will take steps to increase their sense of self-worth, and one way to accomplish this is by making other children feel inferior to them, hence they may become aggressive and bullying. Other children may become unusually interested in electronics, or police work, or anything else that they think represents power and authority. Again, such tendencies are not uncommon in preschool children, and clinicians needs to weigh their observations against what is normal for a child's age group.

The Shy Child

Quite a few young stuttering children are described by their parents as "shy." Although it may seem to anyone watching that a child who is easily intimidated by social situations and says little or hides, is shy, not all stuttering children who behave this way are "shy." Adult stutterers often complain that people have always told them they were shy, when in fact they didn't feel shy but only wanted not to have to talk so much. So, sometimes a child's "shy" behavior may be an attempt to diminish the frustration of trying to speak with a mechanism that seems not to want to work well. On the other hand, a child who really is shy will feel far more discomfort in a new social situation, and if he or she is at risk for a fluency problem, the new or unfamiliar social situation will almost surely exacerbate the difficulty in talking. Children whose social anxiety and stuttering are related typically show a sharp increase in disfluency when they talk to strangers and adults. Also, their stuttering often seems to be focused on specific pragmatic situations that elicit their social anxiety. Some social anxiety is normal in every human being, and clinicians need to balance the behavior that leads parents to label their child in this way against the normal tendency of preschool children to be "shy."

The Child with Specific Brain Anomaly

In the past few years, we have become increasingly aware of the possible relation between specific brain anomalies, such as seizure disorder or Tourette's syndrome, and stuttering. Seizure disorder is usually discovered as a result of a seizure episode. Occasionally, however, a child presents to the speech pathologist with an unusual stuttering pattern or some other aspect of behavior, and the clinician then makes a neurological referral. Sometimes children who just don't look right end up with this diagnosis.

Tourette's syndrome is seldom diagnosed in children younger than 6 years of age, but in some cases, speech pathologists first see these children when they are as young as 3 or 4. They seem to make more vocal sounds than other children, grunting as they get up from the floor or making other extraneous vocal noises. Stuttering may also be present, but in some cases the parents have considered stuttering a possibility because of extraneous facial movements or vocalizations. A neurological referral is necessary, although the neurologist may not feel comfortable making the diagnosis at a very young age.

As with ADD children, a child with a specific brain anomaly who stutters may not respect the personal boundaries of parents or clinician. I recall, for example, the child who pulled a clinician's face around with his hand to command full attention. Few normally developing children would do that. Such children may also be difficult to control and present other behavior problems such as aggression, acting out, tantrums, enuresis, sleepwalking, or night terrors.

Language Therapy

A not uncommon track of stuttering development involves language therapy. Typically, the child is delayed in beginning to talk, and the parents seek the help of a speech clinician. Language stimulation is undertaken, and there is usually a substantial amount of improvement, to the point where the child is close to normal levels of language development, when the child starts to stutter. Sometimes, stuttering appears earlier in the sequence, but more often there has been substantial success with language therapy before stuttering becomes a problem.

Although it is obvious that something has gone wrong—either therapy became too demanding or the child was susceptible to a fluency problem—something has to be changed. A different course of action has to be taken. Language therapy can be discontinued or modified, and fluency therapy can be instituted. Some of these children may simply want to please their clinicians or parents and work too hard at getting language right, and in the process start showing excessive amounts of facial, oral, or vocal muscular tension with accompanying blockages or repetitions. Not always, but in many cases, certain language forms appear to prompt stuttering, which may help the clinician understand how the problem arose.

In my experience, a break from language therapy is often the quickest and easiest route. If fluency returns to normal, the break can be extended for a while to give the child some additional experience with fluent speech. But if language development is still lagging, it will be necessary to reinstate some form of language therapy. Therapy that includes the presentation of language forms at a slow rate with minimal demands on the child's performance seems to have the best chance of continuing an improvement in linguistic knowledge without stuttering returning (Goorhuis-Brouwer, Personal communication, 1988).

Articulation Therapy

The child with an articulation disorder presents very much the same picture, except that language acquisition is proceeding normally and in some cases minor fluency problems may have already been noticed. Articulation therapy requires a child to learn how to move the mouth and use the vocal apparatus in new ways that frequently entail some additional muscular tension. Often, fluency deteriorates, sometimes severely.

In most cases it is best to discontinue articulation therapy, since maturation tends to bring some improvement in speech sound production anyway. In contrast, maturation of stuttering may foster a chronic fluency disorder. If the articulation disorder continues and is severe, it will also have to be addressed, but it will be better addressed when chronic stuttering is no longer a risk.

Some children with severe articulation disorders seem to stutter as a consequence of the disorder, not as a consequence of the therapy for the disorder. The crucial question, then, is whether the child's stuttering has emerged from therapy or as one component of the articulation disorder and the child's reactions to it. Children who stutter on sounds they make correctly are more likely to be reacting to therapy training with excessive muscle tension, while those who stutter on error sounds are more likely to be reacting to their own erroneous productions. In the latter case, it is better to continue work on the articulation disorder, since improvement in the ability to communicate will relieve the child's frustration and diminish struggle. As a result, stuttering will also be relieved indirectly.

Although these tracks have been discerned from an examination of a large number of cases, it is important to remember that each child and family are unique. The essential individuality of children and families derives from the uniqueness of their experience. Clinicians should always consider the possibility that they are seeing a new type of case, one that has not been described before in the literature. Stuttering emerges from a rather wide variety of circumstances and combinations of circumstances, which means that new types of cases are likely.

WAYS OF MODIFYING THE ENVIRONMENT TO REDUCE DEMANDS

Motoric

The sharpest demand on the motor system comes from time pressure and for children, time pressure is generally gross rather than fine. Consequently, time pressure demands can be reduced by creating an atmosphere in which there is little pressure to talk rapidly. It is not necessary to slow a child's speech rate; rather, one can create an atmosphere in which rapid speech is not necessary. In fact, if the child's fluency improves with this modification, it is likely that speech rate will increase, rather than decrease. By reducing environmental demands, fluency will be enhanced.

There are two processes for achieving this goal. Stephenson-Opsal and Bernstein Ratner (1988) have shown that a reduction in parental speech rate increases a child's fluency level. Of all the strategies used with very young stuttering children, slowing the parents' speech rate is most likely to produce success. After a hypothesis-testing period to ensure that the process will produce desired results, the parents can be taught to talk more slowly. Some parents show initial resistance to this change, but most do not find it difficult if they are given specific instructions and opportunities to practice, with clinician feedback, before implementing the change while talking to their child. Clinicians should note that better fluency-enhancing effects appear to come from speech that is slowed through slower movements rather than from inserting more pause time within sentences. With all such modifications, clinicians need to verify that parents are able to execute the modification without accompanying tension or embarrassment before they are permitted to use it with the child.

It is also useful to teach parents to insert a very brief (one second) pause between turns. This slows the pace of the conversation and adds to the reduced time pressure of slower speech. This technique seems particularly targeted at the child who has trouble getting started, since time pressure at the very beginning of the utterance seems likely to increase tension at this more than other moments.

This technique is easy for parents to learn and tends to reduce time pressure dramatically.

Linguistic

Episodes of disfluency that accompany language spurts in a child whose language level is advanced may be a sign of language overstimulation. There is nothing that a clinician can or should do to reverse a child's development of language, even though it may seem clear that language development exceeds the child's developing speech motor system. The best that a clinician can do when language overstimulation is suspected is to stop the overstimulation and slow the rate or pace of development. Although empirical evidence is lacking, clinical experience suggests that when parents spend less time in language demanding interactions with their children and more time engaged in less verbal activities, children's fluency improves.

It is, of course, vital when counseling parents to reduce language demands on a child to help them find ways of interacting that are satisfying for both parent and child. The point is not to reduce the amount of parent-child interaction but to reduce the language demands that are used to mediate that interaction. Parental storytelling and TV watching can be noninteractive, and mostly verbal, but if a child watches TV with the parent's arm around him or her, the child is likely to be enjoying a truly interactive, but nonverbal time. Encouraging parents to substitute touch for verbal interaction can be helpful.

Emotional

Sudden emotional changes, positive or negative, seem most disruptive of fluency. Parent counseling is aimed at calming situations that can be calmed, avoiding excitement where possible, and preparing children for those anxious or exciting times that cannot be avoided so as to reduce the suddenness of their arousal. It is not possible, nor would it be desirable, to remove all excitement from a child's life. Parents need to be helped to discover what they can do and to accept the limitations of their control in this area. Still, much can be done to reduce excitement and anxiety.

In preventing the emergence of a significant stuttering problem, clinicians want to help a child develop speaking skills that do not include reactions of shame or fear to disfluency. In early stages, this is easily accomplished by teaching parents to produce occasional disfluencies, of a type appropriate for the child's age, in their own speech. Most often I teach parents how to insert whole-word and whole-syllable repetitions in their speech that are brief, one or two units of repetition and free of tension or discomfort. The latter is important, since it would be counterproductive to have parents model disfluencies if they also model discomfort at the same time. Consequently, it is essential to check out parents' ability to model disfluencies in a casual way before asking them to do so in the home. There is no need to model disfluencies often, just enough to create an atmosphere in which the occurrence of disfluencies is not unusual or cause for concern. If the child comments on the parents' "bumpy speech" it provides an excellent opportunity for the parent to demonstrate a calm and open acceptance of the topic by saying "Yes, I did trip on that word a little, didn't I? It isn't always possible to say things just the way you want to."

Although it is usually best not to change parents' style of discipline with their children, there are some disciplinary actions that may make stuttering worse. These involve requiring the child to speak as part of punishment. Parents can usually find some other way to punish a child than to require confession of a misdeed or an explanation of the behavior. The question "Why did you break the vacuum cleaner?" really has no answer anyway. And when children are already feeling guilty and afraid, such a request is very likely to provoke more disfluency. A better way to handle such a situation is to say "I know you didn't break the vacuum cleaner on purpose, but some time sitting in your room may help you think about how to be more careful in the future."

Cognitive

The request for a narrative account of past events is cognitively demanding, as is the request for an explanation of any event or behavior. These, and other open-ended questions, make it difficult for the child to respond fluently. Information about activities at playschool or an explanation of some experience can usually be obtained without exacerbating fluency problems by commenting or providing some information about a topic and then pausing. When a child is given opportunities to provide the desired information, but is not requested to do so, the information usually is provided at a slightly slower pace. Clinicians often need to help parents find effective ways to get the information they want without increasing the child's disfluency. Questions having short answers are not disruptive of fluency and need not be avoided.

MODIFYING THE CHILD'S BEHAVIOR TO INCREASE CAPACITIES

A child's awareness and acceptance of stuttering behavior should precede direct attempts to modify it. When change is attempted without acceptance, additional avoidance behavior may result, and acceptance may not be achieved in the presence of denial and avoidance. Thus, awareness is the first step, acceptance the second, and change the third. This sequence suggests that increasing the child's emotional capacities should precede attempts to increase motoric capacities.

Emotional

The simplest way to modify the child's behavior so as to increase fluency is to reduce emotional reactions to the experience of being disfluent. As with adults, the process begins with increased awareness and acceptance. For children, awareness and acceptance can be achieved by talking about talking and about stuttering with them in a calm and supportive manner. Most parents need instruction in how to talk to children about stuttering calmly and supportively. Many have heard that they are not supposed to mention stuttering or that they should pretend that nothing is happening. These attitudes undermine good parental support of a child who has a problem, and most parents quickly see the value of being open and reassuring to a child about this, as about any other, problem. In most families, there is a collective sigh of relief when clinicians suggest the utility of being open and have some suggestions about how to achieve greater openness.

The words used are not important except that they should communicate ideas and attitudes effectively. Although the word "stuttering" has no magic power, it is important to use words that are meaningful to the child. I've found it helpful to ask a child if he or she has a word that describes that way of talking, and then use that word in talking about stuttering. Many come up with "bumpy," "echo," or "sticky" speech, and if a child does not yet have a word, those are good words to use. It is best not to talk too long, lest the child concludes that something is wrong even though the parents are saying that nothing is. Whatever is said should be casual, to the point, and brief. "Yes, sometimes it is hard to say what you want to" or, "People sometimes stumble when talking just the way they do when walking." And then the parents can move on to another topic. These brief, casual, but open comments help a child develop an open and accepting attitude toward disfluency that, in turn, prevents the need to struggle with or to hide stuttering behavior.

Clinicians have long proposed to parents that they reduce requests for "demand speech." Initially, this term seemed to mean requests for performance, such as reciting poetry or telling long stories. But a number of other types of demand speech may also make it difficult for the child who stutters. One bilingual family we worked with asked their young stuttering child to interpret for them. He was linguistically able to do this, but it seemed an unusually demanding speech task for a 4-year-old. We have also seen parents who ask their children to talk for them, for example, when the parents are angry with each other and not talking. These uses of speech are demanding in the sense that they are not spontaneous. The child is not saying what he or she feels like saying but rather the words or thoughts of someone else. This kind of speech has some of the characteristics of recitation and performance and seems to be an advanced skill, one that would be better set aside for awhile in a young stuttering child.

Motoric

When children are a little older, around 5 years of age, they become able to slow their rate of speech with proper instruction. This can be a powerful tool in increasing a child's fluency. Meyers-Fosnot (1992) suggested that the concept of slower movement be taught, in a Piagetian way, as a concept, with the use of stories and symbols to concretize the concept, and lots of modeling. It is usually helpful to make it clear that a slower onset of speaking is also important. Often children may learn to slow down after they begin speaking, but still begin too quickly. And, of course, the first few words are particularly susceptible to disfluency.

Linguistic

Although the use of shorter sentences and words promotes fluency, techniques for achieving such changes without altering a child's self-expression in a seriously negative way are not available. It may be, however, that simplified language is a by-product of slowed rate in some children.

Cognitive

As with linguistic behavior, the only feasible way to improve a child's cognitive capacities is to wait for the natural processes of maturation.

SUMMARY

Many clinicians now agree that it is preferable to treat children who are stuttering as quickly as possible. Therapy takes less time and is more effective than is treatment of adults who stutter. With a clear sense of normal fluency and appropriate definitions of fluency and disfluency, clinicians can reliably assess fluency disorders. An important aspect of a fluency evaluation is the assessment of a child's capacities for fluency and of environmental demands that challenge it. These assessments should evaluate motoric, linguistic, emotional, and cognitive capacities, and the demands placed on each of these areas by the child's environment. Such an evaluation provides the clinician with information that is helpful in constructing both a long-term plan of therapy and specific procedures for intervention. It is nonetheless important to test specific procedures as they are implemented. Although there are exceptions, fluency typically responds quickly to environmental changes that are on target in this population.

Clinicians need to keep in mind that stuttering is variable in children, possibly in its etiology, and certainly in its course of development. In addition,

families change in response to a child's stuttering, and the child changes in reaction to the family. Because of these complexities and the number of different etiological possibilities, a child's stuttering is difficult to understand. But when the capacities and demands that affect fluency are assessed in the context of a dynamically changing, reciprocally influential family, a viable strategy for therapy, tailored to a child's individual needs and situation, is feasible. Such a strategy usually includes both direct and indirect treatment, parent counseling and training to increase both the child's and parents' awareness of stuttering, their calm acceptance of the problem as it is, then learning specific techniques for changing it.

REFERENCES

Adams, M.R., & Hayden, P. (1976). The ability of stutterers and nonstutterers to initiate and terminate phonation during production of an isolated vowel. *Journal of Speech and Hearing Research, 19*, 290–296.

Amster, B. (1984). *The rate of speech in normal preschool children.* Unpublished doctoral dissertation, Temple University, Philadelphia, PA.

Amster, B. (1989). *Case studies in language overstimulation and stuttering.* Paper presented at the meeting of the American Speech-Language-Hearing Association, St. Louis, Mo.

Andrews, G., Craig, A., Feyer, A-M., Hoddinott, S., Howie, P., & Neilson, M. (1983). Stuttering: A review of research findings and theories circa 1982. *Journal of Speech and Hearing Disorders, 48*, 226–246.

Andrews, G., & Harris, M. (1964). *The syndrome of stuttering.* London: Heinemann.

Barrett, R.S., & Stoeckel, C.M. (1979). *Unilateral eyelid movement control in stutterers and nonstutterers.* Paper presented at the meeting of the American Speech-Language-Hearing Association, Atlanta, Ga.

Bennett, E.M. (1994). *Shame in children who stutter.* Unpublished manuscript, University of Colorado, Boulder.

Bloodstein, O. (1960). The development of stuttering II. Developmental phases. *Journal of Speech and Hearing Disorders, 25* 366–376.

Bloodstein, O. (1987) *The handbook of stuttering* (4th Ed.). Chicago: National Easter Seal Society.

Bloodstein, O., & Shogan, R.L. (1972). Some clinical notes on forced stuttering. *Journal of Speech and Hearing Disorders, 37*, 177–186.

Boberg, E., & Kully, D. (1984). Techniques for tranferring fluency. In W.H. Perkins (Ed.) *Current therapy of communication disorders,* New York: Thieme-Stratton.

Brauth, S.E., Hall, W.S., and Dooling, R.J. (1991). *Plasticity of development.* Cambridge, Mass.: MIT Press.

Conture, E., & Kelly, E. (1988). *(Non)Verbal behavior of young stutterers and their mothers.* Paper presented at the meeting of the American Speech-Language-Hearing Association, Boston, Mass.

Cordes, A., Gow, M., & Ingham , R. (1991). On valid and reliable identification of normal disfluencies and stuttering disfluencies. *Brain and Language, 40* , 282–286.

Cordes, A., & Ingham, R. (1994). The reliability of observational data: II Issues in the identification and measurement of stuttering events. *Journal of Speech and Hearing Research, 37*, 779–788.

Cross, D.E., & Luper, H.L. (1979). Voice reaction times of stuttering and nonstuttering children and adults. *Journal of Fluency Disorders, 4*, 59–77.

De Nil, L., & Brutten, G. (1988). *Homorganic and heterorganic consonant clusters in stutterers' and nonstutterers' fluent speech.* Paper presented at the meeting of the American Speech-Language-Hearing Association, Boston, Mass.

DiCara, L.V., & Miller, N.E. (1968). Instrumental learning of vasomotor responses by rats: Learning to respond differentially in the two ears. *Science, 159,* 1485–1486.

Franken, M.C., Peters, H.F.M., & Tettero, C.M. (1989). Evaluation of the Dutch version of Webster's Precision Fluency Shaping Program for stutterers. *Logopedie en Foniatrie, Jaargang 61, (11),* 343–345.

Freeman, F., & Ushijima, T. (1978). Laryngeal muscle activity during stuttering. *Journal of Speech and Hearing Research, 21,* 538–562.

Gens, G. (1951). The speech pathologist looks at the mentally deficient child. *Training School Bulletin, 48,* 19–27.

Goorhuis-Brouwer, S. (1987). *Leren praten gaat niet helemaal vanzelf.* Groningen: Akademisch Ziekenhuis.

Gottesleben, R.H. (1955). The incidence of stuttering in a group of mongoloids. *Training School Bulletin, 51,* 209–218.

Gregory, H., & Hill, D. (1984). Stuttering therapy for children. In Perkins, W. (Ed.), *Stuttering disorders.* New York: Thieme-Stratton.

Hutt, D. (1987). *Mother-child differences in rate of speech in Spanish-speaking families.* Paper presented at the meeting of the American Speech-Language-Hearing Association, New Orleans, La.

Ingham, R. (1984). *Stuttering and behavior therapy: Current status and experimental foundations.* San Diego, Calif.: College-Hill Press.

Kagan, J. (1991). Continuity and discontinuity in development. In S.E. Brauth, W.S. Hall, & R.J. Dooling (Eds.), *Plasticity of development.* Cambridge, Mass.: MIT Press.

Kagan, J., & Moss, H.A. (1962). *Birth to maturity.* New York: John Wiley & Sons.

Kline, M.L., & Starkweather, C.W. (1979). *Receptive and expressive language performance in young stutterers.* Paper presented at the meeting of the American Speech-Language-Hearing Association, Atlanta, Ga.

Levelt, W.J.M. (1989). *Speaking: From intention to articulation.* Cambridge, Mass.: MIT Press.

Louko, L., Edwards, M.L., & Conture, E.G. (1990). Phonological characteristics of young stutterers and their normally fluent peers: Preliminary observations. *Journal of Fluency Disorders, 15,* 191–210.

Malecot, A., Johnston, R., & Kizziar, P.-A. (1972). Syllabic rate and utterance length in French. *Phonetica, 26,* 235–251.

Merits-Patterson, R., & Reed, C. (1981). Disfluencies in the speech of language-disordered children. *Journal of Speech and Hearing Research, 46,* 55–58.

Meyers, S., & Freeman, F. (1985a). Interruptions as a variable in stuttering and disfluency. *Journal of Speech and Hearing Research, 28,* 428–435.

Meyers, S., & Freeman, F. (1985b). Mother and child speech rates as a variable in stuttering and disfluency. *Journal of Speech and Hearing Research, 28,* 436–444.

Meyers-Fosnot, S. (1992). Therapy for preschool stuttering children, ASHA Teleconference.

Miller, N.E. (1969). Learning of visceral and glandular responses. *Science, 163,* 434–445.

Peters, H.F.M., & Boves, L. (1987). Aerodynamic functions in fluent speech utterances of stutterers and nonstutterers in different speech conditions. In Peters, H.F.M., & Hulstijn, W., (Eds.) *Speech motor dynamics in stuttering.* Wien/New York: Springer Verlag.

Peters, H.F.M., & Hulstijn, W. (1984). Stuttering and anxiety: The difference between stutterers and nonstutterers in verbal apprehension and physiologic arousal during the anticipation of speech and nonspeech tasks. *Journal of Fluency Disorders, 9,* 67–84.

Peters, T.J., & Guitar, B. (1991). Stuttering: An integrated approach to its nature and treatment. Baltimore, Md.: Williams & Wilkins.

Ramig, P., & Bennett, E. (in press). Working with 7–12 year old children who stutter: Ideas for intervention in the public schools. *Language, Speech, & Hearing Services in Schools.*

Rathburn, C., DiVirgilio, L., & Waldfogel, S. (1958). A restitutive process in children following radical separation from family and culture. *American Journal of Orthopsychiatry, 28,* 408–415.

Shapiro, A. (1980). An electromyographic analysis of the fluent and dysfluent utterance of several types of stutterers. *Journal of Fluency Disorders, 5,* 203–231.

Sheehan, J.G., & Martyn, M.M. (1966). Spontaneous recovery from stuttering. *Journal of Speech and Hearing Research, 9,* 121–135.

Sheehan, J.G., & Martyn, M.M. (1970). Stuttering and its disappearance. *Journal of Speech and Hearing Research. 13,* 279–289.

Starkweather, C.W. (1987). *Fluency and stuttering.* Englewood Cliffs, N.J.: Prentice-Hall.

Starkweather, C.W. (1993). Issues in therapy efficacy research. *Journal of Fluency Disorders, Special issue, Proceedings of the NIDCD workshop on treatment efficacy research in stuttering,* National Institute on Deafness and Other Communication Disorders, NIH, September 21–22, 1992, 18, 2 & 3, 151–168.

Starkweather, C.W., & Gottwald, S.R. (1993). A pilot

project of relations among specific measures obtained at intake and discharge in a program of prevention and early intervention. *American Journal of Speech Pathology, 2,* 51–58.

Starkweather, C.W., Gottwald, S.R., & Halfond, M.H. (1990). *Stuttering prevention: A clinical method.* Englewood Cliffs, N.J.: Prentice-Hall.

Starkweather, C.W., Hirschman, P., & Tannenbaum, R.S. (1976). Latency of vocalization: stutterers v. nonstutterers. *Journal of Speech and Hearing Research, 19,* 481–492.

Starkweather, C.W., & Myers, M. (1979). The duration of subsegments within the intevocalic intervals of stutterers and nonstutterers, *Journal of Fluency Disorders, 4,* 205–214.

Starkweather, C.W., van Lieshout, P.H.H.M., Hulstijn, W., & Peters, H.F.M. (1989). Motoric variations at the linguistic locations of stuttering in the speech of nonstutterers. *Logopedie en Foniatrie, Jaargang 61,* Nr. 11.

Stephenson-Opsal, D., & Bernstein Ratner, N. (1988). Maternal speech rate modification and childhood stuttering. *Journal of Fluency Disorders, 13,* (1) 49–56.

van Lieshout, P.H.H.M., Peters, H.F.M., Starkweather C.W., & Hulstijn, W. (1993). Physiological differences between stutterers and nonstutterers in per-

ceptually fluent speech: EMG amplitude and duration. *Journal of Speech and Hearing Research, 36,* 1, 55–63.

van Lieshout, P.H.H.M., Starkweather, C.W., Hulstijn, W., & Peters, H.F.M. (1995). The effects of linguistic correlates of stuttering on EMG activity in nonstuttering speakers. *Journal of Speech and Hearing Research, 38,* 2, 360–372.

Van Riper, C. (1973). *The treatment of stuttering.* Englewood Cliffs, N.J.: Prentice-Hall.

Wexler, K.B., & Mysak, E.D. (1982). Disfluency characteristics of 2-, 4-, and 6-year-old males. *Journal of Fluency Disorders, 7,* 37–46.

Wieneke, G., & Janssen, P. (1987). Duration variations in the fluent speech of stutterers and nonstutterers. In H. Peters & W. Hulstijn (Eds.), *Speech motor dynamics in stuttering.* Vienna/New York: Springer-Verlag.

Yairi, E. (1981). Disfluencies of normally speaking two-year-old children. *Journal of Speech and Hearing Research, 24,* 490–495.

Young, M. (1984). Identification of stuttering and stutterers. In R. Curlee & W. Perkins (Eds.). *Nature and treatment of stuttering: New directions.* San Diego: College-Hill Press.

Zimmermann, G. (1980). Stuttering: A disorder of movement. *Journal of Speech and Hearing Research, 23,* 122–136.

SUGGESTED READINGS

Bloodstein, O. (1960). The development of stuttering II. Developmental phases. *Journal of Speech and Hearing Disorders, 25,* 366–376. A classical piece of clinical research that provides the details of changes that children go through as their stuttering develops.

Levelt, W.J.M. (1989). *Speaking: From intention to articulation.* Cambridge, Mass.: MIT Press. This book provides a comprehensive overview of all of the processes involved in speaking. It is an invaluable reference.

Peters, T.J., & Guitar, B. (1991). *Stuttering: An integrated approach to its nature and treatment.* Baltimore, Md.: Williams & Wilkins. This book has brought together the disparate approaches to stuttering therapy, and it has done so with such clarity that very few clinicians today practice any form of therapy other than "integrated" therapy.

Starkweather, C.W., Gottwald, S.R., & Halfond, M.H.

(1990). *Stuttering prevention: A clinical method.* Englewood Cliffs, N.J.: Prentice-Hall. This book is written with the practicing clinician in mind and provides enough detail to implement the approach that is used at the Temple University Stuttering Prevention Center.

Starkweather, C.W. (1987). *Fluency and stuttering.* Englewood Cliffs, N.J.: Prentice-Hall. This book integrates the data on normal fluency with the data on stuttering so as to provide a unified theory of normal and disordered fluency.

Starkweather, C.W., & Peters, H.F.M. (in press). *Proceedings of the First World Congress on Fluency Disorders.* This book provides the latest results of research, the most recent therapeutic ideas, and a number of historical and philosophical accounts from individuals who are specialized in stuttering around the world.

CHAPTER 14

THERAPY FOR CHILDREN'S STUTTERING AND EMOTIONS

BARRY GUITAR

INTRODUCTION

In this chapter I will focus primarily on therapy strategies for children who seem resistant to treatment. I will argue that this resistance stems, in many cases, from a strong emotional response to stuttering. This response appears to interfere with these children's progress in traditional fluency shaping or stuttering modification therapy programs, such as those described in Peters and Guitar (1991). Even if these children do make good initial progress in therapy, they have difficulty transferring their fluency gains beyond the clinic. It is likely that they account for some of the 33 percent of children who drop out of clinical studies before completing treatment (Bloodstein, 1995; Costello, 1983; Martin, 1981).

The motivation for this chapter comes from my recent work with two children who have had a difficult time in treatment. They seemed particularly reluctant to engage in either fluency shaping or stuttering modification activities, despite the fact that both enjoyed coming to the clinic. On the basis of this experience, I am proposing a perspective that views strong emotional responses as part of some children's innate temperament. This perspective led me to the specific treatment strategies and procedures that I will describe. The therapy procedures may be generally suitable for children whose emotions relating to their stuttering are strong, and some may be appropriate for other children who stutter, but whose emotional reactions appear less marked.

INTRODUCTORY CLINICAL MATERIAL

In this section I will briefly recount the evaluations and initial attempts at therapy for two children treated in our clinic. After describing our early failures, I will provide a theoretical perspective that motivated us to develop a different approach and then turn to our therapy with these children. The first child, Adam, has been seen for three years, off and on. The second child, Bob, has been in treatment for a year and a half.

Adam was brought to us by his mother when he was 6. In the initial evaluation she tearfully described how she had watched her child become gradually worse over the past two years, as she heeded medical advice to ignore his stuttering because he would outgrow it. When Adam was interviewed, he vigorously denied that he had any difficulty talking and immediately changed the subject. It soon became evident that he was a master at avoiding uncomfortable experiences. Adam's stuttering was characterized by tense,

ACKNOWLEDGMENTS: I am indebted to several individuals for their suggestions about this manuscript: Nan Bernstein-Ratner, Edward Conture, Rebecca McCauley, and Julie Reville. As usual, Richard Curlee's editing has added much to the clarity of my writing. I would also like to thank David Van Buskirk, M.D., Director of Child Psychiatry at the University of Vermont Medical School for many helpful consultations.

silent blocks and repetitions. His escape behaviors were eye blinks and body movements, and he appeared to substitute words or change the topic if he expected to stutter. Once in the evaluation, when the clinician indicated that he helped other kids who get stuck on words, Adam briefly acknowledged that he did have trouble talking sometimes.

At the end of the evaluation, Adam's parents and the clinicians agreed to a plan of once-a-week therapy, in which Adam would be taught to stutter more openly and easily; his parents would be gradually introduced into treatment and counseled about environmental changes in the meantime.

In the beginning I worked with two student clinicians. While one treated Adam directly, the other counseled Adam's mother as they watched treatment through a one-way window. Initial sessions were spectacularly unsuccessful. Adam tried to leave the room whenever the topic of stuttering was introduced. After several sessions in which no progress was made and our relationship with Adam was deteriorating, we changed the direction of therapy to fluency shaping. We then worked with Adam on a hierarchy of fluent words and sentences, using slightly slowed, normal-sounding speech. Adam again reacted with avoidance and began to ask his mother if he could stop therapy. At this point we decided to discontinue therapy for several months but to encourage Adam to come to the clinic for an occasional social visit without any treatment.

The second child, whom I shall call Bob, started stuttering when he was 2 years old. His parents were relatively unconcerned at first, and their pediatrician, like Adam's, had recommended a "wait-and-see" approach. By the time Bob was 5, however, he was still stuttering, and his parents decided to consult us.

During the evaluation, Bob's repetitions and prolongations were often accompanied by pitch rises and abrupt stoppages. Sometimes Bob would have silent, tense articulatory postures, suggesting that he was shutting off voice and airflow. Bob's parents reported that he appeared to be not only aware but also frustrated with his stuttering. This was consistent with our observations of increasing tension in his repetitions and prolongations. Bob also seemed to be showing signs of general frustration. At home he would sometimes throw toys, and at school he would hit other children. Nevertheless, his parents described Bob as a sensitive child, who was devastated when he was punished for something, and reported that he was also sensitive to change and did not adapt easily to new situations.

Because of scheduling problems, Bob's parents and I decided not to begin therapy in the clinic immediately. Instead, I gave them guidance in how to create a fluency-enhancing environment in their home and asked them to provide Bob with 15 minutes of one-on-one attention each day. I suggested that if this did not improve his fluency substantially within six weeks, direct therapy should be considered. Bob's parents were out of touch with us for almost a year before they sought direct therapy. By this time, Bob's stuttering had increased both in frequency and duration. An additional worry was that Bob was being teased about his stuttering and was having some difficulty relating to other children at school. I decided to bring Bob into the clinic for once-a-week therapy sessions.

Our initial approach to treatment combined fluency shaping with stuttering modification. Fluency shaping began with a hierarchy of words, phrases, and sentences that were produced with gentle onset and a slightly slowed rate. Stuttering modification focused on decreasing Bob's fear of stuttering by having him control the length and type of stuttering that the clinicians were simulating. Bob frequently avoided working on therapy tasks by refusing to participate, distracting the clinicians with inappropriate behavior, excessive fantasizing, and frequently talking about "pooping." The first few weeks of therapy were highly frustrating for the clinicians and, apparently, for Bob.

THEORETICAL PERSPECTIVE

My theoretical model for these children's stuttering and their strong emotional reactions is similar to some aspects of Bloodstein's (1995) view of the development of stuttering. In this view, disfluencies arise initially from any of a number of breakdowns in oral communication. Commonly, these are the repetitions and prolongations associated with speech and language development, but may also include disfluencies associated with cluttering, oral reading problems, and other speaking difficulties. Chronic stuttering emerges when these disfluencies (or other difficulties) occur in a child with a sensitive nature and the child reacts to them emotionally, with increased physical tension.

Recent research on the neurophysiology of stress provides a scaffold for speculating about how "sensitivity" may make some children more susceptible to breakdowns in fluency and subsequent maladaptive responses.[1] Kagan's studies (e.g., Kagan, Reznick, & Snidman, 1987) of children's temperament and Gray's (1987) research on the neuropsychology of fear describe factors that can be applied to speech. Kagan and colleagues (1987) hypothesize that some children are born with a greater reactivity to uncomfortable and unfamiliar experiences. Such children respond to threatening stimuli with heightened activation of the limbic system—a part of the brain that mediates emotions and behavior. This heightened activation causes many responses throughout the body, including increases in muscle tension, particularly in the larynx. Gray (1987) provided a neuroanatomical basis for Kagan's theoretical perspective by suggesting that limbic circuits may respond to fear and frustration with muscular contractions that produce tense and silent immobility ("freezing"), an innate response in most species that can be easily classically conditioned. Moreover, innate flight/avoidance responses may be elicited under threatening conditions and may alternate rapidly with "freezing" responses. It may not be too great a leap of imagination to reconceptualize the essential elements of chronic

stuttering—core, escape, and avoidance behaviors—as manifestations of these three responses to fear and frustration: freezing, flight, and avoidance.[2]

The above research and theory may apply to the children discussed in this chapter as follows:

1. Some children who have a predisposition to the motoric and/or linguistic breakdown underlying disfluency may also be predisposed to be emotionally reactive.
2. This reactivity may produce heightened tension (laryngeal tension and perhaps tension in other parts of the speaking mechanism) during conditions of frustration or fear—specifically frustration and fear related to difficulty in talking.
3. This heightened tension may increase the difficulty in talking, thereby increasing frustration and fear and further increasing manifestations of innate freezing, flight, and avoidance responses in speaking situations.
4. A hyper-reactive temperament may make direct work on stuttering difficult for a child, because frustrating and fear-laden stimuli elicit a conditioned flight or avoidance response.

Without supporting data from children who stutter, this model is only speculation; however, it provides an intuitively appealing explanation of why some children develop stuttering rapidly and why, if innate sensitivity renders a child vulnerable to hyperexcitability of limbic circuits, some children find it difficult to maintain fluency under stress and excitement even after they have made great gains in a controlled treatment environment. This vulnerability to emotion may be related to one of the findings that links research on temperamentally inhibited children with research on indi-

---

[1]Some of this speculation about temperament and stuttering in children was foreshadowed in the writings of Conture (1991) and Peters and Guitar (1991).

[2]Core behavior in the chronic stutterer is commonly a stoppage of voicing, air flow, and/or movement, which may be a manifestation of the muscular co-contraction displayed in freezing. Escape behavior—the struggle to break free of the core behavior—may be the extra tension or movement that is used in flight from the painful experience of being caught in a stutter. Avoidance behavior is simply the stutterer's avoidance of anticipated unpleasantness associated with stuttering.

viduals who stutter. Both groups tend to show evidence of greater right hemisphere activation than do normal controls (Calkins & Fox, 1994; Moore, 1993). Calkins and Fox (1994) suggest that this right hemisphere asymmetry may derive from activity of the amygdala, which apparently plays a key role in conditioned fear responses.

This speculative model also provides a possible basis for understanding why some therapy procedures are successful and how they might be improved. Viewing the chronicity of stuttering, at least in some children, as the result of conditioned and innate frustration and fear responses rather than simply a motor speech breakdown, allows us to use the research on conditioned emotional responses.

Mineka's chapter, "Animal Models of Anxiety-Based Disorders" provides a good overview of this literature (Mineka, 1985). Mineka points out, for instance, that fear increases as a sense of lack of control increases and, conversely, that a sense of mastery can reduce fear-based responses. Such a sense of lack of control may be strong in a child whose speech is disrupted by the excess tension resulting from reactivity of the autonomic nervous system. The child may not be aware of the underlying excitation of limbic circuits and the resulting bodily changes,[3] and the feeling of an unknown force affecting speech may heighten fear. Stuttering therapy has the potential to counteract this sense of helplessness. First, children can be given control of the pace and sequence of therapy. Second, therapy can be designed to give them a sense of mastery through awareness of how they are gaining fluency and of how they can regain it when it is temporarily lost.

The emotional learning literature also suggests there are three key variables for treating phobias that may be important in the treatment of

stuttering: (1) long exposure to the feared stimulus, (2) opportunities to explore feared situations, and (3) presence of a nonfearful social partner (Mineka, 1985). These variables are already part of some treatment programs designed to reduce fear of stuttering but could be exploited further. Long exposure to a feared stimulus occurs when voluntary stuttering is used (e.g., Dell, 1979, 1993; Van Riper, 1973). Exploration of the feared situation may occur when the clinician and child discuss the things that make stuttering better or worse. The nonfearful social partner is, of course, the clinician who demonstrates comfort and familiarity with stuttering, whether she or he stutters or not.

APPLICATION OF THEORY TO CLINICAL CASES

Our initial attempts at therapy with Adam had been unsuccessful, and we had temporarily dismissed him from treatment. After several months without therapy but with occasional social visits, Adam's stuttering worsened and he agreed to try therapy again. I was, then, the lone clinician working with him and his parents. To counteract Adam's previous negative feelings about therapy and to provide a context for helping him feel some control in this situation, I structured therapy around a variety of games that Adam chose at the beginning of each session. These included checkers, "Battleship," bowling, and basketball. In early sessions, I inserted easy "fake" stutters in my speech and only asked Adam to insert them before taking a turn at the game. The easy stutters were essentially words produced with a slightly slow onset, which is common to both fluency shaping therapies and to the later stages of stuttering modification. Adam's comfort in therapy seemed related to the fact that he was given a great deal of control over what was done in each session and that the primary focus of our interaction seemed not to be on his speech, but on games, at which he was expert. Perhaps it also helped that Adam was several months older and was experiencing serious difficulty with his speech outside the clinic, which provided a real need for help.

---

[3]Kagan and colleagues (1987) discuss the neural circuitry involved in a child's hyper-reactivity to fear-producing stimuli, making it evident that this is not at a conscious level. Humphrey, in a personal communication, speculated that the cocontraction that may occur in stuttering, if parallel to the muscle cocontraction he has observed in monkeys, may not be conscious to the speaker (cf., Humphrey & Reed, 1983).

Despite Adam's apparent comfort in therapy sessions, signs of negative emotion about stuttering persisted. For example, he refused to work directly on his stuttering or even to acknowledge it. In addition, his mother reported that Adam wouldn't talk about anything that went on in his therapy. I respected Adam's "news blackout" about therapy and allowed him to maintain a division between what he did in therapy and what he did at home and school. I believe that letting Adam decide what to share with his parents was important to his developing a trusting relationship with me and to his feeling in control of some aspects of therapy.

A turning point in treatment came when Adam saw a jar full of candy on my desk and asked for a piece. Adam and I then set up a contingency that allowed him to earn a piece of candy for each easy stutter. This prompted him to fill his speech with easy stutters and walk away with a bag of twenty-two candies. This lucky pairing of shameful stuttering with sweet signs of success may have provided Adam with hope that he could gain some control of his stuttering.

Soon after this session, Adam and I raised the criterion for candy, changing the target from brief, easy stutters to stutters that he held onto and voluntarily prolonged for several seconds and then released slowly. In these stutters, which we called "slideouts," Adam maintained excellent eye contact as he prolonged the moment of being stuck. Eye contact was used so that Adam could see that his listener was comfortable when he was stuttering easily. It also seemed to elicit a more assertive attitude on his part. These slideouts with eye contact were done in the context of games, which continued to keep the major focus off speech and on activities in which Adam could take the role of expert and instructor.

I worked toward having Adam generalize his easy speech and his voluntary stutters to situations outside the therapy room, but progress was slow. Adam seemed comfortable having his mother and father participate in sessions in which he taught them slideouts, so I arranged for him to do some rewarded practice at home with each of his parents, but this was soon discontinued at Adam's request. He told me in no uncertain terms that he would not do this any more. Moreover, the parents reported that he seemed embarrassed and uncomfortable when doing these home assignments.

Direct work on generalization would have to wait, I thought, so I continued having Adam overlearn a way to respond to stuttering by keeping eye contact and releasing the word slowly. We did this in the therapy room and in various parts of the building with a variety of listeners, but Adam would do this only when I accompanied him, and even then he was reluctant.

Occasionally, on forays around the clinic or, more often, when Adam's family took him on vacation or hosted relatives, Adam would still stutter severely. When I tried to talk to him about his difficult times, he would say a few words, but then clam up. Believing it was hard for Adam to express feelings directly, I worked with him on inventing games in which he could express emotions indirectly, such as by drawing stutters on plastic bowling pins and smashing them with a plastic bowling ball. We continued to bring each parent into therapy sessions intermittently, and while his mother was impressed with his speech in the clinic, she reported not much change on the outside.

Therapy continued once a week over the school year, with frequent lapses due to holidays, intervening activities, and minor illness. In the summer Adam asked for a longer vacation from therapy. I agreed, despite his parents' concerns, that he needed a break. In the fall, Adam experienced an increase in stuttering when school started, and with his parents' encouragement he began therapy again. Another leap forward in therapy occurred when a TV station videotaped Adam talking about his stuttering and demonstrating therapy techniques and the show was broadcast locally. He asked to show the video to his class, as well, and then he shared his therapy experiences with them. Afterwards, in therapy sessions, Adam seemed eager to demonstrate his finesse at catching stutters and turning them into slideouts with excellent eye contact. At the same time, he kept a running tally of his slideouts and rewarded himself with a candy after each one. This reward system made Adam eager to use slideouts during therapy sessions. Soon he had fewer real stutters and had to fake some of his stutters to keep the candies rolling in.[4]

With lessening reluctance, Adam agreed to use these slideouts in more public places. By pre-arranging with various people in the building that Adam and I might be "practicing our stuttering," I ensured that Adam would have receptive audiences for carry-over activities close at hand. I also mixed in carry-over activities in a nearby shopping mall, where I would fake easy and hard stutters to store clerks and, with encouragement, Adam would do an occasional voluntary stutter. Progress was slow, and on some days, Adam seemed to be going backwards. Nonetheless, his parents continued to be supportive of his being in therapy and reported that, despite some remaining stuttering, Adam was no longer avoiding situations and seemed to be happy and successful in his relationships with other children.

After another long break from therapy during the following summer, Adam, the clinician in his school, and I presented another "sharing" about his stuttering for the benefit of new classmates. By this time Adam felt he was an expert on stuttering and taught the student clinician in his school about slideouts. In therapy sessions in our clinic, I invited unfamiliar students to sit in with us so that Adam could explain what he was working on and why. Once, when his assignment was to interview three unfamiliar listeners and use several fake slideouts with each, he not only used the slideouts but decided on his own to explain to the individuals what he was doing. Not content with three interviews, he asked to conduct a fourth, with a high school senior who had just arrived for his first stuttering therapy session. As he was doing his voluntary stuttering with this newcomer, Adam stopped momentarily after the high-school student had a bad block and suggested to him how he might handle bad blocks more easily by maintaining eye contact and sliding out of the stutter slowly.

By Christmas, Adam declared he was no longer stuttering. His parents reported this was true at the time, although I believe he continues to show some repetitive stuttering with tension when he is excited or is in an unfamiliar situation.

I will now describe the therapy devised for Bob. This will be shorter than my description of Adam's treatment because Bob has been in therapy for a shorter time. In applying this theoretical perspective to Bob, the changes made in treatment focused first on giving him a strong sense of control. The student clinician and I began each session by telling Bob what we planned to do that day and getting his input on the sequence of activities. When possible, we let him choose activities. Each activity had firm rules, and success was followed by rewards. The increased structure consisted of a firm plan for each activity, with rules for how the activity was done. At the beginning of each session, we described each activity we would do together and got Bob's agreement. In fluency shaping, for example, we had Bob use a gentle onset at the beginning of each phrase as he went through a packet of ten picture cards and described each one. We gave him a clear model at the beginning of the task and kept him at a high level of accuracy throughout. For each successful gentle onset, Bob received a point, and the total number of points went toward a reinforcement at the end of the session—five minutes playing a computer game. An example of a fairly advanced stuttering modification activity would be having Bob produce a long voluntary stutter with good eye contact and a slow ending, which was rewarded immediately by giving him a turn at throwing a ball into a trash can some distance away. Extensive social reinforcement also followed each successful voluntary stutter. The point system was used as well, and Bob's clinicians were given points for their own attempts at voluntary stuttering (successful) and ball-throwing (less successful). Bob, of course, was the scorekeeper for accumulating points.

In consultation with Bob's parents, we began to work on generalizing both Bob's fluency skills

---

[4]Readers who are concerned about the effect of so many candies on Adam's teeth will be relieved to know that Adam's mother brought big bags of uneaten candies back to the clinic every few weeks. Adam enjoyed winning the candies, but often forgot them once he had brought them home in triumph.

and his positive attitude toward handling his speech. I frequently invited Bob's mother and sister into therapy sessions and involved them in role-playing situations that had provoked stuttering at home. Bob and his parents also described those situations, such as on the school bus, in which Bob was teased for his stuttering. With Bob's expert direction, we role played several of these situations, worked out assertive responses for him, and reinforced them with videotaped replays of the role playing.[5] In addition, we adopted a procedure in which Bob constructed small paper "shields" that were filled with drawings of things that made him feel safe. He would then carry a shield into those situations in which he thought he might be teased to increase his self-confidence. Gradually, over the course of eighteen months of treatment, Bob's fluency improved, and with the combination of fluency shaping and stuttering modification, he began to feel some control of his stuttering and a decrease in the shame that was so strongly attached to it. At this writing, we are making a video starring Bob for him to show to his classmates and teacher to enhance his feeling of being an "expert" about stuttering and decrease negative feelings. In addition, we continue to work on Bob's social skills and self-esteem, which I believe are essential for long-term change in his stuttering.

PRINCIPLES ILLUSTRATED IN ADAM'S AND BOB'S TREATMENT

This work with Adam and Bob was built upon many years of treating children and adults who stutter. Some of the therapy strategies used with them emerged from my prior experience, and some were created on the spot to deal with these children's unique needs. I will highlight a few aspects of these approaches that I think are likely to be useful with other children who stutter.

In both cases, hindsight suggests that therapy was focused too quickly on their stuttering. I think both Adam and Bob felt that their stuttering was a

glaring failure that made them unacceptable to others. Attempts to work directly on their stuttering too quickly produced intense discomfort, which was not outweighed by an established supportive relationship. In the future, I would spend more time at the beginning of therapy helping a child feel supported, understood, and accepted, just as he or she is.

Structuring treatment within the context of games or other activities kept therapy sessions from being simply focused on the painful subject of stuttering. I think these two sensitive children felt success and competence in the games format, which opened the way for the direct work on speech that followed. Additionally, because these two children appeared to feel uncomfortable with the unexpected, they probably benefited from beginning sessions by mutually planning the sequence of activities for the day.

Both youngsters showed evidence of shame and avoidance in their early sessions, and they might have benefited from fluency shaping therapy before stuttering modification procedures. Fluency shaping begins, ideally, with clear clinician models of gentle onset of phonation, light articulatory contacts, and a slow overall speech rate. A carefully designed hierarchy should be used to take the child through increases in linguistic and pragmatic complexity. A critical feature of the programmed hierarchy is to give the child a feeling of competence, control, and success.

I think it is unlikely that fluency shaping alone would have been successful for either Bob or Adam. Each had shown considerable anxiety about his stuttering, which was manifested in unwillingness to talk about stuttering and the initial inability to change it in any way. Again, direct work on the moment of stuttering was probably not appropriate at first. However, in both cases, fear of stuttering had to be reduced to increase the likelihood of long-term success.

As with phobias, reducing the fear of stuttering may be aided by clinicians' modeling a non-fearful attitude toward stuttering, by encouraging a child to approach and "explore" rather than avoid the moment of stuttering, and by reinforcing a child for holding on to a stutter for a prolonged

---

[5]Our work on teasing was greatly enhanced by discussions with Bill Murphy who has used role-playing and videotaping to help children combat negative experiences with teasing.

period of time—all of which has to be carried out in a supportive environment (Guitar & Peters, in preparation; Mineka, 1985). With both of these children, the clinician modeled calm, voluntary stuttering with good eye contact, which was ended in a slow, relaxed way. The children were instructed in how to pretend to stutter calmly and then release the word in a slow and relaxed manner. Following this, games and activities were planned with carefully administered rewards for stuttering, whether real or pretend, that approximated the model.

Contact with both children's families also seemed to be important. In establishing and maintaining this contact, it was necessary to balance each child's need for independence with his need for an understanding and supportive home environment. In Adam's case, he quickly resisted plans to have his parents monitor and reinforce his fluency skills at home. We needed to let Adam decide when and how to involve his parents, such as when he let his mother come to school for his "show and tell" about stuttering, and when he decided to bring home videotapes that he had made. For Bob, an initial attempt, after the diagnostic evaluation, to have his parents make changes in how they interacted with him on their own was not successful in reducing his stuttering. Instead, as Bob progressed in therapy, we intermittently brought his parents and sisters into sessions for role playing and for highly structured tasks involving particular fluency skills. Nonetheless, we also followed his lead in making therapy something that was special for him, an island of support away from his family.

I will now integrate my previous experience with children who stutter with the insights I gained from working with these two children whose emotions related to stuttering were strong. The following suggests an approach for school-aged children at the intermediate level of stuttering development. I think it may be most suitable for those children whose stuttering has produced avoidance and shame, but I will also indicate what might be appropriate for children who do not seem to be so emotionally affected by their stuttering.

GENERAL RECOMMENDATIONS FOR PROCEDURES

Begin with a Focus on the Child, Not on Stuttering

1. Talk with the child about his or her interests; engage in activities that allow talking but do not necessarily require it; be an empathic listener for the child's talking (cf., Starkweather, 1994).[6]
2. Share and examine the child's stuttering with him or her. Begin this by asking about experiences of getting stuck on words with different people and in different places. Keep the questions low key and be prepared to move from these topics to activities not focused on stuttering if the child seems uncomfortable. Don't be afraid to make therapy fun for you and for your young client.

At a pace comfortable for the child and the clinician, help the child to talk about listener reactions, the child's feelings about people's reactions, and the experience of "being stuck." At some point, have the child explore what he or she is doing when stuttering. Show matter-of-factness and acceptance of the stuttering. Have the child teach you to emulate his or her stuttering. Assess how much shame and avoidance the child feels by observing the child's attitude in talking about stuttering (observe body language, including eye contact). If a child expresses shame and avoidance, including off-task behavior, plan to work on self-esteem.

Therapy Procedures

1. **Fluency shaping**. *Begin here with children who show considerable shame and avoidance about their stuttering.*

Establishment—in words
   a. easy onset of phonation
   b. stretching of vowels and consonants (slow overall rate)

---

[6]Starkweather's description of "listening therapy" is an excellent tutorial on how to tune in to a child and help him or her develop confidence in his or her communication abilities.

c. "proprioceptive" awareness of speech movements

Transfer

a. use game formats and reinforcements to develop fluency in gradually more complex contexts, from phrases to conversation with the clinician
b. continue format and reinforcements, as parents, siblings, peers are brought into the treatment setting
c. use various formats and fade reinforcements as a child practices fluency in a variety of settings and with a variety of listeners.

2. **Stuttering Modification, with real and voluntary stuttering.** *Begin here with children who do not show shame and avoidance about their stuttering and with those children who have had Fluency Shaping but have residual stuttering in transfer.*

Establishment—In therapy room, in conversation, in various game formats and with reinforcement

a. stuttering slowly, without hurry or tension
b. stuttering with slow, relaxed, fluent endings ("slideout")
c. hold onto stutter longer than needed
d. "play" with stutter before releasing
e. with all of the above, use good eye contact and work for overall comfort and effective communication style

Transfer

a. use reinforcements, which are gradually faded
b. teach the child a variety of ways in which to be open about stuttering, including humor about stuttering, sharing with classmates, appropriate comments in difficult speaking situations
c. use hierarchy, going from structured situations in the therapy setting with parents, siblings, and others to natural settings such as classroom and home
d. teach child about good overall communications skills

General Guidelines

1. Help the child gain a sense of mastery and control, not only over stuttering, but over other aspects of life as well.
2. With both fluency shaping and stuttering modification, help the child become appropriately open about stuttering. This reduces the tendency to avoid or withdraw from anticipated difficult speaking situations.
3. If a child is being teased or has been teased, work on developing responses to teasing. Use role playing and discussion to help the child develop unique and natural responses.
4. Help the child build self-esteem by developing areas in which he or she can excel.
5. If a child appears to be susceptible to stress and excitement, assume there will be relapses and prepare both the child and parents for this. Help such children develop responses to stress, such as slowing the rate of speech. If a child learns to slow his or her overall speech rate during times of anxiety and stress, this may function as a form of self-calming that turns down the "gain" of a hyper-excitable nervous system.

Assessment Criteria

Over the past five years, the criteria for successful outcomes of stuttering therapy have changed. Formerly, clinicians measured outcomes in terms of stuttering frequency and severity (e.g., Guitar & Bass, 1978). Many clinicians, myself included, now believe that children who stutter should, above all, gain from therapy an increased ability to communicate (e.g., Conture & Guitar, 1993; Starkweather, 1993). Reductions in stuttering frequency and severity are usually an important waystation in a child's journey toward improved communication. Such reductions are probably not effective, however, if they are achieved at the expense of naturalness and spontaneity. If children reduce their stuttering by using, for example, an abnormally slow speaking pattern, or one that requires a great deal of conscious attention, communication is usually not improved. Successful therapy should free children to talk spontaneously when and where and how they want.

Formal measures of stuttering that may be used as the child progresses toward more effective communication may include percentage of syllables stuttered and syllables spoken per minute (Andrews & Ingham, 1971), the *Stuttering Severity Index* (Riley, 1972), and two assessments of communication attitudes—the A-19 Scale (Guitar & Grims, 1977) and the Children's Attitude Test (Brutten & Dunham, 1989). All of these measures are described in more detail in Peters and Guitar (1991).

Informal assessments of children's communication abilities include parents' and teachers' reports of how well the children are communicating with others. A child's own report of progress can be extremely valuable, as well. I also try to evaluate children's willingness to stutter voluntarily, as an informal measure of their fear of stuttering. I try to assess, by observation and report, the child's success at using various means of managing stuttering (e.g., use of slideouts) with parents, classmates, and strangers.

When children have learned fluency management techniques, such as slowing overall speech rate, beginning voicing of words gently, and ending stutters slowly and loosely, I begin generalization activities and assess the extent to which these techniques are used outside the clinical setting. If a child is not succeeding at generalizing these techniques, I work with teachers, parents, and the child to create environments that are more conducive to generalization. This involves the techniques that were described earlier with Adam and Bob to decrease their fear of stuttering, to be open about their stuttering, and to make the class and the home comfortable for working on speech.

If children stop making progress, I become mildly concerned. If they also miss sessions or tell me they don't want to come to therapy, I consider two possible courses of action. The first is to change therapy so that it meets the child's needs at the moment. This may be more direct teaching of fluency techniques, if I was working indirectly. Or, it may be to make therapy less direct if I feel that I am pacing therapy too quickly for the child. A second course of action is to give the child a vacation from therapy. Children older than 4 or 5 years of age who demonstrate repeatedly that they don't want therapy should be allowed to wait until they are ready to begin again. However, if they are failing, as well, to make satisfactory progress in school, aren't connecting with peers, or appear to be unhappy and under stress, I consider referral. I discuss this issue at length with the child's parents and sometimes refer the family for counseling with a psychiatrist or psychologist with whose work I am familiar.

Support of Procedures

The procedures I have described are based on therapies developed by Van Riper (1973), Dell (1979), Ryan and Van Kirk Ryan (1983), among others. The specific combinations of these approaches that were described have not been tested, except as reported here. I presented support for the efficacy of these procedures, when used in their "pure" or uncombined form, in a paper prepared for the NINCD Workshop on Treatment Efficacy Research in Stuttering, published in the *Journal of Fluency Disorders* (Conture & Guitar, 1993). In particular, the studies of Ryan and Van Kirk Ryan (1983) and Peters (1991), which were cited in this report, suggest that these therapies can be effective in reducing stuttering, and in some cases, by a considerable amount. No information on the children's improvement in overall communication is available from these studies.

Future studies are needed to assess the extent to which therapy carried out in school or clinic settings by a qualified clinician improves the communicative freedom and competence of children who stutter. In addition, studies are needed to parse out which components of the treatment procedures used are effective for which children. More details on these and other research needs related to the assessment of therapeutic efficacy are available in the report by Conture and Guitar (1993).

SUMMARY

I will conclude by touching on two themes that I think are important. One is the extent to which the techniques of therapy are important, and the other is the applicability of the techniques described here to most children who stutter.

The approach I have described in this chapter has allowed me to help a number of children who stutter gain greater freedom in their communication. However, even though an approach may be effective for a particular clinician, this does not mean it will be effective for another. Clinicians differ in their personal styles, and each needs to find a suitable approach. I am reminded of the time that I wrote Van Riper about the effectiveness of the prolonged speech treatment we were using in Australia; he remarked, "A good clinician can use almost any approach, even patting the client's rear end, and get good results." Thus, I believe that we need to explore not only the techniques that appear to be effective—because these may be only one part of the treatment package—but the needs of various clients for particular attributes of clinicians' personalities and styles.

The therapy I have described was used with two children who were unusually sensitive to their stuttering, and therapy went on for a matter of years, not weeks or months. How applicable is this approach to the "garden-variety" child who stutters? I believe that most children who need treatment for stuttering have negative emotions tangled up with their disfluency. After all, most of those who need help will have been stuttering for more than a year (Andrews, 1984) and have continued to "struggle or avoid because of frustration or penalties" (Van Riper, 1990). These children, then, are reacting emotionally to their stuttering and to their listeners' responses. Frustration, fear, and shame are among the emotions clinicians must deal with, directly or indirectly. Some children will need only a little work on emotions, and most of that can be a by-product of helping them to change their speaking behaviors. Others will need substantial help reducing their emotional responses to their stuttering and may not be able to make clinically meaningful progress until their feelings of frustration, fear, and shame are reduced.

REFERENCES

Andrews, G. (1984). Epidemiology of stuttering. In R. Curlee & W. Perkins (Eds.), *Nature and treatment of stuttering: New directions*. San Diego: College-Hill Press.

Andrews, G., & Ingham, R.J. (1971). Stuttering: Considerations in the evaluation of treatment. *British Journal of Communications Disorders, 6*, 129–138.

Bloodstein, O. (1995). *A handbook on stuttering*. San Diego: Singular Publishing Group.

Brutten, G.J., & Dunham, S. (1989). The Communication Attitude Test: A normative study of grade school children. *Journal of Fluency Disorders, 14*, 371–377.

Calkins, S.D., & Fox, N.A. (1994). Individual differences in the biological aspects of temperament. In J.E. Bates & T.D. Wachs (Eds.), *Temperament: Individual differences at the interface of biology and behavior*. Washington, D.C.: American Psychological Association.

Conture, E. (1991). Young stutterers' speech production: A critical review. In H. Peters, W. Hulstijn, & C.W.

Starkweather (Eds.), *Speech motor control and stuttering*. New York: Excerpta Medica.

Conture, E., & Guitar, B. (1993). Evaluating efficacy of treatment of stuttering: School-age children. *Journal of Fluency Disorders, 18*, 253–287.

Costello, J.M. (1983). Current behavioral treatments for children. In D. Prins & R.J. Ingham (Eds.), *Stuttering in early childhood: Treatment methods and issues*. San Diego: College-Hill Press.

Dell, C. (1979). *Treating the school age stutterer: A guide for clinicians*. Memphis: Speech Foundation of America.

Dell, C. (1993). Treating school-age stutterers. In R. Curlee (Ed.), *Stuttering and related disorders of fluency*, New York: Thieme Medical Publishers.

Gray, J. (1987). *The psychology of fear and stress* (2nd Ed.). Cambridge: Cambridge University Press.

Guitar, B., & Bass, C. (1978). Stuttering therapy: The relation between attitude change and long-term outcome. *Journal of Speech and Hearing Disorders, 43*, 392–400.

Guitar, B., & Grims, S. (1977). Developing a scale to assess communication attitudes in children who stutter. Poster session presented at the American Speech-Language-Hearing Association Convention, Atlanta, November.

Guitar, B., & Peters, T. (In preparation). *Stuttering: An integrated approach to its nature and treatment* (2nd Ed.). Baltimore: Williams & Wilkins.

Humphrey, D.R., & Reed, D.J. (1983). Separate cortical systems for control of joint movement and joint stiffness: Reciprocal activation and coactivation of antagonist muscles. In J.E. Desmedt (Ed.), *Motor control mechanisms in health and disease*, New York: Raven Press.

Kagan, J., Reznick, J.S., & Snidman, N. (1987). The physiology and psychology of behavioral inhibition in children. *Child Development, 58*, 1459–1473.

Martin, R.R. (1981). Introduction and perspective: Review of published studies. In E. Boberg (Ed.), *Maintenance of fluency: Proceedings of the Banff conference*. New York: Elsevier North-Holland.

Mineka, S. (1985). Animal models of anxiety-based disorders: Their usefulness and limitations. In A.H. Tuma & J. Mase (Eds.), *Anxiety and the anxiety disorders*. Hillsdale, N.J.: Lawrence Erlbaum Associates.

Moore, W.H. (1993). Hemispheric processing research (and discussion following paper). In E. Boberg (Ed.), *Neuropsychology of stuttering*. Edmonton: University of Alberta Press.

Peters, T., & Guitar, B. (1994). *Stuttering: An integrated approach to its nature and treatment*. Baltimore: Williams & Wilkins.

Riley, G. (1972). A stuttering severity instrument for children and adults. *Journal of Speech and Hearing Disorders, 37*, 314–322.

Ryan, B.P., & Van Kirk Ryan, B. (1983). Programmed stuttering therapy for children: Comparison of four establishment programs. *Journal of Fluency Disorders, 8*, 291–321.

Starkweather, C.W. (1993). Issues in the efficacy of treatment for fluency disorders. In *Journal of Fluency Disorders, 18*, 151–168.

Starkweather, C.W. (1994). Working with school-age children and adults. *Logopedie en Foniatrie, 9*, 242–253.

Van Riper, C. (1973). *The treatment of stuttering*. Englewood Cliffs, N.J.: Prentice Hall.

Van Riper, C. (1990). Final thoughts about stuttering. *Journal of Fluency Disorders, 15*, 317–318.

SUGGESTED READINGS

Conture, E., & Guitar B. (1993). Evaluating efficacy of treatment of stuttering: School-age children. *Journal of Fluency Disorders, 18*, 253–287. This article discusses some important aspects of measuring the effectiveness of treatment of stuttering. It contains a review of treatment programs that have reported on their long- and short-term outcome.

Costello, J.M. (1983). Current behavioral treatments for children. In D. Prins & R.J. Ingham (Eds.), *Stuttering in early childhood: Treatment methods and issues*. San Diego: College-Hill Press, and Costello, J. (1984). Treatment of the young chronic stutterer: Managing fluency. In R. Curlee & W. Perkins (Eds.), *Nature and treatment of stuttering: New directions*. San Diego: College-Hill Press. These are accounts of fluency shaping with children who stutter. Both give an overview and general recommendations. The first citation also includes a complete version of Costello's program. Compare with Ryan, below.

Dell, C. (1979). *Treating the school age stutterer: A guide for clinicians*. Memphis: Speech Foundation of America, and Dell, C. (1993). Treating school-age stutterers. In R. Curlee (Ed.), *Stuttering and related disorders of fluency*, New York: Thieme Medical Publishers. These two resources present Dell's approaches to therapy with children. Both provide detailed accounts of an excellent stuttering modification treatment.

Guitar, B., & Reville, J. (1996). *Easy talker*. San Antonio: Communication Skill Builders. This is a workbook for young children who stutter. It takes the child and clinician through a program of stuttering therapy aimed at cognitive, behavioral, and emotional aspects of the problem. The therapy presented is similar to the approach described here, but it is given in greater detail.

Ryan, B.P. (1984). Treatment of stuttering in school children. In W.H. Perkins (Ed.), *Stuttering disorders*, New York: Thieme-Stratton. This describes a fluency shaping therapy for children written by an individual who pioneered the approach. Compare with Costello, cited above.

CHAPTER 15

CLINICAL MANAGEMENT OF CHILDREN: DIRECT MANAGEMENT STRATEGIES

PETER R. RAMIG
ELLEN M. BENNETT

INTRODUCTION AND PURPOSE

Treatment of preschool and elementary school-aged children who stutter has historically focused on either indirect, direct, or combined indirect/direct therapy orientations. This chapter will emphasize direct intervention ideas for children 7 to 12 years old. (Indirect and combined direct/indirect intervention approaches are covered elsewhere in this book and will not be revisited here.) Depending on the frequency, type, and severity of stuttering behaviors, and a child's reaction thereto, many of the intervention strategies discussed in this chapter may apply to some younger and older children as well. In general, however, we feel our treatment emphasis is best suited for children in the 7 to 12 year age range. We first introduce several examples of published therapy programs and other structured intervention approaches. Next, we identify components of the therapy process that allow for tailoring or customizing of treatment to accommodate individual differences in stuttering patterns, personality, reactions to stuttering, and concomitant speech and language problems. For each component presented, rationale and research are offered to support its use. Finally, we discuss how these components may be implemented with children who stutter.

DESCRIPTION OF APPROACHES

Intervention may be approached from three general directions: direct, indirect, and an integration of direct/indirect. Although this chapter focuses on direct approaches to stuttering intervention, a brief discussion of these other approaches will provide a clearer understanding of our emphasis. For example, Van Riper (1973), who was an advocate of direct intervention with children, described the indirect approach as follows:

> *Treatment tends to be very indirect and to be focused primarily on removing or reducing the stressful conditions which presumably precipitate the disfluency. Its major rationale is preventative, the therapists generally seeking to keep the child from developing awareness of stuttering or fears of speaking so that the disorder will not progress. Many workers, for example, feel that all their effort should be concentrated on altering parental attitudes, the family milieu and the conditions of communicative stress, with absolutely no interaction with the child himself (p. 372).*

Thus, the emphasis of this form of treatment is not directly with the child but with changes that are recommended to persons in the child's environment and with environmental circumstances that may be sources of stress in the life of the child. The indirect approach to treating children who stutter was influenced by Johnson's view that parents' reactions to normal disfluent speech may cause stuttering, or if stuttering exists, can exacerbate the problem (Johnson, 1955; Johnson & Associates, 1959). Generally, then, interruptions in the child's speech may become a problem if parents and others view it as such and may occur as a consequence of increased attention to the child's speech.

Examples of direct intervention approaches include those developed by Cooper and Cooper (1985), Conture (1990), Meyers and Woodford (1992), Preobrajenskaya (1953), and Shine (1980). As described by Conture (1990), direct treatment of stuttering:

> involves explicit, overt, and direct attempts to modify the child's speech and related behavior. Parents may still be involved but not to the same degree as with the indirect approach. Directly talking to the child about his or her talking, the "bad" as well as "good" parts, is often part of a direct approach (p. 94).

A third treatment option is a combination of indirect and direct intervention strategies such as those reported by Peters and Guitar (1991), Ramig and Bennett (1995), and Ramig and Wallace (1987).

ASSESSMENT

Assessment is a crucial first step to developing the most appropriate intervention plan for a disfluent child. We encourage readers to refer to the chapter by Conture, in this text, for an overview of an assessment protocol that we endorse, as well as the writings on assessment by Adams (1991), Gregory and Hill (1993), Riley (1984), Rustin and Cook (1983), and Wall and Myers (1995). Table 15.1 presents a sampling of assessment procedures currently on the market and a checklist of assessment components that clinicians may be interested in considering or evaluating during the diagnostic process. Individual clinicians, depending upon their clinical style and needs of the child, usually implement these assessment procedures with

whatever variations seem needed. Information reported in test manuals and instruction booklets was used to compile this table.

BASIC TENETS IN WORKING WITH CHILDREN WHO STUTTER

The majority of children who stutter become aware of interruptions in the forward flow of speech early in their experience with stuttering. As awareness and concern grow, complicating avoidance and struggle reactions may develop (Van Riper, 1973). Once reactions to stuttering are evident, we advocate direct intervention. Before discussing the therapy process, there are several principles which, in our opinion, should guide the management of children who stutter.

1. The clinician should have at least a basic understanding of the onset, phenomenology, and treatment of stuttering in children.
2. The clinician should be caring, sensitive, and empathetic.
3. The clinician should allow, encourage, and reinforce the child's expression of feelings with regards to stuttering.
4. Treatment plans should be highly flexible and designed to meet each child's changing needs.
5. The clinician should emphasize positive reinforcement over punitive techniques or consequences for stuttering.
6. The clinician should educate and involve parents and teachers in the therapy process whenever possible.

The reader is referred to Conture and Schwartz (1984), Conture (1990), Gregory (1991), Gregory and Hill (1993), Kelly (1993), Kelly and Conture (1991), Mallard (1991), Perkins (1992), Ramig (1993), Ramig and Bennett (1995), Riley and Riley (1983), Rustin (1987a), and Zebrowski and Schum (1993) for information on parents and stuttering.

With these principles in mind, we will outline and describe intervention strategies that we use when treating some school-aged children who stutter. We say "some" because our suggestions do

TABLE 15.1   Checklist of Assessment Instruments for Stuttering

	SYSTEMATIC FLUENCY ASSESSMENT	STUTTERING PREDICTION INSTRUMENT	STUTTERING SEVERITY INSTRUMENT	COOPER PERSONALIZED FLUENCY CONTROL THERAPY	ASSESSMENT OF FLUENCY IN SCHOOL CHILDREN	SYSTEMATIC DISFLUENCY ANALYSIS	STUTTERING DISFLUENCY ANALYSIS	THE FLUENCY DEVELOPMENT SYSTEM	ASSESSMENT PROGRAM FOR DYSFLUENT CHILDREN
Age Prescribed for:	3–9	2–9	Children-Adults	Children-Adults	Any	Any	3–9	2–9	
Administration/Analysis Time	2.5	?	?	?	3+	4+		?	2–2.5
Manual Provided	♦	♦	♦	♦	♦	♦	♦	♦	♦
Case History Obtained	♦	♦		♦	♦	♦	♦	♦	♦
Audio Recording Required	♦	♦	♦	♦	♦	♦	♦	♦	♦
Video Recording Required						♦		♦	
Verbatim Transcription Required	♦				♦	♦	?	♦	
Number of Samples Obtained	2+	1+	2+	3+	3+	3+	1+	2+	
Monologue Sample Analyzed	♦	♦	♦	♦	♦	♦			
Dialogue Sample Analyzed	♦	♦		♦	♦	♦	♦		
Parent-Child Interaction		□				♦	♦	♦	
Reading Sample Obtained	♦		♦	♦	♦	♦	♦		
Rate of Speech Calculation	♦				♦	□	□	♦	
Duration Measures		♦	♦	♦		♦	♦	♦	
Percentage of Stuttered Words	♦	♦	♦	♦	♦	♦	♦		♦
Percentage Stuttered Syllables	♦			♦		♦		♦	♦
Stuttered Words Per Minute	♦								
Stuttered Syllables Per Minute	♦							♦	
Physiological Factors	♦				♦				
Secondary Behaviors	♦	♦	♦	♦	♦	♦	♦		♦
Attitudes	□	□		♦	♦	○	♦		♦
Personality Factors									♦
Severity Ratings	○	♦	♦	♦		♦	○		♦
Language Factors	♦				♦	♦		♦	
Parent Interview	♦	♦			♦	♦		♦	♦
Teacher Interview				♦	♦	♦	♦	♦	♦
Client Self-Evaluation				♦	♦	○			
Therapy—IEP Information Included	♦			♦	♦	♦	♦	♦	♦
Normative Data Available	?	♦	♦	♦	?	?	♦	?	?

Nine assessment instruments are described according to 29 components that may be considered when choosing an assessment tool. ♦ represents components incorporated in the assessment instrument. ○ indicates that the feature is obtained from other tools and included in the particular instrument. □ denotes items that are indirectly assessed. ? means not indicated in manual. This form is meant to used as a guide during the assessment process. Each instrument may be utilized differently depending upon clinician style and training. The reader is referred to the manuals of these instruments for more details on their procedures.

not apply to all children who stutter. These strategies apply primarily to 7- to 12-year-old children who are displaying a level of stuttering that they are reacting to with frustration, fear, and embarrassment. In most cases, such children are exhibiting one or more vocal/nonvocal, secondary/accessory behaviors as they attempt to avoid or release themselves from the stuttering moment.

INTERVENTION DIRECTIONS

For those readers interested in learning about programmed or general approaches to direct treatment of stuttering, we listed examples of easy-to-use stuttering intervention programs or kits in Table 15.1. These tools provide clinicians a way to begin intervention with specific instructions for assessment through treatment. Most are fluency-shaping approaches wherein a child's fluency is systematically increased until fluency replaces stuttering. The majority increase fluency through fluency-enhancing speaking patterns or modes. Typically, they do not teach control of stuttering, nor do they examine feelings and attitudes. In contrast, clinicians using stuttering modification approaches teach the child to change the form of stuttering in order to reduce stuttering severity, stress elimination of avoidance behaviors, and emphasize reduction of negative feelings and attitudes (Peters & Guitar, 1991). Regardless of the approach used, sensitivity and understanding are essential in dealing with the child's feelings about stuttering and the impact of those feelings on the child's life. Although such issues usually arise in children who display more involved stuttering, they may be less important, or even not an issue, for many younger children exhibiting less involved stuttering.

There are three general paradigms to follow when planning an intervention program for children who stutter: (1) programmed, (2) general or structured, or (3) tailored instruction, which we prefer. Several programs or kits provide step-by-step, easy-to-use activities. Other structured approaches can be found in books, chapters, or professional journals. The majority include worksheets, materials, and record keeping forms. Programmed instruction can help clinicians develop competence and skill in stuttering therapy, and even experienced clinicians may find these approaches helpful when designing treatment plans. Many programs are also applicable to children younger and older than those targeted in this chapter.

Published Programs/Kits

Systematic Fluency Training for Young Children (Shine, 1980) is a highly structured program. It was developed for children from ages 3 to 9 years and includes both assessment and intervention activities. Shine's program follows a fluency-shaping model that includes four major activities: (1) picture identification, (2) storybook, (3) picture matching, and (4) surprise box. It was designed for use in individual therapy, provides step-by-step procedures with reinforcement schedules, and employs linguistic considerations to task sequencing. Parent, sibling, and peer participation in the program is strongly emphasized.

Personalized Fluency Control Therapy (PFC) (Cooper & Cooper, 1985) was designed as a direct, integrated approach to working with children who stutter. It incorporates the use of "FIGs" (fluency-initiating gestures) in fluency training and provides several visual aids ("My Stuttering Apple" and "My Fig Tree") to help children identify characteristics of their stuttered speech and develop coping strategies to handle it. Practice worksheets and structured activities make this a workable program for school clinicians. PFC proceeds through four stages of therapy: (1) Identification and structuring, (2) examination and confrontation, (3) cognition and behavior orientation, and (4) fluency control. The program can also be modified to assist both younger and older school-aged children who stutter in either individual or group settings. Counseling activities are an additional feature of the PFC program.

The *Stuttering Intervention Program* (SIP) (Pindzola, 1987) was developed for dysfluent children from age 3 to grade 3. It includes assessment procedures, parent counseling and training information, a direct fluency shaping intervention program with formatted individualized educational plans, and teacher/parent handouts. Its individual therapy approach incorporates significant others through counseling activities. Linguistic complexity of speaking tasks is controlled and manipulated throughout the program. Pindzola's protocol for differentiating between incipient stuttering and normal nonfluencies is useful and can assist speech-language pathologists in determining a child's eligibility for services.

The Fluency Development System for Young Children (*TFDS*)(Meyers & Woodford, 1992) is a cognitive, fluency-shaping approach for establishing fluent speech production in children up to age 9. Procedures for assessment and intervention are comprehensive, yet easy to follow. Child-centered activities teach the following "fluency rules": (1) Slow versus fast speech concept; (2) smooth versus bumpy speech concept; and (3) turn-taking concepts. These activities incorporate a multi-sensory dimension to treatment, with tactile, motoric, visual, and auditory modalities integrated into therapy tasks to enhance a child's conceptual understanding of the "rules" necessary for fluency development. Dealing with time-pressure, desensitizing difficult speaking situations, and parent education are additional components of this program. Along with materials and task rationales, TFDS provides a flexible, conceptually based paradigm that can be used in either individual or group settings.

Easy Does It-2 (Heinze & Johnson, 1987) approaches therapy with an eclectic combination of stuttering modification and fluency shaping principles for ages 7 through 13 years. Preparing for fluency, distinguishing fluency from stuttering, establishing fluency, desensitizing a child to fluency disrupters, transferring fluency, and maintaining fluency comprise its six phases. In addition, attitudes toward speech and teaching responsibility for improvement are inherent in its philosophy. *Easy Does It-2* provides well-defined activities as well as all of the materials that are needed.

General/Structured Approaches

Ryan's (1979) programmed approach is based on a behavioral, fluency shaping model and the philosophy that stuttering is a learned behavior. The program consists of four management components: (1) programmed traditional, (2) delayed auditory feedback, (3) punishment, and (4) *Gradual Increase in Length and Complexity of Utterance* (*GILCU*). Ryan recommends that the GILCU program component be implemented with younger children having less severe stuttering. Using operant conditioning principles, Ryan targets the production of fluent speech during three phases of therapy: (1) establishment, (2) transfer, and (3) maintenance. Reinforcement schedules and step-by-step instructions are prominent features of this approach to individual therapy.

Costello (1983) developed a fluency shaping program that includes operant learning principles and controlled linguistic complexity. The *Extended Length of Utterance* (*ELU*) program provides structure to therapy and can be used with all ages, but Costello (1983) states that it is particularly useful for children to establish fluent speech. Like the GILCU program, reinforcement schedules and a clearly defined sequence of treatment tasks are used for establishing fluency. In addition, J. Ingham (1993) incorporates parents and significant others in therapy sessions to facilitate fluency generalization, but transfer and maintenance components are not specifically addressed in ELU.

Gregory (1991) discusses a fluency-shaping program for use with school-aged children who stutter. Although known for the "speak more fluently, stutter more fluently" approach, Gregory emphasizes the use of easy, more relaxed speech production initially and, if necessary, addresses any remaining stuttering behaviors. His *Easy Relaxed Approach-Smooth Movement* (*ERA-SM*) fluency shaping procedure of easy initiation of phonation and smooth movements is characterized by a smooth, slower than normal transition on the first two sounds of a word or utterance. Rate, intensity, and inflection remain normal throughout the utterance. Included in this approach are the use

TABLE 15.2 Program Considerations: A Checklist for Comparing Intervention Components

	Published Programs/Kits						General Approaches Reported in the Literature			
	SYSTEMATIC FLUENCY TRAINING SYSTEM	PERSONALIZED FLUENCY CONTROL THERAPY	STUTTERING INTERVENTION PROGRAM PROTOCOL	THE FLUENCY DEVELOPMENT SYSTEM	ASSESSMENT PROGRAM FOR DYSFLUENT CHILDREN	EASY DOES IT-2	GRADUAL INCREASE IN LENGTH AND COMPLEXITY OF UTTERANCE	EXTENDED LENGTH OF UTTERANCE	EASY RELAXED APPROACH-SMOOTH MOVEMENT	FLUENCY RULES PROGRAM
Age Prescribed for:	3–9	All	3–9	2–9	All	7+	All	All	All	7+
Fluency Shaping Approach	●		●	●	●		●	●		
Stuttering Modification Approach					◻					
Integrated Approach		●				●			●	●
Manual Provided	●	●	●	●	●	●				
Materials Provided	●	●	●	●		●				
Clear Definitions and Rationales	●	●	●	●	●	●	●	●	●	●
Type-Token Reinforcement	●	◻	●				●	●	●	
Guided, Step-by-Step Instruction	●	◻	●	◻	●	●	●	●		
Flexible		●	◻	●		●			●	●
Intensive Orientation				◻	●		◻	◻		
Lesson Plans Provided	◻	●	●		●	◻	●	●		
Individual Instruction	●	●	●	●	●	●	●	●	●	●
Group Instruction		●		●	●	●			●	●
Conceptually Based	◻	●	●	●	◻	◻			◻	●
Language/Linguistic Considerations	●	◻	●	●	○	◻	●	●	●	◻
Significant Others Included	●	◻	●	●	●	◻			●	●
Counseling Components Included	◻	●	●	●	●	◻			●	
Transfer Activities Included	◻	●			●	◻	●	◻	○	●
Maintenance Addressed						●	●		◻	
Efficacy Information Available	○	○	◻	○			○	○		○

Published programs/kits/general approaches are described according to certain intervention features.

● represents features that are included in the manual or literature on the individual program.

◻ represents features that are covered to some extent in the particular program.

○ indicates that efficacy data are available either in the manual or research literature.

of behavioral terminology, learning theory principles, and a variable lesson plan format that systematically individualizes the therapy program for each child (Gregory, 1989). This approach can be easily implemented in both group and individual sessions. Transfer and maintenance issues are addressed through manipulation of treatment variables as outlined in the lesson plan format.

The *Fluency Rules Program* (*FRP*) (Runyan & Runyan, 1993) is a fluency-shaping therapy program, having some behavior modification principles, that was designed specifically for implementation in the school environment. The FRP consists of seven rules for fluent speech production: (1) speak slowly, (2) use speech breathing, (3) touch the "speech helpers" together lightly, (4) use only the speech helpers to talk, (5) keep your speech helpers moving, (6) keep "Mr. Voice Box" running smoothly, and (7) say a word only once. It emphasizes teaching the language concepts necessary for implementing fluency rules in individual and group sessions. Self-monitoring and transfer are added components of this concept-based program.

Tailored/Customized Intervention

We believe that clinicians should feel comfortable working with children who stutter and that tailoring intervention affords the clinician more latitude, flexibility, and freedom of choice. There is a certain amount of creative artistry one feels in devising a specific, individualized treatment plan based on the needs of a specific child who stutters.

When designing a tailored intervention plan, the first step is documentation of the child's overt stuttering behaviors, negative feelings toward stuttering, and secondary or accessory behavior patterns. Obtaining an accurate picture of a child's stuttering patterns, in both quantitative and qualitative domains, facilitates understanding of specifically how the child interferes with the initiation or continuation of ongoing speech. It also allows the clinician to choose from the variety of components that best address the child's needs (see Figure 15.1).

Table 15.3 provides a list of speech behaviors and intervention components that may facilitate change in each. This table is meant to help clinicians in problem-solving ways to handle the various behaviors often exhibited by children who stutter. For example, if the child exhibits excessively long prolongations, the clinician may choose from among the following intervention components when designing the child's intervention plan: regulation and control of breathstream, discussion of normal speaking process, discussion of interference with this process, negative practice, voluntary stuttering, cancellations, pullouts and freezing, facilitation of awareness and monitoring, and transfer skills. This list is not exhaustive and strategies often vary in effectiveness across children, so there are other strategies a clinician may need to consider that are not on this list. It is important to note also that these components should be used discriminately—after having assessed a child's individual needs and characteristics and in light of the child's stuttering severity, age, and maturity level. The following section provides an overview of each intervention component, its rationale, research support, and a description of its strategy.

INTERVENTION COMPONENTS

Increased Length and Complexity

Establishing fluency through the systematic manipulation of linguistic complexity is a widely researched topic (e.g., J. Ingham, 1993; Peters & Guitar, 1991; Ryan, 1984). As the length and complexity of utterances increase, so does the likelihood that stuttering will occur in the speech of young children (Riley & Riley, 1983). This component can also be used in conjunction with a hierarchically based framework of fluency enhancing strategies, such as light articulatory contacts, decreased speaking rate, oral motor planning, and self monitoring. As the length and complexity of the child's utterances increase, the motor planning required to say these utterances also increases (Starkweather, 1987). The coordination of respiration, phonation, and articulation becomes increasingly complex and is accompanied by increased cognitive demands. Reducing

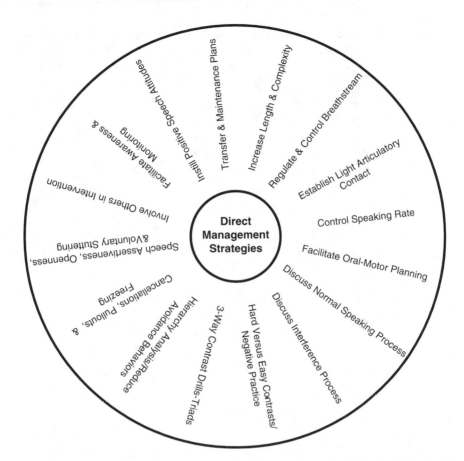

FIGURE 15.1   Direct management strategies that may be selected for inclusion in the treatment plans for children who stutter.

the demands placed on a child's overall speech production system is important when establishing fluency in the speech of children who stutter (Perkins, 1992; Ryan, 1984; Starkweather, 1987).

Conture (1990) recommends an intervention paradigm that moves from simple to complex along a continuum of speech behaviors, for example, beginning intervention at the one-word level and shaping fluency as the length and complexity of responses increase. However, the clinician needs to be aware that the increases in length of utterances do not necessarily produce equivalent increases in complexity (Bernstein Ratner & Sih, 1987). Even at the one-word level, there is a difference in language complexity between repeating numbers and naming an opposite or filling in the blank. After mastery of several single word tasks, the clinician advances through phrase, sentence, multi-sentence, story, conversational levels, and so on. At each level, the clinician needs to be cognizant of the demands placed on the child for both language generation and motor planning.

Regulation and Control of Breathstream

Respiratory management and adequate breath support are important variables to address with some children who stutter. Often, in response to stuttering, a child may develop aberrant breathing patterns in an effort to control speech. Behaviors such

TABLE 15.3   Tailoring Therapy: Intervention Components Selected to Address Observed Speech Behaviors

Observed Speech Behavior	INCREASE LENGTH AND COMPLEXITY	REGULATE AND CONTROL BREATHSTREAM	ESTABLISH LIGHT ARTICULATORY CONTACTS	CONTROL SPEAKING RATE	FACILITATE ORAL-MOTOR PLANNING	DISCUSS NORMAL SPEAKING PROCESS	DISCUSS INTERFERENCE WITH PROCESS	HARD VERSUS EASY CONTRASTS	NEGATIVE PRACTICE	3-WAY CONTRAST DRILLS-TRIADS	HIERARCHY ANALYSIS	SPEECH ASSERTIVENESS & OPENNESS	VOLUNTARY STUTTERING	CANCELLATIONS	PULLOUTS & FREEZING	REDUCE AVOIDANCE BEHAVIORS	FACILITATE AWARENESS & MONITORING	INSTILL POSITIVE SPEECH ATTITUDES	TRANSFER SKILLS	ESTABLISH MAINTENANCE PLAN	INVOLVE OTHERS IN INTERVENTION
Short, Tense Silent Blocks	*	*				*	*	*	*	*			*	*	*	*	*		*		
Excessively Long Prolongations	*					*	*	*	*					*	*		*		*		
Rapid, Tonic Repetitions			*	*		*	*	*	*	*			*	*	*		*		*		
Hard Glottal Attack		*					*	*	*	*				*	*		*		*		
Excessive Fillers and Interjections	*	*				*	*	*	*	*		*	*	*		*	*	*	*		
Distortion of Speech Signal																	*		*		
Quick, Shallow Inhalation	*	*	*	*	*	*		*								*	*		*		
Talking on Exhausted Breathstream	*		*	*	*	*		*									*		*		
Jaw Clenching		*				*	*	*	*	*	*			*			*		*		
Limited Articulatory Movement			*			*	*	*	*	*	*			*			*	*	*		
Negative Comments about Speech												*	*			*	*	*	*		*
Struggle Behaviors		*				*	*	*	*	*			*	*	*				*		
Situational Avoidances/Fear											*	*	*			*	*	*	*		*
Specific Sound or Word		*					*	*	*				*	*		*	*	*	*		
Highly Variable Stuttering	*	*	*									*		*			*		*	*	*
Anticipatory Posturing			*			*	*		*			*	*		*	*	*		*		
Excessive Hesitancies in Speech	*	*	*			*					*	*	*		*	*	*	*	*		
Choppy Quality to Speech	*	*	*	*		*	*							*	*	*	*		*	*	
Difficulty Comprehending Message	*			*	*	*													*	*	*
Limited Oral Expression	*					*	*				*	*				*	*	*	*		*
Expected Language Involvement	*		*	*	*	*	*			*						*	*	*	*		*

Tailored treatment can be achieved by identifying observed speech behaviors and the appropriate intervention component as indicated by the *. This list is not exhaustive and should be viewed as a possible list of components that might be included in therapy. These components have been described elsewhere by Ramig, Stewart, Ogrodnick, and Bennett, 1994.

as talking on exhausted breath, quick shallow inhalations, and talking on inhalatory cycles are sometimes noted. Adams (1980) stated that teaching breathstream management also maximizes a child's chances of competently executing intricate laryngeal behaviors.

Working directly on easy initiation of phonation or inserting easy, voluntary prolongations at the beginning of an utterance may be helpful in managing breathstream difficulties. Teaching children how normal speaking processes (respiration, phonation, and articulation) work together enhances their understanding of this communication breakdown, and Conture (1990), Peters and Guitar (1991), and Ramig and Bennett (1995) provide several age appropriate analogies for school-aged children.

Establishment of Light Articulatory Contacts

Some children who stutter seem to force and push sounds, which results in hard articulatory contacts, increased muscular tension, and impedance of airflow in the oral cavity (Cooper & Cooper, 1985; Gregory, 1991; Van Riper, 1973; Wall & Myers, 1995). In contrast, Peters and Guitar (1991) describe "soft contacts" as movements of the articulators (tongue, lips, jaw) that are slow, prolonged, and relaxed. Practicing light, soft, articulatory contacts provides a child with a way to reduce tension during stuttering moments, thereby facilitating smooth transitions in the production of speech.

Emphasizing the feeling of loose articulatory movements and smooth, continuous airflow can begin at the phoneme level and be incorporated into activities that follow a hierarchy of increased length and linguistic complexity. A useful tool in facilitating practice of light contacts is a delayed auditory feedback (DAF) unit, especially with some older children having more involved stuttering. Voluntary lengthening or prolonging the first syllable of a word requires mastery of soft articulatory contacts. Contrast drills are also helpful for increasing a child's awareness of hard versus soft contacts and for emphasizing kinesthetic awareness. For example, the child reads from a list of words, alternating between hard and soft productions, and is encouraged to feel the physical difference between these contacts. The clinician and child may then engage in a discussion of the differences in the mechanics of each type of speech.

Control of Speaking Rate

Implementation of a slowed speaking rate enhances the spacing and timing of articulatory movements, as well as the coordination and integration of the respiratory, phonatory, and articulatory systems for fluent speech production. Numerous researchers have reported that slowed speech production reduces stuttering (Gregory & Hill, 1980; Meyers & Woodford, 1992; Perkins, 1992; Runyan & Runyan, 1993; Wall & Myers, 1995). Perhaps, slowing speech rate affords the child time to make the adjustments necessary to produce synchronized, fluent speech (Wall & Myers, 1995).

Meyers and Woodford (1992) discuss several ways of building an understanding of slow versus fast movements for young children who stutter. Attaching a name, such as "Turtle Talk" or "Turtling," to slowed speech enhances utilization of this strategy. The clinician provides a continuous model of reduced speaking rate and body movements, allowing the child to see and hear its implementation. Emphasis is placed on smooth articulatory transitions, slightly prolonged consonants and vowels, and natural sounding intonation and stress patterns. Playing "Traffic Cop" with young children is another way of demonstrating the consequences of "going fast" versus "going slow." The child can issue tickets to people at home or in school when they "speed in their speech," thus increasing the child's awareness and sensitivity to speaking rate. Once again, delayed auditory feedback can be used with older school-aged children to facilitate practice and skill of speaking at a slower rate.

Facilitation of Oral-Motor Planning

Current research supports targeting oral motor planning and coordination for those children whose speech is characterized by reduced articulatory movement, reduced jaw opening, and increased velocity of movement. Riley and Riley (1986) use oral-motor planning activities in therapy, if indicated by diagnostic findings, and their research (1983) reveals that a high percentage (87%) of children who stutter also experience difficulty on oral-motor tasks. This, along with the high incidence of phonological disorders among children who stutter (Bloodstein, 1987; Louko, Edwards, & Conture, 1990; Wolk, Edwards, & Conture, 1993), may influence the development of fluency skills in this subgroup of stuttering children.

Therapy for oral-motor coordination may be divided into three areas: accuracy, smooth flow, and rate (Riley & Riley, 1985). Targeting each element separately, and gradually incorporating the three together, may enhance oral-motor skills. With increased awareness and slowed speaking rate, children may better execute their motor speech planning.

Normal Speaking Process Education

Direct intervention also involves helping children to understand what is necessary for initiating and maintaining smooth speech. Teaching a child the symbiotic, yet interactive, relationship among air flow, voicing, and articulation can be a helpful fluency enhancing strategy. Williams (1994) stressed the importance of a child's learning about the normal speaking process before therapy emphasizes how to achieve fluency. In the "Laying the Foundation of Knowledge" stage of the conceptual model "The House That Jack Built," Ramig and Bennett (1995) describe ways to help a child learn as much as possible about speech and the ingredients that make up fluent and nonfluent productions of speech. This learning process is also helpful in paving the way toward removing "the mystery of stuttering" for the school-aged child (Dell, 1993).

Active participation in conceptually based therapy activities helps to establish a knowledge-base that supports behavioral changes. Runyan and Runyan (1993), for example, use various analogies in their *Fluency Rules Program* that build the conceptual understanding necessary for positive speech change. The rules of "Start Mr.

Voice Box Running Smoothly" and "Touch the Speech Helpers Together Lightly" are two examples of how children may be educated. The school librarian is an excellent resource for anatomy books that children can utilize when learning about talking, and talking about talking provides an open atmosphere for children to communicate concerns about their speech.

Normal Speaking Process Interference Education

Closely related to the above component is helping children become aware of how certain of their behaviors interfere with the production of normal speech, and thereby result in stuttering. Williams (1994) eloquently explains to young clients how their blocking, repeating, and tense prolongations tend to disrupt an otherwise smoothly operating system. Many clinicians believe that children need to develop the language needed to describe their moments of stuttering in order to open the door for future discussion about stuttering (Conture, 1990; Dell, 1993; Ramig & Bennett, 1995; Williams, 1994). We believe that assisting children to understand how they interfere with fluent speech production is an important and necessary component of stuttering intervention, and identification plays an integral role. Bennett-Mancha (1992) talks about "clogs" (moments of stuttering) in the child's "pipes" (normal speaking process) and asks a child to experiment with various forms of "decloggers" (therapy techniques) that help to cope with the moment of stuttering. Similarly, Conture (1990) utilizes several analogies that assist children "by breaking the complex task of speaking down into terms and objects that make sense to them" (p. 127). The above references, of course, provide detailed discussions of these analogies.

Hard versus Easy Contacts/Desensitization

Apprehension and fear of stuttering may fuel avoidance of stuttering, people, situations, or specific words. Ham (1986) recommends that clinicians facilitate reduction of fear and anticipatory behaviors, and we believe that clinicians can lessen the impact of stuttering by helping to desensitize a child to feelings of shame, frustration, and embarrassment.

The desensitization process may be aided when a child practices pseudo- or voluntary stuttering in a supportive, accepting, and caring environment. Matter-of-fact practicing of hard contacts in learning to modify and confront stuttering is often helpful when combined with easier forms of voluntary stuttering. Producing a hard contact followed by an easy contact provides the child an opportunity to feel the differences between these two types of speech production patterns. As children develop an understanding of what "hard" feels like, they begin to realize what they are doing when they fear and avoid moments of stuttering. Van Riper (1973) said that an essential but difficult task is to help a child understand what to do differently during stuttering moments. Mass practice drills, in which children voluntarily stutter, help reduce the reaction cycle of stuttering. Ham (1986) recommends repeated exposure to stuttering in a variety of ways, one of which is exposure to what Van Riper called the "stuttering bath" (Bloodstein, 1993). This involves having children insert as much stuttering as possible into their speech during a predetermined period of time. Purposeful stuttering bombardment decreases a child's reactionary behavior toward stuttering and promotes better understandings of ways to change stuttering.

Negative Practice

Practicing undesired stuttering behaviors can help a child identify and learn how to change the moment of stuttering. Gregory (1989) described negative practice with two degrees of tension. A client is asked to stutter purposely on a word, then repeat the word, reducing tension about 50 percent. Emphasis is on feeling the contrast between the two tension levels and monitoring the sensations that both productions evoke. We have found that such "putting your stuttering out on the table" (Gregory, 1989) procedures are particularly applicable for children who are experiencing more involved stuttering.

One adaptation of negative practice drills for children uses an "energy conservation" analogy (Westbrook, 1990). Degrees of energy are equivalent to the level of tension in one's speech or the effort exerted while talking, and the clinician models words produced at various "levels of energy" (e.g., 25, 50, 75, and 100%). Westbrook relates that one of her clients associated these negative practice activities with the rationale for firedrills, you practice what to do when a fire occurs so that you can know what to do when a real fire happens. Through game-oriented activities, the child begins to "play around" with stuttering in a fun, supportive setting. This technique can be desensitizing, in addition to helping a child identify and modify stuttering.

Three-Way Triad Contrast Drills

Triad contrast drills (Ramig et al., 1994) provide mass practice in identifying and modifying hard stuttering and replacing hard with an easier form of stuttering. Van Riper (1973) recommended teaching a child to substitute a new pattern of easy stuttering for the old one with struggle, and Dell (1994) discussed ways of teaching the child that there are three ways of saying a word: the hard stuttering way, the easy stuttered way, and the fluent way. Triad drills follow the same principles. The child first produces a word in the "hard way," then without interruption, produces the word utilizing an easy repetition. The third part of the triad is an easy prolongation. This affords a gradual reduction in tension, improves desensitization, and allows the child to experiment with different forms of easy stuttering such as "bounces" and "slides" (repetitions and prolongations). Such exercises provide clients an opportunity to lessen negative, shame-based emotionality about stuttering that they previously have attempted to hide and avoid.

Hierarchy Analysis

Hierarchies in the therapy process involve the gradual ordering of the difficulty of speaking tasks or activities that must be completed prior to movement to the next stage (J. Ingham, 1993). We refer to hierarchy analysis as the process by which a child identifies easy versus hard speaking situations, people, and topics. Through careful problem solving, the client begins to practice various techniques in easy situations, working towards more difficult ones. The hierarchy structure may vary depending upon the technique being implemented. Particular situations or people may affect the child's ability to use various fluency enhancing strategies and stuttering modification techniques, and clinicians should be cognizant of individual differences among children who stutter (Peters & Guitar, 1991).

Speech Assertiveness and Openness

This component of therapy involves establishing assertive speech behaviors and openness about the disorder of stuttering. Concealment of stuttering—the desire to hide one's stuttering—is an important factor in its maintenance (e.g., Bennett, 1995; Murphy, 1994; Van Riper, 1973). If "stuttering cover-up" continues, interference in the therapy process is a likely outcome. Bennett (in press) noted that "this 'conspiracy of silence' may impact the individual's perception of the problem, exacerbating the motor-speech production, behavioral, and cognitive aspects of stuttering."

Assertiveness in response to teasing and talking with teachers, peers, and parents about stuttering may help to reduce the mystery of stuttering. Openly talking about stuttering with others, inserting easy forms of voluntary stuttering into one's speech, conducting a schoolwide survey on teacher awareness of stuttering, or even presenting a project on stuttering are just a few examples of ways that children can express openness about stuttering. The child who role-plays handling of teasing through assertive responses may have an easier time coping with the feelings of shame and embarrassment when teasing does occur. Murphy (1994) described "Let's Make a Movie" as a strategy for dealing with teasing and ridicule. This activity involves the following steps:

1. Discuss how teasing feels.
2. Discuss why people tease.
3. Consider how we react to teasing.
4. Develop simple scenarios.
5. Videotape scenarios.
6. Watch the scenarios with significant others.
7. Choose "best" one(s).
8. Continue rehearsal.

Murphy (1994) and Bennett (1995) believe that therapy should address stuttering in an open manner to help pave the way for better recovery. As children are able to understand what stuttering is and is not, their coping mechanisms may improve and reduce their adverse reactions to stuttering.

Voluntary Stuttering

The concept of open stuttering is one component of Sheehan's approach-avoidance conflict therapy model (1968). Sheehan advocated that adults practice easy, voluntary stuttering on nonfeared words throughout the day. An easy stutter is a "slide" or easy prolongation on the first sound of the word, with a smooth transition into the second sound. These tactics have also been applied in therapy for older school-aged children (Dell, 1993; Murphy, 1994; Ramig & Bennett, 1995). Dell (1993) reported that voluntary stuttering "reduces rate, and improves proprioceptive ability by getting the child to focus on articulatory movement" (pg. 66). By inserting the "real thing," anxiety is reduced, abnormal stuttering is replaced by easy stuttering, and openness is reinforced. Dell (1993) summarized the rationale for voluntary stuttering as follows: "They are exposing little bits of themselves in a manner that is both comfortable and socially tolerated" (pg. 66).

Typically, a child begins by practicing easy repetitions or prolongations on words and gradually moves up the linguistic hierarchy into conversation. At each step, the clinician reinforces the child's efforts. The clinician and child problem-solve the risks of using voluntary stuttering in various situations and with various people. Together, they come up with a list of opportunities for the child to be open and to insert stuttering into speech.

Gradually, the negative aspects of stuttering begin to be seen in a more positive light as the child experiences successes in openness. After each opportunity, the clinician and child discuss the behavioral, motor, and cognitive aspects of the experience, thereby setting the stage for the next successful openness task.

Cancellations

Van Riper (1973) developed this modification technique to help shape stuttering behavior. "Superficially considered, cancelling is very simple: Once the person emits a stuttered word, he simply pauses deliberately and then says it again before going on" (p. 319). The purpose behind this procedure is to learn a new response to stimuli that triggered the old response, and we have used this procedure with older children who stutter. Cancellations provide an opportunity to revisit the moment of stuttering and dissect its components so that change can occur. It helps clients to become more objectively aware of the features of the moment of stuttering, thus increasing their ability to modify or change their speech.

Drill activities (single word to reading level) are helpful in providing mass practice in cancellations. The clinician models the procedure and the child imitates, followed by a discussion of the cancellation experience. A clinician's caring and supportive attitude plays an important role during initial practice sessions. As a child becomes more familiar with the procedure, modeling is no longer necessary. We have children practice sets of words that begin with the same letter so that they can build up a sensory store of the feelings associated with changing hard stuttering into easy stuttering. Along with Nelson (1991), we feel strongly that children should focus on the feeling part of cancellation and not its auditory component.

Pullouts and Freezing

The skills mastered during cancellation practice enhance a child's ability to learn pullouts. Van Riper noted that "modifications of behavior learned through cancellations tend to move forward in time to manifest themselves during the period of the stuttering itself" (1973, p. 328). From this insight, he developed pullouts, which involve the modification of stuttering during its occurrence. Speakers have to catch themselves in a fluency failure and begin to modify it prior to its completion. These procedures have also been used with older children who stutter (Conture 1990; Dell, 1993; Peters & Guitar, 1991; Ramig & Bennett, 1995).

Again, drill activities are particularly useful during the initial teaching phase of pullouts. The clinician models a hard moment of stuttering, freezes on the moment, and slowly releases with an easy prolongation or repetition. The child then imitates this production. Dell (1993) discussed several ways of teaching a child how to change speech from hard to easy. Clinicians should gradually advance practice into conversational or more unstructured activities in which the child freezes during a moment of stuttering, then slowly releases out of it. The child and clinician then discuss this behavior, talking about "getting stuck and unstuck" (Bennett-Mancha, 1991). This activity empowers children to change as they begin to take charge of their speech and how they stutter.

Reduction of Avoidance Behaviors

If a child avoids stuttering, fear of stuttering often increases. To prevent the growth of stuttering, avoidances must be eliminated (Bloodstein, 1993; Peters & Guitar, 1991; Silverman, 1992). Bloodstein suggested that clients who think they are stutterers expect to stutter, and just the anticipation of stuttering can be enough to produce it.

Avoidance patterns need to be thoroughly investigated by the child, clinician, parent, and teacher. Together, a complete picture can be established prior to establishing a plan for gradually eliminating these behaviors. Characteristics of word and sound avoidances, as well as why the child feels it necessary to avoid, can be problem-solved. Through this process, a child needs to be made aware, in a nonthreatening manner, of the consequences of avoidance behaviors and how they interfere with fluency. Playing games in which the child or clinician inserts various interjections or starter devices, while one person "catches" the other, may assist the child in identifying such patterns. Once these behaviors have been identified, the child is ready to practice eliminating their use. Clients must become comfortable and feel safe with their stuttering through the use of voluntary stuttering, "triad" drills, and easy bounces and slides. As they confront stuttering openly and without fear, the use of this type of avoidance behavior generally declines.

Facilitation of Awareness and Monitoring

We believe that children who stutter have to be able to identify, through training of self-monitoring skills and self-awareness, those elements that interfere with their fluency (Conture, 1990; Ham, 1986; Ramig & Bennett, 1995; Van Riper, 1973). Cooper and Cooper (1985) state that school-aged children who stutter should develop self-awareness of stuttering patterns and associated behaviors as part of their intervention plan. The ability to self-analyze speech behaviors should be part of the client's knowledge and readily accessible during any speaking situation (Ham, 1986).

Use of audiotaped speech samples may be helpful in the initial identification of primary or audible accessory behaviors, and later in the identification of inappropriate speech rates or audible tension. During later stages of therapy, a client may be asked to assess samples of speech for the effectiveness of techniques used outside therapy. Westbrook (1990) described a therapy analogy she called "RSVP" (i.e., rate, smoothness, volume, and pressure) that she used with school-aged children when teaching them to monitor their speech production efforts. Using a checklist of these components, a child may be asked to listen to a segment of speech and make judgments regarding each of these four components. The interrelationships among these factors are discussed (i.e., as rate goes up, pressure increases, and smoothness decreases). Cooper and Cooper (1985) developed

the "My Stuttering Apple" worksheet, which depicts stuttering as the apple core and what the child does because of stuttering as the seeds. This worksheet can be reviewed periodically and updated by the clinician and child as a means of improving awareness of current and past speaking patterns.

Development of Positive Speech Attitudes

A therapy goal for all clients is the development of positive attitudes towards becoming an effective communicator. DeNil and Brutten (1991) found that children who stutter exhibit greater negative communication attitudes than do their nonstuttering peers. Negative attitudes can affect both interpersonal and intrapersonal domains, and both may need attention in the therapy process (Bennett, Reveles, & Ramig, 1993). Several researchers have found that development of positive attitudes about communication is associated with positive treatment outcomes (Andrews & Cutler, 1974; Guitar, 1976; Guitar & Bass, (1978).

To achieve this goal, clinicians should encourage and reinforce a child's strengths through exploration activities, such as an "All About Me Book." Employing hierarchy analysis strategies for therapy tasks increases the chances of success, and success leads to more success. Activities that involve ways of becoming an effective communicator can help children to see that communication is more than just how they speak and includes what they have to say. Addressing turn taking, interruptions, and teaching a child various coping mechanisms broaden a child's concept of communication.

Cooper (1987) emphasized the importance of reinforcing a child's "self-reinforcing behaviors such as expressions of positive feelings toward self" (p. 136). This goal is achieved when the clinician and child agree that the child's self-reinforcement is accurate, positive, and productive. Ramig and Bennett (1995) discuss several ways in which attribution theory can be utilized with children who stutter. For example, clinicians can assist a child to identify "global attributions" through "catch me" and "what does this really mean" activities. They can catch clients when they say "can't" or "never" and spend a few moments discussing how such self-talk may affect behavior. Changing these "stinkin' thinkin'" thoughts into "friendly thinkin'" thoughts (Ramig & Bennett, 1995) is a challenge for both clinicians and children who stutter.

As was noted previously, clinicians should talk openly about stuttering and reduce the "conspiracy of silence" (Bennett, 1995; Murphy, 1994) that often surrounds a child's stuttering. "Talking about talking" and "talking about stuttering" convey an atmosphere of acceptance and promote a child's self-esteem about communicating. An open line of communication is essential to a child's trust and confidence in the clinician's ability to help.

Transfer Skills

The ultimate goal of therapy is to enable a child who stutters to speak fluently or to modify the severity of moments of stuttering in everyday situations. To achieve this goal, the child has to transfer the skills learned within the clinical environment into everyday life. This task is not easy, and transfer activities should be conducted systematically with the cooperation of significant others in the child's school and home settings (Adams, 1991). We, along with Gregory (1979), plan transfer activities from the start of therapy. Establishing a "Speech Folder" that is sent between home and school is one way to involve others in a child's therapy program. Helping the child to remember to implement therapy techniques in settings outside therapy is a special challenge. Westbrook (1994) described an activity to facilitate this process called "Jacob's Secret Speech Bracelet." The child makes a beaded bracelet, and each bead represents a particular strategy to be implemented. The child decides what each bead represents and shares this with someone else. This reminder, worn throughout the day, serves as a subtle cue to transfer speech skills to different settings.

Transfer activities also involve tasks beyond just the practice of techniques with others. They include the exchange of information regarding speech and stuttering; discussing and observing how television personalities speak; or rating others' speech on the components of rate, smoothness, volume, and pressure. Establishing a routine for sharing information, practicing techniques, and exploring aspects of communication within the home and school can act as fluency cues for a child when not in the therapy room. Gregory (1989) discussed several variables of a lesson plan that are excellent ways of promoting transfer at each session. For example, manipulation of listener reactions, physical activity of clinician and child, reinforcement schedules, linguistic complexity, and persons present are several examples of how clinicians can vary each task and foster automaticity in the use of techniques. Defining and using a hierarchy of easy versus difficult speaking situations also assist in the transfer process.

Establishment of a Maintenance Plan

Maintaining fluency and stuttering modification skills that were learned during therapy is an area that needs to be addressed for each child who stutters. Ryan (1974) believes that clients who are enrolled in maintenance programs have better fluency than those who are not. Ramig and Bennett (1995) discuss the establishment of a maintenance plan for children who stutter by "Building a Roof of Fluency" for the child's "House of Fluency." Maintenance plans are as variable as treatment plans for children who stutter. Individual needs and the child's environment influence the type of plan established. Varying the type and frequency of therapy is one way of tailoring a maintenance plan. As the tools (fluency and stuttering modification skills) necessary for fluency are integrated, the child should be gradually phased out of direct intervention, reducing sessions to weekly, biweekly, monthly, and so on. The clinician can provide intermittent home practice through structured and unstructured activities and keep in touch with the child's speech at home. For example, the child might tape record several conversations at home and grade performance in the areas of RSVP (rate, smoothness, volume, and pressure), then discuss the grades with the clinician at the next session.

During this consultative maintenance period,

we have monthly phone contacts with the parents for approximately six months. Additionally, we refer to this phase of therapy as "earned time off" instead of "graduation" from speech therapy. Relapse is common (Boberg, 1981), and it is not something that a clinician can be certain will not occur. A revolving door policy that involves periodic visits with the clinician and discussions of relapse helps children to understand this problem and to cope more effectively should it occur.

Involvement of Others in Intervention

Inherent in working with children who stutter is involvement with their significant others (parents, teachers, siblings, and peers). Stuttering occurs as part of a complex interplay between the environment and the skills and abilities that the child brings to that environment (Botterill, Kelman, & Rustin, 1991; Kelly & Conture, 1991). As a result, clinicians need to incorporate environmental changes that facilitate fluency development into treatment plans (Conture, 1990; Gregory, 1991; Gregory & Hill, 1993; Mallard, 1991; Perkins, 1992; Ramig, 1993; Ramig & Bennett, 1995; Zebrowski & Schum, 1993). These references and other chapters in this text provide additional information on parental involvement and the role of counseling in the therapy process.

Recently, the use of parent support groups has been discussed in the literature (Bennett, 1990; Kelly & Conture, 1991). Establishing evening meetings for parents of children who stutter is one way to reach out to parents and families who cannot attend in-school therapy sessions. Bennett-Mancha (1990) described how one school district organized such meetings, with babysitters and translators, in order to train and educate families about issues surrounding stuttering, environmental factors that can influence a child's speech, and treatment considerations. This atmosphere provides parents an opportunity to share feelings and attitudes with other parents in an accepting environment. However, clinician assertiveness is often needed to achieve the flexible schedules needed to accommodate this extended service.

School clinicians have access to a number of significant others who can be involved in the therapy for the child who stutters. For example, teachers are often willing to collaborate with clinicians on lessons related to communication and language. Working as a team, a clinician can assist in the development of a teacher as a fluency facilitator. During classroom collaboration, peers can become more aware of factors that influence fluency and become better communicators themselves. Lessons that involve pragmatics, ways of becoming an effective communicator, how speech is produced, and handling teasing from others are just a few examples of how clinicians can get involved in the classroom environment and educate others about the disorder of stuttering.

SUMMARY

We have presented practical, usable information about direct intervention procedures for 7- to 12-year-old children who stutter. For those clinicians interested in published treatment programs or other structured approaches, several examples of each were summarized. Additionally, we discussed ways of tailoring treatment procedures to meet the specific needs of an individual child. We emphasized the need to implement direct treatment with children exhibiting more involved stuttering and those who are reacting to their stuttering.

We have found direct intervention to be a viable method in working with children in this age group who stutter as long as the clinician is also committed to being caring, understanding, accepting, and sensitive to the needs of the child and the negative impact that stuttering imposes on many children. As a person who had years of public school speech therapy, the senior author can attest to the positive impact that clinicians played in his life. Even though most were not experts on stuttering, they were considerate and caring and helped in ways no one else could. Carl Dell (1994) eloquently summarized what so many who stutter feel as they reflect on their public school experience in speech therapy:

Let me tell you about some of my own personal feelings as a young stutterer going to speech class, for I have been on both sides of the therapy room table. Although my stuttering was not cured during my school years, the school clinicians did accomplish several very important things. They provided a place where I could come and talk, where no one would laugh at me or scorn me, where I felt free to communicate even if I did stutter. What a great feeling that was! My dog was the only other living creature with whom I felt that way. Here was a place where I could learn something about my stuttering, that mysterious thing that no one else ever mentioned. I needed a safe place where I could touch it and confront it. All of these benefited me a great deal as a young boy. My public school clinicians didn't cure me but they were sorely needed and I believe these experiences laid the foundation for my eventual success. Indeed, I'm certain that, without this early therapy background, my therapy as an adult would have been much more difficult. But most valuable of all was the gift of caring. They cared! I was made to feel some worth as a human being despite my stuttering. Because of this experience, stuttering did not destroy my self-concept the way it does in many young stutterers. The caring and warmth I received from my school clinicians helped me stay together as a person (pg. 9).

Children who stutter usually benefit from interventions that are designed to meet their individual needs. The design process takes clinicians in one of three directions: programmed, general, or tailored approaches. Intervention during this critical time in a child's life can reduce the negative impact of stuttering. Intervention plans that follow a sound rationale, are supported in the literature, and are implemented by trained, dedicated, caring clinicians can significantly and positively influence communication development of children who stutter.

REFERENCES

Adams, M.R. (1980). The young stutterer: Diagnosis, treatment, and assessment of progress. *Seminars in Speech, Language, and Hearing, 1,* 289–300.

Adams, M.R. (1991). The assessment and treatment of the school-age stutterer. *Seminars in Speech and Language, 12,* 279–290.

Andrews, G., & Cutler, J. (1974). Stuttering therapy: The relationship between changes in symptom level and attitudes. *Journal of Speech and Hearing Disorders, 34,* 312–319.

Bennett, E.M. (1995). Shame in children who stutter. In C.W. Starkweather & H.F.M. Peters (Eds.), *1st World Congress on Fluency Disorders,* Vol. I, (pp. 245–248). Nijmegen: University Press Nijmegen.

Bennett, E.M., Reveles, V.N., & Ramig, P.R. (1993). [Speaking attitudes in children: Summer fluency camp]. Unpublished raw data.

Bennett-Mancha, E. (1990, March). *Parent support groups: For parents of children who stutter.* Paper presented at the Texas Speech-Language-Hearing Association Convention, Dallas, Texas.

Bennett-Mancha, E. (1991). *Practical therapy activities for children who stutter.* Paper presented at the Texas Speech-Language-Hearing Association Convention, Houston, Texas.

Bennett-Mancha, E. (1992). The house that Jack built. *Staff.* Aaron's Associates, 6114 Waterway, Garland, Texas 75043.

Bernstein Ratner, N., & Sih, C.C. (1987). Effects of gradual increases in sentence length and complexity on children's dysfluency. *Journal of Speech and Hearing Disorders, 52,* 278–287.

Bloodstein, O. (1987). *A handbook on stuttering.* Chicago, Ill.: The National Easter Seal Society.

Bloodstein, O. (1993). *Stuttering: The search for a cause and cure.* Needham Heights, MA: Allyn and Bacon.

Boberg, E. (Ed.) (1981). *Maintenance of fluency.* New York: North Holland Elsevier.

Botterill, W., Kelman, E., & Rustin, L. (1991). Parents and their pre-school stuttering child. In L. Rustin (Ed.), *Parents, families, and the stuttering child.* San Diego, Calif.: Singular Publishing Group.

Campbell, J.H., & Hill, D. (1989, July). Systematic disfluency analysis. *Stuttering therapy: A workshop for specialists.* Unpublished manuscript, Northwestern University and The Stuttering Foundation of America, Evanston, Ill.

Conture, E.G. (1990). *Stuttering* (2nd ed.). Englewood Cliffs, NJ: Prentice-Hall.

Conture, E.G., & Schwartz, M. (1984). Children who stutter: Diagnosis and remediation. *Journal of Communication Disorders, 9,* 1–18.

Cooper, E.B. (1987). The Cooper personalized fluency control therapy program. In L. Rustin, H. Purser, & H. Rowley (Eds.), *Progress in the treatment of fluency disorders.* London: Whurr Publishers Ltd.

Cooper, E.B., & Cooper, C.S. (1985). *Personalized fluency control therapy.* Allen, Tex.: DLM.

Costello, J.M. (1983). Current behavioral treatments of children. In D. Prins and R.J. Ingham (Eds.), *Treatment of stuttering in early childhood: Methods and issues.* San Diego, CA: College-Hill Press.

Dell, C.W., Jr. (1993). Treating school-age stutterers. In R.F. Curlee (Ed.), *Stuttering and related disorders of fluency.* New York: Thieme Medical Publishers.

Dell, C.W., Jr. (1994). *Treating the school age stutterer: A guide for clinicians.* Memphis, Tenn.: Stuttering Foundation of America.

DeNil, L.F., & Brutten, G.J. (1991). Speech-associated attitudes of stuttering and nonstuttering children. *Journal of Speech and Hearing Research, 34,* 60–66.

Gregory, H.H. (1979). The controversies: Analysis and current status. In H.H. Gregory (Ed.), *Controversies about stuttering therapy.* Baltimore, MD: University Park Press.

Gregory, H. (1989). *Stuttering therapy: A workshop for specialists.* Unpublished manuscript, Northwestern University and The Stuttering Foundation of America, Evanston, Ill.

Gregory, H. (1991). Therapy for elementary school-age children. *Seminars in Speech and Language, 12,* 323–335.

Gregory, H.H., & Hill, D. (1980). Stuttering therapy for children. *Seminars in Speech, Language, and Hearing, 1,* 351–364.

Gregory, H.H., & Hill, D. (1993). Differential evaluation-differential therapy for stuttering children. In R.F. Curlee (Ed.), *Stuttering and related disorders of fluency.* New York: Thieme Medical Publishers.

Guitar, B. (1976). Pretreatment factors associated with the outcome of stuttering therapy. *Journal of Speech and Hearing Research, 19,* 590–600.

Guitar, B., & Bass, C. (1978). Stuttering therapy: The relation between attitude change and long-term outcome. *Journal of Speech and Hearing Disorders, 15,* 393–400.

Ham, R. (1986). *Techniques of stuttering therapy.* Englewood Cliffs, NJ: Prentice-Hall.

Heinze, B.A., & Johnson, K.L. (1987). *Easy Does It-2: Fluency activities for school-aged stutterers.* East Moline, Ill.: LinguiSystems.

Ingham, J.C. (1993). Behavioral treatment of stuttering children. In R.F. Curlee (Ed.), *Stuttering and related disorders of fluency.* New York: Thieme Medical Publishers.

Ingham, R.J. (1993). Transfer and maintenance of treatment gains of chronic stutterers. In R.F. Curlee (Ed.), *Stuttering and related disorders of fluency.* New York: Thieme Medical Publishers.

Johnson, W. (1955). *Stuttering in children and adults.* Minneapolis: University of Minnesota Press.

Johnson, W., & Associates (1959). *The onset of stuttering.* Minneapolis: University of Minnesota Press.

Kelly, E.M. (1993). Speech rates and turn-taking behaviors of children who stutter and their parents. *Seminars in Speech and Language, 14,* 203–214.

Kelly, E., & Conture, E. (1991). Intervention with school-age stutterers: A parent-child fluency group approach. *Seminars in Speech and Language, 12,* 310–322.

Louko, L.J., Edwards, M.L., & Conture, E.G. (1990). Phonological characteristics of young stutterers and their normally fluent peers: Preliminary observations. *Journal of Fluency Disorders, 15,* 191–210.

Mallard, A.R. (1991). Using families to help the school-age stutterer: A case study. In L. Rustin (Ed.), *Parents, families, and the stuttering child.* San Diego: Singular Publishing Group.

Meyers, S., & Woodford, L. (1992). *The fluency development system for young children.* Buffalo: United Educational Services.

Murphy, B. (1994, June). Helping children who stutter: A potpourri of clinical ideas. *Stuttering therapy: Practical ideas for the school clinician.* Workshop sponsored by the Stuttering Foundation of America and the University of Colorado, Boulder.

Nelson, L. (1991). Informal presentation to the Stuttering Foundation of America and Texas Speech and Hearing Association Independent Study Group, Dallas, Texas.

Perkins, W.H. (1992). *Stuttering prevented.* San Diego: Singular Publishing Group.

Perkins, W., Rudas, J., Johnson, L., & Bell, J. (1976).

Stuttering: Discoordination of phonation with articulation and respiration. *Journal of Speech and Hearing Research, 19,* 509–522.

Peters, T.J., & Guitar, B. (1991). *Stuttering: An integrated approach to its nature and treatment.* Baltimore, Md.: Williams and Wilkins.

Pindzola, R. (1987). *Stuttering intervention program.* Austin, Tex.: Pro-Ed.

Preobrajenskaya. (1953). Work with preschool stuttering children. *Experiences in logopedic practices.* Moscow: Institute of Defectology.

Ramig, P.R. (1993). Parent-clinician-child partnership in the therapeutic process of the preschool- and elementary-aged child who stutters. *Seminars in Speech and Language, 14* (3), 226–237.

Ramig, P.R., & Bennett, E.M. (1995). Working with 7–12 year old children who stutter: Ideas for intervention in the public schools. *Language, Speech, and Hearing Services in Schools, 26,* 138–150.

Ramig, P.R., Stewart, P., Ogrodnick, P., & Bennett, E.M. (1994). *Treating the school-age child who stutters.* Unpublished manuscript, University of Colorado, Boulder, Colorado.

Ramig, P.R. & Wallace, M.L. (1987). Indirect and combined direct-indirect therapy in a dysfluent child. *Journal of Fluency Disorders, 12,* 41–49.

Riley, G.D. (1984). *Stuttering prediction instrument for young children.* Tigard, Ore.: C.C. Publications.

Riley, G.D. (1986). *Stuttering severity instrument for children and adults* (Revised). Austin, Tex.: Pro-ed.

Riley, G.D., & Riley, J. (1983). Evaluation as a basis for intervention. In. D. Prins & R.J. Ingham (Eds.), *Treatment of stuttering in early childhood: Methods and issues.* San Diego, CA: College-Hill Press.

Riley, G.D., & Riley, R. (1985). *Oral motor assessment and treatment: Improving syllable production.* Austin, Tex.: Pro-Ed.

Riley, G., & Riley, J. (1986). Oral motor discoordination among children who stutter. *Journal of Fluency Disorders, 11,* 335–344.

Runyan, C.M., & Runyan, S.E. (1993). Therapy for school-age stutterers: An update on the fluency rules program. In R.F. Curlee (Ed.), *Stuttering and related disorders of fluency.* New York: Thieme Medical Publishers.

Rustin, L. (1987a). The treatment of childhood disfluency through active parent involvement. In L. Rustin, H. Purser, & H. Rowley (Eds.), *Progress in the treatment of fluency disorders.* London: Whurr Publishers Ltd.

Rustin, L. (1987b). *Assessment and therapy programme for disfluent children.* Windsor: NFER-NELSON.

Rustin, L., & Cook, F. (1983). Intervention procedures for the disfluent child. In P. Dalton (Ed.), *Approaches to the treatment of stuttering.* London: Taylor & Francis.

Ryan B.P. (1974). *Programmed therapy for stuttering in children and adults.* Springfield, Ill.: Thomas.

Ryan, B.P. (1979). Stuttering therapy in a framework of operant conditioning and programmed learning. In H. Gregory (Ed.), *Controversies about stuttering therapy.* Baltimore, MD: University Park Press.

Ryan, B.P. (1984). Treatment of stuttering in school children. In W. H. Perkins (Ed.), *Stuttering disorders.* New York: Thieme-Stratton.

Sheehan, J. (1968). Stuttering as a self-role conflict. In H.H. Gregory (Ed.), *Learning theory and stuttering therapy* (pp. 72–83). Evanston, Ill.: Northwestern University Press.

Shine, R.E. (1980). *Systematic fluency training for young children.* Tigard, Ore.: C.C. Publications.

Silverman, F.H. (1992). *Stuttering and other fluency disorders.* Englewood Cliffs, N.J.: Prentice-Hall.

Starkweather, C.W. (1987). *Fluency and stuttering.* Englewood Cliffs, N.J.: Prentice-Hall.

Thompson, J. (1983). *Assessment of fluency in school children.* Danville, Ill.: The Interstate Printers & Publishers.

Van Riper, C. (1973). *The treatment of stuttering.* Englewood Cliffs, N.J.: Prentice-Hall.

Wall, M.J., & Myers, F.L. (1995). *Clinical management of childhood stuttering.* Austin, Tex.: Pro-Ed.

Westbrook, J. (1990). Dallas Independent School District Summer Fluency Camp, Camp Curriculum, unpublished document.

Westbrook, J. (1994). Jacob's secret speech bracelet. *Staff.* Aaron's Associates, 6114 Waterway, Garland, Texas 75043.

Williams, D.E. (1994). Discovery: The nuts and bolts of therapy. *Stuttering therapy: Practical ideas for the school clinician.* Workshop sponsored by the Stuttering Foundation of America and the University of Colorado, Boulder, Colo.

Wolk, L., Edwards, M.L., & Conture, E.G. (1993). Co-existence of stuttering and disordered phonology in young children. *Journal of Speech and Hearing Research, 36,* 906–917.

Zebrowski, P.M., & Schum, R.L. (1993). Counseling parents of children who stutter. *American Journal of Speech-Language Pathology, 2,* 65–73.

SUGGESTED READINGS

Bloodstein, O. (1993). *Stuttering: The search for a cause and cure*. Needham Heights, MA: Allyn and Bacon. Provides a historical account of the problem of stuttering, as well as information pertaining to research findings and various treatment approaches.

Conture, E.G. (1990). *Stuttering*. (2nd ed.). Englewood Cliffs, NJ: Prentice-Hall. Presents detailed assessment and treatment information on all ages of children who stutter. Also provides information pertaining to parent involvement and parent counseling.

Curlee, R.F. (Ed.) (1993). *Stuttering and related disorders of fluency*. New York: Thieme Medical Publishers. Offers identification, assessment, and a variety of treatment programs for children who stutter.

Wall, M.J., & Myers, F.L. (1995). *Clinical management of childhood stuttering*. Austin TX: Pro-Ed. Provides chapters on theories, symptomatology, psycholinguistic, and physiological aspects of childhood stuttering. Also includes chapters on assessment and treatment.

CHAPTER 16

MANAGEMENT OF CLUTTERING AND RELATED FLUENCY DISORDERS

KENNETH O. ST. LOUIS
FLORENCE L. MYERS

INTRODUCTION

For at least a generation, cluttering—a condition that rhymes with "stuttering," but doesn't quite fit into the category—was essentially ignored in most textbooks on stuttering. Yet, the fact that cluttering is accorded a chapter in this and other recent books highlights a significant recent development. Cluttering has been rediscovered by mainstream speech-language pathologists as a fluency disorder that exists and demands their attention.

HISTORICAL PERSPECTIVES

Definitions and Terminology

Cluttering has traditionally been classified as a disorder of fluency. However, because of its relatively low incidence and prevalence, the literature on this fluency disorder is sparse. Some (e.g., Preus, 1992) contend that its prominence and prevalence have been underrated and overshadowed by the related fluency disorder of stuttering. A classic and one of the more broadly-based definitions of cluttering was proposed by Deso Weiss (1964, p. 1) who said that cluttering is "the verbal manifestation of Central Language Imbalance, which affects all channels of communication (e.g., reading, writing, rhythm, and musicality) and behavior in general." Weiss, along with other phoniatrists and logopedists trained in the European tradition, viewed cluttering from a gestalt per-

spective that emphasizes the coexistence of communication and non-communicative problems. Freund (1952) and Luchsinger (1963), for example, saw cluttering as a "dysphasia-like disability." The multifaceted nature of cluttering was also noted by deHirsch, (1961) who considered cluttering to be a "disturbance of motor integration suggestive of dyspraxia," as well as by Van Riper (1982) who included articulatory, rate, and linguistic anomalies as characteristics of his Track II stutterers, a group of stutterers having strong cluttering components.

In recent years, several attempts have been made to provide a working definition of cluttering. For example, in the interest of offering an essential definition of this multifaceted disorder, one that delineates only its necessary and sufficient traits, St. Louis (1992, p. 49) defined cluttering as a speech-language disorder characterized mainly by "(1) abnormal fluency which is not stuttering and (2) a rapid and/or irregular speech rate." Daly (1992, p. 107) considered cluttering to be "a disorder of speech and language processing resulting in rapid, dysrhythmic, sporadic, unorganized, and frequently unintelligible speech. Accelerated speech is not always present, but an impairment in formulating language almost always is." Myers (1992) emphasized the coexistence of rate, fluency, articulatory, and language anomalies in clutterers, in the context of a communication system that is impaired in self-monitoring skills.

Behavioral Symptoms

While nearly all speech-language pathologists and logopedists underscored speech rate anomalies (e.g., Dalton & Hardcastle, 1989; Seeman & Novak, 1963), Weiss interestingly did not. The symptoms that Weiss (1964) considered to be obligatory revolve around the notion of perceptual/cognitive disorganization and their sequelae: perceptual weakness and poorly organized thinking, short attention span, lack of awareness of difficulty, and speech repetitions.

Table 16.1 lists the signs and symptoms most often associated with cluttering. These characteristics were culled from the classic as well as more recent literature and organized according to speech, language and "other" behaviors not directly linked to communication (e.g., Dalton & Hardcastle, 1989; Myers & Bradley, 1992; St. Louis, Hinzman, & Hull, 1985; Weiss, 1964).

Physiological Characteristics

The organic or physiological bases of cluttering have been inferred largely from clinical histories of clutterers and their families. A number of reports indicated that cluttering runs in families (e.g., Luchsinger & Arnold, 1965; Weiss, 1964). Relatives of clutterers often report that various members of the family, dating back to the grandparents' generation, spoke disfluently or spoke very quickly or indistinctly. Family members may say, "His uncle also speaks very quickly, but you can understand him." or, "Her aunt used to stutter a lot as a child, but she's much better now." Many parents of clutterers also recall that their child seemed to be disinhibited and impulsive in both verbal and nonverbal behaviors. One parent even approached one of the authors to see if medication, such as that prescribed for children with attention deficit/hyperactivity disorder, might be helpful in curtailing some of the child's troublesome behavioral problems. One should be mindful, however, that not all clutterers exhibit behaviors associated with hyperactivity, impulsivity, or short attention span. Still, when such symptoms are present, one

is inclined to infer some underlying organicity. For example, EEG abnormalities occur more frequently in clutterers than stutterers (Moravek & Langova, 1962; Langova & Moravek, 1964), and cluttering occurs four times more frequently in males than females (Arnold, 1960). Some authors attribute clutterers' fast and irregular speech rate to neurologic changes (Seeman, 1970) and the linguistic and cognitive disorganization to dysphasic-like symptoms (deHirsch, 1961).

Treatment

A historical perspective of the treatment of cluttering comes largely from European trained clinicians. Most authors urge clinicians to take into consideration the stuttering component versus the cluttering component of the fluency problem. The modification of rate and rhythm, however difficult this goal may be, is of paramount importance for the clutterer. Weiss (1964) as well as Dalton and Hardcastle (1989) advocated use of syllable-timed speech, whereas Smith (1955) described an accent method in which relative linguistic stress is appropriated to stressed versus nonstressed syllables. Weiss (1964) also recommended the recitation of poems and paraphrasing stories, anecdotes, and jokes. Rationale for the former is that poetry imposes rhythm on the clutterer's speech and for the latter is that storytelling activities enhance the clutterer's narrative and language formulation abilities.

RELATED FLUENCY DISORDERS

Rapid Speech Rate (Tachylalia)

The term tachylalia means rapid speech and has been used considerably in the European literature. Weiss (1964) wrote that even though some authors considered tachylalia to be an essential feature of cluttering, he did not view it as an obligatory symptom. He pointed out that rapid speech could occur without the usual disfluencies and coexisting articulation or language difficulties so often observed in clutterers. "Pure" tachylalia may be of peripheral interest to speech-language clinicians, but it seems worthwhile to consider excessively rapid speech

TABLE 16.1   Symptoms Characteristic of Cluttering.

Rate

Fast/irregular rate

"Robotic" speech characterized by monotone festination (i.e., talking faster and faster)

Minimal pausing between linguistic phrases and thought units

Discoordination between pauses and breath groups

Fluency

Repetitions of words and phrases*

Little physiological tension or struggle

Incomplete phrases

Revisions, fillers, and interjections

Circumlocutions

Language

Run-on, disorganized utterances

Poor syntax

Word retrieval difficulties

Problems with reading and academic achievement

Reduced coherence of narratives

Overuse of nonspecific words

Articulation/Speech intelligibility

Multiple misarticulations (e.g., elision of sound and syllables, neutralization of vowels, slurring of sounds and syllables)

Indistinct valving of consonants

Weak syllable deletion

Cluster reduction

Reduced speech intelligibility

Other

Poor sensory feedback

Poor sense of timing

Short attention span (particularly on topics not of interest)

Fine-motor discoordination

Family history of stuttering/cluttering

Neurologic soft signs

Poor musical ability

Diffuse EEG abnormalities

Little inhibition, hesitancy, or anxiety related to speech

---

*Sound or syllable repetitions comprise an ambiguous case. Typically, these disfluencies are considered characteristic of stuttering—not cluttering. Even though sound or syllable repetitions have been reported to occur at a higher than normal level in possible clutterers (St. Louis, Hinzman, & Hull, 1985), such repetitions are relatively much higher in the speech of stutterers.

rate, when it occurs in isolation, as a fluency phenomenon that is related—but not identical—to cluttering. Such individuals would manifest speaking rates substantially faster than normal, but would otherwise have no more disfluencies or other difficulties communicating than do normal speakers.

The average speaking rate is generally considered to range from 190 to 210 syllables per minute (spm) in adult spontaneous speech (Ingham, 1984). An earlier normative report, which measured adult oral reading rate in words per minute (wpm) placed the average (50th percentile) at 170 wpm (Fairbanks, 1960). Of course, these values are averages, and it is clear that normal speakers vary considerably in speaking rates. Fairbanks, for example, considered readers who were above the 90th percentile (exceeding 192 wpm) as "too fast." In contrast to the notion that excessive speech rate per se might indicate deviancy, Starkweather (1987) considered rate to be an essential aspect of fluency, along with continuity and ease. He argued that the ability to speak rapidly without breakdown is a sign of enhanced fluency, which implies that a faster than normal rate is not a disorder at all.

To our knowledge, this issue has not been seriously addressed, probably because rapid rates are typically accompanied by compromised articulatory precision, language coherence, and disfluency levels. For example, Beebe (1960) demonstrated that when normal speakers were instructed to read or speak spontaneously as fast as possible, they generally produced disfluency symptoms resembling cluttering, whether or not they actually increased their rates. Yet, some people have heard speakers whom they would judge difficult to understand only because they talk faster than a listener can easily process language. Such speakers are frequently misunderstood unless conditions are optimal and maximal attention is given by listeners. Whereas some might argue that this is a problem for listeners, the fact is that such atypical speakers will be viewed as if they have the problem by most family members, friends, and colleagues. In any case, communication is compromised. For this reason, we believe that individuals with "pure" tachylalia have a clinically significant condition and are candidates for therapeutic intervention.

Therapy for individuals with tachylalia who are free of other problems should involve rate reduction strategies, which will be reviewed later in this chapter. The goal would be to get such persons to slow down so that listeners can follow the conversation with relative ease. Once that is achieved, they should be dismissed.

Cluttering with Coexisting Learning Disabilities and Attention-Deficit/Hyperactivity Disorders

In a frequently cited article, Tiger, Irvine, and Reis (1980) identified numerous similarities between cluttering and learning disabilities (LD). In 1987, the Interagency Committee on Learning Disabilities (ICLD) recommended the following somewhat confusing definition to the U.S. Congress:

> *Learning disabilities is a generic term that refers to a heterogeneous group of disorders manifested by significant difficulties in the acquisition and use of listening, speaking, reading, writing, reasoning, mathematical abilities, or of social skills. These disorders are intrinsic to the individual and presumed to be due to central nervous system dysfunction. Even though learning disabilities may occur concomitantly with other handicapping conditions (e.g., sensory impairment, mental retardation, social and emotional disturbance), with socio-environmental influences (e.g., cultural differences, insufficient or inappropriate instruction, psychogenic factors) and especially with attention deficit disorder, all of which may cause learning problems, a learning disability is not a direct result of those conditions or influences (ICLD, 1987, p. 222).*

This and other definitions of LD regard language impairments as central to the problem. Somewhat surprisingly, language disability per se is not mentioned in the most recent version of the *Diagnostic and Statistical Manual of Mental Disorders*, 4th edition (DSM-IV), (American Psychiatric Association, 1994). It provides a framework for different types of "learning disorders," which are further classified as: "reading disorder" (most common), "mathematics disorder," "disorder of written expression," or "learning disorder not otherwise specified." Diagnoses are based on depressed (standardized) performance relative to the person's chronological age, measured intelligence, and education that significantly interferes with academic achievement or daily living and is not due to a sensory deficit. LD is reported in approximately 5 percent of public school students and in males 1.5 to 4 times more often than in females.

Daly (1992) compared cluttering with the syndrome known as attention deficit disorder (ADD). Most recently identified in the DSM-IV as Attention-Deficit/Hyperactivity Disorder (ADHD), this condition, which was mentioned in the above 1987 definition of LD, also shares many of the symptoms often seen in clutterers. The diagnosis of ADHD is made when a specified number of nine symptoms have been present in at least two settings (e.g., home, school, or work) for at least six months. Specifically, a diagnosis requires observation of at least six of nine symptoms of inattention (e.g., "often fails to give close attention to details or makes careless mistakes in schoolwork, work, or other activities"; "often has difficulty organizing tasks and activities"; "is often easily distracted by extraneous stimuli") and/or six of nine symptoms of hyperactivity or impulsivity (e.g., "often fidgets with hands and feet or squirms in seat"; "often talks excessively"; "often interrupts or intrudes on others [e.g., butts into conversations or games]"). In addition, some symptoms must have been present before the age of 7 years, and there must be clear evidence of a "clinically significant impairment in social, academic, or occupational functioning." There are four types of ADHD: predominately inattentive type, predominately hyperactive/impulsive type, combined type (the most common), and otherwise unspecified (American Psychiatric Association, 1994, pp. 78-85). ADHD is present in a substantial proportion of learning disabled individuals, that is, 20 to 25 percent (American Speech-Language-Hearing

Association, 1992), and LD is present more often among those with ADHD, with estimates ranging from 27 to 80 percent (Cantwell & Baker, 1991; Epstein, Shaywitz, Shaywitz, & Woolston, 1991). ADHD runs in families, occurs in 3 to 5 percent of the population, and has a sex ratio that ranges from 4 : 1 to 9 : 1 males to females (American Psychiatric Association, 1994).

Even casual inspection of the symptoms of LD and ADHD indicates clearly that individuals with these disorders frequently have many of the same associated symptoms as clutterers. Indeed, Freeman (1982) went so far as to suggest that "cluttering may describe the specific speech production characteristics of a subgroup of language-learning disordered children" (p. 686). We hypothesize that there are important differences between cluttering and LD or ADHD in the areas of disfluency and speech rate. Fluency problems are central, whether stated or not, in definitions of cluttering; however, it is important to recognize that disfluency can be one characteristic of LD. For example, Wiig and Semel (1984) list a number of disfluency types (e.g., excessive fillers, interjections, pauses, and repetition of words and phrases) that characterize the speech of LD children. These disfluencies are hypothesized to occur as a result of language problems, such as word finding deficits. It is possible, therefore, that some of these disfluent LD children might be regarded more appropriately as clutterers.

At least one attempt to remediate a group of stutterer-clutterers with learning disabilities was reported in Scotland in 1992 (Wallace, 1992). The program focused on teaching adult clients to recognize breakdowns in their communication attempts and to repair them. Although it was reported that the program was effective, specific data were not provided.

Stuttering with Coexisting Cluttering

It is widely accepted that cluttering frequently coexists with stuttering (Daly, 1986, 1993; Freund, 1952; Myers & St. Louis, 1992; Preus, 1992; Weiss, 1964, 1967, 1968). In fact, authors agree that "pure" cluttering (i.e., without stuttering) is less common than are coexisting varieties. The prevalence of cluttering and stuttering combined has been the subject of considerable speculation.

Freund (1952) reported that cluttering was present in 22 percent of 513 stutterers, ranging from young children to older adults. When only those stutterers with onsets after the age of 10 years were considered, the percentage increased to 47 percent. Data from 121 of these stutterers, for whom family history information on stuttering and tachylalia was available, indicated that 84 percent of the families of stutterer-clutterers reported tachylalia (alone or in combination with stuttering) among relatives, compared to only 21 percent for relatives of "pure" stutterers.

Preus (1981) studied 100 stutterers and reported that 32 percent showed, or had earlier shown, symptoms of cluttering. In this study, he attempted to replicate Van Riper's (1971) subgrouping of stutterers into four tracks (Track II representing stutterers with a cluttering component). Preus identified a Track II subgroup of eighteen stutterers (the same percentage as reported by Van Riper) who clearly manifested speech characteristics of cluttering, articulation disorders, and delayed language development. Using several factor analyses, he identified abnormal neuropsychological findings, low levels of anxiety, mild severity ratings, and lack of beneficial effects of delayed auditory feedback as other characteristics of this subgroup. Preus (1992) later reviewed these and seven other studies of stutterers and concluded that about 35 percent (range 18 to 67%) manifested coexisting cluttering. Daly (1981) described a similar attempt to identify Track II stutterers from 138 stutterers, ages 8 to 20 years. Twenty-four percent were placed in Track II. Of these, 85 percent had a history of articulation disorders and 97 percent a history of language delay.

Weiss (1964, 1967) pointed out that persons with cluttering-stuttering[1] comprise the majority of individuals with fluency disorders who seek professional help. He referred repeatedly to a figure that showed that one-sixth or fewer of this client population were pure stutterers and about one-sixth were pure clutterers. The rest evidenced, in varying degrees, combinations of stuttering and cluttering.

The nature of the relationship between stuttering and cluttering has also been the subject of considerable speculation. Weiss (1964) left no doubt about his view of the importance of this issue when he wrote that "the relationship between cluttering and stammering can be considered the most important single relationship in the field of speech pathology" (p. 68). Citing earlier work, he concluded that stuttering and cluttering both develop from the same physiological imbalance and that stuttering inevitably evolves from cluttering. Therefore, in his view, cluttering is frequently observed prior to stuttering and is also seen when, after successful therapy, a stutterer has eliminated most stuttering symptoms.

Most authors do not assume this degree of interaction. We agree with Preus (1992) that stuttering and cluttering are "related" disorders of fluency but that the two disorders are "different," that is, they can be differentiated, albeit with difficulty in some individuals. We think his third tenet, that cluttering and stuttering are "antagonistic" (i.e., the two disorders are on opposing ends of continua of such dimensions as reactions to delayed auditory feedback or degree to which speech samples manifest coarticulation) is an intriguing notion that requires further empirical study.

Stuttering with Coexisting Articulation and/or Language Disorders

We pointed out that most definitions of cluttering refer to articulation and/or language components. Even St. Louis (1992), whose working definition excludes consideration of these areas, recognized that phonologic, morphologic, syntactic, semantic, and pragmatic deficits are frequently observed in clutterers. This has led to a somewhat confusing state of affairs: When stuttering is accompanied

---

[1]Weiss (1964) actually used the term "cluttering-stammering" because he argued that "stammering" was less ambiguous in meaning and referents than the term, "stuttering."

by articulation or language problems, the person is often regarded, by definition, as having a cluttering component. The influence of this line of reasoning is seen, for example, in the a priori classifications of Van Riper (1971) and Preus (1981). We believe that this is likely to lead to the misdiagnosis of stutterers who have such coexisting disorders but who do not clutter.

Using a national database with accompanying tape recorded speech samples of nearly 39,000 randomly selected schoolchildren, St. Louis and colleagues studied a number of samples of children having fluency disorders (St. Louis, 1992; St. Louis, Chambers, & Ashworth, 1991; St. Louis, Hansen, Oliver, & Buch, 1992; St. Louis & Hinzman, 1988; St. Louis et al., 1985; St. Louis, Ruscello, & Lundeen, 1992). These investigations showed that articulation, language, voice, and even hearing problems are present in a large percentage of stuttering individuals, and in even larger proportions among severe stutterers. In addition, a group of "possible clutterers" were found to manifest more comparable coexisting articulation or language disorders than did samples of either pure or random stutterers, but not groups of stutterers who had overall severity ratings of either moderate or severe. Clearly, many stutterers manifest significant coexisting articulation and language problems just as clutterers do. The extent to which these disorders are similar or different in the two groups has not been systematically investigated in recent years.

Conture and his colleagues recently reported a series of investigations of the coexistence of articulation disorders in young stuttering clients (Conture, Louko, & Edwards, 1993). Consistent with other reports, (e.g., Bloodstein, 1987), these investigators stated that approximately 40 percent of stuttering children have articulation disorders. Recently, they postulated that this subgroup of stutterers with articulation disorders should be viewed as persons whose speech performance is compromised by below average speech ability (Yaruss, Logan, & Conture, 1994).

Figure 16.1, which is speculative but draws from our experiences as well as the literature (e.g.,

Daly, 1992; Diedrich, 1984, St. Louis & Myers, 1995; St. Louis, et al., 1992; Tiger et al., 1980), illustrates the hypothetical overlap among the following conditions: cluttering, stuttering, learning disabilities, attention-deficit/hyperactivity disorders, articulation disorders, and language disorders. Cluttering cuts across the area of greatest overlap among the other disorders, which accounts for the myriad symptoms used to describe the disorder. Cluttering does occur, but rarely, in pure form, and it can occur with or without stuttering, although the two disorders more often coexist. Figure 16.1 does not attempt to depict the relationship of these six disorders with either rate or other fluency disorders, because to include them would render the figure excessively "cluttered." We speculate that rate disorders greatly overlap—but differ from—fluency disorders, a position that is not universally shared (e.g., Starkweather, 1987). We further propose that fluency disorders comprise all of the cluttering and stuttering cases. Rate disorders are hypothesized to include all clutterers as well as small percentages of those having some coexisting combination of stuttering, articulation, language, learning, and attention-deficit/hyperactivity problems. And, rarely would rate disorders (e.g., pure tachylalia) occur in pure form.

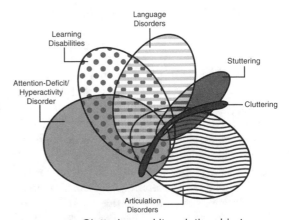

Figure 16.1 Cluttering and its relationship to stuttering, articulation disorders, language disorders, learning disabilities, and attention-deficit/hyperactivity disorders.

DIFFERENTIAL DIAGNOSIS OF CLUTTERING, STUTTERING, AND RELATED FLUENCY DISORDERS

Special Considerations

The assessment and diagnosis of cluttering requires careful, detailed testing in most of the areas for which clutterers are reported to have deficits. Inasmuch as cluttering is a fluency disorder, the evaluation process outlined in Conture's chapter is relevant for young children suspected of cluttering. Typically, the evaluation battery for cluttering begins with a protocol that was developed for stuttering that is supplemented by other components that are deemed important, because, in addition to fluency problems, the clinician needs to identify other areas of strength and weakness. As will be seen, often it is the other symptoms that are targeted for therapy. This means that the evaluation process is usually more protracted than for the typical stuttering client, frequently requiring several sessions. In addition, the expertise of other professionals, such as special education teachers, psychologists, and audiologists may be required in the evaluation process.

The following sections briefly discuss areas that should be considered for testing with a suspected clutterer. Clinicians must decide, however, on a case-by-case basis, which components to include and which may not be necessary.

Case History

In addition to the usual information about fluency problems (e.g., onset, development, and symptoms), the case history (questionnaire and interview) for cluttering should explore a child's developmental landmarks for speech, language, motor, and related behavior. The clinician needs to determine whether the child's development was normal, delayed, accelerated, or mixed. Similarly, it is important to know whether fluency problems occurred after the onset of language, as typically occurs in stuttering, or concurrent with language, a characteristic of Track II stutterers (Van Riper, 1971). Since cluttering appears to have a strong ge-netic influence, particular attention should be directed to queries about family history of fluency problems, followed by questions to isolate family history of cluttering symptoms and other communication, academic, or learning problems. Because intelligibility—not fluency—is often the reason for the referral of a suspected clutterer, clinicians should explore thoroughly the events that led up to the referral. For example, it may have been motivated by a teacher, or in the case of the older clutterer, an employer, who simply has difficulty understanding the client's rapid, disorganized speech.

Case history questions should also determine the extent to which a client manifests heightened activity levels (e.g., fidgeting) or problems in coordination and whether parents, teachers, or the client have noticed problems of attention or distractibility.

Fluency and Rate Assessment

Audio or video recordings should be obtained of the suspected cluttering client in a variety of speech tasks. These generally include rote or "automatic" tasks (e.g., counting, reciting days of the week, or reciting a memorized nursery rhyme, prayer, or pledge), imitated speech (short monosyllabic to long polysyllabic words, phrases, and sentences), oral reading (words, phrases, and sentences) if the client can read, and spontaneous/conversational speech.

It is important to obtain samples of the client's usual rate of speech, as well as samples in which rate is slowed. The client should be asked to speak slowly and carefully to determine the extent to which speech rate can be changed voluntarily. Also, speech tasks that can only be carried out at a slower rate (e.g., giving a series of instructions to the clinician in which each direction must await a response to the previous one) can provide useful information for comparing slowed and usual speech rates.

Once completed, the tape can be analyzed quantitatively and qualitatively. Most fluency assessment protocols include measures of frequency (e.g., percent syllables stuttered or disfluent) and severity (e.g., duration and type of disfluency symptoms, accessory behaviors, or evidence of struggle). In addition, the following measures should be included when cluttering is suspected: rate of speech (i.e., syllables per minute in utterances having no disfluency and containing a minimum number of words, perhaps 10), regularity of speech rate (e.g., on a 1–9 perceptual rating scale), naturalness ratings (i.e., on a 1–9 scale),[2] and the client's awareness of having fluency problems (from a series of questions). If the client's speech sounds quite unnatural, a sample should be analyzed further in terms of such prosodic elements as primary and secondary syllabic stress, intonation, and pauses.

As was noted in Table 16.1, the disfluencies most likely to occur in clutterers are repetitions (especially of phrases or words), revisions, fillers, and interjections, all without excessive tension or struggle. By contrast, stutterers are likely to manifest sound or syllable repetitions, sound prolongations, or complete blocks as well as evidence of forcing, struggle, or tension. The speech of clutterers, even when not excessively disfluent, is more likely to sound unnatural because of insufficient prosodic variability (monotone) and an irregular speaking rate.

Self-perception of speech difficulty is also important and should be included in the cluttering evaluation, particularly since clutterers are reported to be less concerned about their problems than are stutterers. Paper-and-pencil measures that have been widely used with stutterers are the Andrews and Cutler (1974) S-24 Scale and the Woolf (1967) *Perceptions of Stuttering Inventory*. In spite of some attempts,[3] there are no widely accepted standardized measures of awareness of speech. Nevertheless, the examiner should attempt, by observation and questioning, to determine the degree to which a clutterer is—or can be—aware of speech characteristics.

---

[2]St. Louis (1994) reported that regularity of rate and naturalness were highly correlated.

[3]Atkins and St. Louis (1988) reported preliminary normative information on an inventory designed to assess speakers' awareness of various aspects of their speech as well as the speech of others. The inventory was not administered to fluency disordered groups.

Articulation Assessment

An articulation test should be part of the assessment battery for clutterers. In addition to a single-word test, clinicians should analyze a tape recorded sample of spontaneous speech at the client's usual speaking rate for articulation errors or simplifications. A written transcript of the sample, perhaps twenty-five consecutive utterances, should be prepared, and every incorrect word analyzed for articulatory errors, and if relevant, phonological processes. Clinicians should be alert not only for phonemic distortions, omissions, substitutions, and additions, but also for deletions of unstressed syllables (e.g., "caldar" for "calendar"), sound or feature transformations (e.g., Spoonerisms such as "pasketti" for "spagetti" or "ponato" for "tomato"), and cluster simplifications (e.g., "spash" for "splash").

Language Assessment

We recommend that the battery include measures of: morphology (e.g., vocabulary and inflections), syntax, semantics, and pragmatics. This will entail standardized and nonstandardized measures of expressive and receptive language. Analysis of a language sample should also include consideration of mazes (Loban, 1976), that is, parts of utterances containing such unessential verbiage as false starts and unsuccessful revisions.

If samples of voluntarily or prompted slowing of speech are available, the language characteristics of these samples should be compared to those of the client's usual speech output. This information will help to determine to what extent the language difficulties observed are primary linguistic deficits versus the results of attempting to speak at a rate that exceeds the speaker's linguistic capacity.

Auditory Skills Assessment

A complete audiological evaluation is recommended for suspected or confirmed clutterers. This typically includes thresholds for pure tones and speech, speech discrimination, and tympa- nometry. In addition, standardized measures of central auditory skills to identify deficits that may be related to cluttering symptoms can help deter- mine whether auditory processing is affected. Such tasks usually include perception and dis- crimination tasks in difficult listening circum- stances, such as dichotic stimulation or competing messages.

Psychoeducational Assessment

Clutterers often have coexisting learning disabil- ities (LD) or attention-deficit/hyperactivity dis- orders (ADHD). Cluttering children in public schools may have already been diagnosed with either condition, and, if so, the speech-language pathologist should review reports in the child's school records or from the diagnostic center where the testing was done. Ideally, this review precedes the diagnostic evaluation for cluttering, so that duplication of effort—and expense—can be avoided and any additional testing can focus on filling in missing information or verifying ex- isting deficits. If a client has not received such special testing, screening for typical LD or ADHD deficits should be included in the com- plete diagnostic assessment for suspected clut- tering.

Cognitive Assessment

Suspected clutterers in schools may occasionally be labeled as "mentally retarded" if their full-scale intelligence quotient (IQ) falls below a specified number, generally 70. Several authors have re- ported that stuttering in the mentally retarded pop- ulation often resembles cluttering (e.g., Canabas, 1954; Cooper, 1986), especially in Martin-Bell Fragile X Syndrome (Adesman, 1989; Hanson, Jackson, & Hagerman, 1986). If communication deficits, such as various language errors, are sus- pected to be caused by or significantly related to deficits in cognition, clinicians should review find- ings from IQ or related tests. Generally, however, this will not be the case.

Motor Skills Assessment

A variety of motoric symptoms commonly ac- company cluttering (Daly, 1986, 1992; Weiss, 1964). These include hyperactivity, excessive fid- geting, clumsiness, and poor handwriting. A com- plete diagnostic assessment of cluttering should, therefore, include assessment of handwriting (from a writing sample), general body coordina- tion and manual dexterity (from general observa- tion or standardized testing), and overall activity level (from observation of the client's activity level in the diagnostic setting and from reports of family, teachers, co-workers, and peers).

Summary

Table 16.2, adapted from Daly, Myers, and St. Louis (1992) and St. Louis and Myers (1995) and Daly (1986; 1992; 1993), Myers (1992), (St. Louis (1992), Tiger et al. (1980), Weiss (1964), and Wiig and Semel (1984), provides a summary of the di- agnostic information discussed in this section and lists signs that are suggestive or pathognomonic of cluttering and three other diagnostic categories. Like Figure 16.1, this table clearly illustrates the substantial overlap among symptoms of clutter- ing, stuttering, learning disabilities, and attention- deficit/hyperactivity disorders.

SYNERGISTIC APPROACH TO THERAPY FOR CLUTTERING AND RELATED FLUENCY DISORDERS

The clinical approach adopted here, and in several other of our writings (Myers, 1992; Myers & Bradley, 1992; St. Louis & Myers, 1995), has been termed a synergistic approach. Several constructs provide the framework for this therapy perspective: the coexistence of speech-language functions, syn- ergism, synchrony, coherence, and cohesion. Briefly, coexistence of speech-language functions refers to the interrelatedness of different aspects of the communication system. There is increasing ev- idence that two or more communication disorders coexist (Cullinan & Springer, 1980; Louko, Con- ture, & Edwards, 1990; St. Louis et al., 1992), and

TABLE 16.2   Differential Diagnosis of Cluttering

	Key	
CL	Cluttering	*X* Obligatory in diagnosis (Symptoms in italics)*
ST	Stuttering	x Optional symptom frequently present
LD	Learning Disability	? Symptom that may or may not be present
ADHD	Attention-Deficit/Hyperactivity Disorder	

	CL	ST	LD	ADHD
FLUENCY AND RATE ASSESSMENT				
Excessive sound-syllable repetitions, prolongations, and blocks or avoidance of these		*X*		
Excessive whole word repetitions, phrase repetitions, and fillers	*X*		x	
Accessory behaviors		x		
Rapid articulatory rate (excluding pauses)	*X*			
Irregular rate (arhythmic)	*X*		?	?
Improvement in fluency when instructed to slow down and concentrate	x		?	?
ARTICULATION ASSESSMENT				
Presence of developmental errors	x	?	x	?
Presence of vowel neutralization	x			
Presence of telescoping of syllables	x			
Presence of cluster reduction	x			
Presence of prosodic errors	x			
ORAL/AUDITORY LANGUAGE ASSESSMENT				
Reduced comprehension of vocabulary	?		x	
Lexical (word-finding) errors	x		x	
Syntactic errors	x	?	x	?
Disorganized sentences ("mazes")	x		x	x
CASE HISTORY				
Specific onset of fluency disorder identified		x		
Significant changes in the form of disfluencies after onset		x		
Family history of fluency disorder	x	x		
Family history of speech/language disorder	x	x	?	?
Family history of attention-deficit/hyperactivity disorder	?		?	x
Delayed speech/language development	x	x	x	x
Delayed/inadequate motor development	x		x	?
History of academic difficulties	x		x	x
Aggressive, hasty, untidy, impulsive personality	x		x	*X*
History of limited attention span/distractible/hyperactive	x		x	*X*
History of lack of awareness/concern about disorder	x		?	?
PSYCHOEDUCATIONAL ASSESSMENT				
Reading comprehension problems	x		*X*	x
Oral reading difficulties	x		*X*	x
Writing problems	x		*X*	x
Arithmetic problems			*X*	x
Handwriting problems	x		x	?
COGNITIVE ASSESSMENT				
Distractibility/limited attention span	x		x	*X*
Impaired awareness of the problem	*X*		?	
Perceptual deficits	x		x	x
Deficits not due to reduced general intelligence	*X*	*X*	*X*	*X*
MOTOR ASSESSMENT				
Reduced general motor coordination	x		x	x
Reduced diadochokinetic rates	x	?	?	?
Hyperactivity	x		x	*X*

*Authorities do not consistently agree that all symptoms are obligatory.

relationships between the concomitant disorders may be associative or causal. For example, difficulties with word finding may lead a language-disordered child to use a number of fillers such as "um . . . uh . . . well, you see," rendering speech highly disfluent, disjointed, and somewhat incohesive. This interrelation between two or more areas of speech and language is highly pertinent to constructs of synergism and synchrony.

Synergism has to do with different parts of the communication system working together in a highly coordinated and well timed or synchronous manner. One consequence of this synergistic and synchronous interaction is that different parts of the system affect others. When rate is too fast or not well modulated with linguistic or thought units, discourse loses coherence and cohesion. This is why it can be so enervating to carry on a conversation with a clutterer. Listeners rely on clarity of articulation, pauses, falling and rising intonation contours, as well as syntactic/semantic markers to derive meaning. At its worst, clutterers' speech contains a paucity of such markers for increasing speech intelligibility or linguistic clarity. Moreover, many clutterers are often unaware of conversational breakdowns. We have found that most clutterers have a difficult time evaluating their speech on-line, even after they have made behavioral strides in therapy. Table 16.3 illustrates how different aspects of speech and language may affect the speech intelligibility, coherence, and cohesion of discourse.

The major components within the oral communication system (i.e., rate, fluency, articulation, and language) affect each other as well. Other aspects of communication, such as voice, are considered of secondary importance for most clutterers. Speech rate and fluency are related, and both govern the rhythm or flow of speech and language. Viewpoints differ regarding whether rate and fluency should be considered separately or together. Starkweather (1987), for example, views rate and fluency to be so intrinsically linked that the two cannot be separated. In the case of cluttering, however, we prefer to deal with rate and fluency separately, while acknowledging that the two are interrelated, because rate anomalies appear to be a prominent etiologic factor for many of the other symptoms of cluttering. For example, rate that is too fast can lead to multiple misarticulations; language formulation problems can lead to disfluencies; and poor self-monitoring skills can lead to or aggravate existing problems in discourse coherence and cohesiveness.

Special Considerations

We have found the following set of therapy principles and specific therapy techniques to be helpful in the treatment of cluttering. Other chapters in this volume discuss treatment approaches to stuttering. Because clients often evidence elements of both stuttering and cluttering, respective elements of each disorder should be considered and a therapy program designed accordingly. With few exceptions, successful transfer and maintenance has been notoriously difficult to come by, especially with severe clutterers. This latter subgroup may be likened to chronic stutterers who fail to show sustained improvement even with the best of therapy guidance. Prognosis has traditionally been considered guarded with severe clutterers due to difficul-

TABLE 16.3   Aspects of Speech and Language Affecting Speech Intelligibility and Linguistic Coherence/Cohesion

	ARTICU-LATION	LANGUAGE	FLUENCY	SELF-MONITORING	RATE
Speech Intelligibility	YES	—	YES	YES	YES
Linguistic Coherence/Cohesion	—	YES	YES	YES	YES

ties with self-monitoring, or perhaps because of some intrinsic deficit in their sense of timing or various modalities of sensory feedback. Clearly, more systematic research is needed to improve therapy approaches and thereby change the long-held notion that prognosis is less than favorable.

In keeping with the major components framework for the speech and language system just outlined, the following therapy principles and techniques are organized in terms of rate and rhythm, fluency, articulation-phonology, and language functions.

Principles and Techniques for Improvement of Rate and Rhythm of Speech

1. The clinician should systematically modulate the speaking context, starting with contexts that are highly structured and nonpropositional, and encourage the client to use simple and short utterances. The clinician might start with reading lists of words or short phrases first, then longer passages, marked for pauses that coincide with phrase or clause junctures. The next step would be extemporaneous speech using short responses to questions followed by extemporaneous speech using utterances with simple syntactic structures. Clutterers seem to gain better control of their speech faculties, particularly rate, under these step-by-step conditions.

2. If necessary, the clutterer should be provided with the rhythmic scaffolding or structure needed to coordinate respiratory with articulatory and linguistic junctures and to produce appropriate stress patterns within words. Many clutterers speak in run-on sentences with a monotone inflectional contour. Not only is this uninteresting to listeners, but such speech is sometimes difficult to understand. By appropriately stressing syllables, the clutterer eliminates the monotone (by increasing pitch and loudness on the stressed syllables) and slows rate (by adding duration to stressed syllables). Other scaffolding measures include the recitation of poetry, singing, and reading simple scripts from plays, because

these passages have built-in cadences to slow the rate and improve rhythm.

3. Another strategy that can be used involves a delayed auditory feedback (DAF) device to slow speech rate, enhance the intelligibility of speech, and provide clutterers with the sensory feedback associated with slower, smoother speech. It is important that clients keep pace with the preset delay and not attempt to ignore it. The clinician might tape record their speech and play it back to demonstrate that they can slow their rate. Some clutterers dislike having to connect syllables by prolonging (primarily) vowels; others may demonstrate respectable success but need a "booster shot" of DAF if progress is not maintained.

Principles and Techniques for Improvement of Articulation

1. Clutterers typically exhibit multiple misarticulations that are not phoneme-specific. Rather than having a consistent /r/ distortion or a lisp, the more common types of misarticulations include elision of unstressed syllables, cluster reduction, neutralization of vowels, and generally indistinct production of sounds. These characteristics are likely to result from speaking at a rate faster than the clutterer can handle. Therefore, probably the single most powerful principle of therapy for decreasing these misarticulations is to slow speaking rate and use more effective phrasing and pausing.

2. Most clutterers have a tendency to rush through the endings of words and utterances and need help to prolong the endings of words.

3. Some discussion appealing to a clutterer's metalinguistic intuition may also be helpful if the client is old enough to understand. It may be helpful to explain that a fair proportion of intended "information" is lost because of missing sounds and syllables. Because these omissions are not phoneme-specific, listeners have less chance to predict a message correctly. Sometimes it is useful to provide clut-

terers with a transcription of a speech sample that specifies the various omissions of sounds and syllables. This way, they can see the degradation of the intended message, as they listen to a recording of the sample.

4. If a clutterer also happens to evidence a phoneme-specific misarticulation or a phonological process, these sounds/processes can be targeted in conventional ways.

Principles and Techniques for Improvement of Language

1. Some clutterers have word-finding problems. This may be due to a basic language deficiency or to momentary difficulties in organizing and encoding thoughts in a coherent manner. One clutterer reflected, "Sometimes several thoughts would come at the same time, and I don't know how, which to say first and which to say next." We have found that by slowing speech rate (rather than using run-on sentences), the clutterer is more likely to find the time needed to put his or her thoughts in order.

2. Some clutterers need therapy for semantics and syntax, particularly for more linguistically complex utterances. We have found it useful to emphasize relational words that serve to connect thoughts and clauses. Such words include because, unless, therefore, however, nevertheless, but. These relational words require certain logical operations that need to be explained before having a client put them into use.

3. Clutterers can be asked to outline the essential components of narratives. An outline serves to focus on essential elements and to bring out the hierarchical relations of a message. Perhaps the clinician could have a client use the outline as an aid in telling a story, then play back the recorded narrative to demonstrate the increased cohesion and coherence of language when using an outline.

4. Loban's (1976) maze behaviors are often present in clutterers' speech. These include incomplete phrases and revisions, fillers, and

word and phrase repetitions. As was suggested for articulatory errors, a written transcription of recorded discourse, containing all the maze behaviors, may be useful for the clutterer to see. Maze behaviors serve only to "clutter" a message, and like household clutter, should be cleaned out, because they are unessential and only confound messages. An example of Loban's system of transcription for the intended message, "Last Sunday afternoon we went to grandma's house for a picnic with all my cousins" is:

[Last] last [Satur—, I mean,] Sunday afternoon [we] we went to grandma's house for a picnic [um, um] with [my,] all my cousins.

To highlight such errors, the clinician might have the clutterer read his utterance first with all the maze behaviors or clutter included. After reading the transcription, the client can be helped to paraphrase the same story using similar wording but with minimal maze behaviors.

5. Many clutterers can benefit from improving their pragmatic skills. Pragmatics can be viewed as social competence, which reflects an important aspect of "social cognition." Clutterers' pragmatic difficulties appear to be a lack of social awareness. Whereas most people instinctively repair conversational breakdowns when listener feedback indicates such need, clutterers often need to learn the techniques of conversational repair, much as a language-disordered child or adolescent needs such therapy. Role-playing and video playback of conversations and interactions have been useful and effective for us in this regard.

Principles and Techniques to Improve Fluency

1. As was noted earlier in this chapter, fluency and rate are highly related in function. In the case of cluttering, we propose that rate and language are the primary determinants of fluency. Thus, clutterers are less likely to ex-

hibit maze-like behaviors or experience difficulties in formulating thought into language and speech when they are taught to slow their speaking rate.

2. The clinician should determine whether a clutterer needs to practice linguistic fluency or speech fluency. Linguistic fluency has to do with the flow of words and propositions, and when one has difficulty in this area, various forms of disfluency may surface. If linguistic fluency is targeted, the clinician might attempt to broaden the clutterer's semantic network by eliciting and using various synonyms and antonyms for a word and words having multiple meanings. Another strategy involves having the client practice transforming simple-active-affirmative-declarative sentences into other syntactic structures. For example, the sentence, "The girl hugged the boy." can be transformed into such forms as: "Did the girl hug the boy?" "The girl did not hug the boy." "The boy was hugged by the girl." "It was the girl who hugged the boy." "The girl hugged the boy, didn't she?" In this exercise, the aim is improved fluidity of language use. In addition to linguistic fluency, some clutterers also have difficulty with speech fluency. Largely due to an overly fast rate of speech, the sequencing of sounds and syllables becomes disturbed, resulting in elision of sounds and unstressed syllables, cluster reduction, and vowel neutralization. It sometimes seems that speech becomes so fluid that it gushes out of control. Dalton and Hardcastle (1989) used the term "overcoarticulation" to characterize clutterers' sound-to-sound transitions. This contrasts with the speech disfluency of "pure" stutterers, who typically exercise great deliberation, effort, and even struggle to go from one sound or syllable to the next. If a clutterer exhibits "overcoarticulation" that is apparently due to a fast speaking rate (e.g., "telephone" becomes "tephon"), the clinician could have the client underline the stressed syllable but also attend to the unstressed syllables or the smaller words of an utterance such as "a" and "the."

3. If a client exhibits stuttering types of disfluencies, appropriate therapeutic techniques include teaching easy voice onset and loose contacts to counteract the physiological tension often associated with stuttering blocks. This type of client may also need help to reduce avoidance or postponement behaviors. Such behaviors are not common in "pure" clutterers, but many disfluent individuals manifest both cluttering and stuttering. In such cases, a judicious blend of fluency therapy for both disorders is warranted.

Principles and Techniques to Improve Self-Monitoring

1. Improving self-monitoring skills is absolutely essential in therapy for cluttering. This area of therapy can be divided into two phases. First, at least for older children, what is needed is a thorough discussion (with many examples) of the nature of cluttering and how various behaviors reduce the speech and language intelligibility of a clutterer's speech. Many clutterers are not even remotely aware of their communication breakdowns in conversation. Many also have singular difficulty in detecting when they are speaking at a rate faster than they can handle. The analogy of losing control when a car is going too fast and skids on wet pavement can be helpful. Some clutterers seem so "energized" that the analogy of an overheated engine might also be used by encouraging clients to "cool the engine" or "shift to a lower gear" when they sense that their speech and language mechanism is too agitated. After achieving an intellectual appreciation of the effects of cluttering on communication, the second phase should focus on specific techniques to improve self-monitoring skills.

2. The following are specific techniques for improving self-monitoring skills:
   a. using negative practice: purposely contrasting appropriate rate with fast rate

b. developing and using a list of "danger signs" of when speech "gets into trouble": repeating words, beginning to have an irregular rate, producing run-on sentences, seeing listeners' nonverbal or verbal feedback (e.g., a frown or "What did you say?") following a communication breakdown, dropping of sounds and syllables, and mumbling or slurring of speech

c. closing the eyes in order to focus on other senses (tactile, kinesthetic, or proprioceptive) associated with articulation rate

d. varying the rate of movement of other parts of the body (e.g., raising and lowering the arms at various rates) to get a feel of the relative rapidity of movement in larger muscle groups

e. listening to recorded examples of desired rates as well as speech spoken too rapidly

Principles and Techniques to Improve the Client's Cognitive/Attitudinal/Emotional Components Associated with Speech

We agree with Daly (1992) about the importance of cultivating a positive attitude toward speech. Because most clutterers are not aware that they have a speech problem—or even acknowledge that there are frequent communication breakdowns, a situation that presents an even greater clinical challenge—cognitive and attitudinal training is essential. Both clinician and client need to assess what goals might be set. These often involve a realistic acceptance of certain aspects of the client's speech and language behaviors or acknowledging that rate control cannot be achieved with uniform success all the time. We try to strike an appropriate balance between being realistic and being positive. After an initial "honeymoon" period, some clients express resistance to making changes and need help to reaffirm a more positive attitude. We give clients only those homework assignments that we know can be carried out without undue difficulty, so that they can experience success. When friends

or colleagues remark on positive changes (many times, they simply say "Gee, Johnny's speech is more understandable now!"), we pass along these sincere and unsolicited compliments to the client.

Some clutterers may also show elements of impulsivity, not only in speech but also in nonspeech behaviors. For example, upon hearing a car pulling up the driveway, a client may interrupt the lesson by going to the window to see who is arriving at the door. Clutterers often exhibit a divergent style of thinking and problem-solving and may need help to focus on the task at hand. In turn, the clinician can be strategically selective in teasing out the key words of a reading passage, or eliciting the major points of a story to be told, or pointing out the crux of a mathematics problem. If necessary, the clinician should help a client tune out unimportant stimuli in the environment. Many of these techniques should be conveyed to parents and family members so that they can help as well. Cognitive training techniques might be shared with family and close associates so that they have a better understanding of the complex of speech and nonspeech problem behaviors that may coexist with cluttering.

Conconcluding Comments on Management

This discussion of therapy principles and techniques focused largely on the communication problems of clutterers. Other chapters in this volume discuss in detail the clinical management of people who only stutter. The therapy approach we presented adopts a synergistic framework to take into account coexisting speech-language difficulties of clutterers. The ultimate aim of therapy is to enable a clutterer to produce extemporaneous speech that is coherent, cohesive, intelligible, and fluent. Some of the techniques we discussed might also be applied to the speech and language disfluencies present in other disorders, such as those of LD clients. Various clinicians have at one time or another applied one or more of these principles and techniques to therapy, with varying degrees of success.

CHALLENGES FOR THE FUTURE

Nearly every recent presentation, article, chapter, or book on cluttering that we cited ends with a "call to arms" for researchers to address this long-ignored communication disorder. We do so again, but with slightly more hope than before. The reason for hope is that, after a generation, cluttering is once again appearing in most academic texts on stuttering (as in this book, which did not address the topic of cluttering in its first edition [Curlee & Perkins, 1984]), sessions on cluttering are being presented with some regularity at professional meetings, and efforts are underway to devote an issue of a well known journal to a collection of case studies on the disorder.

In spite of the progress that has been made and the efforts that are ongoing, at least two challenges for future research bear highlighting. The first is developing better classifications of fluency disorders.[4] Currently, the term "fluency" has a variety of meanings, ranging, of course, from the flow of speech in a stutterer or clutterer to the expertise one may have in a foreign language. Whereas scientists and clinicians probably cannot be expected to agree on all aspects of classification and nomenclature, agreement to use the same terminology would greatly enhance mutual understanding. Efforts are underway to improve classifications and terminology (e.g. from the Special Interest Division on Fluency and Fluency Disorders of the American Speech-Language-Hearing Association), but it is too soon to tell how successful they will be. In the area of cluttering, a consensus is needed on such questions as: "Is a fluency disorder different from a rate disorder?" "What are the necessary and sufficient signs and symptoms to diagnose cluttering?" and "What should—and should not—be taken as evidence that stuttering and cluttering coexist in the same individual?"

The second challenge is the need for treatment efficacy studies. Such research is difficult to do, for all the reasons that clinical research is always difficult in any disorder, but also because large groups of clients who clutter are typically not available for study. Consequently, we agree with Attanasio (1994) that small group or single-subject clinical research studies offer the best promise for generating useful, meaningful data on what works, and why, as well as what doesn't work, and why not, with this population.

SUMMARY

This chapter has summarized the elusive disorder called cluttering. There is disagreement about the definition, although most authors highlight rate and fluency problems, often associated with articulatory or language difficulties. To complicate matters further, cluttering often is confused with—or coexists with—other disorders such as tachylalia, learning disabilities, attention-deficit/hyperactivity disorders, and stuttering. Therefore, it is important that clinicians carry out careful diagnostic procedures to isolate cluttering from other related speech, language, educational, cognitive, or motoric disorders or disabilities.

The authors recommend a synergistic approach to therapy for cluttering clients. Such an approach focuses on the interrelatedness of various aspects of communication, that is, rate, fluency, articulation, and language. For example, targeting and reducing speaking rate in therapy can and often does have beneficial effects on fluency, language, and articulation as well. Within each of these areas, specific suggestions for therapy with cluttering clients are provided.

Cluttering has apparently been rediscovered by mainstream speech-language pathologists. Nevertheless, there are important challenges that future research must address, including a need for more precise terminology and classifications and for treatment efficacy studies.

---

[4]It is disappointing that those who wrote the DSM-IV revision (American Psychiatric Association, 1994) chose not to include cluttering, even though the DSM-III-R (American Psychiatric Association, 1987) did include a useful definition.

REFERENCES

Adesman, A.R. (1989). Fragile X syndrome. *Children's Hospital Quarterly*, *3*, 69–74.

American Psychiatric Association. (1987). *Diagnostic and statistical manual of mental disorders* (3rd ed., Revised). Washington, D.C.: Author.

American Psychiatric Association. (1994). *Diagnostic and statistical manual of mental disorders* (4th ed.). Washington, D.C.: Author.

American Speech-Language-Hearing Association. (1992). *Attention deficit hyperactivity disorder* (Let's Talk, No. 41). Rockville, MD: Author.

Andrews, G., & Cutler, J. (1974). Stuttering therapy: The relation between changes in symptom level and attitudes. *Journal of Speech and Hearing Disorders*, *39*, 312–319.

Arnold, G. (1960). Studies in tachyphemia: I. Present concepts of etiologic factors. *Logos*, 3–23.

Atkins, C.P., & St. Louis, K.O. (1988). Speech awareness questionnaire (SAQ). *Communiqué* (Journal of the West Virginal Speech-Language-Hearing Association), 8–11.

Attanasio, J.S. (1994). Inferential statistics and treatment efficacy studies in communication disorders. *Journal of Speech and Hearing Research*, *37*, 755–759.

Beebe, H.H. (1960). Voluntary tachylalia. *Folia Phoniatrica*, *12*, 223–228.

Bloodstein, O. (1987). *A handbook on stuttering*. (4th ed.). Chicago: National Easter Seal Society.

Canabas, E. (1954). Some findings in speech and voice therapy among mentally deficient children. *Folia Phoniatrica*, *6*, 34–37.

Cantwell, D.P., & Baker, L. (1991). Association between attention deficit-hyperactivity disorder and learning disorders. *Journal of Learning Disabilities*, *24*, 88–95.

Conture, E.G., Louko, L.J., & Edwards, M.L. (1993). Simultaneously treating stuttering and disordered phonology in children: Experimental treatment, preliminary findings. *American Journal of Speech-Language Pathology*, *2*, 72–81.

Cooper, E.B. (1986). The mentally retarded stutterer. In K.O. St. Louis (Ed.), *The atypical stutterer*. New York: Academic Press.

Cullinan, W.L., & Springer, M.T. (1980). Voice initiation times in stuttering and nonstuttering children. *Journal of Speech and Hearing Research*, *23*, 344–360.

Curlee, R.F., & Perkins, W.H. (Eds.). (1984). *Nature and treatment of stuttering: New directions*. San Diego, CA: College-Hill.

Dalton, P., & Hardcastle, W. (1989). *Disorders of fluency and their effects on communication*. London: Elsevier-North Holland.

Daly, D.A. (1981). Differentiation of stuttering subgroups with Van Riper's developmental tracks: A preliminary study. *Journal of the National Student Speech-Language-Hearing Association*, *9*, 89–101.

Daly, D.A. (1986). The clutterer. In K.O. St. Louis (Ed.), *The atypical stutterer: Principles and practices of rehabilitation*. New York: Academic Press.

Daly, D.A. (1992). Helping the clutterer: Therapy considerations. In F.L. Myers & K.O. St. Louis (Eds.), *Cluttering: A clinical perspective*. Kibworth, Great Britain: Far Communications.

Daly, D.A. (1993). Cluttering: Another fluency syndrome. In R.F. Curlee (Ed.), *Stuttering and related disorders of fluency*. New York: Thieme Medical Publishers.

Daly, D.A., Myers, F.L., & St. Louis, K.O. (1992). *Cluttering: A pathology lost but found*. Paper presented at the annual convention of the American Speech-Language-Hearing Association, San Antonio, Texas.

deHirsch, K. (1961). Studies in tachyphemia: 4. Diagnosis of developmental language disorders. *Logos*, *4*, 3–9.

Diedrich, W.M. (1984). Cluttering: Its diagnosis. In H. Winitz (Ed.). *Treating articulation disorders: For clinicians by clinicians*. Baltimore: University Park Press.

Epstein, M.A., Shaywitz, S.E., Shaywitz, B.A., & Woolston, J.L. (1991). The boundaries of attention deficit disorder. *Journal of Learning Disabilities*, *24*, 78–86.

Fairbanks, G. (1960). *Voice and articulation drillbook*. New York: Harper & Row.

Freeman, F.J. (1982). Stuttering. In N.J. Lass, L.V. McReynolds, J.L. Northern, & D.E. Yoder (Eds.), *Speech, language, and hearing: Pathologies of speech and language, Vol. 2*. Philadelphia: W.B. Saunders.

Freund, H. (1952). Studies in the interrelationship between the stuttering and cluttering. *Folia Phoniatrica*, *4*, 146–168.

Hanson, D.M., Jackson, A.W. III, & Hagerman, R.J.

(1986) Speech disturbances (cluttering) in mildly impaired males with the Martin-Bell Fragile X syndrome. *American Journal of Medical Genetics, 23*, 195–206.

Ingham, R.J. (1984). *Stuttering and behavior therapy: Current status and experimental foundations*. San Diego, CA: College-Hill Press.

Interagency Committee on Learning Disabilities. (1987). *Learning disabilities—A report to the U.S. Congress*. Washington, D.C.: Department of Health and Human Services.

Langova, J., & Moravek, M. (1964). Some results of experimental examinations among stutterers and clutterers. *Folia Phoniatrica, 16*, 290–296.

Loban, W. (1976). *The language of elementary school children*. Champaign, Ill.: National Council of Teachers of English.

Louko, L.J., Conture, E.G., & Edwards, M.L. (1990). *Co-morbidity co-occurrence: Research and clinical considerations*. Paper presented at the annual convention of the American Speech-Language-Hearing Association, Seattle, Washington.

Luchsinger, R. (1963). *Poltern: Erkenung, ursachen und behandlung*. Berlin-Charlottenburg: Marhold Verlag.

Luchsinger, R., & Arnold, G.E. (1965). *Voice-speech-language: Clinical communicology: Its physiology and pathology*. Belmont, Calif.: Wadsworth.

Moravek, M., & Langova, J. (1962). Some electrophysiological findings among stutterers and clutterers. *Folia Phoniatrica, 14*, 305–316.

Myers, F.L. (1992). Cluttering: A synergistic framework. In F.L. Myers & K.O. St. Louis (Eds.). *Cluttering: A clinical perspective*. Kibworth, Great Britain: Far Communications.

Myers, F.L., & Bradley, C.L. (1992). Clinical management of cluttering from a synergistic framework. In F.L. Myers & K.O. St. Louis (Eds.). *Cluttering: A clinical perspective*. Kibworth, Great Britain: Far Communications.

Myers, F.L., & St. Louis, K.O. (1992). Cluttering: Issues and controversies. In F.L. Myers & K.O. St. Louis (Eds.) *Cluttering: A clinical perspective*. Kibworth, Great Britain: Far Communications.

Preus, A. (1981). *Identifying subgroups of stutterers*. Oslo: Universitetsforlaget.

Preus, A. (1992). Cluttering and stuttering: Related, different or antagonistic disorders? In F.L. Myers & K.O. St. Louis (Eds.) *Cluttering: A clinical perspective*. Kibworth, Great Britain: Far Communications.

Seeman, M. (1970). Relations between motorics of speech and general motor ability in clutterers. *Folia Phoniatrica, 22*, 376–378.

Seeman, M., & Novak, A. (1963). Ueber die motorik bei polterern. *Folia Phoniatrica, 15*, 170–176.

Smith, S. (1955). Den paedagogiske behandling of stammen og lobsk tale. In N.Rh. Blegvad (Ed.), *Nordisk laerebog for talepaedagoger*. Copenhagen: Rosenkilde & Bagger.

Starkweather, C.W. (1987). *Fluency and stuttering*. Englewood Cliffs, N.J.: Prentice-Hall.

St. Louis, K.O. (1992). On defining cluttering. In F.L. Myers & K.O. St. Louis (Eds.). *Cluttering: A clinical perspective*. Kibworth, Great Britain: Far Communications.

St. Louis, K.O. (1994). *Investigations of speech naturalness ratings*. Paper presented at the First World Congress on Fluency Disorders, Munich, Germany.

St. Louis, K.O., Chambers, C.D., & Ashworth, M.S. (1991). Coexisting communication disorders in a random sample of school-aged stutterers. *Journal of Fluency Disorders, 16*, 13–23.

St. Louis, K.O., Hansen, G.G.R., Oliver, T.L., & Buch, J.L. (1992). Voice deviations and coexisting communication disorders. *Language, Speech and Hearing Services in Schools, 23*, 82–87.

St. Louis, K.O., & Hinzman, A.R. (1988). A descriptive study of speech, language, and hearing characteristics of school-aged stutterers. *Journal of Fluency Disorders, 13*, 331–356.

St. Louis, K.O., Hinzman, A.R., & Hull, F.M. (1985). Studies of cluttering: Disfluency and language measures in young possible clutterers and stutterers. *Journal of Fluency Disorders, 10*, 151–172.

St. Louis, K.O., & Myers, F.L. (1995). Clinical management of cluttering. *Language, Speech, and Hearing Services in Schools, 25*, .

St. Louis, K.O., Ruscello, D.M., & Lundeen, C. (1992). *Coexistence of communication disorders in school-children*. ASHA Monograph No. 27. Rockville, Md. American Speech-Language-Hearing Association.

Tiger, R., Irvine, T., & Reis, R. (1980). Cluttering as a complex of learning disabilities. *Language, Speech, and Hearing Services in Schools, 11*, 3–14.

Van Riper, C. (1971). *The nature of stuttering*. Englewood Cliffs, N.J.: Prentice-Hall.

Van Riper, C. (1982). *The nature of stuttering* (2nd ed.). Englewood Cliffs, N.J.: Prentice-Hall.

Wallace, S. (1992). *Getting the whole picture: A total*

communication approach to group therapy for dys-fluent adults who have learning disabilities. Unpublished manuscript.

Weiss, D. (1964). *Cluttering.* Englewood Cliffs, N.J.: Prentice-Hall.

Weiss, D. (1967). Similarities and differences between cluttering and stuttering. *Folia Phoniatrica, 19,* 98–104.

Weiss, D. (1968). Cluttering: Central language imbalance. *Pediatric Clinics of North America, 15,* 66–76.

Wiig, E.H., & Semel, E. (1984). *Language assessment and intervention for the learning disabled* (2nd ed.). Columbus, OH: Charles E. Merrill.

Woolf, G. (1967). The assessment of stuttering as struggle, avoidance, and expectancy. *British Journal of Disorders of Communication, 2,* 158–177.

Yaruss, J.S., Logan, K.J., & Conture. E.G. (1994). *Comparing speaking performance and speaking ability of children who stutter.* Paper presented at the annual convention of the American Speech-Language-Hearing Association, New Orleans, LA.

SUGGESTED READINGS

Daly, D.A. (1993). Cluttering: Another fluency syndrome. In R.F. Curlee (Ed.), *Stuttering and related disorders of fluency.* New York: Thieme Medical Publishers. David Daly is widely known for his work on the treatment of clutterers. This chapter summarizes his basic approach to diagnosis and therapy and complements a similar chapter written in the Myers and St. Louis book.

Myers, F.L., & St. Louis, K.O., Eds. (1992). *Cluttering: A clinical perspective.* Kibworth, Great Britain: Far Communications. This book, edited by authors of the current chapter, is the only recent book devoted entirely to cluttering. It contains recent literature, theoretical views, and practical suggestions for diagnosis and treatment of cluttering. (The book has been reissued and will henceforth be available from Singular Publishing Group of San Diego, Calif.).

Weiss, D. (1964). *Cluttering.* Englewood Cliffs, N.J.: Prentice-Hall. This book by Deso Weiss presents a comprehensive historical perspective on cluttering, primarily from the European phoniatrics traditional perspective. Until recently, it was the most widely accepted and cited source on cluttering.

PART FIVE

CLINICAL MANAGEMENT OF ADULTS

Children who continue to stutter into adulthood are unlikely to achieve complete, permanent relief from the symptoms of a chronic stuttering disorder. In addition to disruptions in flow of speech, most adults who stutter find their lives to be disrupted in a variety of others ways. As was noted earlier by Starkweather, most also acquire a number of sound, speaking task, and situational fears related to their stuttering experiences. Complex escape and avoidance behaviors, lowered expectations, and diminished self-concepts often follow as if one's life is revolving around adaptations to stuttering. Management of this panoply of problems usually begins with either a focus on modifying a person's affective, cognitive, and behavioral reactions to stuttering or on behavioral procedures that attempt to prevent or reduce the occurrence of stuttering.

Prins's chapter provides a historical perspective and attempts a conceptual integration of treatment methods developed by Johnson and Van Riper into principles of learning proposed by behaviorists such as Bandura. As a result, clinical procedures that evolved from the etiological views and clinical experiences of early speech pathologists are provided the respectability accorded to theories of learning. It is interesting to note, also, how differently Perkins and Prins interpret the same early period in the history of stuttering theory and treatment, and how differently they view the contributions of those individuals who influenced it.

Next, Onslow and Packman contrast methods that rely on prolonged speech training, which often involve intensive treatment in a group setting, with operant methods that attempt to eliminate stuttering without first teaching stutterers unusual or unnatural speech patterns and which are suitable for nonintensive, individual treatment schedules. It is one of few recent chapters that devotes any space to the operant-based treatment methods that were dominant in the late 1960s and 1970s.

The three chapters that follow are all concerned with aspects of measurement. Bakker discusses the explosive development of objective, instrumental methods for assessing numerous dimensions of speech and fluency. It is apparent that future generations of clinicians will have enormously complex instrumentation to augment that most basic, delicate, and crucial instrument—the clinician's own ears and perceptual skills.

Then, Schiavetti and Metz review the relatively recent development of formal measures for scaling speech naturalness. This scale, as first proposed by Martin, Haroldson, and Triden, was intended to assess the extent to which the speech of people who stutter sounds as natural as that of nonstuttering speakers. Later, of course, it has been incorporated into an operant method that modifies as well as evaluates the speech of stutterers.

Ingham and Cordes conclude this section and the text with a thoughtful discussion of treatment efficacy and its measurement. In recent years, they have been especially active in proposing the use of interval judgments of stuttering as a more reliable alternative to conventional counts of nonfluencies. Here, they propose methods for incorporating self-measurement to assess treatment outcomes, an approach that echoes Perkins's insistence on the stutterer being the only valid arbiter of his or her own behavior.

CHAPTER 17

MODIFYING STUTTERING— THE STUTTERER'S REACTIVE BEHAVIOR: PERSPECTIVES ON PAST, PRESENT, AND FUTURE

DAVID PRINS

INTRODUCTION AND OBJECTIVES

"There is no such thing as <u>the</u> method for treating stuttering" (Johnson, 1939, p. 170). This statement is as true today as it was in 1939. Evidence to support it abounds in the literature (Baer, 1989) and, more particularly, in the variety of treatments that purport to provide a modicum of success (Ingham, 1984; Perkins, 1993). The challenge for clinicians, therefore, is to select methods that unite their expertise with the specific needs and complaints of their clients.

This chapter concerns an approach that has come to be called the *management of stuttering*. It bears this title because treatment focuses on changing the stutterer's reactive responses *during* stutter events. Its origins go back to the 1930s, to the ideas of Johnson and Van Riper, who asserted that stuttering consists primarily of *avoidance* reactions to the expectation of fluency failure during speech. According to Johnson and Van Riper, these reactions, sustained by the chronic stutterer's belief that he or she cannot cope effectively with failures of fluency, were the logical focal points of treatment (Prins, 1984, 1993a,b).

Today, the premise for management of stuttering is that *defensive* reactions, triggered by cues that forecast the interruption of fluency, constitute most of the observable behavior associated with stutter events. Supported by current cognitive learning and self-efficacy theories (Bandura, 1977a,b, 1986), a basic tenet of treatment is that chronic stutterers must learn to react with expectations of self-efficacy in the face of cues that formerly threatened fluency failure (Prins, 1984, 1993a).

After briefly characterizing behavior disorders and behavior modification therapies, this chapter will focus on the evolution of ideas that undergird the management of stuttering. Our concern will be with the concepts, more than with the tactics, of therapy; with understanding the why of treatment more than what to do. Examples of procedures will be used, however, to illustrate principal treatment components.

BASIC CONCEPTS

Stuttering as Behavior Disorder

Human behavior disorders have been characterized by essential features at three levels: impairment, disability, and handicap (Frey, 1984). *Impairment* concerns conditions of loss or deficit that may underlie the evidence of disability. For example, in stuttering this could be a central nervous system that is inadequate to meet the encoding or motor execution demands of fluent speech; demands that result in astounding rates of syllable (5–6/sec) and phone (14–15/sec) production. *Disability* refers to the observable breakdown in performance. In the case of stuttering in adults it includes the observable features of stutter events: part-word repetitions; postural fixations with and without sound; and frequently co-occurring muscular tension revealed in facial grimaces, tremor-like movements of lips, jaw, and tongue; and extraneous bodily movements. Other responses that stutterers may use to postpone or avoid anticipated stutter events may also be a part of the disability, including interjections, word repetitions and substitutions, and circumlocution. *Handicap* concerns the effect of the disability on attitudes and feelings, and thereby on the individual's personal, social, educational, and vocational adjustment. Among persons who stutter, the extent of handicap varies enormously and may have little correspondence with degree of disability. Clients who stutter infrequently and with little overt evidence may represent the extremes of handicap. However irrational, they may blame stuttering for virtually all their self-perceived shortcomings. In such cases the disability, however slight, is a fundamental impediment to self-image, social adequacy, and vocational attainment. Others who stutter frequently with severe tension and erratic speech movements sometimes show no evidence of handicap. They regard stuttering as an obstruction to speaking but not an impediment to personal achievement.

To be successful, the clinician must discover the levels and features that are most critical in sustaining an individual client's disorder, and adapt the treatment program accordingly.

Behavior Modification and the Treatment of Stuttering

By their nature, behavior modification therapies ameliorate disorders by focusing directly on the disability. Depending on their emphases, they may also, directly or indirectly, ameliorate conditions associated with impairment and/or handicap.

Applied to the disorder of stuttering, the term "behavior modification" is usually limited to treatments that became popular beginning in the 1960s

and that accompanied the flood of operant research and theory of that period. These treatments emphasize the achievement of fluency; that is, the elimination, rather than the modification, of stuttering. At the outset, they were based on evidence from research suggesting that stutter events could be extinguished or markedly reduced by the appropriate arrangement of stimulus/response conditions. Accordingly, treatment consisted of manipulating these conditions to reduce the frequency of stutter events and thereby induce fluency rather than modify stuttering reactions.

I will assert, however, that behavior modification therapies for stuttering actually began with the ideas of Wendell Johnson and Charles Van Riper, substantially before the 1960s. The bases for their concepts about the nature of the disorder and its treatment were characteristic of what we have come to call the behavior modification therapies (Bandura, 1969). They viewed the deviant behavior of stuttering, not as symptomatic of disease, but as resulting from the stutterer's learned reactions to environmental and self-imposed demands. Similarly, their approaches to treatment were based on behavioral research and motivational learning theory in vogue at the time.

To understand the management of stuttering as it is conceived today, it is necessary to appreciate the historic contributions of Johnson and Van Riper. By absorbing this history, we not only assure a better understanding of the present, but enhance the possibility of developing more effective treatments in the future.

MANAGEMENT OF STUTTERING—ORIGIN AND EVOLUTION OF IDEAS

Contributions of Wendell Johnson

Theory.   In the late 1920s and early 1930s the theory of Orton (1927) and Travis (1931) dominated thinking about the nature and treatment of stuttering. They believed it to be a symptom of insufficient cerebral dominance that, during speaking, was reflected in the neuromuscular disintegration of speech movements. Accordingly, treatment focused on the impairment source and thereby on improving the stutterer's margin of dominance. After assessment revealed a client's "native" sidedness tendencies, programs were set up to retrain that side's unilateral control of a variety of neuromotor acts including speech.

In a paper titled "An Interpretation of Stuttering," Johnson (1933) began to break with these ideas. Here, he first conceptualized the stuttering moment, and viewed it as an event comprising pre-, during-, and post-spasm stages. Still embracing some of Travis's ideas, Johnson concluded that behavior during the spasm needed to be accounted for in terms of "muscle and nerve physiology" (p. 71). However, the spasm's frequency of occurrence, its intensity, and its duration depended also on pre- and post-spasm reactions or attitudes on the part of the speaker. Pre-spasm reactions included fear, anxiety, and dread. Post-spasm reactions included feelings of disgrace. Johnson allowed that a degree of nervous system instability was a necessary underlying cause of the spasm, but that it was not sufficient in most cases to precipitate the spasm. For that to happen, the stutterer's reactions also had to be considered.

Shortly thereafter, Johnson (Johnson & Knott, 1935, 1936) coined the term "moment of stuttering." He asserted that the fundamental problem in understanding the disorder was to account for the precipitation, duration, and termination of these moments. To help account for precipitation and duration, he proposed that the stutterer had a general inhibitory attitude to avoid stuttering. Specific cues from words, sounds, or levels of muscular response then aroused a specific inhibitory attitude to avoid stuttering at that instant. The stutterer then tried to retreat while simultaneously trying to progress, and this motivational and motor response conflict created what we observe as the stutter event. It terminated when the stutterer gave way fully to either the retreating or progressing responses, thus ending the conflict. Johnson asserted that his ideas accounted for the "psychological factors involved in stuttering" (Johnson & Knott, 1935, p. 26). He left open the idea that there might be underlying neurophysiological factors, but then posed an intriguing question: "Of those factors operating prior to

and during the moment of stuttering, are the psychological factors sufficient and necessary to account for that moment?" (p. 32). As we shall see, he concluded later that they were.

In the meantime, Johnson had already contributed the new and provocative idea that the moment of stuttering (in addition to being objectively observable) had a subjective reality for the speaker—a meaning in terms of the speaker's attitudinal set, or beliefs: "Subjectively, stuttering is the experience of conflict resulting from a desire to speak, operating in opposition to a desire to avoid expected stuttering" (Johnson & Knott, 1935, p. 32).

By 1938, Johnson appeared to have repudiated completely the ideas of Travis. Johnson pointed to research showing that virtually all stutterers are fluent most of the time, that stuttering episodes are usually short, and that they occur in relation to "certain sounds, words, and other spatial, situational, and experiential elements or cues" (Johnson, 1938, p. 85). Any explanation had to account for this systematic intermittency, and Johnson believed that theories proposing a constant causal factor could not. He stated that observations of stutter events showed the stutterer was not "organically unable" to proceed, but did not do so because "he is *doing* something that clearly prevents him from producing the next sound" (p. 86). In other words, the behavior during stuttering moments was purposeful: "The stutterer's reaction to expected-stuttering-to-be-avoided" (Johnson & Knott, 1935, p. 31).

These ideas—and later research concerning the adaptation, consistency, and spontaneous recovery of the stuttering response—led Johnson (1955a) to conclude that stuttering was a learned

anxiety motivated avoidant response. Anxious or apprehensive expectation comes to be associated with and to be elicited by the sounds, words, listeners, and other cues or features of situations in relation to which stuttering has been experienced in the past. Such cues, then, function as reminders, and so as storm signals, warning of danger ahead. (p. 23)

Johnson's explanation of the moment of stuttering accounted for its occurrence in the already chronic stutterer. But, how did the motivation to react this way originate and develop? To answer this question, he offered the "interaction hypothesis" (Johnson, 1959). In the beginning, he proposed that the child's responsible listeners (most often the parents) are unusually sensitive to disfluencies and are prone to evaluate them as something abnormal in the child's speech. This leads them to interact with the child by labeling the otherwise normal behavior as unacceptable. In turn, the child internalizes the parents' definition of "unacceptable" as it applies to his or her own speaking behavior. The child begins to evaluate his or her disfluencies negatively, doing things to prevent their occurrence, and so on. This "interaction," the child's internalization of the parents' negative evaluation of speech behavior, was critical in Johnson's conceptualization. Through it, the child symbolized and stored negative disfluency experiences so as to motivate and perpetuate stuttering behavior. With this concept, Johnson explained the disorder, a chronic condition due to the maladaptive beliefs of the speaker that were a common and continuing source for both disability and handicap.

According to Johnson, the interaction sequence was affected by three variables: (1) the listeners' sensitivity, (2) the speaker's degree of disfluency, and (3) the speaker's sensitivity. Johnson believed that the listeners' reactions were crucial at the outset, but ultimately the speaker's sensitivity and reactions as a perceiver of his own speech "determines whether he makes an issue of his nonfluencies and creates a problem around them" (Johnson, 1959, p. 242). Thus, for Johnson it was not the interruption of fluency that made the stutterer unique as a speaker, but the stutterer's reactions because of what the interruption, or its threat, meant.

Treatment.   Johnson's fascination was with the ideas, more than the techniques, of therapy. He stated this explicitly: "The most fundamental step is that of formulating clearly the underlying principles. Once this step has been accomplished, the working out of specific techniques is a quite simple and easy task" (Johnson, 1937, p. 441).

Based on the assumption that stuttering is learned, and in concert with then-popular theories of learning and principles of semantics, Johnson asserted that changes in the speaker's beliefs were crucial to changes in speaking behavior. By emphasizing change in the stutterer's beliefs, Johnson focused his treatment on what he affirmed was the common source of disability and handicap. He proposed two treatment principles: the descriptional principle, and the principle of static analysis (Johnson, 1937).

The goal of the descriptional principle was to help stutterers replace inferential with descriptional terms when talking and thinking about their speaking behavior. Later, Johnson called this the language of responsibility: "Learning to describe clearly and in detail what you do and what the outcomes are, of being specific, not vague" (Johnson, 1961). The descriptional principle was based on Johnson's idea that stuttering reactions are triggered by false assumptions rather than factual observations about talking. To test and renounce these assumptions, stutterers were immersed in experiences involving analysis of their verbal behavior; for example, examining the meaning of such statements as, "The word is stuck in my throat." What does that mean; what are the assumptions? What properties does the "word" have that gives it "stickiness?" Such inferential statements were then replaced by descriptive ones such as, "I tensed the muscles of my tongue and held it to the roof of my mouth." By using descriptive language, stutterers would adopt new, factual inferences about the relationship between what they do and the outcomes for speaking. Eventually, although Johnson spelled out few procedural details, stutterers would begin to react "as quickly as ordinary speech requires" in response to factual inferences derived from insights associated with descriptive language. They would respond by doing things to progress rather than retreat when speaking.

In his principle of static analysis, Johnson described a process through which the objectives of descriptional therapy could be achieved. In his words, "The Principle of Static Analysis is the statement of a method by which we check and revise the relevant hypotheses, and then build up new and more nearly true and dependable inferences" (Johnson, 1937, p. 440). Clients were guided through experiences in which they arrested speech at any point they, or the clinician, identified as stuttering. Clients examined, felt, and evaluated what they were doing in relation to what they assumed happened and what they were intending at that instant. In turn, this led to new, more nearly true inferences on which more effective responses depended, and so on.

Johnson decried the notion of teaching the stutterer to talk without stuttering, or to speak "perfectly," believing this would lead to speech that was free of "stuttering" but was otherwise more "grotesque" because of its artificiality. He believed these approaches heightened the avoidance motivation that was the crux of the problem. Johnson outlined a general treatment sequence: Convince stutterers that they are physically able to speak normally, and can stutter without excessive struggle and tension; then teach them to imitate deliberately their own stuttering and, finally, to develop a "streamlined" pattern of "nonfluency" to replace the stuttering. This pattern could be a simple syllable repetition (bounce) or prolongation (Johnson, 1946).

Somewhat later, Johnson (1955a) spoke of the need for "massed practice" under "consistent conditions" until "plateaus of improvement" were reached, ideas that hint at later-developed behavior modification techniques. But his primary concerns were in changing the stutterer's beliefs about stuttering and about speaking. He made this clear in 1957: "It is as a listener, a perceiver, an evaluator, quite as much—probably, in fact, far more than—as a speaker that the person who stutters is to be treated" (Johnson, 1957, p. 913). Johnson seemed almost to assume that performance change would take care of itself when he wrote: "One need not be too concerned over the question of how one is to change overt behavior" (Johnson, 1939, p. 172). Of course, others, including Van Riper and those who developed performance-based treatments beginning in the 1960s, would not agree with this assumption.

Before leaving Johnson, we should consider briefly the contributions of three of his students. Williams (1957, 1979, 1982) expanded Johnson's ideas to include the entire speaking process rather than behavior associated only with the moment of stuttering. However, he retained Johnson's fundamental view: "Direct the stutterer's attention from what he evaluates is happening to him and toward (1) those things he is doing to interfere with talking and (2) those things he is doing to facilitate it" (Williams, 1979, p. 254). Wischner and Sheehan fully embraced Johnson's ideas but clothed them in the language of motivational learning (Wischner, 1950, 1952) and approach-avoidance conflict theory (Sheehan, 1953, 1958, 1970, 1975).

Johnson's major contributions to the management of stuttering were conceptual. He remained convinced that changes in beliefs were fundamental to changes in performance; that there was "something peculiarly lacking in those concepts of habit or conditioning which fail to stress duly . . . the meaningful aspects of the stimuli" (Johnson, 1955b, p. 441). Here, Johnson had captured an idea that was to become a fundamental tenet of cognitive learning theory: That "outcomes change behavior in humans largely through the intervening influence of thought" (Bandura, 1977b, p. 18).[1]

Contributions of Charles Van Riper

A colleague of Johnson's, Charles Van Riper, made contributions decidedly more to treatment than to theory concerning the nature of stuttering. In fact, he dedicated his life to a quest for the problem's resolution (Van Riper, 1990). In the 1930s, Van Riper wrote of his dissatisfaction with then-popular objectives of treatment: "We measure the success of our treatment in terms of the decreased number of spasms in the stutterer's speech. The permanent results of such therapy are discouraging, and I believe that in the near future we will base our treatment on a totally different set of principles" (Van Riper, 1937b, p. 149).

---

[1]In this paper, the terms social cognitive learning, cognitive learning, social learning, and observational learning are used interchangeably.

Preparatory Set and the Moment of Stuttering.
Van Riper's approach to treatment was based on
Johnson's idea that the moment of stuttering was
primarily an avoidance reaction (Van Riper, 1947).
Like Johnson, Van Riper believed that a cue warns
of the expectancy to stutter on a word. However,
rather than a vague abstraction, the cue invokes a
preparatory set: A "pre-stimulus neuromuscular
adjustment which selects, determines and controls
the response" (Van Riper, 1937b, p. 150). It is important to understand that this definition of
preparatory set was Van Riper's statement about
the nature of the stutter event. Later, it was also to
become a foundation for his approaches to the
management of stuttering.

According to Van Riper, when the stutterer
experiences a feeling of being blocked, the
preparatory set is released: "The stutterer feels he
has no control over this stuttering performance"
. . . because of . . . "the power of the preparatory
set to determine and control the response to the
signal . . . The form of the overt stuttering is laid
down and determined before the speech attempt
is made" (Van Riper, 1937b, p. 151). With his explanation of preparatory set, Van Riper provided
the motor equivalent of what Johnson described
as the stutterer's perceptual and evaluative set as
a listener. In so doing, Van Riper focused more
on performance failure than Johnson did; more
on the disability of stuttering than on the stutterer's handicapping beliefs. Moreover, Van Riper's
notions about preparatory set were remarkably
prescient (by more than thirty years) of ideas that
would later become a cornerstone for current
motor learning theory (see Schmidt, 1988).

Van Riper based his treatment procedures on
findings from research of the day:

1. The threat of penalty for stuttering was shown
   to increase its frequency, supporting his, and
   Johnson's, concept of stuttering as an avoidance reaction (Van Riper, 1937a).
2. Anticipatory breathing patterns, small rehearsal movements, and levels of tension appeared to premodel response patterns during
   actual stuttering moments (Van Riper, 1936).

3. Stutterers could predict the duration of stuttering moments (Milisen & Van Riper, 1934),
   and they could perform new preparatory sets
   that, after practice, seemed to generalize to
   other similar, though not identical, forms of
   reaction (Van Riper, 1937b).

The Moment of Stuttering—Focal Point of Treatment.

If stuttering was predetermined in its
form and duration by the preparatory set, then it
followed that treatment would need to break down
this set and gradually change the accompanying
reactions. It would no longer be valid for treatment to seek an immediate elimination of stuttering episodes. More so than Johnson, Van Riper
emphasized performance change through the mastery of motor reactions during the stuttering moment. This would be the vehicle for subsequent
change in attitudes and beliefs.

Van Riper avowed that the stutterer should learn
to "stutter with a minimum of abnormality." He
could do so by using effortless stuttering to replace
the "habitual devices . . . to avoid . . . or release himself from the blocks he feels." Van Riper believed
that fluency would be a by-product of this "controlled stuttering" and that by approaching treatment
in this way, "the fear of stuttering and most of the
blocks would disappear" (Van Riper, 1947, p. 332).

Just as important, Van Riper assumed that
adults who stutter chronically will have difficulty
freeing themselves entirely from speech fears in
all situations, no matter what treatment is provided. Since fear was presumed to be at the heart of
maintaining stuttering reactions, fear reduction
and modified stuttering would not only make relapse less frequent, but would also provide stutterers with a method of controlling stuttering
reactions if they did resurface.

Preparatory Set and Treatment.

Van Riper ap-
plied the notion of preparatory set to treatment in the
following way. At the instant when a stutter event is
threatened, the stutterer should rehearse and reject
the old reaction pattern, then assume a new set for
planning and executing the replacement response.
Stutterers should (1) start from a state of "quies-

cence" (not tension), (2) initiate "air flow simultaneously with the speech attempt," and (3) utter the first sound with loose contacts and a deliberate transitional "movement leading directly into the succeeding sound" (Van Riper, 1947, p. 359).

Van Riper worked on one subcomponent of preparatory set at a time and clients achieved certain levels of performance skill before progressing to the next subcomponent. The essence of the new response and its mental imagery was movement that "flows into sound." It had three criteria for successful achievement: "The mouth must be kept in motion, the contacts must be light . . . ("so loose as scarcely to deserve the name") . . . and the succeeding sound must be prepared for in mouth and mind so that the movement may have direction" (Van Riper, 1947, p. 368). It is remarkable how similar these are to target responses that were reasserted during the so-called behavioral revolution in stuttering treatment (Curlee, 1993). A principal difference is that Van Riper was helping the speaker control or replace, rather than prevent, stuttering.

Van Riper reported the development and evolution of his procedures covering a period of more than thirty-five years (Van Riper, 1958, 1973). He described a three-stage sequence for achieving a new preparatory set based on principles of learning (Van Riper, 1954, 1957). Stage 1 was *cancellation*. Stutterers were to come to a complete halt after uttering a stuttered word, then return, and utter the word again, this time stuttering voluntarily in a different way. Van Riper believed cancellation interfered with the self-reinforcing tendency of stuttering reactions—their coincidence with fear reduction at the completion of the episode and their seeming success at achieving utterance of the word. Cancellation also allowed the stutterers to illustrate to themselves (i.e., model) a replacement response that was a "symbolic goal" of behavior acceptable to themselves and others.

Pull out was the second stage. It amounted essentially to moving the cancellation response forward in time by interrupting the old stuttering reaction before it ran its course and replacing it at that point. Based on learning theory, controlled voluntary actions (rather than old stuttering reac-

tions) were now reinforced by the successful utterance of the word.

After completing these stages, stutterers moved on to *preparatory set* itself. "Viewed from the vantage point of learning theory, new competitive responses [were] conditioned to the stimuli which formerly set off the whole stuttering volley of behavioral and emotional reactions" (Van Riper, 1957, p. 893). Van Riper believed this three-stage sequence provided an important insurance policy for dealing with episodes of relapse that were bound to occur in most cases. If stutterers failed at preparatory set, they would try pull out. If still unsuccessful, they would employ cancellation.

Van Riper urged that these ideas were "based upon assumptions urgently in need of experimental verification" (Van Riper, 1957, p. 894). Unfortunately, such experimentation has never been done in a coherent way, and in a moment we shall consider some of the reasons.

Somewhat later, Van Riper labeled two additional phases of treatment that generally preceded the direct modification of stuttering reactions (Van Riper, 1973). These were *identification* and *desensitization*. In the identification phase, Van Riper essentially described procedures for actualizing Johnson's descriptional principle: To bring stutterers to an understanding of their stuttered speech and an acceptance of responsibility for it and for change. In desensitization, Van Riper developed a host of procedures for reducing the intensity of emotional arousal during stuttering events, sufficiently so that the motor responses of speech would become manageable. In this phase, Van Riper emphasized the use of vicarious modeling whereby the clinician takes the role of stutterer in real situations in order to demonstrate that stutter-like responses can be performed calmly without excessive emotionality. Van Riper based his use of modeling on then-emerging applications of social learning theory to behavior modification: "Virtually all learning phenomena resulting from direct experiences can occur on a vicarious basis through observation of other persons' behavior and its consequences on them" (Bandura, 1969, p. 118).

In his "Final Thoughts," Van Riper (1990)

restated the rationale for management of stuttering. He asserted that at its core stuttering consisted of "tiny lags and disruptions" in the timing of speech movements. Those who, for whatever reason, react to these lags by struggling or avoiding their expected consequences become the chronic stutterers. Here, Van Riper reiterated what has come to be the commonly held two-component explanation of stutter events: an interruption of fluency (experienced as a loss of control), and the speaker's reaction thereto (Bloodstein, 1987; Perkins, Kent, & Curlee, 1991; Prins, 1991; Rosenfield & Nudelman, 1987; Van Riper, 1971). Van Riper went on to state that the struggle-avoidance reactions are learned and can be modified, but the lags cannot. Therefore, treatment should not try to reduce the frequency of stuttering episodes directly. Rather, the goal of therapy should be to teach the stutterer to stutter "easily and briefly," and thereby gain adequate speaking skill while reducing or eliminating negative emotion that may be present.

THE BEHAVIORAL REVOLUTION

For a period of twenty years beginning in the 1960s, treatments for behavioral disorders became dominated by what has been called "radical behaviorism" (Bandura, 1977b). This so-called behavioral period was characterized by a dramatic shift in causal explanations of human behavior from internal to external factors, to a strict view of the "determinants of behavior as residing not within the organism but in environmental forces" (Bandura, 1977b, p. 6).

Concerning treatment of stuttering, the climate was right for a shift in emphasis. There were problems with Johnson's anxiety-motivated-avoidant-response model as well as with the treatment procedures it spawned.

Failure of the Model

Two papers launched what Ingham (1984) has called a revolution (Flanagan, Goldiamond, & Azrin, 1958, 1959). While involving only a few

subjects, these studies appeared to demonstrate unequivocally that by selective presentation of consequential stimuli, stuttering could be isolated and manipulated as a response class. More significantly, an aversive consequence for stuttering was shown to decrease rather than increase the frequency of its occurrence. These outcomes, coupled with findings that discredited parent diagnosis as a necessary cause of stuttering, and showed no consistent relationship between anxiety and stutter events (Berlin, 1960; Bloodstein, Jaeger, & Tureen, 1952; Gray & Brutten, 1965; Reed & Lingwall, 1976; Ritterman & Reidenbach, 1975), seriously damaged the anxiety-motivated-avoidant-response model upon which Johnson and Van Riper developed their concepts of treatment.

Limitations of the Stuttering Management Approach

After almost thirty years, the management of stuttering approach proved unsatisfying in many ways:

> *The goal of treatment itself, to "stutter fluently" (Van Riper, 1973), seemed a semantic conundrum, not naturally appealing to client or clinician (Prins, 1984).*
>
> *With a few exceptions, there had been little emphasis on developing and implementing objective measures of treatment outcome (Ingham, 1984). Van Riper spoke mainly of subjective evaluation (1958, 1973), and issues of replicable procedures and reliable measurement were not seriously considered. In part, this resulted from the goal of treatment itself: To modify the client's physical and mental reactions to stutter events, not to reduce or eliminate their occurrence directly. Now, however, results of the Flanagan, Goldiamond, and Azrin studies led quite naturally to, as well as legitimized, an objective, measurable treatment goal: "Total primacy to the achievement of fluent speech" (Ingham, 1984, p. 9). This was attractive to client and clinician alike.*
>
> *There were a disheartening array of treatment procedures from which to choose (Van Riper, 1973). Many techniques might be used, but how should the*

clinician determine which ones, how much, and in what order? In short, treatment seemed an uncertain labyrinth of trial and error, too idiosyncratic, too dependent on the individual therapist's art. Moreover, treatment seemed to require a daunting level of knowledge, expertise, motivation, positive character traits, and heroic dedication on the part of both clinician and client (Van Riper, 1958, 1973, 1975). Professionals and their clients longed for a simpler and less ambiguous way. As suggested by the Flanagan, Goldiamond, and Azrin procedures, systematic manipulation of stimulus/response conditions with a defined effect on the occurrence of stuttering, seemed to provide it (Perkins, 1993).

Finally, even though the management of stuttering was designed to offset post-treatment relapse, it clearly had not solved that problem (Prins, 1970; Van Riper, 1973).

Management of "Fluency"—Rebirth of Old Techniques

Buttressed by the initial response contingent papers of Flanagan, Goldiamond, and Azrin (1958, 1959) and a host of subsequent studies (see Prins & Hubbard, 1988), the goal of treatment shifted to eliminating the occurrence of stutter events rather than modifying the stutterer's reactions during them. Procedures induced fluency by substituting a novel speech pattern, or directly attenuating or extinguishing stutter events (Martin, 1993).[2] Concerning novel speech patterns, a group of fluency-inducing techniques emerged that were based substantially on the work of Goldiamond (1965). Singly or in combination, these techniques included variants of prolonged, continuous phona-

tion; slow articulatory rate; and easy voice and articulatory onset (Ingham, 1993). Although they had had a prior history in treatment (Van Riper, 1973), the techniques were now embedded in more carefully managed behavior modification programs than had been the case earlier.[3] But more than that, they received support from an unexpected quarter: New explanations of stuttering that focused on speech motor control failures as the precipitants of stutter events (e.g., Wingate, 1976; Zimmerman, 1980). According to these explanations, stuttering reveals the disruption of processes by which speech is encoded and its movements executed. Now the effects of fluency-inducing techniques such as slow articulatory rate, continuous phonation, and gentle voice and articulatory onset could be rationalized and their use in treatment justified; they helped to offset conditions of impairment that underlie the loss or interruption of fluency.

Treatment Outcomes of the Behavioral Period

There were many positive outcomes of the behavioral period. Overall, it was marked by attention to the relationship between procedure and outcome:

1. Treatment parameters and sequences were more carefully described and arranged so as to be replicable.
2. Performance-contingent progress, lacking in most of the stuttering management programs, became a requisite feature to help assure that behavior changes occurred and were the basis for client advancement through treatment.
3. The goal of treatment—stutter-free speech— was stated clearly and was measurable.
4. Outcome assessment became a more integral part of treatment, its termination, and the study of long term effects (Ingham, 1984).

However, these positive outcomes did not come without a price—trivialization of the problem and its clinical management, a natural out-

---

[2]At about this same time, reciprocal inhibition treatment also enjoyed a brief period of popularity as a behavior therapy for stuttering. Its use was based on the notion that stuttering was a behavioral accompaniment to learned anxiety reactions during speaking (Gray & England, 1969). The principal treatment procedure paired relaxation with hierarchically arranged images of speaking situations. Because little evidence was provided for treatment effectiveness or for a causal role of anxiety in stuttering (Ingham, 1984), these approaches sustained less interest than operant-based procedures.

---

[3]An apparent exception to this is the rather detailed fluency shaping sequence described by Hahn (1943).

growth of heightened emphasis on accountability and objective measurement (Siegel, 1975):

> *The problem of stuttering and the focus of treatment tended to be limited to the sum of stutter events. And clearly the occurrence of stuttering was not the only dimension of the disorder or of many clients' needs in treatment (Cooper, 1986; Prins, 1993b).*
>
> *Though stutter events were eliminated during treatment (and perhaps because they were eliminated), the client's speech pattern often was substantially deviant and unacceptable (Ingham, 1984; Perkins, 1992).*
>
> *Performance change during treatment was taken as evidence of learning, disregarding data that had been accumulating for some time to show that human learning involves change in the way people think and on internal (covert) as well as external (overt) conditions (Bandura, 1977b).*

In addition to these factors, two others served to lessen enthusiasm for treatments based on radical behaviorism: (1) the operant model's limitations in explaining effects of response contingent stimuli on stutter events (Ingham, 1984; Martin & Ingham, 1973; Prins & Hubbard, 1988), and (2) the persistent problem of relapse following treatment (Boberg, Howie, & Woods, 1979).

During this period the implications for behavior modification of Johnson's and Van Riper's ideas were largely overlooked (Prins, 1984). This was unfortunate for, as we shall see, their models are quite compatible with current approaches to behavior therapy based on cognitive learning and self-efficacy theories (Bandura, 1969, 1977a, 1986).

BEHAVIOR MODIFICATION—COGNITIVE MODELS FOR THE TREATMENT OF STUTTERING

We turn now in sequence to: (1) certain key findings from research of the behavioral period that bear on cognitive learning, (2) some basic concepts of social cognitive and self-efficacy theories, and (3) cognitive models for defensive behavior and stuttering reactions. Together, this information

provides evidence to support the management of stuttering approach and thereby to link Johnson's and Van Riper's ideas to contemporary theories of learning and behavior therapy.

Key Findings from the Behavioral Period

Martin and Haroldson (1977) published results of a fascinating study that illustrates the positive effect of observation on speech fluency. Twenty stutterers showed a significant decrease in stuttering frequency as a consequence of watching a videotape of another stutterer whose stuttering frequency was attenuated dramatically when followed by response contingent time out (RCTO). Using the operant model, Martin and Haroldson viewed this outcome as a demonstration of vicarious punishment. However, from the perspective of social cognitive learning, the results would be viewed as evidence of the effects of vicarious modeling or, using Martin and Haroldson's own words, "observing another client responding dramatically to a treatment procedure" (p. 25). Vicarious modeling is a cornerstone of cognitive behavior therapy. Observation allows people to form ideas about how to perform complex acts without having to acquire them gradually by trial and error (Bandura, 1977b).

A puzzling and provocative finding from the behavioral period is that time out remains the only contingent stimulus that consistently reduces the frequency of stuttering (Ingham, 1984; Prins & Hubbard, 1988). Within the operant model, this outcome is attributed to the effect of time out as a punisher. However, other research reveals that aversive stimuli generally do not consistently attenuate stuttering frequency (Prins & Hubbard, 1988). Moreover, in violation of a principle of operant conditioning, the time-out effect appears to be independent of accurate consequation of stutter events (James, 1983; Martin & Haroldson, 1982). These findings invite an alternative model to explain the RCTO effect, a cognitive one provided by social learning theory: "A vast amount of evidence lends validity to the view that reinforcement serves as an informative and motivational operation" (Bandura, 1977b, p. 21). In other words, time out may have its effect because it means something to stutterers. It may inform them about their unwanted behavior and thereby motivate them to exercise their capacity to speak fluently, a capacity that virtually all persons who stutter have (Bloodstein, 1987).

Studies of contingent self-stimulation and self-evaluation of stuttering, while explainable within the operant framework, also fit nicely within the social cognitive model. Ingham (1982) reported that the introduction of self-evaluation contingencies into a treatment program improved the maintenance of its effects. Martin and Haroldson (1982) showed that stutterers who provided their own time out for stuttering had less recovery of stuttering frequency following the time out condition and, even more important, showed significantly greater generalization to an untreated telephone situation than stutterers who received experimenter-delivered time out. The findings of these studies not only suggest procedures that may enhance treatment effectiveness for persons who stutter, they also suggest the reasons: That is, by thought processes, people preserve experiences to motivate and guide future responses and to control their behavior by creating internal consequences (Bandura, 1977b). This explanation of learning invites a revised model for the nature and treatment of stuttering within cognitive theory.

Concepts of Social Cognitive and Self-Efficacy Theories

The fundamental tenets of social cognitive learning theory are that "most human behavior is learned observationally through modeling" (Bandura, 1977b, p. 22) and that "to alter how people behave one must alter how they think" (Bandura, 1986, p. 519). These principles also undergird self-efficacy theory, proposed by Bandura to explain the unifying mechanism that accounts for behavior changes resulting from different modes of treatment, particularly in relation to defensive reactions (Bandura, 1977a). Self-efficacy theory holds that people change their defensive behavior because they alter their expectations of personal efficacy; they come to expect that they can execute successfully the responses required to achieve a satisfactory outcome.

Defensive Behavior, Social Cognitive Theory, and Stuttering Reactions

Seen in light of social cognitive and self-efficacy theories, a defensive behavior model for stuttering reactions provides the current foundation for management of stuttering. This model corresponds with Bloodstein's anticipatory struggle hypothesis (1987), and its conceptual origins go back to Johnson and Van Riper (Prins, 1984).

According to social cognitive theory, defensive behavior occurs when a person perceives cues that warn of aversive events. The cues are represented cognitively by vivid images and symbols that not only motivate the defensive reactions, but are the source for their perpetuation and resistance to extinction as well (Bandura, 1986).

For chronic stutterers, the cues are hypothesized to be speech stimuli that signal an imminent loss of fluency control. As in an emergency, stutterers react to these signals defensively by tensing, forcing, struggling, retreating, and so on, thereby producing most of the observable behavior of stuttering and its most debilitating features. Though the cues are represented in memory cognitively, the reactions to them are reflexive in nature, comparable to one's self-protective reactions in response to catching the outside edge of a ski or accidentally touching a moist glass at a dinner table (Prins, 1984, 1993a,b). Physiological arousal and the experience of negative emotion (i.e., anxiety) are viewed as co-effects of such reactions rather than causal, and "after people become adept at self-protective behaviors, they perform them in potentially threatening situations without having to be frightened (Bandura, 1977b, p. 209).

In chronic stutterers, cues that activate defensive reactions are presumed to be perceived aberrations in speech production processes. For example, when stutterers detect subtle timing lags or degrees of tension in the vocal tract they are threatened because of what they have come to expect: the stutter event. As long as this expectation is held, so long will the cues be a warning and the defensive responses be activated. According to this model and to self-efficacy theory, treatment is effective when individuals come to believe in their capacities to cope successfully in the face of cues that formerly threatened stutter events. This idea is completely compatible with the treatment concepts of Johnson and Van Riper.

MANAGEMENT OF STUTTERING

As currently conceived, the management of stuttering approach comprises three basic components: exploration, desensitization, and modification. A summary of the rationale and objectives will be given for each component, followed by illustrations of modeling procedures to accommodate the processes that govern observational learning and the sources of information by which individuals achieve positive self-efficacy expectations.[4]

Exploration

Rationale and Objectives.   "Habitual patterns of behavior become so routinized that people often act without much awareness of what they are doing . . . Systematic self-observation provides a self-diagnostic device for gaining a better sense of what conditions lead one to behave in certain ways" (Bandura, 1986, p. 338). The essence of exploration in treatment is to help stutterers become aware of, and responsible for, what they do as they speak. This idea was basic to Johnson's concept of treatment in the mid-1930s, and it is a cornerstone for the management of stuttering today.

The first experiences of treatment focus on self-observation, putting clients in touch with their behavior so that they understand themselves as speakers, understand what they do and feel as they talk that inhibits and facilitates fluency. The objectives are to discover, and accept responsibility for, speaking behavior; to objectify and understand the relationship between performance and feelings; and to begin setting personalized goals for treatment. We emphasize discovery of the cues for stuttering reactions, details of the reactions themselves, and the feelings that accompany them.

Applications of Modeling.   It is usually difficult for clients to capture the idea of meaningful self-observation. They have a tendency to observe and describe generalities of performance and thereby fail to identify crucial details (see Bandura, 1986, p. 55). Early in treatment, the language they use is often vague rather than descriptive of behavioral events. To offset these problems, we begin with vicarious modeling. Clients observe videotape segments of other stutterers who are observing themselves on videotape and describing their speaking behavior in various situations.[5] Initially, the clinician points to positive discoveries the videotaped clients are making and to their use of language to describe what they are doing, rather than what is happening, as if they were victims. Later, participant modeling allows clients to observe and describe their speaking behavior from videotapes recorded earlier. Tapes are viewed in real-time and then in slow motion. These activities direct individuals to attend to, internalize, and retain the relevant aspects of their behavior.

Clients finally tape themselves while describing the video samples of their speech recorded earlier, or, while they speak before a mirror. They review these tapes to evaluate the accuracy of their descriptions, observations, and insights. Based on these discoveries, they prepare preliminary outlines of goals they would like to achieve in treatment. By having clients actively involved in setting, and later refining, treatment goals, clients become motivated to achieve treatment objectives.

---

[4]While this chapter focuses principally on models for treatment, two others describe and illustrate in greater detail clinical procedures for achieving performance and cognitive change within the management of stuttering approach (Prins, 1984, 1993a,b).

---

[5]The availability of affordable optical disc recorder/playback devices will significantly enhance these vicarious modeling procedures.

Successful completion of this component of treatment sets the stage for self-regulating behavior (see Bandura, 1986, ch. 8). Clients have begun (1) to make self-observations by which they can set internal standards for achievement, and (2) to develop judgmental skills in order to self-motivate, evaluate, and internally reinforce their behavior.

Desensitization

Rationale and Objectives.   "Because high arousal usually debilitates performance, individuals are more likely to expect success when they are not beset by visceral arousal" (Bandura, 1977b, p. 82). Persons who stutter may vary enormously in the degree of emotional arousal they experience as an accompaniment to stutter events and speaking situations. However, laboratory studies over a substantial period report that stuttering is usually accompanied by evidence of "visceral correlates of tension, exertion, or emotional arousal" (Bloodstein, 1987, p. 23). In fact, the very essence of the difference between stutterers' perceptions of faked and real stutter events is the sense of tension and being out of control that accompanies real moments of stuttering (Bloodstein, 1987).

Clients lay the foundation for perceptions of self-efficacy by demonstrating their ability to "lessen the severity of aversive events" (Bandura, 1986, p. 440). This is the essence of the desensitization component as conceived and developed by Van Riper: "Our purpose in desensitization therapy is to reduce the strength of the attendant emotional upheaval enough to *enable* the stutterer to learn new ways of coping with the expectancy and experience of broken words" (Van Riper, 1973, p. 267). Clients must learn that it is possible to react calmly during stutter events. When they do, they create less tension and experience reduced emotional arousal. Their movements are slower and less effortful; their thoughts become more realistic about what they are doing and what they might do to respond more effectively.

Applications of Modeling.   Lessening physiological arousal during stuttering is a gradual process. First, clients illustrate and calibrate the difference between their intense and calm stuttering episodes. Then they establish their ability to remain at relatively calm levels of stuttering in speaking situations of varying difficulty.

Initially, clients experience vicarious modeling by observing videotapes of other stutterers as they display, rate, and comment on their episodes of stuttering that range from relatively effortless (calm) to extremely effortful (tense). These tapes are of clients who not only illustrate a range of effort in their stutter events, but also comment meaningfully on how they feel and whether their feelings correspond with what they are doing. Tapes of these same stutterers are then observed as they achieve calm stuttering in speaking situations that are increasingly difficult. The clinician draws special attention to the fact that stuttering can be quite effortless, and when done in this way, much of its abnormality subsides. Particular emphasis is placed on eye contact during stutter events and its calming effects on both speaker and listener.

Participant modeling follows as clients proceed to make their own videotapes, first demonstrating and calibrating their range of effortful/effortless stuttering. These tapes are evaluated repeatedly until clients are able to rate their stuttering episodes reliably and, by verbalizing what they are doing and feeling, internalize a different meaning for the cues that trigger stuttering reactions. In a hierarchy of situations, clients make and self-evaluate tapes, progressing after they are able to remain consistently at low levels of arousal and effort during moments of stuttering. Within the clinic setting, taped situations range from controlled and open dialogue with the clinician to similar situations with other individuals, more than one listener, and the telephone.

Before clients attempt effortless stuttering in outside situations, the clinician usually serves as a model. In selected situations (often store settings), the clinician will simulate stuttering and, while doing so, will sustain eye contact and remain emotionally calm. The clinician emphasizes that this will be difficult, and it may be necessary to enter a number of situations before calm, effortless stuttering is achieved. Clients observe and help to evaluate the clinician's performance. When both are satisfied that the response criteria have been met, clients enter previously selected situations until they consistently achieve their target level.

Achieving calm stuttering reactions in difficult speaking situations may depend on successful completion of the modification component of treatment. However, consistently calm stuttering in clinical situations that are videotaped, and in selected outside modeling situations, is usually necessary before proceeding with the remainder of the program.

Modification

Rationale and Objectives. "Cognitive events are induced and altered most readily by experiences of mastery arising from successful performance" (Bandura, 1977b, p. 79). In the modification component of treatment, stutterers learn to respond with the movements necessary to produce speech smoothly and effortlessly when they perceive cues that formerly activated stuttering reactions. Earlier, during desensitization activities, they observed and perceived the effect that remaining calm had on their reactive behavior. Now, they do something that successfully replaces residual stuttering reactions and thereby induces expectations of self-efficacy.

For most clients, the target response is similar to that described by Van Riper in his application of preparatory set to treatment: Starting from an appropriate posture to initiate the syllable's first sound, clients simultaneously initiate air flow with light articulatory contacts and a slightly exaggerated transitional movement to the succeeding sound. This basic response is adapted for the individual to help to assure that it: (1) is clearly contrastive to, and more appealing than the client's typical stuttering reactions; (2) is simple, with subcomponents that can be readily identified and perceived; (3) moves speech forward, emphasizing the movements required for normal utterance; (4) results in completion of the syllable or word without unnecessary tension.

Applications of Modeling.   Preceding activities in which the replacement response is established, a three-step sequence is used that requires accurate detection, interruption, and variation of stutter events. For each of these steps, as well as for replacement activities proper, vicarious and performance modeling are the principal treatment vehicles. Clients observe videotapes of other stutterers who accurately identify, interrupt by pausing, then restart stuttering reactions. Clients make their own tapes in which they detect and interrupt episodes of stuttering. With help from the clinician, they evaluate the tapes until both are satisfied that detection and interruption are done reliably. Clients observe tapes of others who vary their performance during stuttering moments by slowing repetitions or prolonging sounds in ways that contrast with their habitual stuttering reactions. Clients then make their own tapes and, with the clinician's help, evaluate their variation responses.

After these steps have been completed successfully, clients progress to establishing responses that replace residual stuttering reactions. As before, observation of others on videotape precedes clients videotaping and observing their own performance. Real time and slow motion analyses are used during tape observations.

Initially, tapes of other stutterers' pre-, during-, and post-treatment speech samples illustrate varying levels of achievement in replacing stuttering reactions. According to Bandura (1977b), "By observing a model of the desired behavior, an individual forms an idea of how response components must be combined and sequenced to produce the new behavior" (p. 35). The clinician uses visual images and labels to isolate and highlight subcomponents of replacement responses and to discuss their characteristics when done successfully. Clients rehearse and perform subcomponents, and the response as a whole. Tapes of client performance provide feedback on relevant aspects of behavior and build cognitive representations that serve as a source of self-motivation, self-control, and self-reinforcement.

Clients evaluate and meet performance and self-efficacy criteria as they progress through a hierarchy of speaking tasks and situations. Throughout the program, experiences enhance the processes that govern observational learning: attention to significant subcomponents of behavior; retention through imaging, symbolization, and rehearsal; response production with gradual refinement from feedback and self-evaluation; and motivation from observing positive outcomes for others and themselves.

Clients are likewise exposed to the sources of information by which self-efficacy expectations are achieved: reduced physiological arousal, verbal persuasion, observation of others and themselves performing successfully, and performance mastery through repeated success (Bandura, 1986). Recently, a number of other programs have described similar cognitive strategies for working with chronic stutterers: Craig and Howie (1982), Emerick (1988), Maxwell (1982), Webster and Poulos (1989).

PERENNIAL OBSTACLES TO SUCCESSFUL TREATMENT

Motivation

"Self-motivation requires standards against which performance is evaluated . . . Once individuals have made self-satisfaction contingent upon goal attainment, they tend to persist in their efforts until their performances match what they are seeking to achieve" (Bandura, 1977b, p. 161). No greater obstacle thwarts successful treatment of chronic stutterers than weak motivation and the attendant failure to persist in achieving and sustaining treatment objectives. The adult who seeks to resolve the problem of stuttering, therefore, must be internally motivated to take risks, to encounter discomforting experiences, and to persevere when success is not immediately apparent.

From the outset of treatment, client and clinician together design self-therapy activities that are directed to achieving the objectives of each treatment component. These activities promote self-observation, self-judgment to internalize performance standards, and self-evaluation to create motivational incentives and the source for internal

reinforcement. Performance is verified and evaluated through use of video and audio recordings and protocols that the client completes.

As a part of this feature of the program, clients are taught to operate equipment in a clinical laboratory room containing a video camera, VCR, and telephone. On their own, they observe tapes of other clients who are working to achieve similar objectives, and they video record and self-evaluate their performance and self-efficacy status using protocols designed for this purpose. At subsequent client-clinician sessions, the tapes and self-evaluation protocols are re-evaluated to verify progress, revise procedures, and (as necessary) modify treatment objectives.

"According to social learning theory, self-regulated reinforcement increases performance mainly through its motivational function. By making self-reward conditional upon attaining a certain level of performance, individuals create self-inducements to persist in their efforts until their performance matches prescribed standards" (Bandura, 1977b, p. 130). In relation to stuttering, we not only have this theoretic foundation for emphasizing self-regulation, we also have empirical evidence for its importance (Ingham, 1993).

Automatization of Modified Speech

If it is to be effective, the response that replaces old stuttering reactions must become automatic, done without special attention or effort. This requirement for automatization of speech performance change plagues the successful treatment of stuttering (Perkins, 1992). It is typified by the frequent statement of clients: "I can modify my speech in the clinic, but outside, when I have to think about what I'm going to say, I can't take the time or make the effort to think about how I'm going to say it."

Bandura (1986) identifies three processes that accompany and account for the automatization of new skills: (1) gradually merging from elements to the whole response, from slow and awkward to effortless; (2) linkage to specific contexts by practice in various conditions in which the response is required; (3) shifting the locus of attention to the outcomes and effects of the behavior. Videotape observations of other stutterers who illustrate these processes help to encourage and persuade clients that automatization can and does take place. Evidence for it abounds in many acquired complex motor tasks; for example, in skiing. When an adult takes lessons for the first time, elements of the whole response are almost painfully labored and awkward. Later, through practice in specific contexts, the elements are fused into a graceful, natural whole; done at high speed, without observable details; automatically, by feel, and with attention to outcome.

Similarly, in the modification component of treatment, new responses are broken into their elements, identified, and practiced, slowly and awkwardly at first. Gradually, with practice in structured clinical situations and in various circumstances of daily living, the response is executed effortlessly as a whole. To help achieve this, we employ a procedure called voluntary disfluency on nonstuttered words. First, clients observe videotaped models of other stutterers. These models illustrate how brief disfluencies at word onsets, done awkwardly at first, are later done so smoothly and effortlessly that they are scarcely noticeable to the average listener. Clients then demonstrate and establish their ability to modify nonstuttered words, in isolation and in contextual speech, and evaluate their performance on videotape. These activities accommodate processes that Bandura identifies to account for automatization. They also give stimulus value to the response, priming it for replacement of stuttering reactions, and they allow the stutterer to lose sensitivity to doing something that at first seems unnatural and calls attention to itself.

Client Selection

At the beginning of this chapter, we quoted Wendell Johnson on the theme that there is no known best treatment approach for adults who stutter. It is clear that all stutterers do not suffer the same disorder in terms of possible impairment source factors, disability characteristics, and handicapping effects. Hence, they do not come to treatment with the same needs or complaints (Baer, 1989).

With regard to speech disability characteristics, the management of stuttering is not equally applicable to all clients. It is usually most effective for those whose moments of stuttering are discrete, readily and easily identifiable, clearly contrastive to their so-called fluent speech, and that usually show a clear onset and offset. These clients often can associate stuttering with specific words, types of words, and speaking situations. They may have specific word and situation fears, and they sometimes show signs of careful speech monitoring that allows them to anticipate and postpone or prevent stutter events by using pauses, interjections, word substitutions, circumlocution, and other devices.

Clients whose stutter events are difficult to isolate from their nonstuttered speech are poorer candidates for the management of stuttering approach. In these clients, episodes of stuttering are often fleeting in duration and are embedded in what may be described as a chaotic overall speech pattern. This pattern is usually identified as a combination of cluttering and stuttering. Speech is generally dysrhythmic, characterized by a rapid, irregular speaking rate, and lacking in syllabic and articulatory clarity (see Daly, 1993). These clients seem to monitor their speech poorly, and approaches that focus on the management of fluency may be more appropriate. Later, during treatment, if discrete moments of stuttering remain, procedures for the management of stuttering may be useful.

VALIDATION

Van Riper's assertion of more than thirty-five years ago requires restating in relation to the models and procedures for treatment presented in this chapter: They are "based upon assumptions urgently in need of experimental verification" (Van Riper, 1957, p. 894).

Studies of treatment procedures from the behavioral period have already provided a foundation of evidence to support the importance of observation and self-regulation to treatment outcome (see Key

Findings from the Behavioral Period). However, we need to understand more about these procedures as they are currently viewed within a cognitive learning framework (Bandura, 1986). And, more specifically, we need to test the defensive behavior model and self-efficacy theory as applied to the nature and treatment of stuttering. For example:

> *Do vicarious modeling procedures (watching others gradually achieve behavioral change objectives) have a significant treatment effect when used with different approaches or in different phases of treatment?*
>
> *Do self-efficacy-based criteria for progress in treatment affect the generalization and maintenance of speech change?*
>
> *When treatments are equated for modeling and self-efficacy achievement, do outcomes vary for different approaches; for example, for management of stuttering versus management of fluency?*

The first two questions may be applied to basic components of the management of stuttering approach (exploration, desensitization, modification) and to other treatment approaches as well. The last question is concerned particularly with the defensive behavior model of stuttering reactions.

Experiments to answer questions like these are easier to suggest than to design, but there is an excellent model in Martin and Haroldson (1982). In a one-hour experiment, they demonstrated different outcomes for two experimental treatments and a control condition. Differences were apparent, moreover, because the authors measured outcome in an untreated telephone situation as well as during the treatment task. As a consequence, they were able to draw conclusions about the generalization of treatment effects that otherwise would have been impossible. By adding short, post-experiment time intervals in studies of this type, then reassessing outcome in a generalization task (or by providing degrees of difficulty in that task), the durability of effects over time and situational complexity also could be ascertained. In turn, this would further delineate treatment effects by suggesting their maintenance potential.

Experiments like Martin and Haroldson's provide an excellent opportunity to differentiate the clinical potential of treatment procedures. But more than that, they can shed light on the nature of the disorder itself. It is for this reason that such experiments should test explanatory models for the nature of the disability and the processes of change. By so doing, we achieve Siegel's (1993a) admonition: "In the long run the research that has greatest impact on treatment will be research that looks to the underlying nature of a communication disorder" (p. 37).

SUMMARY AND CONCLUSIONS

This chapter traces the evolution of behavior therapy for stuttering during the modern era, the period beginning about 1930 with the first academic research program in speech pathology at the University of Iowa. Its purpose has been to illuminate ideas from the past in order that we may better understand the present and how to proceed into the future. This is an important task, for in the words of Santayana, "Those who cannot remember the past are condemned to repeat it."

The focal point has been an approach called management of stuttering. It originated with, and continues to utilize, many of Wendell Johnson's and Charles Van Riper's pioneering ideas concerning the nature and treatment of stuttering: Ideas that, although they were transmitted with a different vocabulary, are compatible with current theories of cognitive learning and behavior therapy.

Today, management of stuttering views most of the observable features of stutter events as defensive reactions—what stutterers do to save themselves in a perceived emergency of fluency failure. Contemporary social cognitive and self-efficacy theories provide the models of learning and treatment on which this approach is based. According to these theories, chronic defensive behavior is motivated and perpetuated by the meaning of cues that forecast aversive events. Such cues serve to activate defensive reactions as long as they evoke images of disastrous consequences. Long-standing behavior of this type is extraordinarily difficult to extinguish.

Successful behavior therapies for defensive reactions are believed to provide experiences of performance mastery that induce cognitive change in the form of self-efficacy expectations. From this perspective, performance experiences are the vehicles for change, but the medium for change is cognitive. Applied to the management of stuttering, clients, as a result of successful performance experiences during stuttering episodes, develop the conviction that they are capable of producing speech smoothly and effectively in the face of cues that formerly threatened fluency catastrophe.

Self-efficacy expectations can be achieved by the management of fluency as well as by the management of stuttering, or by a combination of the two approaches. The approach of choice for an individual client depends on the nature of the problem: the specific features of impairment (if any), disability, and handicap; the client's needs and complaints; the clinician's expertise.

The defensive behavior and self-efficacy mod-els for nature and treatment of stuttering require experimental verification. If they are shown to be valid, we probably should not expect to improve treatment by discovering a new technique for modifying speaking performance. Rather, we should expect to improve therapy for chronic stutterers by developing more effective ways to bring about cognitive change; to alter their expectations of self-efficacy as speakers (see Perkins, 1993; Prins, 1993a,b). Evidence already exists to support this expectation. It comes from the enormous array of speech modification techniques that are known to ameliorate temporarily the occurrence of stuttering (Bloodstein, 1987; Martin, 1993; Van Riper, 1973), and the improvement in generalization and maintenance of treatment effects that follows observation of others, self-stimulation, self-evaluation, and self-perception (Craig & Andrews, 1985; Craig & Howie, 1982; Ingham, 1982; Martin & Haroldson, 1977, 1982; Owen, 1981).

REFERENCES

Baer, M.B. (1989). *The critical issue in treatment efficacy is knowing why treatment was applied: A student's response to Roger Ingham.* Paper presented at the Conference on Treatment Efficacy, American Speech-Language-Hearing Foundation, San Antonio, Tex.

Bandura, A. (1969). *Principles of behavior modification.* New York: Holt, Rinehart, & Winston.

Bandura, A. (1977a). Self-efficacy: Toward a unifying theory of behavioral change. *Psychological Review, 84*, 191–215.

Bandura, A. (1977b). *Social learning theory.* Englewood Cliffs, N.J.: Prentice-Hall.

Bandura, A. (1986). *Social foundations of thought and action.* Englewood Cliffs, N.J.: Prentice-Hall.

Berlin, C.I. (1960). Parents' diagnoses of stuttering. *Journal of Speech and Hearing Research, 3*, 372–379.

Bloodstein, O. (1987). *A handbook on stuttering* (4th ed.). Chicago: The National Easter Seal Society.

Bloodstein, O., Jaeger, W., & Tureen, J. (1952). A study of the diagnosis of stuttering by parents of stutterers and non-stutterers. *Journal of Speech and Hearing Disorders, 17*, 308–315.

Boberg, E., Howie, P., & Woods, L. (1979). Maintenance of fluency: A review. *Journal of Fluency Disorders, 4*, 93–116.

Cooper, E.B. (1986). Treatment of disfluency: Future trends. *Journal of Fluency Disorders, 11*, 317–329.

Craig, A., & Andrews, G. (1985). The prediction and prevention of relapse in stuttering. *Behavior Modification, 9*, 427–442.

Craig, A., & Howie, P.M. (1982). Locus of control and maintenance of behavioral therapy skills. *British Journal of Clinical Psychology, 21*, 65–66.

Curlee, R.F. (1993). The early history of behavior modification of stuttering: From laboratory to clinic. *Journal of Fluency Disorders, 18*, 13–27.

Daly, D. (1993). Cluttering: Another fluency syndrome. In R.F. Curlee (Ed.), *Stuttering and related disorders of fluency.* New York: Thieme Medical Publishers.

Emerick, L. (1988). Counseling adults who stutter: A cognitive approach. *Seminars in Speech, Language and Hearing, 9*, 257–267.

Flanagan, B., Goldiamond, I., & Azrin, N. (1958). Operant stuttering: The control of stuttering behavior through response-contingent consequences. *Journal of the Experimental Analysis of Behavior, 4,* 45–56.

Flanagan, B., Goldiamond, I., & Azrin, N. (1959). Instatement of stuttering in normally fluent individuals through operant procedures. *Science, 130,* 979–981.

Frey, W. (1984). Functional assessment in the '80s. In A. Halpern & M. Fuhrer (Eds.), *Functional assessment in rehabilitation.* Baltimore: Paul H. Brookes.

Goldiamond, I. (1965). Stuttering and fluency as manipulatable response classes. In L. Krasner & L.P. Ullmann (Eds.), *Research in behavior modification.* New York: Rinehart & Winston.

Gray, B.B., & Brutten, E.J. (1965). The relationship between anxiety, fatigue, and spontaneous recovery in stuttering. *Behavior Research and Therapy, 2,* 251–259.

Gray, B.B., & England, G. (Eds.). (1969). *Stuttering and the conditioning therapies.* Monterey, Calif.: Monterey Institute for Speech and Hearing.

Hahn, E.F. (1943). *Stuttering: Significant theories and therapies.* Palo Alto: Stanford University Press.

Ingham, R.J. (1982). The effects of self-evaluation training on maintenance and generalization during stuttering treatment. *Journal of Speech and Hearing Disorders, 47,* 271–280.

Ingham, R.J. (1984). *Stuttering and behavior therapy: Current status and experimental foundations.* San Diego: College Hill Press.

Ingham, R.J. (1993). Current status of stuttering and behavior modification—II: Principal issues and practices in stuttering therapy. *Journal of Fluency Disorders, 18,* 57–81.

James, J.E. (1983). Parameters of the influence of self-initiated time-out from speaking on stuttering. *Journal of Communication Disorders, 16,* 123–132.

Johnson, W. (1933). An interpretation of stuttering. *Quarterly Journal of Speech, 19,* 70–76.

Johnson, W. (1937). The descriptive principle and the principle of static analysis. Reprinted in W. Johnson & R.R. Leutenegger (Eds.), *Stuttering in children and adults* (1955). Minneapolis: University of Minnesota Press.

Johnson, W. (1938). The role of evaluation in stuttering behavior. *Journal of Speech Disorders, 3,* 85–89.

Johnson, W. (1939). The treatment of stuttering. *Journal of Speech Disorders, 4,* 170–173.

Johnson, W. (1946). *People in quandaries: The semantics of personal adjustment.* New York: Harper & Brothers.

Johnson, W. (1957). Perceptual and evaluational factors in stuttering. In L.E. Travis (Ed.), *Handbook of speech pathology.* New York: Appleton-Century-Crofts.

Johnson, W. (1959). *The onset of stuttering.* Minneapolis: University of Minnesota Press.

Johnson, W. (1955a). The time, the place, and the problem. In W. Johnson & R. Leutenneger (Eds.), *Stuttering in children and adults.* Minneapolis: University of Minnesota Press.

Johnson, W. (1955b). The descriptive principle and the principle of static analysis. In W. Johnson & R. Leutenneger (Eds.), *Stuttering in children and adults.* Minneapolis: University of Minnesota Press.

Johnson, W. (1961). *The language of responsibility.* Commencement address, The State University of Iowa, Iowa City, Ia.

Johnson, W., & Knott, J.R. (1935). A systematic approach to the psychology of stuttering. Reprinted in W. Johnson & R.R. Leutenegger (Eds.), *Stuttering in children and adults* (1955). Minneapolis: University of Minnesota Press.

Johnson, W., & Knott, J.R. (1936). The moment of stuttering. *Journal of Genetic Psychology, 48,* 475–479.

Martin, R. (1993). The future of behavior modification of stuttering: What goes around comes around. *Journal of Fluency Disorders, 18,* 81–109.

Martin, R., & Haroldson, S.K. (1977). Effect of vicarious punishment on stuttering frequency. *Journal of Speech and Hearing Research, 20,* 21–26.

Martin, R., & Haroldson, S.K. (1982). Contingent self-stimulation for stuttering. *Journal of Speech and Hearing Disorders, 47,* 407–413.

Martin, R., & Ingham, R.J. (1973). Stuttering. In L. Lahey (Ed.), *The modification of language behavior.* Springfield, Ill.: Charles C. Thomas.

Maxwell, D. (1982). Cognitive and behavioral self-control strategies: Applications for the clinical management of adult stutterers. *Journal of Fluency Disorders, 7,* 403–432.

Milisen, R., & Van Riper, C. (1934). A study of the predicted duration of the stutterer's blocks as related to their actual duration. *Journal of Speech Disorders, 4,* 339–345.

Orton, S.T. (1927). Studies in stuttering. *Archives of Neurology and Psychiatry, 18,* 671–672.

Owen, N. (1981). Facilitating maintenance of behavior change. In E. Boberg (Ed.), *Maintenance of fluency.* New York: Elsevier.

Perkins, W. (1992). Fluency control and automatic fluency. *American Journal of Speech-Language Pathology, 1,* 9–10.

Perkins, W. (1993). The early history of behavior modification of stuttering: A view from the trenches. *Journal of Fluency Disorders, 18,* 1–13.

Perkins, W., Kent, R.D., & Curlee, R.F. (1991). A theory of neurolinguistic function in stuttering. *Journal of Speech and Hearing Research, 34,* 734–752.

Prins, D. (1970). Improvement and regression in stutterers following short-term intensive therapy. *Journal of Speech and Hearing Disorders, 35,* 123–135.

Prins, D. (1984). Treatment of adults—managing stuttering. In R.F. Curlee & W. Perkins (Eds.), *Nature and treatment of stuttering: New directions.* San Diego: College-Hill Press.

Prins, D. (1991). Theories of stuttering as event and disorder: Implication for speech production processes. In H.F.M. Peters, W. Hulstijn, & C.W. Starkweather (Eds.), *Speech motor control and stuttering.* Amsterdam, The Netherlands: Elsevier Science Publishers B.V.

Prins, D. (1993a). Management of stuttering: Treatment of adolescents and adults. In R.F. Curlee (Ed.), *Stuttering and related disorders of fluency.* New York: Thieme Medical Publishers.

Prins, D. (1993b). Models for treatment efficacy studies of adult stutterers. *Journal of Fluency Disorders, 18,* 333–351.

Prins, D., & Hubbard, C.P. (1988). Response contingent stimuli and stuttering: Issues and implications. *Journal of Speech and Hearing Research, 31,* 396–709.

Reed, C.G., & Lingwall, J.B. (1976). Some relationships between punishment, stuttering, and galvanic skin responses. *Journal of Speech and Hearing Research, 19,* 197–205.

Ritterman, S.I., & Reidenbach, J.W. (1975). Inter-digital variability in the palmar sweat indices of adult stutterers. *Journal of Fluency Disorders, 1,* 33–46.

Rosenfield, D., & Nudelman, H. (1987). Neuropsychological models of speech dysfluency. In L. Rustin, H. Purser, & D. Rowley (Eds.), *Progress in the treatment of fluency disorders.* New York: Taylor & Francis.

Schmidt, R.A. (1988). *Motor control and learning: A behavioral emphasis* (2nd ed.). Champaign, Ill.: Human Kinetics Publishers.

Sheehan, J.G. (1953). Theory and treatment of stuttering as an approach-avoidance conflict. *Journal of Psychology, 36,* 27–49.

Sheehan, J.G. (1958). Conflict theory of stuttering. In J. Eisenson (Ed.), *Stuttering: A symposium.* New York: Harper & Row.

Sheehan, J.G. (1970). *Stuttering: Research and therapy.* New York: Harper & Row.

Sheehan, J.G. (1975). Conflict theory and avoidance-reduction therapy. In J. Eisenson (Ed.), *Stuttering: A second symposium.* New York: Harper & Row.

Siegel, G.M. (1975). The high cost of accountability. *Asha, 17,* 796–797.

Siegel, G.M. (1993a). Research: A natural bridge. *Asha, 26,* 36–37.

Siegel, G.M. (1993b). Stuttering and behavior modification: Commentary. *Journal of Fluency Disorders, 18,* 109–115.

Travis, L.E. (1931). *Speech pathology.* New York: Appleton-Century.

Van Riper, C. (1936). Study of the thoracic breathing of stutterers during expectancy and occurrence of stuttering spasms. *Journal of Speech Disorders, 1,* 61–72.

Van Riper, C. (1937a). The effect of penalty upon frequency of stuttering spasms. *Journal of Genetic Psychology, 50,* 193–195.

Van Riper, C. (1937b). The preparatory set in stuttering. *Journal of Speech Disorders, 2,* 149–154.

Van Riper, C. (1947). *Speech correction: Principles and methods* (2nd ed.). New York: Prentice-Hall.

Van Riper, C. (1954). *Speech correction: Principles and methods* (3rd ed.). New York: Prentice-Hall.

Van Riper, C. (1957). Symptomatic therapy for stuttering. In L.E. Travis (Ed.), *Handbook of speech pathology.* New York: Appleton-Century-Crofts.

Van Riper, C. (1958). Experiments in stuttering therapy. In J. Eisenson (Ed.), *Stuttering: A symposium.* New York: Harper & Row.

Van Riper, C. (1971). *The nature of stuttering.* Englewood Cliffs, N.J.: Prentice-Hall.

Van Riper, C. (1973). *The treatment of stuttering.* Englewood Cliffs, N.J.: Prentice-Hall.

Van Riper, C. (1975). The stutterer's clinician. In J. Eisenson (Ed.), *Stuttering: A second symposium.* New York: Harper & Row.

Van Riper, C. (1990). Final thoughts about stuttering. *Journal of Fluency Disorders, 15,* 317–318.

Webster, W.G., & Poulos, M.G. (1989). *Facilitating fluency: Transfer strategies for adult stuttering treat-*

ment programs. Tucson, Ariz.: Communication Skill Builders.

Williams, D.E. (1957). A point of view about "stuttering." *Journal of Speech and Hearing Disorders*, *22*, 390–397.

Williams, D.E. (1979). A perspective on approaches to stuttering therapy. In H. Gregory (Ed.), *Controversies about stuttering therapy*. Baltimore, Md: University Park Press.

Williams, D.E. (1982). Stuttering therapy: Where are we going and why? *Journal of Fluency Disorders*, *7*, 159–170.

Wingate, M.E. (1976). *Stuttering: Theory and treatment*. New York: Irvington.

Wischner, G. (1950). Stuttering behavior and learning: A preliminary theoretical formulation. *Journal of Speech and Hearing Disorders*, *15*, 324–335.

Wischner, G. (1952). An experimental approach to expectancy and anxiety in stuttering behavior. *Journal of Speech and Hearing Disorders*, *17*, 139–154.

Zimmermann, G. (1980). Stuttering: A disorder of movement. *Journal of Speech and Hearing Research*, *23*, 122–136.

SUGGESTED READINGS

Bandura, A. (1977). *Social learning theory*. Englewood Cliffs, N.J.: Prentice-Hall, Inc. This short, readable book is an excellent primer on cognitive theory and behavior therapy. Topics include: The relationship of cognitive to stimulus-response explanations of learning, the functions of modeling, and the treatment of defensive behavior.

Brutten, G.J. (Ed.). (1993). *Journal of Fluency Disorders*, *18*(1). The entire volume consists of papers written by six recognized authorities on behavior modification and stuttering. They provide an informative overview of the history, current status, and future of behavioral therapies for this complex disorder.

Johnson, W. (1955). The descriptional principle and the principle of static analysis. In W. Johnson, & R.R. Leutenegger (Eds.), *Stuttering in children and adults* (pp. 432–447). Minneapolis: University of Minnesota Press. Written in 1937, this paper summarizes the principles and procedures of treatment that flow from Johnson's concepts about the nature of stuttering. His ideas about self-analysis and self-evaluation, about the importance of internalized beliefs to maintaining and changing behavior, are at the core of current cognitive approaches to behavior modification.

Prins, D. (1993). Management of stuttering: Treatment of adolescents and adults. In R.F. Curlee (Ed.), *Stuttering and related disorders of fluency*. New York: Thieme Medical Publishers. This chapter reviews procedures for the management of stuttering. It emphasizes the stutterer's achievement of self-efficacy expectations through the use of modeling and related techniques for behavioral self-regulation and self-evaluation.

Van Riper, C. (1937). The preparatory set in stuttering. *Journal of Speech Disorders*, *2*, 149–154. In this remarkable five-page paper, Van Riper sets the stage for his prodigious contributions to treatment that spanned more than fifty years. Providing evidence from experimental research, and using ideas that are consistent with current explanations of motor and cognitive learning, he explains his shift in the goal of therapy from elimination to modification of stuttering.

CHAPTER 18

DESIGNING AND IMPLEMENTING A STRATEGY TO CONTROL STUTTERED SPEECH IN ADULTS

MARK ONSLOW
ANN PACKMAN

INTRODUCTION

Behaviorism prompted the development of two separate procedures to control stuttering; those that rely on prolonged speech (PS) and those that rely on operant methodology. Single subject experiments comprised the early research in these areas, yet the literature suggests that behavioral treatment for adults who stutter is often conducted in groups using PS. One reason for the predominance of group treatment is that groups lend themselves to efficacy research incorporating group-comparison designs (Ingham, 1993). However, such research assumes that members of a group are more similar than different and that uniform therapy is appropriate for all members of the group (Ingham, 1993).

Both of us have worked extensively in PS group programs and we do not believe that they are the ideal behavioral treatment format for all adults who stutter. Additionally, a study by James, Ricciardelli, Hunter, and Rogers (1989) demonstrated that an intensive group format may not be necessary. Nor are group treatments ideal for generalist clinicians who wish to manage stuttering clients in a more traditional setting. In our clinic, we use a range of behavioral approaches, incorporating group and individual treatment with PS and operant procedures. In this chapter we explore the merits of various approaches and suggest ways of

designing intervention for individual clients. Thus, we hope that generalist clinicians will be encouraged to consider treatment of individual clients with PS as well as intensive PS group treatment.

THE DEVELOPMENT OF PROLONGED-SPEECH TREATMENT PROGRAMS

Techniques similar to PS were known from at least the eighteenth century. However, the bulk of modern clinical developments of this speech pattern to control stuttering can be traced to Goldiamond's (1965) report on the use of delayed auditory feedback (DAF). It was known that DAF was a speech-disruptive stimulus with some ameliorative effects on stuttering (see Ingham, 1984). Because of its aversive properties, Goldiamond (1965) reported using DAF as a punishing stimulus during a series of laboratory experiments on behavioral control of stuttering. In those single-subject experiments, Goldiamond established that DAF could be used to generate a clinically useful speech pattern that could replace stuttered speech.

Ingham (1984) noted that Goldiamond's experiments foreshadowed the development of modern PS treatment programs. This is not surprising, given the clinical value of Goldiamond's discovery. A machine-governed technique (DAF) was rapidly able to establish stutter-free speech and then shape it to resemble normal speech. The salient features of Goldiamond's methodology were establishment of a slow and unnatural sounding speech pattern with DAF, systematic reduction of the DAF, and systematic increase of speech rate. Since that time, four distinct treatment programs have emerged that were based on Goldiamond's methodology (see Ingham, 1984). Modern published treatment programs reflect Goldiamond's procedure in that they describe establishment of a slow and unnatural speech pattern, followed by attempts to shape that speech pattern to natural sounding speech with programmed instruction (Boberg & Kully, 1985; Ingham, 1987; Neilson & Andrews, 1993; Perkins, 1984; Ryan, 1974; Shames & Florance, 1980; Webster, 1980). In many cases, Goldiamond's DAF procedure has been replaced by clinician instruction in speech patterns referred to variously as "smooth speech," "smooth motion speech," "slow motion speech,"[1] and containing components referred to as "soft contacts," "gentle onsets," "light articulatory contacts," and "continuous vocalization."

The development of specialized treatment facilities has been part of the history of PS. Typically, such facilities have their equipment and operations built around the conduct of intensive group treatment, and their staffs specialize in the conduct of that treatment. During the past decades, such specialized treatment programs have become prominent. For example, the Webster (1980) and Boberg and Kully (1985) programs attract clients from across the United States and Canada. In Australia, variants of the Ingham and Andrews (1973) program have proliferated in major cities, with four such variants currently existing within Sydney, where the original program was developed. At one stage this situation was so pervasive that, during one year, it was reported that 88 percent of adult Australians diagnosed by speech pathologists to be stuttering were referred to such specialist treatment facilities (Onslow & Ingham, 1989).

The documented history of the treatment programs cited above shows that their development has not been rapid, principally because of the concern for thorough evaluation shown by those who developed them. All programs have been systematically evaluated over many years, with modifications introduced in response to those evaluations. Within this evaluation process, it is necessary that clinical procedures remain constant for long periods as they are administered to groups of clients. An example of this time-consuming process can be seen in the recent publication of Boberg and Kully's (1994) study of outcomes of a program that was described nine years earlier (Boberg & Kully, 1985). In our own case, at present there is an outcome evaluation report for the Ingham (1987) program (Onslow, Costa, Andrews, Harrison, & Packman, in press) that contains a single major revision to procedures in an earlier version of that program (Ingham, 1981).

There is no doubt that the steady and painstaking evolution of specialized, group-based, intensive PS treatment services throughout the world is a necessary component of research and development in this field. Such developments provide a proven means by which those who stutter can control their condition. But we suggest that such developments also have a legacy; published details of specialist programs are virtually the only existing clinical documentation of procedures for the control of stuttered speech with PS. Yet, as we have stated, one of the limitations of specialist PS treatments is the slow rate of their development because of the need to remain constant for long periods. Consequently, that published clinical material does not always reflect the full range of creative development that may be stimulated by treatment research and clinical thought. This is problematic for those who administer PS treatments in other than specialist settings; for example, clinicians who see stuttering clients once or twice a week as part of a general caseload. We believe that such clinicians can adapt the clinical procedures of intensive group treatments for their own needs in the generalist clinic. In our view, such freedom to experiment clinically is the major benefit of conducting PS treatment with individual

---

[1]In this chapter we use the term "prolonged speech" (PS), coined by Goldiamond, to refer generically to these speech patterns.

clients in standard clinical settings. Every client can be managed with variations on the fundamental concept of replacing stuttered speech with PS, but at present there is little documentation to assist clinicians in formulating those creative variations.

ADAPTING PROLONGED-SPEECH PROGRAMS

In this section we discuss possible variations on the traditional techniques of using PS to establish, generalize, and maintain control over stuttering. In so doing, we draw on available research and clinical demonstrations. We indicate when we feel that techniques developed in intensive group programs are and are not empirically and conceptually justifiable. We argue that some such techniques qualify as standard procedures that should apply to every client and that some do not. The issues that are discussed in this section are programmed instruction, speech naturalness, generalization, and maintenance.

Programmed Instruction

The intensive group PS program (Ingham, 1987) that we have conducted is fairly typical. Clients learn to speak without stuttering by using PS at increasing speech rates; 40 syllables per minute (SPM), 70 SPM, 100 SPM, and so on. Such programmed attempts to shape natural sounding, stutter-free speech have their origin in Goldiamond's initial DAF procedure. One response of the speaker to DAF is to reduce speech rate, hence the need to restore normal rate. However, it is worth questioning whether there is any need to reduce a client's speech rate so much in the first place. It is likely that, for many clients, reduced speech rate contributes to the control of stuttering and therefore is a useful component of a PS pattern. However, the clinician might establish a rate that exerts control over stuttering but is similar enough to normal speech rate for functional communication. Ingham and Packman (1977) reported a laboratory procedure for establishing the speech rate most

conducive to stuttering reduction, and Onslow (1996) outlined a clinical procedure in which a "tradeoff" speech rate is established by means of a set of brief speaking trials with varying speech rate. If it were the case that such a trade-off rate for a client was 170 SPM, there seems little need for that client to learn to speak at 40 SPM as a preliminary step. In our experience, it is not problematic to specify a target speech rate range and to train a speaker to stay within that range through intermittent or continuous feedback (Onslow, 1996).

One possible justification for the use of greatly reduced speech rate and subsequent shaping is that this is an integral part of learning the various components of PS. However, this concept has some limitations also. It is clear that skills such as "soft contact," "gentle vocal onset," and "easy phrase initiation" are best modeled by the clinician and learned by the client at a reduced rate. This permits clients to observe the clinician's model and learn those skills as precisely as possible. Further, reduced rate allows the clinician to observe the client's productions and determine whether the skills have been mastered. But it is open to question whether speech drills at varying rates contribute to the client's capacity to use these skills to produce natural sounding, stutter-free speech in everyday situations. Consequently, rate-based programmed instruction procedures with PS need to be questioned when—according to published reports—they occupy a large proportion of treatment time.

In short, there are some serious conceptual limitations to the traditional speech rate increment procedure for establishing natural sounding speech, and there has been no treatment research to demonstrate the value of that procedure. In that regard, Webster's (1980) outline of his "Precision Fluency Shaping" program is of interest. Webster's program has moved away from the shaping of stutter-free speech by the step-wise increments in speech rates described by Goldiamond. Instead, Webster's current program begins with clients learning the various target behaviors of the speech pattern in single-syllable words. Establishment of stutter-free speech proceeds in increments—from two- to three-syllable words, then to phrases and sentences.

Thus, there is more than one kind of programmed instruction that can be used to teach clients a novel speech pattern. There is no need to adhere to the method of programmed instruction that was instigated by Goldiamond. We often use a procedure similar to Webster's with clients treated in nonintensive conditions. It is based on Ryan's (1974) Gradual Increase in Length and Complexity of Utterance (GILCU) procedure, and most closely resembles an Extended Length of Utterance (ELU) variant of that technique (Costello, 1983; J.C. Ingham, 1993). Our clinical materials are many sheets of single-syllable words with every consonant occurring in many CVC contexts. Using these stimuli, clients are taught the components of the PS speech pattern (soft contacts, gentle onsets, extended vocalization) to criterion. When the client is able to read the single-syllable word list to criterion, with zero stuttering and satisfactory PS, the next clinical task is to read the same number of two-syllable words and syntactic strings. Subsequently, the client is required to read three-syllable through ten-syllable utterances to criterion. During this procedure, the utterance lists enable us to know the precise location of each consonant that should be articulated with a soft contact, and each vowel that should be initiated with a gentle onset and spoken with extended vocalization. In our view, during the learning of PS skills, this allows the clinician to give more detailed feedback than is possible if training tasks are based on connected speech at varying speech rates.

When our clients have mastered the ten-utterance lists to criterion, we continue the ELU process using time as the basis of programmed instruction. The steps are designed specifically for individual clients, but 10 seconds, 20 seconds, and 30 seconds are typical increments in early stages of this instruction, with subsequent 1-minute increments up to a target of 5 minutes of stutter-free speech. We impose no speech rate criteria during this shaping process from one syllable to 5 minutes of speech. Throughout, the client is free to speak at any rate, provided that there is no stuttering and that PS skills are satisfactory. Typically, the client chooses a slow speech rate during the early stages of instruction and gradually settles into a comfortable rate as the program approaches 5 minutes of stutter-free prolonged speech.

A recent study (Packman, Onslow, & van Doorn, 1994) provides some support for the idea that programmed instruction is not a necessary part of PS treatment, and that not all clients require all elements of the PS pattern to control stuttering. In that study, three adults who stuttered, but who had never received treatment, learned to speak with PS at 40 SPM, which is the first stage of the Ingham (1987) program. The subjects practiced 40 SPM PS for 5 minutes, after which they resumed customary speaking conditions for a 5-minute monologue. In this speaking condition (Phase B), all subjects showed clinically significant stuttering reductions, with the stuttering of one subject approaching zero. In a subsequent speaking condition (Phase C), subjects were informed that PS is the basis of a treatment procedure and were instructed to use whatever features of PS they liked to eliminate stuttering. Two subjects achieved near-zero stuttering rates in this condition and maintained that for a number of speaking sessions. In Subject 2, who stuttered severely, stuttering reduced significantly but not to zero. An analysis showed that stuttering reductions occurred without compromising speech naturalness. The findings of this study are presented in Figure 18.1.

These findings demonstrate that, for some subjects, systematic instruction in PS may not be necessary. Some may be able to learn PS skills and then use those skills immediately to produce stutter-free, natural-sounding speech. In such cases, treatment procedures might then concentrate on consolidating the client's skill at PS and generalizing its use to everyday situations.

Many clients can achieve stutter-free speech after around 10 minutes' practice with the procedure illustrated in Figure 18.1, that is, by teaching them a slow and exaggerated PS pattern and then instructing them to use that speech pattern to control stuttering. Nonetheless, even clients who benefit from this procedure require considerable practice at their new-found skill for it to be of functional use to them. The clients in Figure 18.1

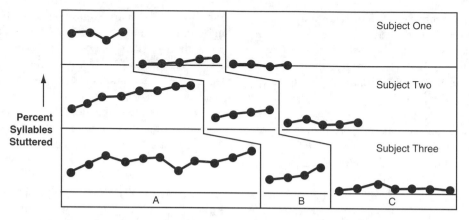

Figure 18.1   Results from Packman, Onslow, and van Doorn (1994), adapted by permission of the American Speech-Language-Hearing Association. See text for explanation. The solid dots represent %SS scores in 5-minute monologues. Three subjects were studied under three conditions. A represents the baseline condition, B represents the condition where subjects practiced Stage 40 prolonged speech before each speaking session, and C represents the condition where subjects were told to use the speech pattern to eliminate stuttering.

achieved only several minutes of natural-sounding, stutter-free speech, and it is clinically realistic to have clients maintain that for a number of stutter-free 5-minute trials before deciding that this is an appropriate procedure for instating stutter-free speech that might generalize outside the clinic. One procedure to help such clients achieve that goal is ELU (Costello, 1983; J.C. Ingham, 1993); however, for the type of client for whom this approach may be successful, it may still be the case that programmed instruction is not necessary.

Figure 18.2 illustrates a clinical procedure to increase the duration of stutter-free speech that a client is able to produce. Treatment sessions—conducted in the clinic or by the client at home—consist of speaking trials during which the client attempts to increase the duration of periods of stutter-free speech. Measures are minutes and seconds of stutter-free speech. In the example in Figure 18.2, only the client's successful attempts have been recorded, along with the number of trials that were required to increase duration of stutter-free speech from the previous target. The clinician has measured speech rate to ensure that the client did not increase the durations of stutter-free speech merely by reducing rate. If the client succeeds at a

target of 5 minutes of monologue, one option is to repeat the procedure with conversational targets. Often, we then repeat the procedure with the client making all decisions about whether stuttering occurs and with the clinician correcting any errors in self-evaluation.[2] This is not a programmed instruction procedure because there are no predetermined steps for the client to progress through. A clear advantage is that the client need not complete any predetermined steps that are superfluous to achieving the eventual target.

Speech Naturalness

One of the recurring problems with PS treatments is that they reduce stuttering at the expense of natural-sounding speech. Perceptual studies have confirmed this observation (see Onslow & Ingham, 1987, for a review), and scores on a speech naturalness scale developed by Martin and colleagues (

---

[2]We have found that this procedure is very successful for children because they enjoy constructing their graphs and seeing performance rise during home and clinic sessions. Children also enjoy tokens awarded for achieving predetermined durations of stutter-free speech.

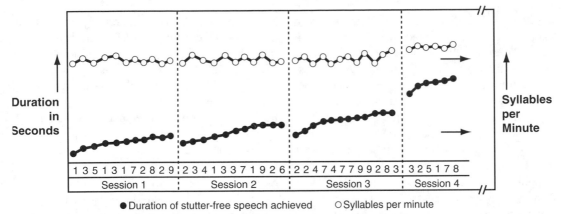

Figure 18.2   Shaping the duration of stutter-free speech in a client without programmed instruction (adapted from Onslow, 1993). See text for explanation. Solid data points represent durations of stutter-free speech achieved in each clinical trial, and the open data points represent speech rate at each clinical trial. The numbers recorded below the data points represent the number of attempts required for the client to improve on the duration of stutter-free speech in the previous trial.

Martin & Haroldson, 1992; Martin, Haroldson, & Triden, 1984;) show that speech at the completion of a PS treatment is more unnatural than that of control speakers (Onslow, Hayes, Hutchins, & Newman, 1992; Ingham, Gow, & Costello, 1985). Further, it appears that there is a positive relation between pretreatment stuttering severity and listener-judged unnaturalness after treatment (Kalinowski, Noble, Armson, & Stuart, 1994; Onslow et al., 1992; Packman et al., 1994). The extent of this problem was highlighted in the recent report by Kalinowski et al. (1994) on the posttreatment naturalness of clients in an adaptation of Webster's (1980) precision fluency shaping program. These authors found that the posttreatment speech of clients classified with severe stuttering was assigned a mean listener naturalness rating of 7.92. Considering that the range of naturalness scores for controls is in the range 2–4 (Ingham et al., 1985; Martin et al., 1984; Metz, Schiavetti, & Sacco, 1990; Onslow et al., 1992; Runyan, Bell, & Prosek, 1990), this suggests that this group's speech had little in common with normal speech. In fact, these clients' posttreatment naturalness scores were higher than their pretreatment scores, indicating that their posttreatment speech sounded more unnatural to listeners than their stuttered speech.

It is worthwhile trying to eliminate this problem. We have met clinicians who are prepared to accept extremely unnatural sounding speech in the interests of eliminating stuttering, but in our experience few clients are prepared to tolerate such speech, long-term, in everyday life, and those who do are extraordinary in some way. As Martin, Haroldson, and Triden (1984) stated, unnatural posttreatment speech is one likely contributor to the well-known problem of posttreatment relapse. *We aim for a natural-sounding speech pattern, and we do nothing clinically that trains the client to the contrary unless we have reason to believe that such is necessary.*

Some of the clinical procedures described earlier are examples of how PS training may encourage natural-sounding speech. The programmed instruction procedure based on Costello's ELU procedure contains no speech rate targets or any other specification about speech naturalness. The same can be said of the techniques illustrated in Figures 18.1 and 18.2. The technique in Figure 18.1 simply gave the clients free reign to use PS to eliminate stuttering, and the results of that study (Packman et al., 1994) show that such an action may result in elimination of stuttering with little compromise to speech naturalness. And in Figure

18.2, all that was required of the client was zero stuttering, at whatever speech rate or speech naturalness level the client selected. We have found with this procedure, too, that clients typically establish optimal use of PS to achieve a tradeoff between stuttering control and speech naturalness.

Such clinical management scenarios apply to clients who have an aptitude for PS and who show signs of being able to use it in a functional manner after a short period of instruction. For clients with whom this is not the case, it may be necessary to shape speech naturalness with programmed instruction that incorporates systematic stepwise drills. Such clients may include those who have a history of failed PS treatment, particularly severe stuttering, or limited cognitive capacity. However, we cannot predict which clients will require programmed instruction to achieve natural-sounding speech and which will not. As we indicate in a final section on designing a management strategy, the only way to settle the matter is through clinical investigation.

Historically, intensive PS programs have attempted to shape natural-sounding speech with progressive speech rate increments, but there are good reasons to believe that this procedure is not successful. As we indicated above, unnatural sounding speech is often the end product of such programs. Ingham, Martin, Haroldson, Onslow, and Leney (1985) raised the possibility of a clinical solution to this problem by showing that a clinician could use Martin, Haroldson and Triden's (1984) naturalness scale with adequate reliability and that reliable naturalness ratings could be fed back to assist a speaker to improve speech naturalness. This approach to shaping speech naturalness was refined by Ingham and Onslow (1985) with a study of clients who had established stutter-free speech in a PS program, but whose speech was quite unnatural sounding. Ingham and Onslow used ratings from a clinician to program steps in a hierarchy of speech naturalness that clients were required to follow to achieve natural-sounding speech.

Figure 18.3 presents the results from one subject in this study. After this subject had established stutter-free speech in the program, speech naturalness scores indicated extremely unnatural-sounding speech. The client was required to speak for several trials with zero stuttering, and when speech naturalness was stable over a number of speaking trials, a lower range of speech naturalness was prescribed for the client on the naturalness scale. The client was fed back a clinician's naturalness score every 15 seconds and instructed to modify speech naturalness to the prescribed range. Figure 18.3 shows that the client was able to modify speech naturalness to that level, at which point a final target range of speech naturalness—similar to normal speech—was prescribed. Figure 18.3 shows that the client achieved this final level of naturalness.

One of the strengths of PS treatments is that they have incorporated measurement within their operations (Onslow & Ingham, 1987); clients progress contingent on their achievement of criterion measures of stuttering and speech rate. The point of the Onslow and Ingham study is that a measure of speech naturalness may be included in a PS treatment, and these measures can be used to program the acquisition of speech that is as natural as possible.

This procedure was incorporated into the latest revision of the intensive group PS program that we have conducted (Ingham, 1987). The first part of the procedures, which establish stutter-free speech, remains unchanged from a previous version (Ingham, 1981). After clients have learned PS skills, they progress through programmed steps, each of which requires a new speech rate—40 SPM, 70 SPM, and 100 SPM (plus or minus 20 SPM)—in addition to zero stuttering. Each of these steps requires that clients achieve six consecutive speaking trials to criterion. Changes in the PS speech pattern occur across these three steps, and this is the start of the shaping process towards natural-sounding speech. Subsequently, clients progress through three further steps, during which they may speak at any rate they wish as long as their speech is stutter-free. However, an additional target behavior is included: criterion or below-criterion speech naturalness in addition to zero stut-

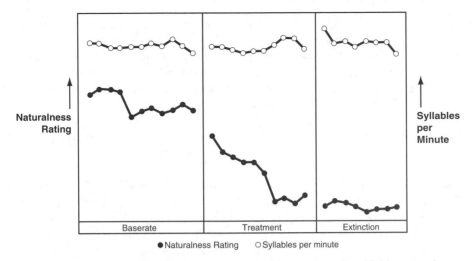

Figure 18.3   The use of fed-back speech naturalness ratings (1 = highly natural, 9 = highly unnatural) to shape natural-sounding, stutter-free speech. Results for one subject from Ingham and Onslow (1985), adapted by permission of the American Speech-Language-Hearing Association. See text for explanation.

tering. These steps are conducted in the same manner as the previous three, with the exception that clients' speech naturalness is measured using naturalness scale. The clinician scores speech naturalness and presents this score to the client during speaking trials after every minute of speech. During this procedure, clients may exaggerate or minimize features of PS, providing they remain stutter-free and maintain their target level of speech naturalness.

During these three steps, referred to as Na, Nb and Nc, naturalness scores are reduced systematically to a score of 2, or as close to this level as the client can achieve. The naturalness criteria for steps Na, Nb and Nc are calculated with reference to the client's mean naturalness scores during the last speaking trial at 100 SPM. The goal is a naturalness score of 2, which is subtracted from the mean naturalness score during the last 100 SPM speaking trial. The result is divided by three to form the naturalness criteria for Na, Nb, and Nc. For example, if the mean naturalness score for the last 100 SPM trial is 7.0, then 5.0 is divided by 3, which rounds to 1.7. This value, 1.7, is used to set naturalness targets for Na, Nb, and Nc (i.e., the target for Na is 5.3 or below, the target

for Nb is 3.7 or below, and the target for Nc is 2.0 or below).

When a client has completed a succession of six stutter-free speech trials at stage Na, the clinician calculates the mean naturalness score for those six trials. If it is equal to or below the Na target naturalness, the client progresses to stage Nb. If not, the client attempts another sequence of six speaking trials in an effort to achieve the Na target. Clients are allowed three sets of six trials to achieve target speech naturalness. If a client fails to achieve a speech naturalness target at any point in the program after three sets of six trials, the target for that client becomes the mean naturalness score during the last set of six trials.

We have found this procedure to be particularly effective with clients who are treated individually in nonintensive conditions, because, to a considerable extent, the naturalness shaping procedure is individualized. It does not pressure clients to achieve speech naturalness targets in a set period of time, permitting them to achieve targets at differing rates. With some clients it is not possible to achieve satisfactory naturalness and zero stuttering, because attempts to reduce speech naturalness scores result in the reappearance of stuttering. With such clients, this procedure enables clinicians to establish the point at which there is a tradeoff between stuttering and speech naturalness. Such clients may, in fact, improve naturalness scores some time after they have established stutter-free speech. However, it is critical to identify those clients for whom it is best not to attempt to establish near-normal levels of speech naturalness.

In our experience, speech naturalness scores on a 9-point scale are an excellent means to communicate how natural a client's speech pattern sounds. When a client and clinician work together, they gain full agreement about the meaning of certain scale values, so that it is possible for clients to manipulate their speech patterns on-line in response to the clinician's instructions to speak at different naturalness levels. Invariably we find that, with practice, clients are able to alter their speech patterns immediately from "three" to "five" to "four," and so on. This is an important clinical achievement for several reasons. First, it facilitates clients' self-assessment of how natural they sound in various situations. It also is an effective way to instruct clients in how they should practice PS when they are alone; in many cases it is useful for clients to practice their speech pattern at a less natural level than they would normally use in everyday situations. The naturalness scale can be used, for example, to prescribe periods of practice at naturalness level "six," followed by "five," "four" and then "three" or "two." Finally, speech naturalness scores assist clients to cope with problematic speaking situations. Many published PS programs recommend that the client use an exaggerated, unnatural sounding PS pattern for a period to cope with such situations. The speech naturalness scale can help the clinician and client determine exactly what level of speech naturalness provides optimal control in those speaking conditions.

Generalization

There are advantages and disadvantages of intensive group treatment formats, and it is not our intention to explore that issue here. However, *one disadvantage of group PS treatment is that it is con-*ducted under conditions that are contrary to what is believed to facilitate the transfer of treatment gains to everyday speaking environments.* The results of clinical research have demonstrated little about how to facilitate generalization apart from the obvious value of self-evaluation of performance (Ingham, 1980), which has been incorporated into many programs. Most of the information about facilitating generalization is contained in the well-known discussion of Stokes and Baer (1977), who outlined clinical techniques that reflect common sense more than research findings. All of the active strategies recommended by these authors involve agents that exist in the everyday speaking environments of clients, such as people and speaking situations. Yet, by necessity, the establishment of stutter-free speech in intensive, group PS programs occurs in conditions that remove clients from those agents in everyday speaking environments. To overcome this problem, intensive PS programs incorporate a set of formal speaking tasks designed to extend stutter-free speech, after it has been established, from the clinic to beyond the clinic. In most cases, these tasks are organized into a hierarchy of difficulty, and the client tape records speech in each of these tasks progressively. This procedure is referred to by Stokes and Baer as "sequential modification."

Although intensive PS treatments must attempt to achieve generalization in this manner, it is not necessary when clients are treated individually with PS in nonintensive conditions. We emphasize this point, because it is easy to be misled into believing that the generalization procedures described in published PS intensive programs are the only way to facilitate generalization of stutter-free speech; that the generalization component of management is nothing more than a set of hierarchical speaking tasks. In fact, such "sequential modification" is only one of many techniques for generalization available to clinicians who conduct individual, nonintensive PS treatments.

When treating clients individually, we have found that adapting some of Stokes and Baer's techniques is valuable for easing the client, week by week, into the use of PS during daily life. The technique, *introduce to natural maintaining contingen-*

cies, is based on the idea that naturally occurring reinforcers of clinical procedures can be found in the client's environment. In the case of PS treatment of adults, those reinforcers are mostly support and encouragement. Intuitively, such naturally occurring reinforcers would better facilitate generalization than would contrived or unnatural reinforcers that are associated with the clinic. It also seems intuitively correct that clients are unlikely to succeed in the task of controlling stuttering for a lifetime without the support and encouragement of people close to them. It is true that some adult stuttering clients are powerfully motivated and will succeed no matter what, but we are sure that the majority will not succeed if the only maintaining contingencies come from the clinician during clinic contacts.

Stokes and Baer's technique, *train sufficient exemplars*, involves teaching PS in some of the speech settings that are typical of the client's speaking life. This technique is no more than clinical commonsense. If the goal of treatment is to have the client stutter-free in everyday situations, then it may impair treatment if training of stutter-free speech occurs only in a clinic that bears little resemblance to those situations. As far as possible with each client, we insist that a substantial portion of the work we prescribe in learning the PS pattern occurs in different speaking situations, most typically with family and friends. We also insist that, wherever possible, family and friends attend some treatment sessions. Related to this technique is *train loosely*, which is a technique designed to overcome the well-known effects of discriminated learning. This effect occurs when a clinically learned response is elicited by some things or people but not others. This can be a powerful effect in stuttering treatment. Clinicians in the intensive PS program we conduct use an instrument for counting syllables and stutterings online, and in cases of posttreatment relapse, the mere sight of that device may trigger stutter-free speech. To offset the effects of discriminated learning, we recommend that PS training occur not only during speech to various people, but also in a variety of speaking situations. It inhibits generalization if all training occurs in the same place

with the same person—even more so if that place and person are the clinic and clinician.

However, in some situations, discriminated learning may assist with generalization. Such situations occur when learning of stutter-free speech is yoked to things in the client's environment rather than things in the clinic. In effect, this is the *program common stimuli* technique suggested by Stokes and Baer. Whenever possible, we attempt to have a significant person in the client's life be present and actively involved at every clinic session and every practice session at home. We suspect that much of the successful generalization we have reported for operant treatments with children (Lincoln, Onslow, Wilson, & Lewis, in press; Onslow, Andrews, & Lincoln, 1994, Onslow, Costa, & Rue, 1990) arises from the fact that parents are inextricably involved in treatment; in fact, they conduct it from start to finish under our guidance.

The *sequential modification* procedure described by Stokes and Baer is the practice of arranging therapy tasks in an order of increasing difficulty. Although this practice is common in the "transfer" portions of all published PS programs, there is no empirical evidence for its value. Further, it is logistically difficult to design and execute this procedure, and it is labor intensive for clinicians who need to assess tape recordings made by clients. It is also an example of programmed instruction, which we believe may be an unnecessarily elaborate procedure for many clients. For these reasons, we avoid this procedure whenever possible. However, there is one type of client who, more often than not, will benefit from programmed, hierarchical generalization procedures. Such clients are those who experience significant state anxiety—even reluctance—about talking in everyday speech situations. This condition may be present before treatment or it may develop after the client has learned stutter-free speech and attempts to enter speaking situations that previously were avoided. For such anxiety-related conditions, exposure is likely to be a key to management, and a hierarchy of anxiety-provoking speaking situations is often a productive clinical strategy.

Maintenance

There is general agreement that relapse after PS treatment is a major management difficulty. There have been several attempts to quantify this problem (Craig & Calver, 1991; Howie, Tanner, & Andrews, 1981; Martin, 1981), but it would be misleading to accept an overall percentage rate of relapse because of the many different ways that relapse may be defined and also because these studies involved specialized PS programs that are likely to attract clients who may be predisposed to succeed. As indicated previously, clients may travel across the United States and Canada to enroll in such programs. In Australia, the status of the Neilson and Andrews (1993) program is conveyed by Mooney's (1990) description:

> *People have to be highly motivated to take part in the intensive course. The typical patient is . . . in his mid to late twenties with a moderately successful to very successful career. He is usually either facing a promotional block or has reached it. (p. 26)*

Relapse is probably more of a problem for generalist clinicians who may deal with less motivated clients. Unfortunately, there is little research about facilitating maintenance of stutter-free speech that generalist clinicians might draw on to counter this problem. There have been two data-based reports suggesting that a series of formal maintenance visits to the clinic are a hedge against relapse after PS treatment (Boberg, 1981; Ingham, 1980), and several reports that cognitive variables such as "attitude to communication" and "locus of control" are critical to relapse prevention (Andrews & Craig, 1988; Andrews & Cutler, 1974; Craig, Franklin, & Andrews, 1984; Craig & Howie, 1982; Guitar, 1976; Guitar & Bass, 1978). In the remainder of this section we explore some of the implications of this information for generalist clinicians who conduct PS treatments.

The key to productive maintenance is to regard it as a part of the treatment process, not as a supplementary procedure for use when "treatment" is finished. For clients, maintaining treat-

ment gains is the hardest part of treatment. We regard maintenance as one of several behavioral responses involved in a client's stuttering treatment. Just as one client response during treatment may be stutter-free speech in the clinic, during maintenance the client response may be stutter-free speech in everyday situations for a clinically significant period. With this notion, maintenance can be managed systematically in the same way as any other behavioral response of clients in stuttering treatment. Criteria can be specified, goals can be programmed, contingencies can be arranged, and shaping procedures can be implemented if needed.

The first step in managing maintenance as a client response is to specify the criteria that indicate a client has succeeded in achieving that response. In cases where the client response involves zero or near-zero stuttering, the task is straightforward. In such cases, maintenance criteria might be something like this:

> *On six consecutive assessments separated by 2 months, stuttering rate will be below 1%SS and mean speech naturalness will be below 3.5 in three 1,000-syllable within-clinic conversations and three tape-recorded 1,000-syllable beyond-clinic conversations with different people.*

In effect, these maintenance criteria replicate criteria for successful treatment, but make them applicable to maintenance by specifying that they must remain in place for twelve consecutive assessments over a period of one year. Having established performance criteria for maintenance, there is the creative option of programmed or nonprogrammed instruction to facilitate that client response. A study by Ingham (1980) was designed to show the relative merits of programmed and nonprogrammed maintenance. Nine clients were assigned to a group that participated in a programmed maintenance schedule or to a group that participated in a nonprogrammed maintenance schedule. The group in programmed maintenance progressed though a series of assessments as long as their speech performance met certain criteria. If those criteria were met at an assessment, the client progressed to the next assessment. If the criteria were not met at an assessment, the client was required to return to the first of the series of maintenance assessments. The other group progressed through a set number of steps regardless of their speech status. Although all stuttering rates were low in this study, the clients in the programmed maintenance group achieved better results in the long term than did those in the other group.

We favor Ingham's procedure with group and individual treatments because it manages maintenance as a client response by attaching contingencies to it, similar to any other response in treatment. Clinically significant periods during which treatment goals remain in place are rewarded. An innovative aspect of this procedure is that part of the contingency for meeting maintenance criteria is increasing the period until the next assessment is scheduled. Clients are rewarded for maintaining stutter-free speech with an increased interval until their next assessment, which shapes the client response of long-term maintenance. This has the practical advantage that clients consume clinical time according to their needs during the maintenance phase of treatment. If they continue to meet program targets, they consume progressively less clinical time. If they fail to meet program targets, they see their clinician more regularly. In contrast, a maintenance schedule that is independent of client performance might expend much clinician effort on clients who do not need it to maintain their treatment targets.

In the case of nonintensive, individualized treatments, there is flexibility in selecting the goals of treatment that is not normally available in intensive, group treatments. The structure of group treatments is built around achieving zero or near-zero stuttering in all speaking situations; however, such a goal does not suit the needs of all clients. Many clients only want to achieve the capacity to control their stuttering in certain situations. We find clients—often those whose stuttering is not severe—who are willing to stutter while they speak with family and friends, but who require stutter-free speech in certain situations. One recent case is

a woman with mild stuttering who often socialized with her husband's work colleagues. Such situations caused considerable speech anxiety. For this client, it was inappropriate to establish a client response target of zero stutterings in all speaking situations; the effort could not be justified. Instead, together with the client, we decided the criterion would be to produce stutter-free, natural sounding speech on demand. Accordingly, her maintenance targets were as follows:

> *On six consecutive assessments separated by 2 months, stuttering rate is to be zero and mean speech naturalness is to be below 3.0 in one 1,000-word within-clinic conversation, and one recorded 1,000-syllable conversation with a stranger. Additionally, ten 10-syllable word lists will be read in prolonged speech with soft contacts, gentle onsets, and extended vocalization judged by the clinician to be satisfactory.*

There are some similarities between these maintenance requirements and those outlined previously. However, there is an important conceptual difference. The former maintenance criteria are designed to establish near-zero stuttering in everyday speaking situations. But in the case of the woman just discussed, the *skill* of using PS to speak on demand without stuttering is what is required to be retained. In this case it was not of concern if she came to a maintenance session stuttering openly, provided that she had the capacity to speak without stuttering on demand, and had retained the correct use of the components of prolonged speech.

Virtually all research into the effect of cognitive variables on maintenance of treatment gains has dealt with "attitude to communication" and "locus of control" (Andrews & Craig, 1988; Andrews & Cutler, 1974; Craig, Franklin, & Andrews, 1984; Craig & Howie, 1982; Guitar, 1976; Guitar & Bass, 1978). This body of research culminated with a report by Andrews and Craig (1988) on relapse in eighty-four clients. They found that clients who had not relapsed had zero stuttering, an internalized locus of control, and normalized attitude about communication at the conclusion of their intensive treatment. Relapse was defined as more than 2%SS during a 600-syllable telephone call to a stranger ten to eighteen months after the conclusion of the program. Andrews and Craig reported that the success rate of the clients related to how many of three treatment goals were achieved, and that 97 percent of the clients who had achieved all three treatment goals did not relapse.

There is certainly no argument with the substance of Andrews and Craig's conclusion. Clients can't be expected to control stuttering in the long term unless they have an appropriate attitude about verbal communication and feel that they are able to control their disorder rather than being a victim of it. But the context of Andrews and Craig's conclusion may be misleading for clinicians who use PS to treat clients individually. *We believe that the role of cognition in self-regulation during maintenance is a complex matter;* however, Andrews and Craig focused on only two of many variables and, by showing their relevance, implied that the matter is a simple one. Their findings can be interpreted as showing a causal relationship between internalized locus of control and normalized attitude to communication, and successful treatment, but the reverse may be true; those cognitive variables may be determined by speech performance. Clients may feel in control of their speech and have healthy attitudes about communication when they are no longer bothered by stuttering. And there may be other variables that contribute to long-term stuttering reduction and the cognitive changes that were studied, and it is likely that these variables differ across clients.

A second problem with Andrews and Craig's conclusion is that it pertains to one particular specialized treatment program. Neilson and Andrews's (1993) outline of this program supports our previous argument that specialized treatment programs select specialized clients. Such programs, because of the nature of their caseload, may screen out clients on the basis of cognitive variables that hinder maintenance of long-term treatment gains.

Those . . . who view 3 weeks of intensive work on their speech as too great an investment, usually decline treatment and do not present a problem in case selection. The second group of people, who do not manage well in other aspects of their lives, will have similar difficulty in managing the rigors of a demanding treatment program and the ensuing self-care during maintenance. When this is apparent, we choose not to offer treatment. Although the program may bring short-term gains to such clients, there is little chance of long-term success. . . . The best chance for such people is individual therapy. The program we run today is aimed firmly at those stutterers in the third group, who manage life well but who find their stutter has become an unacceptable handicap in reaching otherwise feasible goals. These clients come well motivated and well prepared for the long hours of hard work that are required by our treatment. (pp. 143–144)

In our own efforts with PS treatment we agree with Neilson and Andrews's contention that elimination of stuttered speech may only be permanent if the client has something to gain from that achievement. Too often, we have worked with a client to eliminate stuttered speech only to witness relapse simply because that client's life stayed the same as before, with no benefits accruing from stutter-free speech. We also agree with another of Neilson and Andrews's points that some clients, who have failed to achieve goals in life, misguidedly blame such failures on their stuttering.

In summary, research on clinically relevant cognitive variables has implied that, in order to solve the problem of relapse, clients need only achieve stutter-free speech, an internalized locus of control, and normalized attitudes toward communication. While this may be appropriate for selective clinical caseloads, it is not useful for those clinicians who treat all types of clients, including those who have been found unsuitable for intensive group treatment. There are many cognitive variables that seem likely to affect maintenance. In our final section on assessment we draw attention to the role of pretreatment counseling in determining those cognitive variables that may affect maintenance of stutter-free speech.

DECIDING WHEN TO USE OPERANT STRATEGIES

An important skill for a clinician who favors a behavioral approach is deciding which technique for controlling stuttering is appropriate for an individual client. This is an important issue considering the long-term rigors involved in successful PS treatment; between 50 and 100 hours of training (Andrews, Guitar, & Howie, 1980; Perkins, 1984; Webster, 1980) followed by frequent speech practice and continuous attention to the act of speaking. Before making a commitment to such a regime, the client needs to be aware of treatment choices. This issue has been brought into focus with mounting evidence that many children respond extremely well to operant treatments that rely on contingent stimulation of stuttering rather than replacement of stuttering with a novel speech pattern. There are approximately twenty treatment reports of operant methods that have been used successfully with school-aged children (for example, Browning, 1967; Johnson, Coleman, & Rasmussen, 1978; Leach, 1969; Manning, Trutna, & Shaw, 1976; Martin & Berndt, 1970; Reed & Godden, 1977; Rickard & Mundy, 1965; Ryan, 1974; Ryan & Van Kirk-Ryan, 1983; Salend & Andress, 1984), and children younger than 5 years (Martin, Kuhl, & Haroldson, 1972; Onslow, Andrews & Lincoln, 1994; Onslow, Costa, & Rue, 1990; Reed & Godden, 1977),[3] who seem to achieve long-term generalization and maintenance of treatment effects with little effort more completely than do adults, in fewer clinical hours. A long term follow-up study in progress shows that clients in two of these re-

ports (Onslow et al., 1994, Onslow et al., 1990) have maintained such treatment gains from four to seven years.

There is general agreement that the stuttering of young children is markedly tractable in comparison to adults' stuttering. This suggests that, from the onset of the condition, many who stutter are on a temporal path from tractable stuttering to intractable stuttering: *A path that will lead from a time when operant methods are an effective intervention to a time when they are less likely to be effective.* For many clients, the latter time is when PS is the only effective way to offset the condition. Most likely, changes in the tractability of stuttering are related to the maturation of the speech motor system. In our clinical experience this change begins in clients around 7–11 years old. For example, we have conducted a clinical trial with children that age using the operant procedure reported by Onslow, Andrews, and Lincoln (1994; Lincoln, Onslow, Wilson & Lewis, in press). We found that children in this age range responded to treatment but took a little longer to generalize stutter-free speech and experienced more problems with relapse than did 5-year-olds.

Older children and some adults may respond clinically to operant treatments, but empirical support is lacking, because much of the research on response-contingent stimulation of stuttering has been confined to the laboratory. There is only one report with speech data on a single subject to suggest that treatment benefits were maintained after twelve months (James, 1981a). Data showing the maintenance of treatment benefits in PS programs nine to twelve months posttreatment are overwhelming by comparison (Andrews & Feyer, 1985; Andrews & Ingham, 1972; Boberg; 1981; Boberg & Kully, 1985, 1994; Howie, Tanner, & Andrews, 1981; Ingham, 1980; Webster, 1980). The sheer weight of the findings on PS has tended to divert attention from the potential benefits of operant methods in treating adult stuttering. This state of affairs may not be in the best interests of clients and is problematic for two reasons. First, outcome evaluations of intensive PS programs inspire only limited confidence, and second, there

---

[3]Studies were considered clinically relevant only if speech data were presented in support of claims of treatment effects. Laboratory studies of RCS and stuttering were counted if they either showed evidence of generalization of treatment effects to outside the laboratory or demonstrated near-zero stuttering levels achieved for many experimental sessions with apparatus that clinicians would be able to obtain and use.

are reasons to believe that operant methods may have clinical value with some adult clients.

One problem that detracts from PS outcome evaluations is that none convincingly measured speech under conditions free of association with the clinic. This is obviously the case for the within-clinic speech sampling used in many evaluations. Some sampled speech away from the clinic but nonetheless retained the problem of association with the clinic. In the Ingham (1980) study, for example, data came from tape recordings made mostly with the knowledge of subjects, who presumably also knew the purpose of those recordings. In Webster's (1980) report, clinic staff telephoned the clients, and Howie, Tanner, and Andrews's (1981) telephone assessments were conducted by a psychologist who mentioned the treatment program and discussed future assessment. Boberg and Kully's (1985) telephone assessments were made while the clients were in the clinic, and their (1994) clients were assessed during a surprise telephone call from a clinic staff member. These studies may indicate the extent to which clients were capable of producing stutter-free speech at significant posttreatment intervals, but it is uncertain that they indicate the extent to which clients did during their everyday lives.[4] PS outcome research is critically in need of speech data from many everyday situations to explore this issue.

Considering that clients who are treated with PS are likely to use an unnatural-sounding speech pattern, it is disturbing that not one of these reports determined how natural clients sounded after treatment. Some studies did not include measures of speech rate. Hence, the impression conveyed by these reports may be misleading, because clients may have been controlling stuttering by using an extremely unnatural speech pattern such as that described by Kalinowski et al. (1994). This is particularly problematic considering that assessments were linked to the clinic. Under such conditions

clients may be prepared to use speech that sounds unnatural but that they may be reluctant to use in everyday life. We do not advocate natural-sounding speech as the only acceptable goal for PS treatments, but we do believe that if clinicians have clients control stuttering with unnatural-sounding speech, that should be made clear to readers of outcome studies. Generalist clinicians may be particularly vulnerable to such misleading research because they need to choose between PS and operant treatments, and the latter procedures are not intended to alter speech quality.

There is another reason why PS outcome research may be misleading for a generalist clinician choosing between PS and operant methods. Such research has limited external validity; outcomes from specialized, intensive PS programs may not be as easy to achieve in other settings. For example, it is not straightforward for clinicians not having specialized training to replicate the targets of the various PS patterns used by specialist clinicians. Just as problematic, advanced clinical skill is used to teach a client to use PS to establish, generalize, and maintain stutter-free speech. Results achieved with PS by a group of specialist clinicians working closely together are unlikely to be representative of those achieved by clinicians in other settings. Furthermore, as discussed, client selection for intensive PS treatment is likely to be highly selective.

In short, PS outcome findings are most relevant to clinical settings in which such studies are done, and their findings cannot be confidently generalized elsewhere. This reflects the difference between clinical research and program evaluation; clinical research is generalizable but program evaluation pertains only to the clinical setting in which treatment is conducted. This is not meant as a denigration of program evaluation. Any reputable treatment program should be accountable in this way, but program evaluation of PS may be misinterpreted and may reinforce the idea that such treatment is superior to other forms of treatment and foster the notion that all clients should be treated with PS.

Although the outcome of operant treatments for adolescents and adults who stutter has not been comprehensively assessed, there are aspects of this

---

[4]A report by James, Ricciardelli, Hunter, and Rogers (1989) involved repeated assessments in several beyond-clinic settings with substantial speech samples. However, data were only reported for a six-month posttreatment period, hence this study did not fit the criteria for posttreatment assessments at nine- to 12-month intervals that we used to cite reports.

methodology that make it attractive to clinicians who treat clients individually. It is clear from laboratory studies that time out (TO) from conversation has strong clinical potential (see Costello & Ingham, 1984, for a review), because it can control stuttering more readily than any other clinically viable stimulus. Other positive features of TO are that the duration of the TO period seems flexible (James, 1981b), self-imposition of TO need not be accurate (James 1981c; Martin & Haroldson, 1982), and when TO is self-imposed, its effect appears to generalize (Martin & Haroldson, 1982). This latter finding makes self-imposed TO during everyday conversation an attractive procedure, because the client is able to self-administer a contingency that has powerful control over stuttering during any daily speaking situation. In effect, this gives clinicians an alternative way to "mediate generalization" (Stokes & Baer, 1977). There is a report (James, 1981a) of a client being taught this procedure and maintaining treatment effects for twelve months posttreatment. We have found that operant procedures alone are not successful with all clients, and sometimes require supplementation with either PS or rate control. Studies such as those of Ingham and Packman (1977) and James, Ricciardelli, Rogers, and Hunter (1989) demonstrate the value of such clinical combinations.

The advantages of self-imposed contingent stimulation are substantial. The procedure does not require an unnatural speech pattern, it requires fewer clinical hours than PS training, and it is simple enough for any client to learn to do in selected situations in daily life. Consequently, if there is a chance that such procedures can control stuttering, it would be unwise to select PS as the treatment of choice. The number of clients for whom operant treatment will be effective may be small, but they can be identified in clinical practice, and it would be a mistake to overlook them.

DESIGNING A MANAGEMENT STRATEGY

In this section we tie together previous discussions in suggesting a protocol for designing a client's management procedure. This protocol is intended for clinicians who work with individual clients. The first step in designing a management strategy is pretreatment interviewing to establish, among other things, whether reducing stuttering is a suitable treatment goal. Intensive PS programs cater to a special type of client, but we believe individual treatment is a viable option for most clients. There are many factors to consider when deciding which approach is suitable for an individual client, and such decisions can only be made after discussion with the client. Hence, we recommend that, when a client comes for individual treatment, behavioral procedures are not implemented until the client is known quite well. Considering the time that may be expended in PS training, a few sessions devoted to establishing a relationship with the client is a small and worthwhile investment, because it lays the groundwork for positive treatment outcome.

One goal of pretreatment interviewing is to identify the client's complaint (Baer, 1988) and to establish with the client whether stuttering reduction is the desired outcome. On most occasions, this will be the case. However, pretreatment counseling may raise issues such as (1) whether the client's quality of life will improve as a result of controlling stuttering, (2) whether the client has the drive and determination to succeed with the task of controlling stuttering, (3) whether anxiety rather than stuttering is the predominant problem, (4) whether the client is sufficiently organized in lifestyle for a commitment to treatment, and (5) whether it is the client or others who are the motivating force for seeking treatment. Even if these issues are not resolved prior to treatment, they may be clarified during treatment, and this should guide decisions about the remainder of management. In our view, a major advantage of individual stuttering treatment over group treatment is that the elimination of stuttering can be yoked productively to a counseling relationship. Curlee (1984) overviews the processes that might occur during such a relationship.

Some of our clients who begin a behavioral program designed to eliminate stuttering are later redirected to management routes that do not include behavioral control of stuttered speech. This does not imply that behavioral control will not be an option for them in the future. We have found as many reasons for counseling a client as there are clients. One reason may be that the clinician finds the client has "maladaptive cognitions" (Curlee, 1984) that are not sufficiently tractable to permit establishment and generalization of stutter-free speech. Another common reason to abandon behavioral control of stuttering is that anxiety proves to be a problem that does not subside with the establishment of stutter-free speech, in which case specialized management procedures are necessary before further behavioral control procedures can be instigated. Finally, we take care not to overlook the possibility that a client will benefit from learning to live with stuttering. We find wisdom in a comment made by one of our clients that "stuttering is not the worst thing in the world." There are many ways that a client can learn to live with it. For example, Schloss, Espin, Smith, and Suffolk (1987) report assertiveness training procedures that can assist clients to participate freely in conversations without penalty for their stuttering. *It becomes apparent during the early stages of treatment that in some cases—especially clients with mild stuttering—learning to cope with the condition may be far more productive and less onerous than spending a lifetime trying to control it.*

If the decision is made to proceed with a plan to eliminate stuttering, we believe that either PS or, for a small number of cases, operant methods, are justifiable treatment approaches, because the value of these procedures has been demonstrated empirically to some extent. There are two reasons why we may decide that PS is a suitable treatment for a client. One reason is that a client's case history information leads us to believe that operant methods will not be effective. Commonly, an adult with several failed therapy attempts over many decades will prompt such a decision. Another reason we may decide that PS is a suitable treatment is that after testing operant methods initially (see below) we found that they are not beneficial for the client. In both of these cases, the choice of format for PS treatment is either programmed or nonprogrammed. Faced with this decision, our first step is

to teach PS targets of "soft contacts," "gentle onsets," and "extended vocalization" using single-syllable word lists as teaching materials. After a short period of such instruction, we decide whether we will attempt to establish stutter-free PS with programmed or nonprogrammed instruction. We base such decisions on the client's rate of progress in learning PS targets, our judgment of the client's understanding of the concepts underlying PS, and how quickly the client masters PS skills.

In cases where the client rapidly achieves a good conceptual and practical grasp of PS, we proceed with the nonprogrammed instruction procedure summarized earlier (Packman et al., 1994). Such a client can quickly attain the skill of maintaining PS targets for a monologue of several hundred words. Then, we give instructions to use that speech pattern to control stuttering in whichever way the client chooses. In many cases the client is able immediately to produce a long monologue of stutter-free speech. In cases where subsequent speaking trials show that the client is spontaneously heading toward natural sounding speech, shaping speech naturalness will not be necessary. On other occasions, we use systematic instruction to shape speech naturalness (see below).

In some cases we decide at pretreatment interview that the client will require programmed instruction to learn how to eliminate stuttering with PS. There are many reasons for such a decision, but most common are clients who do not acquire the PS techniques in a short period of time and those who perform much better on systematically structured tasks. Our preference is nearly always to use a variant of GILCU to shape stutter-free speech, and we rarely use traditional speech rate shaping procedures for this purpose, for reasons discussed previously. One exception is when we see a client who has relapsed after an intensive treatment program that taught PS with speech rate increments. In many such cases, the most efficient clinical route to re-establishing stutter-free speech is to reconstruct those speech rate increments.

We recommend a trial of operant methods for late adolescent or young adult clients who are seeking treatment for the first time and have no history of attempting to control stuttering. Such a trial is based on James's (1981a) self-imposed TO procedure, in which the client is trained to self-impose TO contingent on stuttering in some speaking situations and for some portion of the speaking day. We believe one of the reasons for positive results from operant interventions with children is that those procedures (Lincoln et al., in press; Onslow et al., 1994) combine TO from conversation with self-correction of stuttered utterances and reinforcement for stutter-free speech. When we try operant procedures with older clients, we have the client pair self-correction with TO and select suitable rewarding stimuli or activities in conjunction with the client. It requires several weeks to determine whether a client will benefit from such a procedure. We do not attempt operant treatments with programmed instruction, because there is not sufficient empirical evidence to justify it; in addition there are data that support the nonprogrammed use of TO.

The decision to instigate programmed procedures to shape natural-sounding speech is based solely on whether they are necessary. One advantage of self-imposed operant methods is that they do not rely on a novel speech pattern, and hence there is not a problem with unnatural-sounding speech. In contrast, PS procedures often require the use of programmed instruction to assist the client to control stuttering while sounding as natural as possible. However, in our experience, two procedures maximize the chance that natural-sounding speech will occur spontaneously when PS is used to control stuttering. The first is using a nonprogrammed approach to PS establishment. More often than not with this procedure, clients will find their own optimal use of the speech pattern to maximize stuttering control and speech naturalness. The second procedure is using GILCU and its variations; in our experience clients find optimal use of the speech pattern as the target duration of response increases. It is normally apparent a short time into the establishment phase of treatment whether a client will require shaping of natural-sounding speech. When this is necessary, we use the procedure described previously (Ingham, 1987).

It takes a little longer into management to determine whether treatment gains are generalizing. Again, operant procedures carry a distinct advantage. Treatment is self-administered during everyday speaking situations, so, by definition, generalization is part of any treatment effect. There is virtually no chance that the client will isolate learning of the treatment effect to the clinic and the clinician. For PS management, we believe that one of the more important differences between standard group and individual treatments lies in the generalization phase. During individual treatments, the clinician has an opportunity to assess whether spontaneous generalization is occurring. This assessment occurs with clients' self-reports, the reports of significant others, and the customary beyond-clinic speech measures that allow the effects of treatment to be evaluated. In our experience, there are two reasons why spontaneous generalization may fail to occur. The first is that the client is reluctant to enter speaking situations that were previously avoided, in which case, programmed instruction using hierarchical situations would be indicated. The second reason why generalization may fail to occur spontaneously is that the client is simply not prepared to use the new speech pattern. It may feel or sound too unnatural for functional communication or, worse, it may not control stuttering in real-life situations. During individual treatment with PS, there is ample opportunity to rectify this problem by reconstructing a speech pattern. It would be unwise to attempt generalization with programmed instruction if a PS pattern is unsatisfactory to the client.

Programmed instruction during maintenance is a hedge against posttreatment relapse. For this reason we always manage maintenance in a systematic manner. After generalized treatment effects are in place, the client response of maintenance is carefully defined. Then a schedule of assessments is designed over a period of one to two years, through which the client progresses contingent on meeting maintenance criteria. A failure to meet maintenance criteria at any step returns the client to the initial assessment procedures. Our fundamental contingency arrangement incorporates Ingham's (1980) procedure of increased periods between assessments as one of the contingencies for meeting assessment criteria. This approach utilizes clinical time effectively, but is suitable only for those clients whose maintenance period is trouble-free. Some clients never wane in their drive to sustain control over stuttering, they manage their practice regimes without guidance, and they recover from inevitable bad days through their own resources. For other clients, maintenance is a period when regular contact with a clinician is required. These are clients whose motivation to continue a practice schedule wanes, who become despondent and fail to respond constructively if their speech begins to deteriorate, and who are prone to lack confidence and to be apprehensive about their speech. These are the kinds of clients whom Neilson and Andrews (1993) identify as suitable targets for individual therapy. For them, well-constructed, programmed maintenance, coupled with regular counseling support from a clinician, gives them the best chance of learning what is necessary to cope with their disorder.

SUMMARY

In our clinic we manage stuttering from a behavioral perspective. In this chapter, we have described how we design and implement treatment strategies for individual adult clients. We base intervention on procedures that research has shown can control stuttering, but we adapt these procedures to suit the needs of individual clients. For example, we believe that operant procedures are preferable to some clients, while using a new speech pattern such as prolonged speech is more suitable for others. Also, when we use prolonged speech with individual clients we do not rely on the lengthy speech-rate shaping procedures that typify intensive group programs. We design our intervention strategies to maximize natural-sounding speech and we believe that strategies to maintain improvement in the long term are an important component of treatment.

REFERENCES

Andrews, G., & Craig, A. (1988). Prediction of outcome after treatment for stuttering. *British Journal of Psychiatry*, *153*, 236–240.

Andrews, G., & Cutler, J. (1974). Stuttering therapy: The relation between changes in symptom level and attitudes. *Journal of Speech and Hearing Disorders*, *39*, 312–319.

Andrews, G., & Feyer, A.M. (1985). Does behavior therapy still work when the experimenters have departed? *Behavior Modification*, *9*, 443–456.

Andrews, G., Guitar, B., & Howie, P. (1980). Meta-analysis of the effects of stuttering treatment. *Journal of Speech and Hearing Disorders*, *45*, 287–307.

Andrews, G., & Ingham, R.J. (1972). An approach to the evaluation of stuttering therapy. *Journal of Speech and Hearing Research*, *15*, 296–302.

Baer, D. (1988). If you know why you're changing a behavior, you'll know when you've changed it enough. *Behavioral Assessment*, *10*, 219–223.

Boberg, E. (1981). Maintenance of fluency: An experimental program. In E. Boberg (Ed.), *Maintenance of fluency*. (pp. 71–111). New York: Elsevier.

Boberg, E., & Kully, D. (1985). *Comprehensive stuttering treatment program*. San Diego: College-Hill Press.

Boberg, E., & Kully, D. (1994). Long-term results of an intensive treatment program for adults and adoles-

cents who stutter. *Journal of Speech and Hearing Research*, *37*, 1050–1059.

Browning, R. (1967). Behavior therapy for stuttering in a schizophrenic child. *Behaviour Research and Therapy*, *5*, 27–35.

Costello, J.M. (1983). Current behavioral treatments for children In D. Prins & R. Ingham (Eds.), *Treatment of stuttering in early childhood: Methods and issues* (pp. 69–112). San Diego: College-Hill Press.

Costello, J.M., & Ingham, R.J.(1984). Stuttering as an operant disorder. In R.F. Curlee & W.H. Perkins (Eds.), *Nature and treatment of stuttering: New directions* (pp. 187–213). San Diego: College-Hill Press.

Craig, A.R., & Calver, P. (1991). Following up on treated stutterers: Studies of perceptions of fluency and job status. *Journal of Speech and Hearing Research*, *34*, 279–284.

Craig, A.R., & Howie, P.M. (1982). Locus of control and maintenance of behavioural therapy skills. *British Journal of Clinical Psychology*, *21*, 65–66.

Craig, A.R., Franklin, J.A., & Andrews, G. (1984). A scale to measure locus of control of behaviour. *British Journal of Medical Psychology*, *57*, 173–180.

Curlee, R.F. (1984). Counseling with adults who stutter. In W.H. Perkins (Ed.), *Stuttering Disorders* (pp. 153–159). New York: Thieme-Stratton.

Goldiamond, I. (1965). Stuttering and fluency as manipulatable operant response classes. In L. Krasner & L.P. Ullman (Eds.), *Research in behavior modification* (pp. 106–156). New York: Holt, Rinehart & Winston.

Guitar, B. (1976). Pretreatment factors associated with the outcome of stuttering therapy. *Journal of Speech and Hearing Research, 19,* 590–600.

Guitar, B., & Bass, C. (1978). Stuttering therapy: The relation between attitude change and long-term outcome. *Journal of Speech and Hearing Disorders, 43,* 392–400.

Howie, P.M., Tanner, S., & Andrews, G. (1981). Short- and long-term outcome in an intensive treatment program for adult stutterers. *Journal of Speech and Hearing Disorders, 46,* 104–109.

Ingham, J.C. (1993). Behavioral treatment of stuttering children. In R.F. Curlee (Ed.), *Stuttering and related disorders of fluency* (pp. 68–100). New York: Thieme Medical Publishers.

Ingham, R.J. (1980). Modification of maintenance and generalization during stuttering treatment. *Journal of Speech and Hearing Research, 23,* 732–745.

Ingham, R.J. (1981). *Stuttering therapy manual: Hierarchy control schedule.* Sydney, Australia: Cumberland College Press.

Ingham, R.J. (1984). *Stuttering and behavior therapy: Current status and experimental foundations.* San Diego: College-Hill Press.

Ingham, R.J. (1987). *Residential prolonged speech stuttering therapy manual.* Santa Barbara: Department of Speech and Hearing Sciences, University of California.

Ingham, R.J. (1993). Stuttering treatment efficacy: Paradigm dependent or independent? *Journal of Fluency Disorders, 18,* 133–149.

Ingham, R.J., & Andrews, G. (1973). Details of a token economy stuttering therapy programme for adults. *Australian Journal of Human Communication Disorders, 1,* 13–20.

Ingham, R.J., Gow, M., & Costello, J.M. (1985). Stuttering and speech naturalness: Some additional data. *Journal of Speech and Hearing Disorders, 50,* 217–219.

Ingham, R.J., Martin, R.R., Haroldson, S.K., Onslow, M., & Leney, M. (1985) Modification of listener-judged naturalness in the speech of stutterers. *Journal of Speech and Hearing Research, 28,* 495–504.

Ingham, R.J. & Onslow, M. (1985). Measurement and modification of speech naturalness during stuttering therapy. *Journal of Speech and Hearing Disorders, 50,* 261–281.

Ingham, R.J., & Packman, A. (1977). Treatment and generalization effects in an experimental treatment for a stutterer using contingency management and speech rate control. *Journal of Speech and Hearing Disorders, 42,* 394–407.

James, J.E. (1981a). Behavioral self-control of stuttering using time-out from speaking. *Journal of Applied Behavior Analysis, 14,* 25–37.

James, J.E. (1981b). Punishment of stuttering: Contingency and stimulus parameters. *Journal of Communication Disorders, 14,* 375–386.

James, J.E. (1981c). Self-monitoring of stuttering: Reactivity and accuracy. *Behavior Research and Therapy, 19,* 291–296.

James, J., Ricciardelli, L., Hunter, C., & Rogers, P. (1989). Relative efficacy of intensive and spaced behavioral treatment of stuttering. *Behavior Modification, 13,* 376–395.

James, J., Ricciardelli, L., Rogers, P., & Hunter, C. (1989). A preliminary analysis of the ameliorative effects of time-out from speaking on stuttering. *Journal of Speech and Hearing Research, 32,* 604–610.

Johnson, G.F., Coleman, K., & Rasmussen, K. (1978). Multidays: Multidimensional approach for the young stutterer. *Language, Speech and Hearing Services in Schools, 9,* 129–132.

Kalinowski, J., Noble, S. Armson, J., & Stuart, A. (1994). Pretreatment and posttreatment speech naturalness ratings of adults with mild and severe stuttering. *American Journal of Speech-Language Pathology, 3,* 61–66.

Leach, E. (1969). Stuttering: Clinical application of response-contingent procedures. In B.B. Gray & G. England (Eds.), *Stuttering and the conditioning therapies* (pp. 115–127). California: Monterey Institute of Speech and Hearing.

Lincoln, M., Onslow, M., Wilson, L., & Lewis, C. (in press). A clinical trial of an operant treatment for stuttering school-age children. *American Journal of Speech-Language Pathology.*

Manning, W., Trutna, P., & Shaw, C. (1976). Verbal versus tangible reward for children who stutter. *Journal of Speech and Hearing Disorders, 41,* 52–62.

Martin, R.R. (1981) Introduction and perspective: Review of published research. In E. Boberg (Ed.), *Maintenance of fluency* (pp. 1–30). New York: Elsevier.

Martin, R.R., & Berndt, L.A. (1970). The effects of

time-out on stuttering in a 12-year-old boy. *Exceptional Children*, *36*, 303–304.

Martin, R.R., & Haroldson, S.K. (1982). Contingent self stimulation for stuttering. *Journal of Speech and Hearing Disorders*, *47*, 407–413.

Martin, R.R., & Haroldson, S.K. (1992). Stuttering and speech naturalness: Audio and audiovisual judgments. *Journal of Speech and Hearing Research*, *35*, 521–528.

Martin, R.R., Haroldson, S.K., & Triden, K.A. (1984). Stuttering and speech naturalness. *Journal of Speech and Hearing Disorders*, *49*, 53–58.

Martin, R.R., Kuhl, P., & Haroldson, S. (1972) An experimental treatment with two preschool stuttering children. *Journal of Speech and Hearing Research*, *15*, 743–752.

Metz, D.E., Schiavetti, N., & Sacco, P.R. (1990). Acoustic and psychophysical dimensions of the perceived speech naturalness of nonstutterers and posttreatment stutterers. *Journal of Speech and Hearing Disorders*, *55*, 516–525.

Mooney, J. (1990). Stutterers master smooth speech. *Australian Doctor Weekly*, *26–27*, June.

Neilson, M., & Andrews, G. (1993). Intensive fluency training of chronic stutterers. In R.F. Curlee (Ed.), *Stuttering and related disorders of fluency* (pp. 139–165). New York: Thieme Medical Publishers.

Onslow, M. (1996). *Behavioral management of stuttering*. San Diego, Calif.: Singular Publishing Group.

Onslow, M., Andrews, C., & Lincoln, M. (1994). A control/experimental trial of an operant treatment for early stuttering. *Journal of Speech and Hearing Research*, *37*, 1224–1259.

Onslow, M. Costa, L., Andrews, C., Harrison, E., & Packman, A. (in press). Speech outcomes of a prolonged-speech treatment for stuttering. *Journal of Speech and Hearing Research*.

Onslow, M., Costa, L., & Rue, S. (1990). Direct early intervention with stuttering: Some preliminary data. *Journal of Speech and Hearing Disorders*, *55*, 405–416.

Onslow, M., Hayes, B., Hutchins, L., & Newman, D. (1992). Speech naturalness and prolonged-speech treatments for stuttering: Further variables and data. *Journal of Speech and Hearing Research*, *35*, 274–282.

Onslow, M., & Ingham, R.J. (1987). Speech quality measurement and the management of stuttering. *Journal of Speech and Hearing Disorders*, *52*, 2–17.

Onslow, M., & Ingham, R. J. 1989). Whither prolonged speech? The disquieting evolution of a stuttering therapy procedure. *Australian Journal of Human Communication Disorders, 17*, 67–81.

Packman, A., Onslow, M., & van Doorn, J. (1994). Prolonged speech and the modification of stuttering: Perceptual, acoustic, and electroglottographic data. *Journal of Speech and Hearing Research*, *37*, 724–737.

Perkins, W.H. (1984). Techniques for establishing fluency. In W.H. Perkins (Ed.), *Stuttering disorders* (pp. 173–181). New York: Thieme-Stratton.

Reed, C.G., & Godden, A.L. (1977). An experimental treatment using verbal punishment with two preschool stutterers. *Journal of Fluency Disorders*, *2*, 225–233.

Rickard, H., & Mundy, M. (1965). Direct manipulation of stuttering behavior: An experimental clinical approach. In L.P. Ullmann & L. Krasner (Eds.), *Case studies in behavior modification* (pp. 268–277). New York: Holt, Rinehart and Winston.

Runyan, C.M., Bell, J. N. & Prosek, R.A. (1990). Speech naturalness ratings of treated stutterers. *Journal of Speech and Hearing Disorders*, *55*, 434–438.

Ryan, B.P. (1974). *Programmed therapy for stuttering in children and adults*. Springfield, Ill.: Charles C. Thomas.

Ryan, B.P., & Van Kirk Ryan, B. (1983). Programmed stuttering therapy for children: Comparison of four establishment programs. *Journal of Fluency Disorders*, *8*, 291–321.

Salend, S., & Andress, M. (1984). Decreasing stuttering in an elementary-level student. *Language, Speech and Hearing Services in Schools*, *15*, 16–21.

Schloss, P., Espin, C., Smith, M., & Suffolk, D. (1987). Developing assertiveness during employment interviews with young adults who stutter. *Journal of Speech and Hearing Disorders*, *52*, 30–36.

Shames, G., & Florance, C. (1980). *Stutter-free speech: A goal for therapy*. Columbus: Charles E. Merrill.

Stokes, T.F., & Baer, D.M. (1977). An implicit technology of generalization. *Journal of Applied Behavior Analysis*, *10*, 349–367.

Webster, R.L. (1980). Evolution of a target-based therapy for stuttering. *Journal of Fluency Disorders*, *5*, 303–320.

CHAPTER 19

INSTRUMENTATION FOR THE ASSESSMENT AND TREATMENT OF STUTTERING

KLAAS BAKKER

INTRODUCTION

Since the inception of speech pathology as a discipline, speech-language pathologists have mostly relied on subjective, behavioral, and intuitive judgments regarding the acceptability of speech (Baken, 1987). Especially in fluency disorders, where judgments by the client and significant others are often considered factors that, at least, contribute to the problem, these types of assessment have prevailed. The current influx of instruments for speech analysis has created new options for measurement, clinical feedback, and manipulation of aspects of speech to enhance fluency and reduce stuttering. Although the ramifications of this development have not been fully determined, the new options are expected to benefit both clinicians and researchers in improving services to individuals who stutter.

The purpose of this chapter is to (1) discuss measurable aspects of fluency, dysfluency, and associated symptoms; (2) discuss instrumentation for the measurement, clinical feedback, and manipulation of these aspects; and (3) provide new instrument-based solutions for a number of cumbersome clinical procedures.

The scope of this chapter is deliberately broad. As a result, its content is limited in certain ways. The applications of these procedures, for example, are not discussed in detail. Also, clinical goals and methods selected by clinicians often depend on their private clinical philosophies. This chapter is insensitive to such differences in clinical preference. Finally, some of the procedures await empirical support for their validity and reliability. They were included only to stimulate research and discussion of their potential for assisting clinicians who work with stutterers.

FLUENCY

Current stuttering treatments often target aspects of both fluent and dysfluent speech. To understand stuttering implies a notion of what comprises normally fluent speech. Starkweather (1987, p. 12) defined fluency as "the ability to talk with normal levels of continuity, rate, and effort." As a result, measurable aspects of fluency, such as continuity, rate, segmental (and subsegmental) features, and prosody have now become routine targets of many fluency evaluations. The following sections discuss how instrumented procedures may be used to evaluate most of these aspects of fluency or to arrange effective client-oriented feedback.

CONTINUITY

Acoustic Continuity of Speech

Absolute continuity of speech production, of course, is physiologically impossible. The perception of continuous speech, however, can be approximated by prolonging intervals of audible speech (i.e., acoustic segments) while reducing breaks and pauses. The clinical rationale for this approach is that a reduction of speech initiations also reduces the number of loci at risk for stuttering.

There are different opinions regarding the recommended lengths and durations of acoustic segments that are practiced in fluency enhancement therapies. According to some authors, acoustic segments should have a restricted length varying between three and eight syllables (e.g., Curlee and Perkins, 1969; Perkins, 1973 a,b). Others have recommended the use of prolonged acoustic segments by deleting the unnecessary breaks and pauses (e.g., Apel, Masterson, Mathers-Schmidt, & Bakker, 1993; Haynes & Christenson, 1994). While the overall number of pauses may be reduced, there may be an increased need for planning and preparation time during the pauses that remain. Unfortunately, there is little, if any, evidence to support the use of either restricted or prolonged durations of acoustic segments, or the pauses between them, to establish speech that is perceptually fluent.

Durations of acoustic segments and their pauses can be examined from sound intensity envelopes. This display form is available on most current comprehensive speech analysis stations. When employed for clinical feedback to clients, a real-time display is preferred (e.g., walking display) and is available only on some of these systems (e.g., the Visipitch, DSP 5500, and CSL—extended with the real-time Pitch program—by Kay Elemetrics; the PM-Pitch Analyzer by Voice Identifications; IBM's SpeechViewer II, and Video-Voice). Real-time feedback informs the client about the immediate consequences of behavioral adjustments and thus maximizes learning of continuity related skills.

Graphical or numerical displays associated with continuity feedback are not appropriate, or effective, with all clients. Youngsters who stutter, for example, are not able to interpret this type of representation. For them, computerized animations are preferred in situations where continuity and phrasing skills are targets for therapy (e.g., by employing a Visipitch, SpeechViewer II, or Video Voice). Options are available on all of these systems for expressing the acoustic presence (and thus continuity) of speech in a simple and entertaining way.

When computers or the required hardware peripherals for speech analysis are unavailable to clinicians, meaningful feedback concerning the continuity of phrases, and durations of pauses that separate them, may still be obtained with the VU-meters of recording equipment and sound level meters. Also, the Voice Lite I system (Behavioral Controls, Inc.), which indicates the intensity level of speech through a light that varies in brightness, is helpful for this purpose. Voice Lite I, like most current sound level meters, has an advantage in that its response rate can be adjusted for maximizing the effectiveness of continuity related feedback. However, this and the previous alternatives for computerized feedback forms do not lead to quantified or objective measures concerning the status of continuity related goals of therapy.

It is unfortunate that the form of continuity feedback available on most systems for speech analysis allows for merely a global (visual) inspection of the relative durations of individual acoustic phrases and pauses. Measurement of the actual duration of each pause and phrase are either impossible or too cumbersome to be practical for routine clinical applications. Nevertheless, descriptive statistics concerning continuity related goals in the long range (e.g., aspects of central tendency and variability) would be valuable for objective and quantified evaluations of therapeutic progress.

The development of a system that provides numerical-statistical (or graphically oriented) feedback regarding continuity targets is straightforward. Figure 19.1 displays a simple design for a speech timer that would be sufficiently accurate for this purpose. Its resulting signal permits real-time visual feedback regarding the client's ability to produce acoustic segments that are continuous and of a desired duration. Moreover, the decision of whether pause durations allowed sufficient planning and adjustment time is comparatively easy.

From data acquired with the feedback system shown in Figure 19.1, statistical analysis of the client's ability to approximate continuous speech production is possible. Among the available measures are: numbers and durations of acoustic segments and pauses, and proportion (or percentage) of time engaged in speech production. Moreover, when based on oral readings—and thus the total number of syllables is known ahead of time—two additional continuity-related measures may be estimated from these data: average phrase length in syllables and fluent speaking rate (in SPM or WPM) employing articulatory time as its temporal reference. Such measures are also available for extemporaneous speech if the number of syllables produced by the client is counted by the clinician. A solution for obtaining all of these measures for speech that is contaminated by stuttering follows.

Although not widely available on a commercial basis, CASPER[1] (Computer Aided SPeech Evaluation and Remediation, Till, 1990) allows for the measurement of a number of continuity targets. Analysis protocol 1 of this assessment and therapy system contains procedures for the determination of percent articulatory and pause time of a sample of up to 30 seconds. Among the remaining measures available with this protocol are mean phrase (and pause) duration, and number of syllables per phrase.

[1]CASPER (Computer Aided SPeech Evaluation and Remediation, Till, 1990) may be available upon request from the developer:
James Till, Ph.D.
Veterans Administration Medical Center
Division of Speech Pathology (126)
5901 East Seventh Street
Long Beach, CA 90822

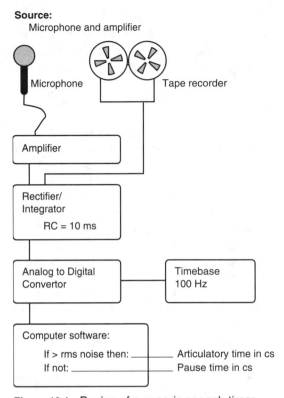

Figure 19.1 Design of a generic speech timer capable of measuring articulatory time, pause time, and average phrase and pause duration.

Continued Phonation

The establishment of continued phonation (e.g., Shames and Florance, 1980) has found widespread acceptance as a clinical goal for fluency enhancement. Continued phonation, of course, is a relative term and impossible in an absolute sense. The perception of continued phonation may be approximated by allowing one's voicing to cross word boundaries (blending), or by prolonging steady states of voiced continuant sounds. These procedures result in an increase of prolonged phonation intervals, or PIs (Ingham, Montgomery, & Ulliana, 1983).

The extent to which the client employs continued phonation may be reflected in results obtained with a design similar to the hypothetical speech timer displayed in Figure 19.1. However, for this analysis the speech signal is filtered (a bandpass could be created at the fundamental frequency range; e.g., 50 Hz < × < 350 Hz at –24 dB/octave). Rather than filtering acoustic waveforms, one could also consider methods that reveal vocal fold oscillations directly, such as electroglottography (Gow & Ingham, 1992) or the use of contact microphones positioned over the larynx. The latter, unfortunately, introduce movement artifacts (Hubbard & Prins, 1994). Electroglottography, furthermore, does not work equally well for all clients (e.g., Baken, 1987) and suffers when employed with some children, women, or individuals with relatively large neck diameters.

After rectification, integration (e.g., 10 ms integration time), and analog-to-digital conversion, the voicing related data are processed by computer software, and a number of continued phonation related measures may be derived. The average duration of phonation intervals, for example, reflects the extent to which a client is successful in prolonging voiced continuant sounds and word blending. On the other hand, the number of phonation intervals reflects the extent to which the client blends words. When measured during oral reading this information may be used, in addition, for determining the average length of phonation intervals expressed in number of syllables. The latter provides a check to establish whether prolongations of phonatory intervals were the result of a reduction in rate, or of the successful use of continued phonation skills targeted in therapy.

By combining continued phonation related data with those available from a speech timer (Figure 19.1), two additional measures can be determined: articulatory time (based on the acoustic presence of speech) broken down into a percentage of voiced and voiceless time (e.g., Horii, 1983; Till, 1990; Walker, 1988). The proportion of voiced articulatory time primarily reflects a client's ability to extend durations of voiced continuant sounds.

Aerodynamic Continuation Targets

A number of authors have suggested procedures for modifying airflow management during speech as a means of achieving fluency (e.g., Adams, 1974; Azrin & Nunn, 1974). Airflow may be present during moments when neither speech nor

phonation are acoustically evident. This measure reflects features of speech-continuity not available from acoustic recordings. The measurement of airflow through pneumotachographs, however, presents conditions that may impede the naturalness of speech production and are impractical for routine clinical application. Among the limitations are the need to wear a face mask and the client's efforts invested in maintaining a proper seal. The difference in speech related sensory feedback caused by the face mask is also important.

Fortunately, the extent to which clients maintain a steady continuous flow of air during speech production may be examined indirectly through pneumographic methods (e.g., bellows system, Whitney strain gauges, magnetometers, or pneumo-plethysmographs; see Baken, 1987). Pneumographs are less invasive than pneumotachographs and allow speech to progress more or less normally. They are also capable of visualizing patterns of coordination between thoracic and abdominal breathing, and additional aspects that may be important to the treatment of stuttering.

Pneumographic feedback makes up part of the CAFET[2] system (Goebel, Hillis, & Meyer, 1985), which has become a popular choice for many stuttering therapists. CAFET is unique in that it visualizes the coordination of respiration and phonation in preparation for and during speech production. The producers of CAFET suggest the following potential clinical goals for fluency enhancement: diaphragmatic breathing (operationally defined as an increased intake of air), pre-voice exhalation, continuous airflow, slow expiration, syllable stretch, syllable-timed speech, and continuous phonation.

CAFET reveals a client's respiratory adjustments for speech only through measuring diameter changes at the lower part of the chest cavity. Presumably, this reflects diaphragmatic breathing and is used to help clients increase their available respiratory supply for speech production. However,

[2]CAFET, Inc.
4208 Evergreen Lane, Suite 213,
Annandale, Virginia 22003

CAFET does not differentiate the individual contributions of the thoracic, abdominal, and diaphragmatic subsystems. Neither does it reveal the interactions among these systems in building a sufficient power supply for speech production (Borden, Harris, & Raphael, 1993). Because of its one respiratory channel orientation, CAFET may be misleading during moments when, due to discoordination between thoracic and abdominal breathing, the flow and available air supply for speech are impeded. Moreover, it is questionable that the recommended placement of the transducer singles out the diaphragmatic contributions to speech breathing. It would seem that CAFET is suited only for its own unique clinical objectives and cannot be considered a replacement for pneumographic feedback in general. The therapeutic procedures associated with CAFET are, however, well developed and discussed in a thorough manual delivered with the system. The producers of CAFET recommend specialized training for those interested in using their system for fluency enhancement.

Comprehensive pneumographic feedback implies simultaneous monitoring of thoracic and abdominal breathing. Visual inspection of these components of breathing reveals the unique interactions that occur between these subsystems of the respiratory function. By combining both signals into one, a reasonable estimate of changes in pulmonary volume associated with speech breathing may be obtained. It should be noted, however, that pneumographic devices suffer from movement artifacts and are useful only for global visual inspections of respiratory behaviors. They are too crude to permit statistical analyses of aerodynamic continuity targets. Accurate and direct measurements of changes in pulmonary volume can be obtained with spirometers (volume) and pneumotachographs (volume and flow). Because these methods either preclude or hinder speech production, their utility for fluency enhancement is limited.

The measurement of aeromechanic aspects of speech clearly facilitates one's ability to track continuity related targets not available from acoustic applications. Nevertheless, there is a lack of empirical data concerning the effectiveness of aero-mechanically derived measures in stuttering therapy. The studies that have been conducted have suggested the presence of anomalies in the respiratory-laryngeal coordinations just prior to or during speech production in individuals who stutter (e.g., Dembowski & Watson, 1991; Peters & Boves 1988; Williams & Brutten, 1994).

Recently, there has been a call for multichannel physiological feedback procedures (Borden & Watson, 1987). This approach was recommended because of its potential for revealing the subtle aspects of coordination within and among speech-related systems and subsystems. Unfortunately, there are no therapy-ready multichannel feedback systems. A recent expansion of CSL (Kay Elemetrics) to allow for multichannel monitoring of a desired mixture of physiological and acoustic data, however, has paved the way for such a development.

RATE

Manual Speech Rate Determinations

Many current stuttering therapies require routine determination of fluent speaking rate. Whether rate is targeted as a goal by itself, or as a vehicle for achieving fluency, its measurement is necessary throughout therapy. Rate is usually measured by counting the number of syllables produced per unit time. This is a cumbersome clinical task. Moreover, manual speech rate determinations may have questionable reliability when near normal rates are targeted (Bakker & Gregg, 1994). Extended periods of on-line counting and timing, furthermore, detract from implementing additional clinical goals (e.g., the client's successful use of gentle voice onsets or soft articulatory contacts), and cause therapeutic interactions to be unnatural.

Manual speech rate determination requires the use of a stopwatch and counter. Depending on the clinician's preference, either syllables or words are counted during a predetermined time interval. The resulting counts are converted to rate measures (syllables per minute, or SPM) by dividing them by their corresponding sample durations (in minutes). Unfortunately, due to the nature of this procedure, feedback to clients tends to be delayed. This weakens the link between performance and its resulting feedback, a condition counterproductive to learning.

A potential solution for reducing the delays caused by manual speech rate determinations is to follow a "time by count" procedure, such as was initially suggested for the determination of verbal diadochokinetic rates (Fletcher, 1972). A predetermined number of syllables (or words) is counted during representative intervals of speech production. The time necessary for completing the targeted number of syllables (e.g., the first twenty syllables) is then converted to its corresponding rate. To make this conversion easy, one could employ conversion tables that may be prepared ahead of time.

The accuracy of the time-by-count procedure depends on the clinician's skills in manipulating a stopwatch (Starkweather, Armson, & Amster, 1987). It is also sensitive to natural variations in the rate of producing phrases and sentences. This measure, then, is no solution when precision or consistency are essential. It is useful only as a means of providing snapshots of a client's current performance for establishing intermediate rate adjustments during practice drills.

The increased popularity of rate modification therapies in speech pathology has created a need for convenient automated rate assessment procedures. Rate modifications are now routinely targeted in the treatment of stuttering (Andrews, Neilson, & Cassar, 1987), cluttering (Daly, 1986), foreign dialects (Driscoll, 1981), and a number of motor speech disorders (Yorkston, Hammen, Beukelman, & Traynor, 1990). There is a need for efficient, accurate, and reliable ways to measure speech rates during diagnostic evaluations, and for ongoing assessments of therapeutic progress.

Automated procedures for speech rate determination would have a number of advantages over manual approaches. They ensure consistency of rate-related feedback to clients. Moreover, ongoing or intermediate feedback can be easily arranged to inform clients about their most recent rate-related performance. After all, the immediacy of conse-

quences following a response is considered an essential factor in the acquisition of new behavior.

Any automated method for determining speech rate hinges on the availability of some discrete aspect in the speech signal predictive of rate expressed in syllables per minute. Unfortunately, current speech recognition technology does not permit reliable counting of such perceptual units of speech production as syllables and words. Automated counts of stressed syllables and voice initiations, however, have been achieved and were found to have useful properties for the development of instrument-based speech rate measurements (Bakker, Brutten, & McQuain, 1995). These measures predicted the numbers of syllables and words determined from transcription. Stressed syllable counts were achieved by identifying and counting the steep acoustic rises characteristic for the onsets of vowel nuclei in stressed syllables. Voice initiations were determined by identifying onsets of acoustic energy in the fundamental frequency range of phonation.

In the most recent version of Video Voice, a syllable counting protocol has been adopted that follows a paradigm similar to one employed by Bakker et al. (1995). Furthermore, a phrases-per-minute rate and a semi-automatic syllables-per-minute rate are included in protocol 1 of CASPER (Till, 1990). Despite the availability of these options, the functionality of automated or semi-automated feedback on rate during speech that is severely slowed or prolonged has not been determined and is potentially problematic.

Irrespective of the counting strategy chosen, rate-related results depend at least in part on the procedure for measuring speaking time. The possibility that speech rates, whether they were measured through manual or instrument-based procedures, are confounded by the occurrence of pauses (e.g., for breathing, speech planning, and language formulation) poses threats to their validity. To reduce this type of confounding it is recommended that articulatory time is used as a replacement. A recent study has revealed that the need for employing articulatory time is particularly evident during episodes of extemporaneous speech production (Bakker & Gregg, 1994).

Articulatory time can be determined manually with a stopwatch for pauses that exceed 2 seconds (Perkins, 1975). This aspect has been considerably simplified in a recent timing/counting program (STRR, Fowler & Ingham, 1986). In the STRR, accumulation of articulatory time stops automatically after no new syllables are entered for a specified duration following the last entry. Nearly exact articulatory time may be obtained with timers that are acoustically triggered and thus accumulate articulatory time only when speech is acoustically evident. Voice- (or speech-) triggered timers are easy to develop and offer many opportunities for improving the accuracy and validity of speech rate measures, but they still do not reflect moments during which quiet physiological adjustments and preparations for speech are being made.

Recently, Bakker and Gregg (1994) have assessed the relationship between rate measures that are based on articulatory time (manual and automatic) or total sample duration during oral readings and monologues. Their results revealed that these measures were only weakly correlated, particularly when monologues were the source of the

analysis. These findings call into question the practice of employing overall sample durations for speech rate determinations. They also imply that speech rate cannot be manually determined by clinicians. Obviously, there is a need for implementing voice-actuated speech timers for achieving accurate and consistent results in rate modification therapies.

The author has experimented with a number of methods for computerized determination of speech rate and in arranging intermediate feedback to clients. Figure 19.2 displays the feedback screen of one such program (Bakker, 1994b). It has three options. Speech rate may be estimated from automated counts of voice initiations, stressed syllables (Bakker, Brutten, & McQuain, 1995), or directly from the numbers of syllables (or words) as they are entered through pressing keyboard keys (see also the description of the STRR system, Fowler & Ingham, 1986). A preferred timing method may be selected (i.e., total sample duration or total articulatory time) to concur with preferred standards for rate measurement.

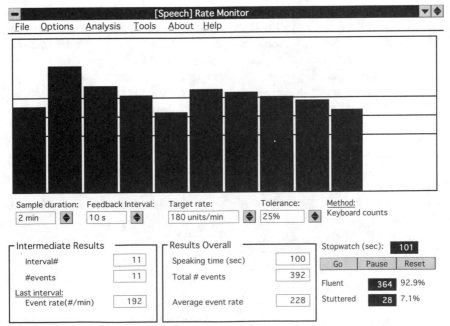

Figure 19.2   Speech rate feedback program based on syllable input procedure.

The Use of DAF for Speech Rate Modification

Many clinicians who pursue speech rate modification as a vehicle for achieving fluency rely on delayed auditory feedback (DAF) as their primary means of intervention (e.g., Curlee & Perkins, 1969). In addition to reducing rate, DAF has been observed to produce other speech changes that are now known to be fluency enhancing in their own right, including continued phonation (Shames & Florance, 1980) and the establishment of a prolonged speaking pattern.

The use of DAF for speech rate reductions has a number of practical advantages. Its effect on rate is consistent and almost automatic. The desired degree of this effect may be manipulated by adjusting the delay that is applied (usually varying between 50 and 250 ms, in steps of 50 ms). Little is known, however, about the speech rates that result and some speakers are able to resist its effect altogether. This problem became apparent in two recent studies in which DAF was employed for manipulating speech rates of normal speakers (Bakker & Rader, 1992; Bakker & Dugan-Feldt, 1993). The rates differed substantially across subjects. Also, the extent to which DAF reduced rate varied differentially across the settings of delay. This implies that, despite predictable effects on some subjects, additional interventions (e.g., instruction, or modeling) may be needed for others. Furthermore, it is necessary that rates are frequently checked by the clinician.

Additional problems associated with sustained use of DAF have been reported. For DAF to be effective, a client's hearing is subjected to sound intensities that exceed normal levels. Moreover, the distracting nature of a DAF signal may be a nuisance for some clients. The effectiveness of DAF is vested in its ability to perturb one's system for speech discrimination. Moreover, as Ingham (1993) concluded recently, it may not be DAF per se, but rather prolonged speech that helps produce fluency enhancement. Prolonged speech, according to this author, may well be established without DAF.

DAF is not the only solution to achieve speech rate reduction. Perhaps its greatest value rests in its ability to achieve rate reductions in clients for whom other methods have failed, or in situations where fluency has been difficult to obtain otherwise.

Regardless of the rate modification procedure chosen, the client ultimately is expected to control rate voluntarily. Self-control in achieving rate modifications is the sine qua non for promoting maintenance and generalization to out-clinic speaking situations. Procedures that employ DAF are characterized by an external locus of control and may impede this important step in therapy. Though successful in reducing speech rate in many clients, the responsibility to turn such changes into voluntary and lasting adjustments still rests with the client and clinician.

Modeling Speech Rate with Metronomes

On occasion, rate modifications have been established with metronomes, typically presented in the form of some auditory stimulus (e.g., a click or electronic beep). When used strictly for rate modification, a number of variations could be considered for adjusting to unique clinical needs. For example, rather than through the auditory modality, speech rate may be guided by rhythmic light pulses or a computer program that produces animations that move at a rate targeted by the client. Visual metronomes would be particularly beneficial for rate modification in children.

Although the traditional use of metronomes for fluency enhancement requires clients to speak rhythmically, they can be used more liberally in rate modification therapies. One version of a computerized metronome visually cues words and syllables, one at a time, for establishing target rates during oral reading (Goldojarb and Secor[3]). Another such program (Beukelman,

---

[3]Goldojarb, M., and Secor, J., Slow speech rate drill for dysarthric speakers. Sunset Software, 11750 Sunset Blvd., Suite 414, Los Angeles, CA 90049.
Reviewed by Arthur Schwartz (1988). *Journal for Computer Users in Speech and Hearing, 4* (1), 62–63.

Yorkston, & Tice[4]), in addition, allows words or phrases to be printed at a predetermined rate for oral reading. Rather than presenting (or cueing) words or syllables one at a time, a moving focus that highlights sequential words in the text (e.g., five subsequent words) could also be arranged. The latter form of metronomic feedback is less compelling because it marks only roughly where one needs to be if a targeted rate is followed successfully. Such "soft metronomes" allow for variations in rate characteristic of normal speech production. By allowing the client to interrupt a metronome's action when it is not needed (for example, at the end of an utterance or at a conversational turn), its disruptive effect may be reduced.

Current developments in speech synthesis have created new options for the production of models for speech rate modification. By employing digitized or LPC-converted speech samples, rate models can be generated that are identical in quality. By determining LPC-related parameters from the client's own speech, such models could be made to sound much like the client. LPC-generated models are also useful in rate modification strategies that employ chorus reading (while the sound intensity of the model is gradually faded) or imitation (sequentially or delayed).

SEGMENTAL AND SUBSEGMENTAL ASPECTS OF SPEECH FLUENCY

The temporal and spatial patterns of individual speech sounds and their transitions affect the overall impression of a speaker's fluency (Starkweather, 1987). In fact, it is at this level that essential stuttering behaviors occur (i.e., audible or silent sound repetitions, prolongations, and broken words). Molecular aspects of speech sounds and their transitions have been infrequently measured

[4]Beukelman, D.R., Yorkston, K.M., and Tice, R.L., Pacer/Tally for pacing or tallying responses. Communication Skill Builders, 3830 E. Bellevue, PO Box 42050, Tucson, AZ 90049. Reviewed by Arthur Schwartz (1989). *Journal for Computer Users in Speech and Hearing, 5* (1), 40–43.

or manipulated as an approach to fluency enhancement. Only a few such changes have been described in the literature.

Among the segmental (or subsegmental) targets of fluency enhancement therapy are the establishment of vowel prolongations and word blending (continued phonation), gentle voice onsets (GVOs), and soft articulatory contacts (e.g., Curlee & Perkins, 1969). Durations of vowels (and other voiced continuant sounds) and the use of word blending can be examined from spectrographic displays available on a number of acoustic speech analysis stations. Such clinical targets do not require spectrographic displays, however. Continued phonation skills are also reflected by continuity measures such as those discussed on previous pages. Continuity feedback, in fact, has a number of advantages over current spectrographic approaches. It measures this aspect automatically and may provide on-line feedback as well as summary statistics for entire periods of speech production.

The establishment of GVOs (e.g., Webster, 1974, 1979) and soft articulatory contacts (Curlee & Perkins, 1969) has received much attention in recent literature concerning fluency enhancement. GVOs, for example, may be established with feedback from such systems as the Voice Onset Monitor (or VOM), a device used in the Hollins College Fluency Shaping Program. The VOM signals to clients when, during phonatory onsets, a selected criterion of abruptness is exceeded. Voice initiations may also be visually examined with sound intensity envelopes available on most acoustic speech analysis stations (e.g., CSL or SoundScope). The nature of the displays provided by these products, however, limits measurements at the segmental level and makes quantification of therapeutic progress a lengthy and tedious process.

One way of quantifying abruptness of voice initiations is through measurement of their vocal rise times (Koike, 1967; Peters, Boves, & van Dielen, 1986), defined as the period during which sound intensity raises from threshold to 90 percent of the steady state. When used for evaluating the relative abruptness of phonatory onsets in stutterers, this measure has a number of limitations. Vocal rise time depends on the intensity level during the steady state portion of the sound. Because vowels differ with respect to the amount of sound radiation at the oral opening and the loss of acoustic energy due to degree and type of constriction along the vocal tract, GVO-related feedback is not consistent across vowels. Furthermore, by including almost all of the onset slope, the actual phonatory onset that comprises only its earliest aspect may not be measured at all. Thus, when extension of vocal rise time is targeted as a means of establishing gentle voice onsets, it may potentially be responsible for perceived abnormality of speech following therapy.

There is a need for standards in evaluating the relative abruptness of phonatory onsets, as well as specific guidelines for identifying the most relevant aspects of GVO-related skills for the treatment of stuttering. There appear to be two options for standardizing this type of feedback. Exacting results could be obtained, for example, by measuring the slope of phonatory energy during a brief fixed time interval following the first glottis stroke of the phonation interval (e.g., 50 ms). In contrast, one could measure the time interval between phonatory onset and the moment when a predetermined vocal intensity level (expressed in dB SPL) is reached. Research is needed to establish if such procedures significantly enhance the consistency and effectiveness of GVO-related feedback to clients. The results of such studies would lead to important decisions about achieving an optimal balance between fluency enhancement and preserving normalcy of speech production.

Aside from the apparent lack of clinical guidelines, measurement of vocal rise time is cumbersome with most systems for speech analysis. The assessment of voice onset related targets during longer speech utterances or running speech is currently impractical for clinical applications. To develop a system for on-line GVO-related feedback in running speech, the author has experimented with a new form of feedback (Bakker, 1994a) in which abruptness of phonatory onsets is measured by differentiating the sound intensity envelope of phonatory energy real-time. Abrupt onsets are reflected by sharp positive peaks, while negative peaks mark abrupt reductions in phonatory energy. This type of feedback allows clinicians to set target lines for evaluating whether a specified criterion of abruptness is exceeded. By applying auditory rather than visual feedback, the client need not continuously watch a computer monitor. Auditory feedback during later phases of therapy facilitates generalization of GVO-related skills to normal interactive situations. Summary statistics describing one's average abruptness of voice onsets across entire periods of speech production are also available. They express the incidence of abruptness violations per minute articulatory time. A more complete discussion of the technique may be found in Bakker (1994b). The efficacy of abruptness feedback for establishing fluent speech is currently under investigation.

Although the recent literature on the therapeutic use of prolonged speech has capitalized on abruptness of phonatory onsets, smooth articulations and soft articulatory contacts are considered significant agents in fluency enhancement by some authors (e.g., Curlee & Perkins, 1976). Acoustic abruptness associated with consonantal productions is not easily established. Although abruptness would be apparent from abruptness feedback such as that applied with voice onsets (but without bandpass filtering), it tends to be nondistinct. Consonants are lower in sound intensity than are vowels and their sound intensity levels vary, depending on manner and place of articulation. Perhaps consonantal abruptness can be effectively measured with feedback based on airflow measurements. This is a hypothetical possibility, however. Aside from the many practical difficulties associated with using a pneumotachograph for sustained periods of time, its usefulness for fluency enhancement has not yet been determined.

An increasing body of research is focusing on detailed aspects of speech motor control and timing during fluent speech productions. Among the techniques employed in this research are electromyography (Adams, Freeman, & Conture, 1984; Shapiro, 1980), strain gauges, and transducers of force. Currently, only peripheral and movable articulators are targeted in kinematically oriented investigations, while EMG has been employed on occasion to measure activity in the laryngeal musculatory (e.g., Adams, Freeman, & Conture, 1984). The measurement protocols followed in these investigations have not led to clinical applications because they are too time consuming, invasive, or costly. This, of course, is a problem not limited to the area of fluency disorders.

PROSODY

The possibility that prosody and dysfluency are functionally related has been entertained for some time (e.g., Wingate, 1976). Recently, this interest has taken on a new meaning, because many clients who have completed a fluency enhancement therapy are judged to sound abnormal with regard to prosodic expression. Clinicians who have a need for modifying patterns of intonation, loudness, and rhythm to achieve normalcy in their clients have a broad range of available instruments to support this work. Molar aspects of intonation (overall changes in F_0, loudness, and rhythm) are represented well in feedback displays provided by a Visipitch (Kay Elemetrics), CSL (expanded with its real-time option; Kay Elemetrics), Dr. Speech Science (Tigard Electronics), the PM Pitch Analyzer (Voice Identifications), IBM's SpeechViewer, and Video Voice. A system for prosodic feedback should be able to display results real time; variations in pitch, loudness, and duration should be expressed in quantified form. While the former is essential for the efficient acquisition of new prosodic patterns, the latter ensures consistency in goal setting, treatment evaluations, and clinical reports.

MEASURABLE ASPECTS OF DYSFLUENCY

Despite the behavioral complexity of a fully developed stuttering problem, dysfluency often plays a primary, or exclusive, role in differential diagnostic decisions and treatment evaluations. Unfortunately, dysfluency is a perceptual term and presents few options for developing equipment that may assist clinicians in stuttering identification and measurement. A system for stuttering recognition requires a common set of measurable criteria robust enough to differentiate stuttered and normally fluent speech. Without this fundamental information, it is perhaps impossible to develop a system that can replace clinician judgments regarding the presence or absence of stuttering.

Traditionally, the assessment of dysfluency and normal forms of fluency failure has occurred through observational procedures that involved transcription in vivo, or from audio- or videotaped speech samples. The role of equipment in this process was limited to augmenting, rather than replacing, clinician judgments. Few attempts have been made to rely entirely on objective characteristics of speech for determining whether stuttering occurred and to what extent. There is only one report of a computerized methodology for stuttering recognition. Howell and Sackin (1994) employed a neural networks technology for establishing automated stuttering recognition. However, their procedure required exposure to prototypes of the client's stuttering before it was capable of recognizing future stuttering moments. The use of neural networks for stuttering identification and measurement is in an initial exploratory stage and awaits thorough and systematic evaluation of its potentials for clinical application.

Despite the limited role of equipment in stuttering identification, it has great potential for measuring detailed aspects of dysfluencies after they are identified by clinicians. Clinicians often use counters for determining the frequency of stuttering moments in general, frequencies of specific dysfluency types, and even the incidence of nonverbal stuttering-related behaviors (e.g., Brutten, 1975; Johnson, 1961).

Stuttering counts are easily obtained with self-prepared tracking forms. This type of recording allows for a number of useful variations not possible with manual counters. For example, one could tally syllables spoken while using a special symbol for syllables that were stuttered. The use of a set of symbols for representing dysfluency types ensures that the original sequence of behaviors is retained and available for future inspections. An example of a useful tracking sheet is the scoring form that accompanies the Stuttering Severity Instrument, SSI-3 (Riley, 1994). Fluently spoken syllables are marked with periods, while each stuttered syllable is represented with a slash. After completion, the clinician can quickly determine the percentage of syllables stuttered (%SS), the most commonly used measure in treatment evaluations of today.

Results obtained with counters and tracking sheets do not reflect aspects of duration or variability (Figure 19.3). Durations of stuttering dysfluencies also reflect severity. They contribute importantly to diagnostic decisions and impart information that has been shown to be independent of frequency measures, at least among stuttering children (Zebrowski, 1994). Furthermore, duration may be among the earliest and most sensitive indices of therapeutic change (Conture & Caruso, 1987). Durational measures are an integral part of a number of current assessment protocols (e.g., the Stuttering Severity Instrument-3, Riley, 1994; Costello & Ingham, 1984). They are typically measured with hand-held timing devices (e.g., a stopwatch).

A number of therapies measure progress in terms of the average length of fluent intervals between stuttering moments (e.g., the GILCU program, Ryan, 1974; Conversational Rate Control Therapy, Curlee & Perkins, 1969; Stutter Free Speech, Shames & Florance, 1980). Measurement of a client's three longest intervals of fluent speech has been suggested by Costello and Ingham (1984).

Unfortunately, a number of potentially useful clinical measures exceed the normal attentional and reaction time skills of clinicians when determined with hand-held timers and counters. With current improvements of the timing capabilities of personal computers, new opportunities have emerged for the development of sophisticated and comprehensive timing/counting programs. One is

encouraged to monitor the availability of such programs because they permit interpretations and analyses that are not currently feasible with hand-held timers and counters. Among the anticipated gains with such programs are the clinician's ability to: (1) track multiple behaviors simultaneously, (2) retain aspects of individual behavioral instances (e.g., time of occurrence and duration), (3) measure durations of intervals between targeted behaviors, (4) examine sequential patterns of behaviors (e.g., variations in occurrence, duration, or sequence), (5) display intermediate results to clients or analyze trends throughout sessions, and (6) generate hard copies for clinical reports.

There are three emergent input strategies for the computerized assessment of stuttering. One such strategy assists clinicians in differential diagnostic decisions that are based on counts and durations of specific dysfluency types (e.g., Adams, 1980). Rather than employing manual counts (or tallies), the user may select dysfluency types with a computer mouse, and hold down a button for the duration of each behavior. While this strategy is cumbersome when conducted on-line with clients, it is feasible from recorded speech samples that allow the clinician to replay parts of a tape. Among the available results are frequency of dysfluency types, percentage of stuttering-type dysfluencies, and average duration of stuttering-type dysfluencies. It should be noted, however, that a clinician's ability to identify and time individual stuttering moments is currently questioned by some authors (e.g., Cordes & Ingham, 1994; Ingham, Cordes, & Gow, 1993).

A second input strategy is geared towards therapeutic procedures that target increased durations of fluent periods of speech production (or reductions in stuttering durations). The only action needed here is to hold down a mouse button (or a key on the keyboard) for the perceived durations of stuttering moments, while a shift-key may be optionally pressed for marking the periods when speech is audible or attempted. Among the available results are numbers and durations of stuttering moments and periods of fluent speech production. Also, the distributional aspects (mean, standard de-

COUNTS

Dysfluencies

# of stuttering events (use of counters, tallying, or tracking sheets)
# of specific types of stuttering, or normal, dysfluencies (frequency tables; percentages)
# of units of repetitions (part-word repetitions only)

Nonverbal behaviors

# of behaviors secondary to stuttering

Syllables   (total #; or percentage of syllables stuttered: %SS)
Words   (total #; or percentage of words stuttered: %WS)

Length of fluent intervals

(average # of syllables, or words, produced between moments of stuttering)

OVERALL DURATIONS

The entire sample duration broken down into:

a. *Pause time*	(% time when speech is not attempted)
b. *Total articulatory time*	(% time when speech is audible, or attempted, including stuttering)
1. *Fluent articulatory time*	(% of total articulatory time when fluent speech is audible, or attempted)
2. *Stuttering time*	(% of total articulatory time engaged in audible or silent stuttering)

SEGMENTAL DURATIONS

Durations of:

- individual stuttering events (or specific dysfluency types)
- periods of fluent speech production (expressed in fluent articulatory time)
- periods between nonverbal stuttering related behaviors
- pauses (silent moments free of stuttering)

Additional optional statistics for segmental durations:

.. measures of central tendency (e.g., mean duration)
.. measures of variation (e.g., standard deviation)
.. mean duration of longest three (or "typical") incidences
.. frequency distributions (e.g., tables, histograms, pie charts)

Figure 19.3 Measurable aspects of dysfluency and related behaviors.

viation, mean of longest three instances) of stutterings and periods of fluent speech are available, as well as the percentage of speaking time that was stuttered by the client. The need to mark articulatory time is obviated when an automated speech timer is integrated into the design. For the latter, the clinician need only hold down a mouse button for the perceived durations of stutterings.

A third input strategy emphasizes aspects of fluent and stuttered speech at the syllabic level. This creates the opportunity to enter data one syllable at a time, employing one mouse button for the fluent syllables and another for the stutterings. This method is not new, and has proven useful for measuring clinical progress (the STRR program; Fowler & Ingham, 1986). Among the results obtained with STRR are percentage of syllables stuttered and speech rate, while results are updated in an interval fashion. The STRR method could be taken one step further by incorporating a timing procedure for stuttering duration and an automated speech timer. This recording process presents an optimal opportunity for integrating a broad range of quantifiable dimensions of fluent and dysfluent speech into one measurement protocol: frequency and duration of stuttering, as well as their effects on speech rate. Among the most valuable measures available with the latter type of recording are:

- Percentage of syllables stuttered (%SS)
- Average stuttering duration (in seconds)
- Percentage of articulatory time stuttered
- Estimated fluent speaking rate and rate reduction due to stuttering
- Average duration of fluent intervals (in seconds)
- Average length of fluent intervals (in syllables)

The behavioral counting and timing strategies described provide a number of useful options for computerized counting and timing in clinical practice that do not require more skill than is already necessary for hand-held timers and counters. They may ultimately play an important role in many stuttering therapies, but aspects of their validity, accuracy, and reliability are in need of empirical investigation.

In addition to the counting and timing strategies discussed, many current speech analysis stations contain options for quantifying and measuring aspects of dysfluency in a more rigorous and exacting way than was previously thought possible. Research has since initiated the use of such systems for measuring aspects such as stuttering duration (e.g., Zebrowski, 1991, 1994) and acoustic characteristics of the transitions between units in repetition.

Current speech analysis workstations allow for exacting ways to capture individual moments of dysfluency. Selections of stuttering moments can be verified by replaying marked sections of digital recordings. Also, additional analyses are available, including spectrograms and sound intensity envelopes. The extent to which these methods are practical for clinical application, however, is still undetermined. The suspicion is that the operation

time involved in capturing relevant parts of recorded speech, selecting details with cursors, and conducting measurements and calculations may be too lengthy for routine clinical applications. The accuracy gained with such systems, then, is offset by the additional operation time required from the user.

All of these acoustic analyses can be conducted from tape-recorded speech. In fact, one is encouraged to have clients bring in taped samples reflecting their use of clinical targets in designated out-clinic situations. The value of such post-hoc analyses depends on the quality of these recordings.

Finally, spectrographic displays may be used to verify the presence of schwas in segmental repetitions, a sign of true stuttering according to many authors (e.g., Van Riper, 1982). To conduct this analysis in a meaningful way, one should verify that the system produces wide band spectrograms (a bandpass of around 300 Hz) of up to at least 4000 Hz (or 5000 Hz for young children) that have a sufficient timing resolution (reveals changes in steps of 5 ms, or less) to reveal these features. Spectrograms that do not meet these standards lead to unreliable results and cannot be compared to published norms.

Measuring Physiologic, Aeromechanic, and Kinematic Characteristics of Stuttering

Over the years there have been many reports involving physiologic, aeromechanic, and kinematic measurements during, or in the proximity of, stuttering moments (e.g., Bloodstein, 1987). These reports have generally attempted to describe discoordination within (or between) the respiratory, phonatory, and articulatory systems for speech production. Through such observations clinicians can be made more aware of what actually occurs internally and motorically when clients stutter.

Aside from being suggestive potential causes of stuttering, discoordination may represent struggle and escape behaviors, or simply attempts to repair (Bloodstein, 1987). It is unlikely that in the midst of a stuttering block a client would be able to use feedback concerning the speech apparatus. It is no surprise, then, that there have been few clinical attempts to utilize physiological, kinematic, or aeromechanic measures of the speech system during stuttering. Of course, stutterers may lack awareness of what goes on motorically and internally during stuttering, and external measurements could lead to improvements of this awareness. To the knowledge of this author, however, this has not been attempted as an approach to the treatment of stuttering.

PRODUCING FLUENT SPEECH THROUGH MANIPULATING SENSORY FEEDBACK

A number of instruments commonly used in stuttering therapy are based on the principle that dysfluency can be manipulated by altering sensory feedback associated with speech production. Delayed auditory feedback (DAF), masking, and syllable-timed speech (produced with metronomes), for example, have been reported to result in either a partial or complete elimination of dysfluency in many stutterers (Andrews, Craig, Feyer, Hoddinott, Howie, & Nelson, 1983). Perhaps because these results are immediate and automatic, and thus reduce the amount of intervention and effort needed from the clinician and client, these systems have been popular over the years. This convenience, however, suggests a potential weakness as well. DAF, Edinburgh Maskers, and metronomes would not likely foster a great degree of self-control in establishing transfer and maintenance of acquired fluency to real-life situations. Rather, the effects of these systems are characterized by an external locus of control for both client and clinician. The effects usually vanish when the instruments are turned off and normal feedback is restored. Nevertheless, these systems largely retain the power to re-establish fluency almost indefinitely. There are no reports that suggest that the fluency inducing effects of DAF or maskers wear off. Silverman (1992) observed, however, that the effects of metronomes seem to decline over time.

The unique fluency enhancing effects of DAF, metronomes, and maskers on the speech of stutterers have made them beneficial partners in differential diagnostic applications. These systems produce nearly opposite effects on the fluency of neurogenic dysfluents and clutterers (Daly, 1986), probably because the latter are more dependent than stutterers on auditory feedback to speak correctly. Speech of malingerers, furthermore, may reveal changes under these conditions that are inconsistent with known facts about any of these disorders.

While it is possible that the fluency-enhancing effects produced by these systems result from blocking the speaker's ability to monitor speech auditorily, a number of authors have argued that it is, rather, the speech changes under these conditions that produce improved fluency (Andrews, Howie, Dozsa, & Guitar, 1982; Wingate, 1976). For a while, DAF, masking, and metronomes were considered laboratory examples for how stuttering could be treated. One speech difference produced by most systems is a reduction in rate. Although this is most clearly obtained with DAF (Wingate, 1976), increased vowel and consonant durations have been observed for syllable-timed speech as well (Brayton & Conture, 1978). Brayton and Conture (1978) also observed slight increases in consonantal durations during masking. Shifts in habitual pitch, loudness, degree of vowel prolongation, and rhythm have all been reported with DAF, masking, and metronomes (Wingate, 1976) and are potentially responsible for the fluency enhancing effects on the speech of stutterers.

A complete account of the fluency enhancing ingredients of sensory feedback modifications, and their associated speech changes, is not available. In fact, there are incidental reports of yet other ways of manipulating auditory feedback to establish fluency. Webster (1991), for example, has experimented with modification of the phase-relationship of auditory feedback of the fundamental frequency of phonation between the left and right ear. Although casual reports of the fluency-enhancing effects of this procedure exist, independent controlled studies of its clinical effectiveness have yet to occur.

Altering speech-related auditory feedback as a method for fluency enhancement seems to be also the principle behind the effects of Edinburgh maskers (Dewar, Dewar, Austin, & Brash, 1979). As a voice-triggered noise generator, this device blocks auditory feedback only during speech production. Because it does not block speech produced by others, it allows communication to proceed more or less normally. Edinburgh Maskers, like DAFs, are available in miniaturized form. Their portability makes them accessible for clients who seek fluency enhancement in specific speaking situations.

There is limited but positive evidence for immediate fluency enhancing effects of masking on the speech of stutterers. Evidence that these devices produce permanent fluency that is maintained independently of their use is missing, however. In fact, there have been individual reports that the dysfluency reductions achieved under the influence of Edinburgh Maskers were surprisingly resistant to generalization (Ingham, 1993). The utility of maskers, then, is limited to producing instant fluency in situations where this is important for, or highly desired by, the client. Edinburgh maskers are useful also when differential diagnostic decisions need to be confirmed through additional observations.

Metronomes have been reported to cause substantial and immediate reductions in dysfluency in many stutterers. Miniaturized metronomes the size of a hearing aid have been available for some time (Silverman, 1992). Among the fluency-enhancing changes are rhythmicity of speech as well as changes in duration, pitch, and loudness. Although most metronomes work in a continuous mode, it would be easy to develop metronomes in a voice- or manually triggered mode, thus facilitating their use in natural communication. Moreover, the user would then be freed from the rhythmic stimulus during the speech of others, or silent intervals. Metronomically induced fluent speech, like the changes obtained with other sensory feedback manipulations, is resistant to generalization and its results have been shown to maintain less well than fluency obtained with either prolonged speech or GVO-related clinical strategies (Andrews, Guitar, & Howie, 1980).

The age of digital processing has paved the way for a recent development in auditory feedback manipulation. Frequency altered feedback (FAF) changes the quality of one's speech by shifting the fundamental frequency of phonation. This manipulation leads to perceptions that have been described as "alien" and robot like, while intelligibility is preserved. The fluency-enhancing effects of FAF have been evaluated in a number of recent reports (Hargrave, Kalinowski, Stuart, Armson, & Jones, 1994; Howell, El-Yaniv, & Powell, 1987). Although the available database is still rather limited, FAF appears to have roughly comparable effects on stuttering as DAF or masking. Importantly, FAF does not result in dramatic changes in rate, or rhythm, of speech, which implies that speech normalcy is relatively well preserved. Little is known about the effectiveness of FAF in establishing a sustained fluent speaking pattern that is resistant to differences in speaking situations. Research into the therapeutic benefits and its use across dysfluent speakers is urgently needed. A miniaturized DAF-FAF unit is currently available at a reasonable price.[5] This particular device has optional adapters for use during telephone conversations.

The fluency enhancing devices based on altering auditory feedback all have in common the potential for miniaturization. Portable versions of these devices are usually available. Because their electronic functions have a great deal of overlap, there is the opportunity to integrate these functions into one electronic unit.

INSTRUMENTATION FOR THE ASSESSMENT AND TREATMENT OF ASSOCIATED SYMPTOMATOLOGIES

In addition to nonverbal stuttering-related behaviors (e.g., eye blinks, head turns, movements with arms or legs), other symptoms associated with stuttering include speech-related anxiety and stut-

---

[5]Clinical Fluency Aid (FAF and DAF)
Casa futura technologies
Biofeedback Systems for Speech Disorders
P.O. Box 7551
Boulder, CO 80306–7551

tering anticipation. These also have aspects that are measurable and permit arrangement of client-oriented biofeedback procedures.

A number of clinicians have targeted speech-related concerns as the primary means of achieving fluency (Brutten & Shoemaker, 1967), while others have referred to reduction of speech-related tension because it was observed to contribute to the problem. Speech-related concerns can be treated by employing relaxation procedures. The client is first taught how to achieve general relaxation, and then practices the skill in the face of fear-provoking stimuli through systematic desensitization. Among possible fear-provoking stimuli are specific sounds, words, or speaking situations.

Because speech-related fears, concerns, and tensions have physiological components, relaxation can be practiced through biofeedback. Traditionally, GSR (galvanic skin response) or SCL (skin conductance level) have been the most popular choices for this type of therapy. These techniques reflect changes in skin impedance (or conductance) due to the differential levels of activation of sweat glands (for example, in the palmar surfaces).

The option of tracking quick (phasic) changes in SCL in response to speech- or situation-specific stimuli (in vivo, or vicariously) appears not to have been considered in the literature. Yet such changes might reflect the occurrence of stuttering anticipations and would allow clinicians to help clients reduce at least this physiological component of their fears and concerns for speech and speaking situations.

Little is known about the efficacy of biofeedback procedures for achieving relaxation in stutterers. Less is known about how this technique would benefit generalization of relaxation to designated out-clinic situations and establish fluent speech. It should be noted, furthermore, that the universal presence of autonomic reactions (such as palmar sweating) as indicators for speech-related anxiety in stutterers has not been confirmed by the literature (e.g., Janssen & Kraaimaat, 1980; Peters & Hulstijn, 1984). Because of this, it is perhaps best to restrict the use of GSR-related biofeedback

to those clients who evidenced strong levels of concern (and palmar sweating) during diagnostic interviews or in response to speech-anxiety related surveys (e.g., Brutten & Shoemaker, 1974; Johnson, Darley, & Spriestersbach, 1952).

Other physiological measures of tension and anxiety may have significance for treatment in some stutterers. Electromyography (EMG) has been shown to be useful for attaining both general relaxation (e.g., frontalis muscle) and differential relaxation of speech-related muscles and muscle groups and is an attractive choice with clients who gave evidence that specific portions of the musculature tensed up during speech production. Among the potentially productive sites for relaxation with surface-EMG are the strap muscles of the neck (Peters & Hulstijn, 1984), muscular floor of the oral cavity (the mylohyoid and anterior digastric muscles are easily accessible with surface electrodes), the masseters, and perioral muscle groups. Intra-oral, pharyngeal, and intrinsic laryngeal muscles are not accessible for routine general or differential relaxation EMG. Other measurable aspects of arousal and tension have been reported, such as heart rate (Baumgartner & Brutten, 1983) and peripheral blood volume (Ickes & Pierce, 1973). These vascularly related measures would also be expected to reflect amounts of physiological arousal or sympathetic activity associated with variations in speech-related concern, but there is no evidence that these forms of measurement are useful for the treatment of stuttering or its concomitant tensions and anxiety.

All aforementioned forms of biofeedback involve (semi)invasive procedures and require accurate electrode placements and relatively time-consuming procedures for calibration. Moreover, no biofeedback procedure promotes automatic transfer of relaxation skills to out-clinic situations. This is partly the result of the nonportable nature of the equipment needed for these procedures. To the extent that relaxation exercises (e.g., progressive muscle relaxation, Jacobson, 1962) are effective, they are more amenable to generalization than most biofeedback applications. They are also characterized by higher levels of self-control on the part of the client. Biofeedback procedures, then, are indicated mostly for clients who cannot learn the necessary relaxation skills through relaxation exercises, and who are dependent on external feedback for developing a sensitivity for their physiological responding to anxiety-provoking speech-related stimuli or situations.

SUMMARY

Like all specializations in communication disorders, clinical work with stutterers faces an increased reliance on instrument- or computer-based procedures and methodologies. Though promising as a trend, this is not necessarily a blessing in all cases. Many technological advances in the past did not produce the results that were initially anticipated. New technological procedures for the diagnostic evaluation, assessment, and treatment of stuttering should be judged with the same known standards that apply to any changes in clinical practice.

The current increase in clinical instrumentation and computer-based applications calls for systematic research to help define their role in routine clinical applications. There are many questions concerning the validity, reliability, and feasibility of many of these products. There are questions, also, concerning when equipment should be introduced in therapeutical sessions, or withdrawn. This is important especially when procedures for generalization or maintenance are planned, and one wishes to ensure that the targeted speech changes can be produced independently from biofeedback. Unfortunately, the science of communication disorders does not have the necessary resources to keep up with all of the technological developments or their upgrades, leaving potential users alone in making decisions concerning clinical utility. It is important that their effectiveness in producing lasting fluency, or reducing their effects of stuttering and its related symptomatologies, is demonstrated before these technologies are considered replacements for or additions to current clinical practices.

REFERENCES

Adams, M.R. (1974). A physiologic and aerodynamic interpretation of fluent and stuttered speech. *Journal of Fluency Disorders, 1*, 35–47.

Adams, M.R. (1980). The young stutterer: Diagnosis, treatment, and assessment of progress. *Seminars in Speech, Language, and Hearing 1.* New York: Thieme Medical Publishers.

Adams, M.R., Freeman, F.J., & Conture, E.G. (1984). Laryngeal dynamics of stutterers. In R.J. Curlee & W.H. Perkins (Eds.), *The nature and treatment of stuttering:* New directions (pp. 89–129). San Diego, CA: College-Hill Press.

Andrews, G., Craig, A., Feyer, A.M., Hoddinott, S., Howie, P.M., & Neilson, M. (1983). Stuttering: A review of research findings and theories circa 1982. *Journal of Speech and Hearing Disorders, 48*, 226–245.

Andrews, G., Guitar, B., & Howie, P.M. (1980). Meta-analysis of the effects of stuttering treatment. *Journal of Speech and Hearing Disorders, 45*, 287–307.

Andrews, G., Howie, P.M., Dozsa, M., & Guitar, B.E. (1982). Stuttering: Speech pattern characteristics under fluency-inducing conditions. *Journal of Speech and Hearing Research, 25*, 208–216.

Andrews, G., Neilson, M., & Cassar, M. (1987). Informing stutterers about treatment. In L. Rustin, H. Purser, and D. Rowley (Eds.). *Progress in the treatment of fluency disorders.* London, UK: Taylor and Francis.

Apel, K., Masterson, J.J., Mathers-Schmidt, B., & Bakker, K. (1993). Clinical ground rounds: Getting to the meat of the matter. Shortcourse at the *Annual Convention of the American Speech Language and Hearing Association.* Anaheim, Calif.

Azrin, N.H., & Nunn, R.G. (1974). A rapid method of eliminating stuttering by a regulated-breathing approach. *Behavior Research and Therapy, 12*, 279–286.

Baken, R.J. (1987). *Clinical measurement of speech and voice.* Boston: Allyn and Bacon.

Bakker, K. (1994a). Gentle voice onset feedback during

running speech: Its design and technical specifications. *First Congress of the International Fluency Association*, Munich, Germany.

Bakker, K. (1994b). Integrating automated speech rate feedback into clinical applications. *First Congress of the International Fluency Association*, Munich, Germany.

Bakker, K., Brutten, G.J., & McQuain, J. (1995). A preliminary assessment of the validity of three instrument-based measures for speech rate determination. *Journal of Fluency Disorders, 20*, 63–75.

Bakker K., & Dugan-Feldt, H. (1993). Speech rate determination employing laryngographic and acoustic voice-initiation counts. Paper presented at the *National Convention of the American Speech-Language-Hearing Association*, Anaheim, Calif.

Bakker, K., & Gregg, B. (1994). Speech rates based on instrumentally, or manually, derived articulation times. Paper presented at the *National Convention of the American Speech-Language-Hearing Association*, Anaheim, Calif.

Bakker, K., & Rader, H. (1992). Does speech rate affect automated counts of voice initiations? Paper presented at the *National Convention of the American Speech-Language-Hearing Association*, San Antonio, Tex.

Baumgartner, J.M., & Brutten, G.J. (1983). Expectancy and heart rate as predictors of the speech performance of stutterers. *Journal of Speech and Hearing Research, 26*, 383–388.

Bloodstein, O.H. (1987). *A handbook on stuttering.* Chicago: National Easter Seal Society.

Borden, G., Harris, K., & Raphael, L.J. (1993). *Speech science primer: Physiology, acoustics, and perception of speech* (3rd ed.). Baltimore: Williams and Wilkins.

Borden, G., & Watson, B.C. (1987). Methodological aspects of simultaneous measurements: Limitations and possibilities. In H.F.M. Peters, & W. Hulstijn (Eds.), *Speech motor dynamics in stuttering.* New York: Springer-Verlag.

Brayton, E.R., & Conture, E.G. (1978). Effects of noise and rhythmic stimulation on the speech of stutterers. *Journal of Speech and Hearing Research, 21*, 285–294.

Brutten, G. J. (1975). Stuttering: Topography, assessment, and behavior-change strategies. In J. Eisenson (Ed.), *Stuttering: A second symposium*, New York: Harper and Row.

Brutten, G.J., & Shoemaker, D.J. (1967). *The modifica-*

tion of stuttering. Englewood Cliffs, N.J.: Prentice-Hall.

Brutten, G.J., & Shoemaker, D.J. (1974). *The speech situations checklist.* Carbondale, Ill.: Speech Clinic, Southern Illinois University.

Conture, E.G., & Caruso, A.J. (1987). Assessment and diagnosis of childhood dysfluency. In L. Rustin, H. Purser, & D. Rowley (Eds.), *Progress in the treatment of fluency disorders.* London, UK: Taylor & Francis.

Cordes, A.K., & Ingham, R.J. (1994). The reliability of observational data: II. Issues in the identification and measurement of stuttering events. *Journal of Speech and Hearing Research, 37*, 279–294.

Costello, J.M., & Ingham, R.J. (1984). Assessment strategies for stuttering. In R.J. Curlee, & W.H. Perkins (Eds.). *The nature and treatment of stuttering: New directions* (pp. 303–333). San Diego, CA: College-Hill Press.

Curlee, R.F., & Perkins, W.H. (1969). Conversational rate therapy control for stuttering. *Journal of Speech and Hearing Disorders, 34*, 245–250.

Daly, D.A. (1986). The clutterer. In K.O. St. Louis (Ed.), *The atypical stutterer.* Orlando, FL: Academic Press.

Dembowski, J., & Watson, B. (1991). An instrumented method for assessment and remediation of stuttering: A single-subject case study. *Journal of Fluency Disorders, 16*, 241–273.

Dewar, A., Dewar, A.D., Austin, W.T.S., & Brash, H.M. (1979). The long term use of an automatically triggered auditory feedback masking device in the treatment of stammering. *British Journal of Disorders of Communication, 14*, 219–229.

Driscoll, J. (1981). Research trends in rate-controlled speech for language learning. *NALLD Journal, 15*, 45–51.

Fletcher, S. (1972)., Time-by-count measurement of diadochokinetic syllable rate. *Journal of Speech and Hearing Research, 15*, 763–769.

Fowler, S.C., & Ingham, R.J. (1986). Stuttering Treatment Rating Recorder (Software and Manual). Santa Barbara: University of California.

Goebel, M., Hillis, J., & Meyer, R. (1985). The relationship between speech fluency and certain patterns of speechflow. Paper presented the *National Convention of the American Speech-Language-Hearing Association*, Washington, D.C.

Gow, M., & Ingham, R.J. (1992). Modifying electroglottograph-identified intervals of phonation:

The effect on stuttering. *Journal of Speech and Hearing Research, 35,* 495–511.

Hargrave, S., Kalinowski, J., Stuart, A., Armson, J., & Jones, K. (1994). Effect of frequency-altered feedback on stuttering frequency at normal and fast speech rates. Research Note. *Journal of Speech and Hearing Research, 37,* 1313–1319.

Haynes, E., & Christenson, S. (1994). The story is in the pause. *First World Congress on Fluency Disorders of the International Fluency Association,* Munich, Germany.

Horii, Y. (1983). Some acoustic characteristics of oral reading by ten to twelve year old children. *Journal of Communication, 16,* 257–267.

Howell, P., El-Yaniv, N., & Powell, D.J. (1987). Factors affecting fluency in stutterers. In H.F.M. Peters and W. Hulstijn (Eds.), *Speech motor dynamics in stuttering* (p. 361–369). New York: Springer-Verlag.

Howell, P., & Sackin, S. (1994). Automatic recognition of stuttering: Preliminary reports. *First World Congress on Fluency Disorders of the International Fluency Association,* Munich, Germany.

Hubbard, C.P., & Prins, D. (1994). Word familiarity, syllabic stress pattern, and stuttering. *Journal of Speech and Hearing Research, 37,* 564–571.

Ickes, W.K., & Pierce, S. (1973). The stuttering moment: A plethysmographic study. *Journal of Communication Disorders, 6,* 155–164.

Ingham, J. C. (1993). Current status of stuttering and behavior modification I: Recent trends in the application of behavior modification in children and adults. *Journal of Fluency Disorders, 18,* 27–55.

Ingham, R.J., Cordes, A.K., & Gow, M. (1993). Time-interval measurement of stuttering: Modifying interjudge agreement. *Journal of Speech and Hearing Research, 36,* 503–515.

Ingham, R.J., Montgomery, J., & Ulliana, L. (1983). The effect of manipulating phonation duration on stuttering. *Journal of Speech and Hearing Research, 26,* 579–587.

Jacobson, E. (1962). *You must relax.* New York: McGraw-Hill.

Janssen, P., & Kraaimaat, F. (1980). Disfluency and anxiety in stuttering and nonstuttering adolescents. *Behavioral Analysis and Modification, 4,* 116–126.

Johnson, W. (1961). Measurements of oral reading and speaking rate and disfluency of adult male and female stutterers and nonstutterers. *Journal of Speech and Hearing Disorders,* Monograph Supplement, No 7, 1–20.

Johnson, W. Darley, F., & Spriestersbach, D.C. (1952). *Diagnostic manual in speech correction.* New York: Harper and Row.

Koike, Y. (1967). Experimental studies of vocal attack. *Practica Otologica Kyoto, 60,* 663–688.

Perkins, W.H. (1973a). Replacement of stuttering with normal speech: I. Rationale. *Journal of Speech and Hearing Disorders, 38,* 283–294.

Perkins, W.H. (1973b). Replacement of stuttering with normal speech: II. Clinical procedures. *Journal of Speech and Hearing Disorders, 38,* 295–303.

Perkins, W.H. (1975). Articulatory rate in the evaluation of stuttering treatments. *Journal of Speech and Hearing Disorders, 40,* 277–278.

Peters, H.F.M., & Boves, L. (1988). Coordination of aerodynamic and phonatory processes in fluent speech utterances of stutterers. *Journal of Speech and Hearing Research, 31,* 352–361.

Peters, H.F.M., Boves, L., & van Dielen, J.C.H. (1986). Perceptual judgment of voice onset in vowels as a function of the amplitude envelope. *Journal of Speech and Hearing Disorders, 51,* 299–308.

Peters, H.F.M., & Hulstijn, W. (1984). Stuttering and anxiety: The difference between stutterers and nonstutterers in verbal apprehension and physiologic arousal during the anticipation of speech, and non-speech tasks. *Journal of Fluency Disorders, 9,* 67–84.

Riley, G.D. (1994). *Stuttering severity instrument for children and adults* (3rd Ed.). Austin, Tex.: Pro-Ed.

Ryan, B.P. (1974). *Programmed therapy of stuttering in children and adults.* Springfield, Ill.: Charles C. Thomas.

Shames, G.H., & Florance, C.L. (1980). *Stutter-free speech: A goal for therapy.* Columbus, Oh.: Charles E. Merrill.

Shapiro, A.I. (1980). An electromyographic analysis of the fluent and dysfluent utterances of several types of stutterers. *Journal of Fluency Disorders, 5,* 203–231.

Silverman, F.H. (1992). *Stuttering and other fluency disorders.* Englewood Cliffs, N.J.: Prentice-Hall.

Starkweather, C.W. (1987). *Fluency and stuttering.* Englewood Cliffs, N.J.: Prentice-Hall.

Starkweather, C.W., Armson, J.M., & Amster, B.J. (1983). An approach to the study of motor speech mechanisms in stuttering. In L. Rustin, H. Purser, & D. Rowley (Eds.), *Progress in the treatment of fluency disorders.* London, UK: Taylor & Francis.

Till, J.A. (1990). Computer-assisted evaluation of speech disorders: Rationale and directions for future development. *Journal of Computer Users in Speech and Hearing, 6,* 134–148.

Van Riper, C. (1982). *The nature of stuttering* (2nd Ed.). Englewood Cliffs, N.J.: Prentice-Hall.

Walker, V.G. (1988). Durational characteristics of young adults during speaking and reading tasks. *Folia Phoniatrica, 40,* 16.

Webster, R.L. (1974). A behavioral analysis of stuttering: Treatment and theory. In K.S. Calhoun, E.E. Adams, & K.M. Mitchell (Eds.), *Innovative methods in psychopathology.* New York: John Wiley.

Webster, R.L. (1979). Empirical considerations regarding stuttering therapy. In H.H. Gregory (Ed.), *Controversies about stuttering therapy.* Baltimore, Md.: University Park Press.

Webster, R.L. (1991). Manipulation of vocal tone: implications for stuttering. In H.F.M. Peters & H. Hulstijn, *Speech motor control and stuttering.* New York: Elsevier Science Publishers.

Williams, D.F., & Brutten, G.J. (1994). Physiologic and aerodynamic events prior to the speech of stutterers and nonstutterers. *Journal of Fluency Disorders, 19,* 83–111.

Wingate, M.E. (1976). *Stuttering: Theory and treatment.* New York: Irvington.

Yorkston, K.M., Hammen, V.L., Beukelman, D.R., & Traynor, C.D. (1990). The effect of rate control on the intelligibility and naturalness of dysarthric speech. *Journal of Speech and Hearing Disorders, 55,* 550–560.

Zebrowski, P.M. (1991). Duration of the speech disfluencies of beginning stutterers. *Journal of Speech and Hearing Research, 34,* 483–491.

Zebrowski, P.M. (1994). Duration of sound prolongation and sound/syllable repetition in children who stutter: Preliminary observations. *Journal of Speech and Hearing Research, 37,* 254–263

SUGGESTED READINGS

Baken, R.J. (1987). *Clinical measurement of speech and voice.* Boston: Allyn and Bacon.

Bloodstein, O.H. (1987). *A handbook on stuttering.* Chicago: National Easter Seal Society.

Borden, G., & Watson, B.C. (1987). Methodological aspects of simultaneous measurements: Limitations and possibilities. In H.F.M. Peters and W. Hulstijn (Eds.), *Speech motor dynamics in stuttering.* New York: Springer-Verlag.

Cordes, A.K., & Ingham, R.J. (1994). The reliability of observational data: II. Issues in the identification and measurement of stuttering events. *Journal of Speech and Hearing Research, 37,* 279–294.

Costello, J.M., & Ingham, R.J. (1984). Assessment strategies for stuttering. In R.F. Curlee and W.H. Perkins (Eds.), *Nature and treatment of stuttering: New directions.* San Diego, CA: College Hill Press.

Orlikoff, R.F., & Baken, R.J. (1993). *Clinical speech and voice measurement.* San Diego, CA: Singular Publishing Group.

Starkweather, C.W. (1987). *Fluency and stuttering.* Englewood Cliffs, N.J.: Prentice-Hall.

Van Riper, C., (1982). *The nature of stuttering* (2nd Ed.). Englewood Cliffs, N.J.: Prentice-Hall.

CHAPTER 20

STUTTERING AND THE MEASUREMENT OF SPEECH NATURALNESS

NICHOLAS SCHIAVETTI
DALE EVAN METZ

INTRODUCTION

Speech production is generally taken for granted as a biological function that takes care of itself. Speakers instantiate their thoughts and ideas verbally with little or no apparent effort. In short, speech is natural. For all its apparent simplicity, however, the use of speech for communication requires an incredibly complex series of biophysical and perceptual events. As Hixon and Abbs (1980, p. 42) stated:

> The wonder is that anyone at all can generate the sounds of normal speech. Talking requires an extremely intricate coordination of three major functional subdivisions of the speech production mechanism, tens of body parts, more than a hundred muscles, and millions of nerve cells.

It is paradoxical that so complex a physiological act appears to be so natural and effortless. Perhaps this natural paradox is necessary for the accomplishment of what might be an impossible task if speakers were to focus conscious attention upon its completion. As the self-proclaimed "biology watcher" Lewis Thomas (1979, pp. 123–124) stated:

> It is conceivable that if we had anything like full, conscious comprehension of what we are doing, our speech would be degraded to a permanent stammer or even into dead silence. It would be an impossible intellectual feat to turn out the simplest

> of sentences. . . . Doing that sort of thing, monitoring all the muscles, keeping an eye on the syntax, watching out for the semantic catastrophes risked by the slightest change in word order, taking care of the tone of voice and expression around the eyes and mouth, and worrying most of all about the danger of saying something meaningless, would be much harder to accomplish than if you were put in charge of your breathing and told to look after that function, breath by breath, forever, with your conscious mind.

For millions of people with communicative disorders, speech behavior is anything but natural in the sense of being a task that they accomplish with ease and economy of effort. The production of stuttered speech, for example, requires great effort and the acoustic consequences (repetitions and prolongations) of stuttered speech sound unnatural and call untoward attention to the speaker. Regrettably, even after these behaviors have been removed by treatment, listeners may perceive unnaturalness in the stutter-free speech samples of treated stutterers compared to what they hear from nonstutterers. The clinical importance of speech naturalness measurement is highlighted by the dilemma of stutterers who go through treatments that reduce their stutterings to near zero but who still may be regarded by themselves and by others as having a problem because their speech sounds unnatural.

During the past decade, the concept of speech naturalness measurement has emerged as a salient and powerful clinical dimension that has great importance to the successful treatment of stuttering. Speech naturalness has clinical utility as an evaluative dimension in both pre- and post-treatment evaluation and as a functional contingency during the treatment process. The general concern of this chapter, then, is the measurement of speech naturalness, a variable of obvious interest for research in a number of areas of speech. The specific focus will be on research concerning the perceived naturalness of speech produced by persons who stutter. The topics to be discussed in this chapter include the definition of speech naturalness, some fundamental principles of measurement, specific scaling procedures for the measurement of speech naturalness, reliability and validity of speech naturalness measures, relationships between instrumental measures of physical speech characteristics and perceptual measures of speech naturalness, clinical application of naturalness measures, and future research directions.

Despite the extensive history of research on instrumental and perceptual measurement of a variety of speech characteristics, the direct quantitative measurement of speech naturalness has a relatively brief history in the fluency disorders literature (cf., Martin, Haroldson, & Triden, 1984). The study of speech naturalness falls within the general category of research on the measurement of "speech quality" (Onslow & Ingham, 1987) and has useful applications in evaluating post-treatment speech of persons with disorders of fluency, voice, or articulation as well as other areas of speech research, such as the evaluation of the quality of synthetic speech (Mirenda & Beukelman, 1987) or of speech produced during simultaneous manual communication (Whitehead, Schiavetti, Whitehead, & Metz, 1993). Although the concept of speech naturalness measurement could be approached from the point of view of both speech production and speech perception and could be examined in relation to a number of acoustical or physiological speech characteristics, the literature review in this chapter will concentrate on perceptual measurement of speech naturalness since it has been the focus of the bulk of the research thus far. The topics of physiological and acoustic characteristics of natural speech production and the relationship between production and perception of natural speech are important, however, and will be discussed with regard to suggestions for future research at the end of the chapter.

DEFINITION OF SPEECH NATURALNESS

Society places a high premium on naturalness: We demand natural ingredients in the food we eat and the beverages we drink. Since natural is perceived as better, advertising has made product names like "Natural Choice" or "Nature's Way" commonplace. Nonetheless, society seems unclear about how to define "natural." For example, manufacturers remove coloration from dish soaps, mouthwash, deodorants, and soft drinks to render their appearance ostensibly more natural. The term "natural" appears to be used on an ad hoc basis to mean "color removed" in such a case. In another example, however, a cosmetic tailored to mask the natural graying of hair brandishes a name like "The Natural Look." The term "natural" appears to be used on an ad hoc basis to mean "color added" in such a case. We must be careful to avoid apparent contradictions in the definition of "speech naturalness" in our scientific literature, especially since the term may often be defined on an ad hoc basis by the observers employed in our experiments.

Experimenters generally have not provided a specific definition of the term "speech naturalness" to the listeners or speakers participating as subjects in their experiments. Martin et al. (1984, p. 54) instructed their original group of naturalness raters:

> *We are studying what makes speech sound natural or unnatural. . . . "Naturalness" will not be defined for you. Make your rating on how natural or unnatural the speech sounds to you.*

A number of studies (Ingham, Gow, & Costello, 1985a; Kalinowski, Noble, Armson, & Stuart, 1994; Martin & Haroldson, 1992; Metz, Schiavetti & Sacco, 1990; Schiavetti, Martin, Haroldson & Metz, 1994; Whitehead et al., 1993) have used these instructions verbatim or in slightly modified form. Ingham, Martin, Haroldson, Onslow, and Leney (1985b, p. 49) instructed a group of talkers who were attempting to modify their own speech naturalness in response to listener feedback (where feedback display indicated that 1 = natural and 9 = unnatural sounding speech) by stating:

> You will not be told how to make your speech sound more natural to the listener. You must discover for yourself how to keep the display numbers as close to 1 as possible.

Finn and Ingham (1994, p. 339) instructed talkers to rate how their speech felt to them:

> We would like you to make judgments at 30-second intervals about how much attention you feel you are paying to the way you are speaking.

and how it sounded to them:

> We would like you to make judgments at 30-second intervals about how natural you think your speech sounds to a listener.

A tacit assumption in perceived speech naturalness research, then, appears to be that listeners and speakers will use their own internal standards concerning what sounds and feels natural. However, it might be appropriate to consider both internal standards of listeners and speakers and external standards imposed on them by experimenters in attempting a definition of speech naturalness. For example, Gerratt, Kreiman, Antonanzas-Barroso, and Berke (1993) compared internal (observer-generated) and external (experimenter-generated) standards used by observers in judging voice quality (vocal roughness) and examined the influence of external standards on reliability and drifting of the absolute values of voice quality ratings. Experienced listeners (speech pathologists and otolaryngologists) were asked to judge the vocal roughness of synthetic stimuli that were systematically varied in voicing source amplitude and noise source amplitude to simulate a range of vocal roughness. The judgments were made under one of two conditions: (1) listeners using their own internal standards of roughness with an "unanchored" five-point equal-appearing interval scale, or (2)

using an external standard of roughness with an "anchored" five-point equal-appearing interval scale on which examples of roughness at the five points were presented to the listeners. Listeners provided with the external standard showed significantly better interrater agreement, higher reliability, and less drift toward more severe roughness ratings over time than the listeners who used their own internal standards on an unanchored scale. In light of these advantages to external standards for vowel roughness judgments, it might be useful to develop a preliminary definition of the construct of speech naturalness and to study the influence of an external definition on the ratings of observers who are asked to scale speech naturalness.

The adjective "natural," derived from the Latin word *naturalis*, meaning "of nature," has fourteen definitions in *Webster's New Collegiate Dictionary*. Among those fourteen definitions, the sense of the term "natural" that may approximate what we have been trying to measure over the last ten years is probably definition thirteen: "true to nature; marked by easy simplicity and freedom from artificiality, affectation, or constraint; having a form or appearance found in nature." This definition connotes a perception by the agent or observer of (1) a customary and inconspicuous behavior, and (2) an economy of effort in the emission of the behavior.

We do not suggest at this point that a dictionary definition of speech naturalness be imposed as an external standard for observers to use, but, rather, offer this preliminary notion to prompt future research on the consequences of judges' usage of different internal and external definitions of speech naturalness. It is unclear at present what the source of a definition for speech naturalness should be. Perhaps the impetus will come from speech science research on physiological characteristics of natural speech or perhaps from naive listeners' reports of what they believe sounds natural. Until experimenters have evidence of the value of a consistently used external definition of speech naturalness, however, the concept of speech naturalness will probably continue to be defined on an individual, ad hoc basis by observers using their own internal standards.

SCALING PROCEDURES FOR MEASUREMENT OF SPEECH NATURALNESS

Martin et al. (1984) completed the first serious research attempt to have observers use a quantitative scale to judge the "naturalness" of speech samples from stutterers and nonstutterers, and several subsequent experiments have employed their naturalness scaling procedure to study a variety of issues in stuttering treatment (e.g., Finn & Ingham, 1994; Ingham et al., 1985a; Ingham, Ingham, Onslow, & Finn, 1989; Ingham et al., 1985b; Ingham & Onslow, 1985; Martin & Haroldson, 1992; Metz et al., 1990; Runyan, Bell, & Prosek, 1990; Schiavetti et al., 1994). In their 1984 paper, Martin et al. demonstrated the utility of a 9-point interval rating scale for the judgment of speech naturalness by unsophisticated listeners. The raters demonstrated satisfactory interrater reliability, interrater agreement, and consistency. They judged the speech of ten stutterers speaking typically and of ten stutterers using stutter-free speech under delayed auditory feedback (DAF) as sounding significantly more unnatural than the speech of ten nonstutterers. Ingham et al. (1985a) followed up the Martin et al. (1984) study with data comparing treated stutterers and nonstutterers and reported that the treated stutterers were judged as significantly more unnatural sounding than the nonstutterers. Both of these studies presented only audio recordings to listeners for judgment of naturalness. Subsequent studies by Martin and Haroldson (1992) and by Schiavetti et al. (1994) demonstrated that observers could make reliable naturalness judgments when presented with audiovisual recordings of speech samples. Martin and Haroldson (1992) found that, for stuttered speech samples, the judges rated the audiovisual samples as somewhat more unnatural than the audio portion of the same sample, suggesting that the scaled dimension of speech naturalness for audiovisual samples may be influenced by both visible variables and audible variables present in the samples.

All of the above studies have employed the speech naturalness scale originally developed by Martin et al. (1984). This scale is a 9-point equal-appearing interval scale presented to observers in the following format:

1	2	3	4	5	6	7	8	9
Highly Natural								Highly Unnatural

Judges are instructed to mark the number 1 on the scale if the speech sounds "highly natural," to mark the number 9 on the scale if the speech sounds "highly unnatural," or to mark the appropriate number in between if the speech sample sounds somewhere between highly natural and highly unnatural. Since lower numbers indicate greater naturalness and higher numbers on the scale indicate greater unnaturalness, the scale is, in a sense, a scale of degree of perceived unnaturalness. As long as the values on the scale are kept consistent across studies, there is no serious problem with the validity of scaling the inverse characteristic of "unnaturalness." As Stevens (1975, p. 123) stated:

> On some kinds of continua it may not be obvious just which end is up, so to say. When you rub your finger on a series of different grades of emery cloth or sandpaper, for example, do you experience roughness or smoothness? And when you squeeze a rubber sample, is it hardness or softness that commands attention? There are several such continua on which we may find it almost as natural to judge in terms of one attribute as its opposite.

Stevens (1975, p. 123–126) reviewed the psychophysical literature on the scaling of several inverse attributes to determine which attribute is the primary and which is the inverse in a pair, and which is easier for observers to judge. This work has not been done with speech naturalness and may be a fruitful avenue for future research that may aid in the definition of perceived speech naturalness.

In addition to the scaling of perceived naturalness by listeners, speakers have also been asked to scale how natural their speech sounds and feels to themselves. Ingham et al. (1989) demonstrated that stutterers could modify the naturalness of their speech and produce reliable ratings of how natural their speech sounded to themselves and that these ratings were generally comparable to ratings of other listeners, especially for speech that was judged more unnatural on the scale. When trying to make their speech sound more natural, however, the stutterers were able to recognize differences in their own speech naturalness by listening for unusual prosody or prolongation, although these subtle changes in speech naturalness went undetected by independent listeners. Finn and Ingham (1994) investigated stutterers' self-ratings of how natural their speech sounded and how natural they felt about the amount of attention they were paying to the way they were speaking. In general, stutterers could produce reasonably reliable self-ratings of speech naturalness. Ratings were more reliable when made while listening to their previously recorded speech than when made while actually speaking, and the stutterers could reliably differentiate between how natural their speech felt and sounded. Evidence for the validity of the self-ratings was demonstrated by significant covariance of speech naturalness, stuttering frequency, and syllable counts across several rhythmic stimulation conditions that varied systematically in patterns of stimulus on- and off-times.

RELIABILITY OF SPEECH NATURALNESS MEASURES

Several studies have reported on the reliability of perceived speech naturalness. Martin et al. (1984), Martin and Haroldson (1992), Metz et al. (1990), and Schiavetti et al. (1994) have reported intraclass correlations (Ebel, 1951) indicating substantial reliability for group mean ratings of listeners judging speech naturalness under a variety of conditions. These conditions included audio and audiovisual stimulus presentation; speech samples of stutterers, nonstutterers, and stutterers speaking under DAF; and experimental tasks such as oral reading, picture description, and spontaneous speaking. In

general, the reliability coefficients for group mean ratings were substantial and were higher than those for average individual raters as is consistent with the psychometric literature on the reliability of ratings (Guilford, 1954). These results indicate that we can expect the group mean ratings in research studies to be more consistent than individual listener ratings gathered under clinical conditions.

In addition to these correlational studies of rater reliability, a number of studies have examined rater agreement. Kreiman, Gerratt, Kempster, Erman, and Berke (1993, pp. 22–26) provide an extensive discussion of the difference between agreement and reliability:

> Listeners are in agreement to the extent that they make exactly the same judgments about the voices rated. Ratings are reliable when the relationship of one rated voice to another is constant (i.e., when voice ratings are parallel or correlated), although the absolute rating may differ from listener to listener (p. 22).

Agreement data should be analyzed to describe both intrarater agreement (what some authors term "consistency" or "test-retest" agreement) and interrater agreement. Martin et al. (1984) presented an extensive evaluation of both intrarater and interrater agreement in their original report of the development of the scale. Their interrater results for audio stimulus presentation indicated that approximately one-third of the 4350 judgments made by the listeners of the different speech samples were identical, about three-quarters were within ±1 scale value, about 95 percent were within ±3 scale points, and all were within ±4 scale points. Their intrarater results for test-retest analysis were slightly better, with about 45 to 50 percent identical, 85-90 percent within ±1 scale value, 97 to 99 percent within ±3 scale points, and 99 to 100 percent within ±4 scale points. Martin and Haroldson (1992) reported similar results for audiovisual stimulus presentation and concluded:

> Although the levels of interrater agreement reported to date are quite high, it should be noted that sufficient interrater disagreement exists so that the

use of a single rater (clinician) to assign absolute naturalness scale values to a single stutterer is a questionable procedure.

This conclusion regarding interrater agreement is consistent with the findings cited above regarding the intraclass correlational analysis of reliability. Mean ratings of a group of observers demonstrate sufficient reliability and agreement for use in research studies of speech naturalness; individual ratings do not. Future research needs to consider the effects of practice, training, and feedback on the reliability and inter- and intrarater agreement of individual ratings.

Other potential effects that may influence rater reliability on a speech naturalness scale have been examined by Onslow, Adams, and Ingham (1992a) and Onslow, Hayes, Hutchins, and Newman (1992b). Onslow et al. (1992a) investigated intrarater reliability of unsophisticated and sophisticated raters who judged speech samples of different speakers at various times during a treatment program. The intrarater and interrater agreement indices for the unsophisticated raters were statistically equivalent to those of the sophisticated raters. Intraclass correlation coefficients, however, indicated a slight superiority of the sophisticated group in their reliability.

Onslow et al. (1992a) also examined the potential effects on judgment reliability of the length of the sample presented to the raters. Significantly higher intrarater agreements were associated with sample lengths of 60 seconds versus samples of 15 and 30 seconds. Onslow et al. (1992b) found that the reliability of speech naturalness judgments using the Martin et al. (1984) scale were stable across different types of speech samples. Their examination of mean speech naturalness scores over multiple listening conditions indicated no differences between conversational and monologue samples.

Martin and Haroldson (1992) have summarized the reliability and agreement data from a number a studies and reached the following conclusions:

1. Group ratings of stutterer speech samples have a high degree of reliability.

2. Group ratings of nonstutterer speech samples are considerably less reliable, although satisfactory for most purposes.
3. Individual rater reliability is marginally satisfactory for stutterer samples but is very low for nonstutterer samples.
4. Although interrater agreement is high, there is sufficient interrater disagreement to make questionable the use of a single rater.
5. Intrarater agreement for groups of judges is sufficient for group studies.
6. Individual rater naturalness judgments can be made with reasonable intrarater consistency for a stuttering subject over time.
7. The absolute scale values of ratings made by one observer may not agree closely with those made by a different observer.

These conclusions imply that we may be reasonably confident about the absolute scale values of group mean judgments, but not the absolute values of individual rater judgments. We may, however, be confident about the *relative* scale values of individual raters who have demonstrated previous consistency (i.e., high intrarater agreement on test-retest tasks).

VALIDITY OF SPEECH NATURALNESS MEASURES

Several sources of evidence that relate to theoretical predictions support the validity of measurements of perceived speech naturalness. First, a valid speech naturalness scale should be sensitive to changes in speech under conditions that disrupt the natural flow of speech production. In the original Martin et al. (1984) study, for example, their speech naturalness scale differentiated between the speech of stutterers speaking typically, stutterers speaking under DAF, and nonstutterers. In addition, Martin and Haroldson (1992) demonstrated that both audio and audiovisual judgments of speech naturalness discriminated between the speech of stutterers and nonstutterers in the expected direction (i.e., more unnatural speech for stutterers). Both of these studies reported strong correlations between stuttering frequency and perceived unnaturalness of speech, and Martin and Haroldson (1992) also reported strong correlations between ratings of stuttering severity and perceived unnaturalness of speech. Ingham et al. (1985a) and Metz et al. (1990) reported differences between the speech naturalness of treated stutterers and nonstutterers. When viewed collectively, these studies indicate a substantial degree of construct validity for the speech naturalness scale by virtue of its ability to distinguish speech that intuitively should sound less natural because it is produced under an artificial listening condition (DAF), because its temporal nature has been altered (post-treatment speech), or because it has been produced nonfluently (stuttering).

Second, a valid speech naturalness scale should reflect logical expectations regarding the perception of naturalness by both the agent and the observer of the behavior. For example, when a speaker is instructed to change parameters like speech rate, listeners ought to perceive changes in speech naturalness. Ingham et al. (1989) presented a partial validation of the scale in their study of the relationships between stutterers' self-perception of speech naturalness and independent listeners' ratings of the same speech samples. When instructed to make their speech sound more unnatural, stutterers made changes in their speech that caused independent listeners to judge their speech as sounding more unnatural. When instructed to make their speech sound more natural, however, the stutterers were unable to influence judges to rate them as more natural, despite the changes in their own self-ratings toward more natural. This result may be more a function of the subtlety of the speech changes (making them detectable by speakers but not by listeners) rather than a function of the invalidity of the naturalness scale. Future research on scale validation needs to examine the effects of more specific instructions to speakers to make speech sound more or less natural (e.g., change overall rate, specific segment durations, pause duration, pitch variability, syllable stress pattern) and the effects of these changes on perceived speech naturalness.

Third, a valid speech naturalness scale should reflect logical expectations regarding the perception of the naturalness of both the sound and the feeling of speech production. In addressing this issue, Finn and Ingham (1994) inferred validity of self-ratings of speech naturalness on three bases of evidence. First, comparisons of data regarding natural feeling and natural sounding self-ratings indicated that speakers used different criteria for these judgments and based feeling naturalness on ability to monitor the process of formulating and producing speech. Second, comparison of on-line and off-line self-ratings indicated good agreement of these judgments across conditions that altered their speech. Third, changes in rhythmic stimulation speaking conditions systematically influenced listeners' ratings of naturalness in the expected directions. Future research on scale validation should examine the effects of more specific instructions to speakers to make speech feel more or less natural to themselves and the effects of these changes on perceived speech naturalness.

In addition to the empirical confirmation of the predictions described above, psychophysical evidence may be used to help validate the form of a specific scale of speech naturalness. Stevens (1968, 1974, 1975) has discussed the validity of specific interval and ratio scaling procedures for the measurement of a variety of physical and social dimensions and has issued cautions regarding the use of equal-appearing interval scales to measure continua that observers cannot easily partition into equal intervals. Metz et al. (1990) addressed the issue of the construct validity of specific scaling procedures used to measure speech naturalness in relation to the psychophysical predictions of Stevens' (1975) theoretical constructs regarding prothetic (additive or quantitative) and metathetic (substitutive or qualitative) continua. Stevens (1975) demonstrated that observers can easily partition a metathetic continuum like pitch into equal intervals using an equal appearing interval (EAI) scale and that the resultant interval scale values have a linear relation to direct magnitude estimates (DME) of the same stimuli. Therefore, either EAI or DME could be used as a valid procedure to scale a metathetic continuum. However, Stevens (1975) has shown that observers cannot achieve a linear partition of a prothetic dimension like loudness because of a systematic bias toward subdividing the lower end of the continuum into smaller intervals than those at the upper end of the continuum. Stevens (1975) concluded that EAI scaling is not valid for measuring a prothetic continuum because the intervals do not demonstrate the equality necessary for the scaling procedure to subdivide the continuum evenly along the range of stimulus values. The large body of Stevens's psychophysical research has indicated that his constructs regarding the scaling of prothetic and metathetic continua apply not only to the scaling of responses to unidimensional metric stimuli, such as sound intensity or frequency, but also to the scaling of responses to nonmetric stimuli as seen in measurements of complex social dimensions such as the perceived seriousness of crimes, aesthetic value of art works, or status of occupations (Stevens, 1966, 1968, 1974).

Metz et al. (1990) used Stevens's method to ascertain if perceived speech naturalness is a prothetic or metathetic continuum by asking observers to assign speech naturalness scale values to audiotaped speech samples from treated stutterers and nonstutterers. Half of the listeners judged speech naturalness using the 9-point interval scale developed by Martin et al. (1984), and the other half made judgments of perceived naturalness using a DME procedure. The graphical and mathematical analysis of Metz et al. (1990) revealed a linear relationship between the two sets of data that is characteristic of a metathetic continuum, leading to the conclusion that either interval scaling or direct magnitude estimation may be used for the valid measurement of speech naturalness. Schiavetti et al. (1994) reached the same conclusion regarding judgments of speech naturalness from audiovisual recordings of speech samples of stutterers and nonstutterers.

RELATIONSHIPS BETWEEN PHYSICAL SPEECH CHARACTERISTICS AND PERCEPTUAL MEASURES OF SPEECH NATURALNESS

Although a great deal is known about physiological and acoustical characteristics of normal speech production, little information has been published on physiological and acoustical correlates of the perceived naturalness of disordered speech produced by stutterers before, during, or after treatment. Such information would be of obvious importance for the description of disordered speech, for the explanation of what makes speech sound (or feel) natural for stutterers in various stages of treatment, and for setting criteria for improvement as a result of treatment. In addition, information on the relationships between physical characteristics of speech production and naturalness could aid in understanding why some stutterers relapse after treatment. The reluctance of some stutterers to maintain a fluency enhancement technique that creates speech that feels or sounds unnatural may be explained by an understanding of the physiological basis of the feeling of unnaturalness and the acoustical basis of the sound of unnaturalness. As Onslow et al. (1992b, p. 274) stated:

> The issue of speech quality in stuttering management is important for a number of reasons . . . including especially the suspicion that unusual speech quality may contribute to the clinical problem of post-treatment relapse.

As a first approximation to measuring the relation of speech production characteristics to perceived naturalness, Martin et al. (1984) reported moderate negative correlations between speech rate in words-per-minute and naturalness ratings for nonstutterers and stutterers speaking under DAF. The correlation was substantial, however, for stutterers speaking typically ($r = -0.83$). These results indicate that temporal characteristics of speech are important first candidates as variables that may influence perceived speech naturalness. Metz et al. (1990) studied acoustical dimensions of the perceived speech naturalness of non-stutterers and treated stutterers. The treated stutterers had been rated as sounding significantly more unnatural than the nonstutterers. Their analysis of six acoustic measures revealed significant differences between nonstutterers and treated stutterers on three temporal characteristics: voice onset time (VOT), vowel duration, and sentence duration. The VOT measure emerged from a multiple regression analysis as the single best predictor of judged speech naturalness for a picture description task and the sentence duration variable emerged as the single best predictor of judged speech naturalness for a paragraph reading task. The correlations between the acoustic characteristics and perceived naturalness were modest (multiple R's of .679 and .637, respectively for VOT and sentence duration) and left a reasonable amount of variance unaccounted for.

These results, linking specific temporal differences to differences in perceived speech naturalness, suggest that studies of physiologic and acoustical correlates of speech naturalness may be a fruitful avenue for future research. Such research may enhance our understanding of what physical parameters make speech sound and feel natural and how fluency enhancing treatment techniques may modify these parameters.

CLINICAL APPLICATION OF NATURALNESS MEASURES

There are several ways in which the measurement of speech naturalness can be applied directly to the clinical enterprise. The measurement of speech naturalness can be readily adopted (1) as an index of posttreatment status, (2) as an instrument for follow-up evaluation, (3) as an index employed for continued modification of speech during treatment, and (4) as an integral component of pretreatment evaluative protocols. Curlee (1993, p.322), in fact, has referred to such use of speech naturalness measurement as "basic" and "obligatory" in the assessment of stuttering.

The use of speech naturalness scores to assess a stutterer's posttreatment speech has obvious ap-

peal as an adjunct to measures of stuttering frequency and scaled stuttering severity. In the same vein, speech naturalness measures can be useful in follow-up evaluation to determine the success of long-term maintenance of treatment gains. Whereas stuttering frequency and scaled stuttering severity measures indicate changes in overt nonfluency, speech naturalness measures contribute information about the quality of fluency that is achieved by the reduction in number of stutterings. Some stutterers may reduce their number of stutterings at the expense of a speech pattern that is stutter-free but not really fluent.

Another compelling reason to consider speech naturalness is related to its potential in feedback during stuttering treatment. Pretreatment naturalness scores might serve as baseline measures in treatments that use naturalness ratings as a functional contingency. Ingham and Onslow (1985) and Ingham et al. (1985b; 1989) have presented clinician-judged naturalness scores to stutterers during prolonged speech or speech rate control treatment regimens. The general findings of these studies suggested that speech naturalness was improved and stuttering was maintained at near zero frequencies by presenting clinician feedback to the stutterers. Although the stutterers' ratings of how natural their speech felt and sounded were not always congruent with independent listener judgments (Ingham et al., 1989), the overall efficacy of such feedback suggests great future promise. An obvious application in future research would be the on-line comparison of the efficacy of different treatment procedures using speech naturalness ratings as another criterion for measuring improvement.

The importance of pretreatment measurements of naturalness is only beginning to emerge in the research literature. Early indications are that pretreatment stuttering severity may have complex interactions with both pretreatment and posttreatment naturalness ratings. Onslow et al. (1992b), for example, reported a significant positive relationship between pretreatment stuttering severity and posttreatment naturalness ratings. The posttreatment naturalness scale values of the most severe stutterers were approximately two scale values higher than those of the least severe stutterers. In addition, Franken, Boves, Peters, and Webster (1992) reported that the speech naturalness scores of thirty-two severe stutterers remained essentially unchanged from pretreatment to posttreatment. Kalinowski et al. (1994) reported that the posttreatment naturalness ratings of stutter-free speech of both mild and severe stutterers were significantly more unnatural than their pretreatment ratings and that severe stutterers had significantly higher posttreatment naturalness scores (i.e., more unnatural speech) than the mild stutterers. But, in contrast, Runyan et al. (1990) reported no pretreatment severity influences on posttreatment naturalness scores.

Such conflicting findings invite further investigation regarding the specific relationship between pretreatment stuttering severity and posttreatment naturalness scores, including consideration of possible sampling differences among the studies, differential effects on posttreatment speech naturalness of different types of treatment programs, differences in internal standards of naturalness judges, and interactions among these factors. It is critical to understand why some stutterers may sound as unnatural after treatment while using stutter-free speech as they sounded when they stuttered before treatment. It is also important to determine if more severe stutterers sound more unnatural after treatment than less severe stutterers do. Finally, we must determine whether milder stutterers emerge from treatment stutter-free and more natural sounding whereas severe stutterers emerge from treatment stutter-free but sounding as or more unnatural than they did prior to treatment.

FUTURE RESEARCH DIRECTIONS

The measurement of speech naturalness has significant potential for further investigation. A dozen specific topics that are immediately apparent may be grouped together under a handful of general issues that are ripe for productive exploration.

First is the general refinement of the speech naturalness scale. Topics for future research on scale refinement include: (1) definition of naturalness; (2) the influence of instructions on observers' performance; (3) the effect of training on listeners' reliability, interrater agreement, and intrarater consistency; and (4) the use of alternative scaling procedures.

As discussed earlier, experimenters have not defined speech naturalness for observers. Future research needs to compare internal and external standards in speech naturalness judgments as Gerratt et al. (1993) have done for voice quality judgments. To understand how the concept of speech naturalness is used by observers, it is important to study criteria used by different observers to define naturalness for themselves in making their judgments. For example, after judging a set of speech samples, judges could be surveyed to develop a list of speech characteristics that they used in judging speech naturalness. It would be important to ascertain what criteria observers believed they used without the influence of an external standard imposed on them by the experimenter. Development of a definition of speech naturalness might start with the "ears of the beholders" so to speak, rather than writing a definition first and imposing it on listeners. An important variable to be examined in analyzing observer generated characteristics would be the type of speech samples that observers had been exposed to. Would listeners who judged stuttered versus nonstuttered speech differ in the speech characteristics identified from listeners who heard treated stutterers versus nonstuttered speech? This possibility arises because both stutterers and treated stutterers have been rated as more unnatural than nonstutterers, yet the speech of treated versus untreated stutterers may differ markedly. In addition, it would be important to examine what speech characteristics would be identified by observers who audited the speech of both stutterers and treated stutterers before being asked to list judgment criteria. In other words, an important research question concerns the influence of listening experience on the speech characteristics that observers may select in making judgments of speech naturalness. Gerratt et al. (1993) have addressed this question in their analysis of the unit of voice quality judgments with internal versus external standards when judges are exposed first to mild and then to moderate vocal roughness samples. Their results indicated more influence of order and carry-over effects on judgments made with internal than with external standards.

Another question concerns whether improvement in the reliability of the naturalness scale would result from attempts to define naturalness for observers, incorporate a definition into instructions, and train listeners to use the definition consistently in judgment trials over time. Such improvement might be most noticeable in interrater agreement and could lead to the development of a training program for making the absolute values of individual ratings more useful for clinical and research studies. For example, an individual could be trained to emulate a previously gathered set of group mean ratings of the naturalness of a large set of speech samples. Gerratt et al. (1993) found that voice quality judgments made with an externally imposed standard were more reliable and showed more intra- and interrater agreement than those made by observers using their own internal standards. Applying their research method to the study of speech naturalness would be an important step toward the improvement of speech naturalness scaling procedures.

Some experimenters may raise objections to use of external standards to train listeners, however. It could be argued that what is perceived to be natural might best be left to the internal standards of the observers. As Young (1969, p. 135) has said:

> A measurement of a speech disorder is primarily a perceptual event, and the observer's response necessarily represents the "final" validation for any measurements.

Objections raised against observer training because it would impose an external definition of speech naturalness on observers might be somewhat reduced if the definition were based on criteria originally suggested by listeners. One problem, however, is that listeners might use widely diverse criteria in setting internal standards for the definition of speech naturalness. For example, Kreiman, Gerratt, and Precoda (1990) found that experienced clinicians and naive listeners used different criteria for judging voice quality and that naive listeners showed more similarity among themselves than the clinicians in the perceptual strategies they adopted for judging voice quality.

Similar problems in measurement of speech intelligibility of deaf persons by experienced and inexperienced listeners have been studied by Monsen (1978) and Boothroyd (1985). Boothroyd devised a novel procedure for eliminating the experienced/inexperienced listener differences with a forced-choice phoneme-identification intelligibility test. Future research should explore experienced/inexperienced listener differences in voice quality and in speech naturalness judgments. If experience is found to be a variable affecting naturalness judgment criteria, several questions must be considered. First is whether short term training can reduce the difference between experienced and inexperienced listeners as Monsen (1978) found with deaf speech intelligibility. Second is what different criteria may be used by experienced and inexperienced listeners. Understanding the ways in which experienced and inexperienced listeners may differ in their naturalness criteria may reveal important information about the identification of stuttering and the evaluation of stutterers' pre- and posttreatment speech quality.

These results raise questions concerning what group of listeners would provide the most useful criteria for defining speech naturalness: the clinicians who treat the stutterers or the everyday listeners encountered by the stutterers in real life. Future research needs to compare experienced versus inexperienced and sophisticated versus unsophisticated judges to ascertain if they use similar criteria in setting internal standards for the definition of speech naturalness. Experienced versus inexperienced judges differ in the degree to which they have had long-term experience listening to stuttering (e.g., speech pathologists and family members of stutterers versus general public) in everyday life and also in the degree to which they have had short-term experience making naturalness judgments (e.g., persons with no judgment experience versus persons who have served in experiments for a certain number of hours). Sophisticated versus unsophisticated judges differ in the degree to which they have knowledge of stuttering and speech production (e.g., speech pathologists versus general public). Onslow et al. (1992a) found statistically significant differences (albeit of limited clinical value) in absolute scale values of speech naturalness assigned to stutterers in treatment by sophisticated versus unsophisticated listeners. The mean difference between the two groups of listeners was only about one-third of a scale value on the 9-point scale. It should be pointed out, however, that their Figure 1 indicates that in some specific conditions of the experiment, unsophisticated listeners judged speech samples to be as much as 2 full scale values higher in unnaturalness than the sophisticated judges did. These results indicate that more comparison is needed of sophisticated and unsophisticated judges to determine under what conditions their naturalness judgments are similar or different. In addition to these findings regarding the absolute scale values assigned by sophisticated and unsophisticated judges, Onslow et al. (1992a) reported that the reliability, interrater agreement, and intrarater consistency were reasonably comparable for the two groups of listeners. Further research is necessary to confirm these results regarding both absolute scale values and reliability and agreement of naturalness ratings and to extend the comparison of listener groups to a variety of listening conditions and types of speech samples in order to study the influence of both listener experience and listener sophistication on speech naturalness judgments.

Exploration of alternative scaling procedures such as sensory modality matching (Dawson, 1974), absolute magnitude estimation (Zwislocki & Goodman, 1980), or what Zwislocki (1991) has recently termed "natural measurement" might also be productive for further validation of the currently employed scale. A large body of evidence has been accumulated over the years (Stevens, 1975) regarding the use of magnitude

production and cross-modality matching procedures for the validation of scale values of a number of social opinion type variables that are similar to speech naturalness judgments. Employment of such ratio scaling techniques could be effective in bolstering the validity of speech naturalness measurements.

A second general issue concerns the identification of parameters that make speech sound and feel natural. The relationship of physiological speech characteristics (e.g., measures of air flow and pressure, force and velocity of articulator movements, respiratory patterns, and laryngeal timing) to the perceived feeling of natural speech is a critical area of research for the description of posttreatment speech patterns and the possible explanation of posttreatment relapse. Although there have been comparisons of self-ratings versus listener ratings (Ingham et al., 1989) and of on-line versus off-line ratings of naturalness (Finn & Ingham, 1994), there have not been any specific comparisons of autophonic versus extraphonic listening for speech naturalness along the lines of the work of Lane, Catania, and Stevens (1961) on perceived vocal loudness. The relative contributions of bone conduction and air conduction to the self-perception of naturalness by the speaker may be interesting to explore in this regard. Another specific topic concerns the relationship of the feeling of speech naturalness to self-perceived physiological parameters like self-ratings of articulatory effort (Parnell & Amerman, 1977) or of vocal effort (Netsell, 1973).

Research is also needed to explore the acoustical characteristics that make speech sound natural and to explore the relationships between the feeling and the sound of naturalness in both physical and perceptual terms. Are the physiological parameters that make speech feel natural the same as those that make it sound natural? Which physiological parameters produce the specific acoustical results that make speech sound more natural? Are there physiological and acoustical parameters of unnatural feeling or sounding speech that are not well tolerated by posttreatment stutterers who demonstrate relapse? These and many other questions may help us to understand the posttreatment speech of stutterers and to explain the possible influence of the feel and sound of naturalness on relapse.

A third general issue concerns the identification of visible parameters of speech naturalness and the interaction of visible parameters with audible parameters influencing observers' judgments. Martin and Haroldson (1992) found that audiovisual presentation yielded higher (i.e., more unnatural) ratings than audio presentation of speech samples of stutterers but not of nonstutterers. An important question concerns the influence of visible characteristics on the judged speech naturalness of posttreatment stutterers. Future research needs to use a research design similar to the one employed by Metz et al. (1990) to study the influence of visible as well as audible characteristics of speakers on perceived naturalness. Such research should employ a systematic approach to the measurement of visible nonspeech behaviors such as the facial action coding system developed by Ekman (1982) and used by Conture and Kelly (1991) to study young stutterers' nonspeech behaviors. Multiple regression analysis could be used to predict speech naturalness from a combination of audible and visible characteristics measured in audio-videotaped speech samples.

A fourth general issue concerns the future use of speech naturalness measures in evaluating the effectiveness of stuttering treatment. Published reports reviewed above have demonstrated the potential utility of speech naturalness measures for on-line modification of speech and for the assessment of posttreatment speech. There is great potential for the use of speech naturalness measures to supplement traditional measures of stuttering frequency, speech rate, and perceived stuttering severity in future research comparing the relative efficacy of various approaches to stuttering treatment (cf., Curlee, 1993). In addition, if future research can identify physiological correlates of natural feeling and sounding speech, it might be possible to discover the variables that predict posttreatment relapse. The ability to predict relapse in advance would be an important first step toward the prevention of relapse by follow-through treatment.

A fifth general issue forces a broader view of speech naturalness as one measurable aspect of speech quality: What other areas of speech research could profit from application of the work reviewed in this chapter? Measurement of perceived speech naturalness and of the acoustical correlates of naturalness has application in the evaluation of the quality of synthetic speech, speech produced during simultaneous manual communication, and speech produced by persons with disorders other than fluency problems. Naturalness measurements might find application in the evaluation of the efficacy of treatment procedures for voice disorders, phonological processing problems, prosodic difficulties associated with deafness or brain injury, or cleft palate. Van Riper's long held notion that "speech is defective when it is conspicuous, unintelligible, or unpleasant" (Van Riper & Emerick, 1984, p. 34) certainly has room to accommodate the concept of speech naturalness within the construct of defectiveness.

SUMMARY

This chapter reviewed literature on the measurement of speech naturalness as a variable of interest in stuttering research and treatment. The topics discussed included definition of speech naturalness, measurement principles, specific scaling procedures for the measurement of speech naturalness, reliability and validity of speech naturalness measures, relationships between instrumental measures of physical speech characteristics and perceptual measures of speech naturalness, and clinical application of naturalness measures. Future research directions are suggested regarding refinement of speech naturalness measurement procedures, identification of parameters that make speech sound and feel natural, interaction of audible and visible speech characteristics that influence perception of naturalness, use of speech naturalness measures in evaluating stuttering treatment efficacy, and the application of speech naturalness measures to other areas of speech research.

REFERENCES

Boothroyd, A. (1985). Evaluation of speech production of the hearing impaired: Some benefits of forced-choice testing. *Journal of Speech and Hearing Research, 28,* 185–196.

Conture, E.G., & Kelly, E.M. (1991). Young stutterers' nonspeech behavior during stuttering. *Journal of Speech and Hearing Research, 34,* 1041–1056.

Curlee, R.F. (1993). Evaluating treatment efficacy for adults: Assessment of stuttering disability. *Journal of Fluency Disorders, 18,* 319–331.

Dawson, W.A. (1974). An assessment of ratio scales of opinion by sensory modality matching. In H.R. Moskowitz, B. Scharf, & J.C. Stevens (Eds.), *Sensation and measurement: Papers in honor of S. S. Stevens* (pp. 49–60). Dordrecht-Holland: D. Reidel.

Ebel, R.L. (1951). Estimation of the reliability of ratings. *Psychometrika, 16,* 407–424.

Ekman, P. (1982). Methods for measuring facial action. In K. Scherer & P. Ekman (Eds.), *Handbook of methods in nonverbal behavior research* (pp. 45–90). Cambridge: Cambridge University Press.

Finn, P., & Ingham, R.J. (1994). Stutterers' self-ratings of how natural speech sounds and feels. *Journal of Speech and Hearing Research, 37,* 326–340.

Franken, C.M., Boves, L., Peter, H.F.M., & Webster, R.L. (1992). Perceptual evaluation of speech before and after fluency shaping therapy. *Journal of Fluency Disorders, 17,* 223–241.

Gerratt, B.R., Kreiman, J., Antonanzas-Barroso, N., & Berke, G.S. (1993). Comparing internal and external standards in voice quality. *Journal of Speech and Hearing Research, 36,* 14–20.

Guilford, J.P. (1954). *Psychometric methods.* New York: McGraw-Hill.

Hixon, T.J., & Abbs, J.H. (1980). Normal speech production. In T.J. Hixon, L.D. Shriberg, & J.H. Saxman (Eds.), *Introduction to communication disorders* (pp. 43–87). Englewood Cliffs, N.J.: Prentice-Hall.

Ingham, R.J., Gow, M., & Costello, J.M. (1985a). Stuttering and speech naturalness: Some additional data. *Journal of Speech and Hearing Disorders, 50,* 217–219.

Ingham, R.J., Ingham, J.C., Onslow, M., & Finn, P. (1989). Stutterers' self-ratings of speech naturalness: Assessing effects and reliability. *Journal of Speech and Hearing Research, 32,* 419–431.

Ingham, R.J., Martin, R., Haroldson, S.K., Onslow, M., & Leney, M. (1985b). Modification of listener-judged naturalness in the speech of stutterers. *Journal of Speech and Hearing Research, 28,* 495–504.

Ingham, R.J., & Onslow, M. (1985). Measurement and modification of speech naturalness during stuttering therapy. *Journal of Speech and Hearing Disorders, 50,* 261–281.

Kalinowski, J., Noble, S., Armson, J., & Stuart, A. (1994). Pretreatment and posttreatment speech naturalness ratings of adults with mild and severe stutterering. *American Journal of Speech-Language Pathology, 3,* 61–66.

Kreiman, J., Gerratt, B.R., Kempster, G.B., Erman, A., & Berke, G.S. (1993). Perceptual evaluation of voice quality: Review, tutorial, and a framework for future research. *Journal of Speech and Hearing Research, 36,* 21–40.

Kreiman, J., Gerratt, B.R., & Precoda, K. (1990). Listener experience and perception of voice quality. *Journal of Speech and Hearing Research, 33,* 103–115.

Lane, H.L., Catania, A.C., & Stevens, S.S. (1961). Voice level: Autophonic scale, perceived loudness, and effects of sidetone. *Journal of the Acoustical Society of America, 33,* 160–167.

Martin, R.R., Haroldson, S.K., & Triden, K.A. (1984). Stuttering and speech naturalness. *Journal of Speech and Hearing Disorders, 49,* 53–58.

Martin, R.R., & Haroldson, S.K. (1992). Stuttering and speech naturalness: Audio and audiovisual judgments. *Journal of Speech and Hearing Research, 35,* 521–528.

Metz, D.E., Schiavetti, N., & Sacco, P.R. (1990). Acoustic and psychophysical dimensions of the perceived speech naturalness of nonstutterers and posttreatment stutterers. *Journal of Speech and Hearing Disorders, 55,* 516–525.

Mirenda, P., & Beukelman, D.R. (1987). A comparison of speech synthesis intelligibility with listeners from three age groups. *Augmentative and Alternative Communication, 3,* 120–128.

Monsen, R.B. (1978). Toward measuring how well hearing impaired children speak. *Journal of Speech and Hearing Research, 21,* 197–219.

Netsell, R. (1973). Speech physiology. In F.D. Minifie, T.J. Hixon, & F. Williams (Eds.), *Normal aspects of speech, hearing, and language* (pp. 211–234). Englewood Cliffs, N.J.: Prentice-Hall.

Onslow, M., Adams, R., & Ingham, R.J. (1992a). Reliability of speech naturalness ratings of stuttered speech during treatment. *Journal of Speech and Hearing Research, 35,* 994–1001.

Onslow, M., Hayes, B., Hutchins, L., & Newman, D. (1992b). Speech naturalness and prolonged-speech treatments for stuttering: Further variables and data. *Journal of Speech and Hearing Research, 35,* 274–282.

Onslow, M., & Ingham, R.J. (1987). Speech quality measurement and the management of stuttering. *Journal of Speech and Hearing Disorders, 52,* 2–17.

Parnell, M. & Amerman, J.D. (1977). Subjective evaluation of articulatory effort. *Journal of Speech and Hearing Research, 20,* 644–652.

Runyan, C.M., Bell, J.N., & Prosek, R.A. (1990). Speech naturalness ratings of treated stutterers. *Journal of Speech and Hearing Disorders, 55,* 434–438.

Schiavetti, N., Martin, R.R., Haroldson, S.K., & Metz, D.E. (1994). Psychophysical analysis of audiovisual judgments of speech naturalness of nonstutterers and stutterers. *Journal of Speech and Hearing Research, 37,* 46–52.

Stevens, S.S. (1966). A metric for the social consensus. *Science, 151,* 530–541.

Stevens, S.S. (1968). Ratio scales of opinion. In D.K. Whitla (Ed.), *Handbook of measurement and assessment in behavioral sciences* (pp. 171–199). Reading, Mass.: Addison-Wesley.

Stevens, S.S. (1974). Perceptual magnitude and its measurement. In E.C. Carterette & M.P. Friedman (Eds.), *Handbook of perception* (Vol. II). New York: Academic Press.

Stevens, S.S. (1975). *Psychophysics.* New York: Wiley.

Thomas, L. (1979). *The medusa and the snail: More notes of a biology watcher.* New York: Viking.

Van Riper, C., & Emerick, L. (1984). *Speech correction* (7th Ed.). Englewood Cliffs, N.J.: Prentice-Hall.

Whitehead, R.L., Schiavetti, N., Whitehead, B., & Metz, D.E. (1993). *Simultaneous communication: Acoustic characteristics and speech naturalness.* Paper presented at American Speech-Language-Hearing Association Annual Convention, Anaheim, Calif.

Young, M.A. (1969). Observer agreement: Cumulative effects of rating many samples. *Journal of Speech and Hearing Research, 12,* 135–143.

Zwislocki, J.J. (1991). Natural measurement. In S.J. Bolanowski & G.A. Gescheider (Eds.), *Ratio scaling of psychological magnitude: In honor of the memory of S. S. Stevens* (pp. 18–26). Hillsdale, N.J.: Lawrence Erlbaum Associates.

Zwislocki, J.J., & Goodman, D.A. (1980). Absolute scaling of sensory magnitudes: A validation. *Perception and Psychophysics, 28,* 28–38.

SUGGESTED READINGS

Curlee, R.F. (1993). Evaluating treatment efficacy for adults: Assessment of stuttering disability. *Journal of Fluency Disorders, 18,* 319–331.

Martin, R.R., Haroldson, S.K., & Triden, K.A. (1984). Stuttering and speech naturalness. *Journal of Speech and Hearing Disorders, 49,* 53–58.

Metz, D.E., Schiavetti, N., & Sacco, P.R. (1990). Acoustic and psychophysical dimensions of the perceived speech naturalness of nonstutterers and posttreatment stutterers. *Journal of Speech and Hearing Disorders, 55,* 516–525.

Onslow, M., & Ingham, R.J. (1987). Speech quality measurement and the management of stuttering. *Journal of Speech and Hearing Disorders, 52,* 2–17.

Stevens, S.S. (1975). *Psychophysics.* New York: Wiley.

CHAPTER 21

SELF-MEASUREMENT AND EVALUATING STUTTERING TREATMENT EFFICACY

ROGER J. INGHAM
ANNE K. CORDES

INTRODUCTION

Current research on the nature and treatment of stuttering has been severely affected by at least three issues related to the definition and measurement of the disorder. First, the features that are necessary and sufficient to define normally fluent speech and to define stuttered speech have not been satisfactorily identified. Second, measurement validity and reliability are problematic for essentially all of the features suggested as important elements of stuttered speech. And third, the recommended procedures for evaluating the efficacy of stuttering treatment have become overwhelmingly complex, while prevailing notions about the nature of stuttering have become increasingly biological. The alarming result of this combination is that most recent studies of stuttering treatment seem to have been conducted without outcome evaluation procedures at all, and treatments are now being recommended with little or no empirical support.[1]

This chapter begins by discussing the problems with five features that have been used or suggested as those elements of stuttering that distinguish this disorder from normal speech. These features include the presence of disfluent moments or events in speech, abnormal speech rate, abnormal speech quality, the presence of abnormal speech-motor processes at a physiologic or neurophysiologic level, and an abnormal capacity to meet demands for fluency. As will become clear, none of these features, as currently defined and measured, can establish a necessary and sufficient difference between stuttered speech and normally fluent speech, or between persons who stutter and those who do not.

The second section of this chapter considers some of the problems inherent in attempting to define normal and abnormal fluency. Recent trends

ACKNOWLEDGMENTS: Preparation of this chapter was supported by grant number DC00060 awarded by the National Institutes of Health. This chapter is based on issues presented in a paper read to the First World Congress on Fluency Disorders, Munich, Germany, August 10, 1994. This paper was prepared while the second author was associated with the University of California, Santa Barbara. Special thanks are due to James Till and Ron Netsell for their suggestions regarding measurement of effort. We also thank Patrick Finn for his helpful comments on this chapter.

[1]A particularly troubling example of this problem is provided by a recent issue of *Language, Speech, and Hearing Services in the Schools* (April, 1995), which included many recommended treatment procedures. Most of these articles provided no data at all, and none provided any data that supported the efficacy of the recommended procedures. Other examples can be found among recent reports on the effects of botulinum toxin injections and other pharmacological treatments (see Brady, 1991; Ingham, 1993b).

away from measures of speech, toward measures of physiological events that may even be described as "subperceptual," appear to have led researchers away from considering stuttering as a disorder of human communication. Some of the disabilities that lead to stuttering are certainly neurological or physiological, but it seems equally true that the handicapping effects of stuttering lie at the level of speech output and the effects of that output on communicative interaction (see Prins, 1991). This chapter will argue that it is not physiological or neurological events that lead stutterers to seek treatment, but the handicapping effects of being unable to produce speech that they perceive as acceptably fluent for their own needs (cf. Baer, 1988, 1990; Perkins, 1990; Prins, 1991). The distinctive difference between normal fluency and stuttering, in other words, may be the speaker's lack of complaint in the former case and the speaker's self-judged problem with fluency in the latter—a possibility that suggests that self-judgments should play a central role in any clinically valid measurement procedure for stuttering.

The third section of this chapter, therefore, incorporates self-judgments of stuttering into one current three-factor model of treatment outcome evaluation. The three-factor model requires that treatment procedures be shown, first, to alter variables that are believed to be relevant in describing stuttering or differentiating it from normal fluency. The model then requires that these changes be measured in multiple speaking situations, and across some clinically meaningful period of time. All three of these factors, as will be argued below, could be significantly enhanced by the adoption of self-judgment procedures for measuring stuttering.

CURRENT STATUS: FIVE FEATURES PROPOSED AS DIFFERENTIATING BETWEEN STUTTERING AND NORMAL FLUENCY

The original attempts to apply behavioral treatments to stuttering identified only two features that appeared to require change: stuttering event frequency and speech rate (Andrews & Ingham,

1972). Many other features have since been proposed as relevant, and the history of stuttering measurement includes an expanding list of features that must be evaluated to determine whether treatment has produced normally fluent speech. The greatest problem with all five of the features discussed here, however, is that none has been shown to be incompatible with the occurrence of normal fluency (with the possible exception of stuttering event frequency). More importantly for the purposes of this chapter, none has been shown to be the source of complaint among persons who stutter.

Stuttering Frequency

The most common measure of stuttering frequency evaluates the number of certain types of behaviorally defined disfluencies, such as repetitions or prolongations, that are identified by a clinician or some other observer (e.g., Ryan, 1974; Wingate, 1964; see Cordes & Ingham, 1994a, for review). A second type of measure depends on a more global or perceptual definition of stuttering events or moments of stuttering (Johnson & Knott, 1936; Martin & Haroldson, 1969, 1979). Both measures are based on a concept of stuttering behaviors as discrete events that occur in the midst of otherwise perceptually normal speech, a concept that has dominated stuttering research and treatment throughout most of its history.

Despite the primacy of these measures, however, many challenges have been raised to the notion of stuttering as occasions of abnormal speech within otherwise normal speech. At a theoretic level, claims have been made that the boundary between the presence and absence of stuttering is artificial, either because the speaker's entire speech production system is dysfunctional (e.g., Smith, 1990) or because the definitive features of stuttering are experiential rather than observable (e.g., Perkins, 1990). There has always been some discomfort about stuttering event measures at a clinical level, because such measures do not include aspects of stutterers' speech such as word avoidance or slow speech rate; because they fail to reflect the magnitude or severity of individual events;

and because they provide only the roughest indication of overall severity of stuttering.

The most damaging challenges to the validity of observer-based stuttering event measurements come from reports that different clinicians and researchers disagree substantially in the number of stuttering events they identify in identical speech samples, and that they may be recording qualitatively different behaviors as stuttering (see Cordes, 1994b; Cordes & Ingham, 1995a; Ham, 1989; Ingham & Cordes, 1992; Kully & Boberg, 1988). Indeed, as the authors have observed (Cordes & Ingham, 1994a; Ingham & Cordes, 1992), the differences between counts reported by workers in different clinics may exceed the pre- and posttreatment differences reported in many therapy studies. Siegel (1990) has cautioned that many experimental effects based on stuttering event counts have been routinely replicated across research centers, suggesting that the differences among judges may not be entirely calamitous after all. That argument may prevail when experimental effects are based on dramatic changes, such as those produced by the so-called fluency-inducing conditions. It is also common in stuttering research, however, for smaller changes or smaller differences to be reported, and smaller differences are precisely those that may be either masked or created by these differences among judges.

Speech Rate

The importance of speech rate measurement stems from early behavioral approaches that used either rhythmic or prolonged speech patterns to instate stutter-free speech (see Ingham, 1984b). This process relied on the use of controlled and relatively slow speaking rates; as treatment progressed, rate was increased, and it was assumed that more normal-sounding speech would emerge as speech rate increased toward normal levels. These procedures were complicated, however, by the tendency for reduced rate alone to cause a decrease in stuttering frequency. Thus, research and treatment outcome reports needed to include speech rate data in order to control for the possibility that any reported decrease in stuttering could have been due to the effect of reduced speaking rates alone. At the very least, lack of speech rate data meant that different treatments could be neither compared nor adequately evaluated (see Bloodstein, 1995; Ingham & Costello, 1984).

In treatment contexts, measures are made of either syllables per minute (SPM) or words per minute (WPM) (see Costello & Ingham, 1984). These measures, which are also widely used in treatment research, are usually obtained by clinicians manually counting syllables or words spoken in real time (e.g., Fowler & Ingham, 1986). Other researchers compute SPM or WPM from transcriptions of speech, a time-consuming procedure that does not appear to be necessary, given the high levels of reliability that are generally obtained for real-time syllable and word counts. Ingham, Martin, and Kuhl (1974), for example, reported differences exceeding 5 percent between a judge's real-time word counts and independent transcriptions for only 8 out of 480 minutes of adult stutterers' spontaneous speech.

Several problems face clinical researchers concerned with measuring speech rate. First, there are no agreed guidelines for complete or representative measurements. Data gathered from 1-minute samples, for example, or from transcribed 300-word speech samples, cannot reflect the striking variations in rate that pragmatic factors demand of normally fluent speakers in different situations. Indeed, it is not clear how to quantify speech rate as unusually slow or fast, or as overly or insufficiently variable, given the wide ranges of speech rates that are used by different speakers and in different situations. Mean conversational WPM values for normal speakers (e.g., Lutz & Mallard, 1986; Walker, 1988; Yorkston & Beukelman, 1980) encompass speech rates from below 140 WPM to above 200 WPM within one standard deviation of the mean (Walker, 1988: mean 172.2 WPM, standard deviation 33.4 WPM), with ranges for individual utterances presumably even greater. It is also not clear from mean data whether rates outside of the given ranges would be considered abnormal, either by a listener or by the speaker.

Similar issues are raised by the consideration of articulation rate (Perkins, 1975). This measure records SPM after intervals of stuttering and excessively long pauses have been removed from the sample. Articulation rate is widely recommended and supposed to provide a more valid estimate of rate than measurements that include time spent in stuttering and in excessively long pauses. It has never been definitively established, however, that stuttering inappropriately influences speech rate or its measurement. The assumption is made that the occurrence of stuttering will decrease speech rate, because time taken up in stuttering cannot be spent in producing speech at a "normal" rate, and this assumption is probably correct if speech rate is defined in terms of the number of new meaningful syllables produced per unit time. It might be equally relevant, however, to define speech rate (and its perception) in terms of the frequency of *all* speech-motor movements, including those produced during intervals of stuttering.

Problems with stuttering measurement also affect the viability and validity of an articulation rate measure that depends on identifying and removing occasions of stuttering and inappropriate pauses. In addition, even if it is possible to calculate speech rate for stutter-free speech only (e.g., by using interval measurement and calculating syllables or words spoken in stutter-free intervals), complex decisions are involved in attempting to exclude inappropriate pauses. Pauses of 100 msec or longer have been excluded by some researchers, with pauses of up to 250 msec included by others (see Kent, 1994, p. 79), yet none of these numbers has any demonstrated relevance to what speakers or listeners consider to be appropriate pauses in connected speech.

Attempts have also been made to measure speech rate automatically with acoustic recognition systems, and syllabic structure can be recognized with reasonable levels of accuracy by some rapid acoustic analysis techniques (Bakker, Brutten, & McQuain, 1995; Jaffe, Anderson, & Rieber, 1973). When the integrity of the syllable boundary is diminished, however, as occurs in prolonged speech and other important stuttering treatment techniques, the accuracy of syllable recognition software diminishes significantly. In fact, Bakker et al. (1995) recently reported that their automated procedure was most accurate, not with normal speech, but with listener-marked stressed syllables—the opposite of the reduced articulatory stress that is so common during stuttering treatments.

Speech Quality

Measures of speech quality or speech naturalness were added to stuttering treatment evaluation because of the need to measure the undesirable monotone speech quality that often results from prolonged speech treatments. A 9-point speech naturalness rating scale presented by Martin, Haroldson, and Triden (1984), for example, provides the means for global measures of perceived speech quality. Franken and colleagues (e.g., Franken, Boves, Peters, & Webster, 1992, 1995) have also used 7-point rating scales of individual dimensions of speech quality in their attempts to isolate the variables that contribute to the unusual quality of prolonged speech. Naturalness ratings have also been fed back to speakers, with the initial results suggesting that subjects who had achieved a typical stutter-free prolonged speech pattern could use this feedback to improve their speech naturalness to within the range of normally fluent speakers (Ingham & Onslow, 1985).

The major problems with the speech naturalness scale are similar to those described for stuttering frequency and speech rate, including differences among observers and a lack of information to define whether any particular naturalness score is necessarily outside the normal range. There are currently neither agreed exemplars of speech to typify particular scale scores nor standardized training procedures to instruct judges about how to use the scale. The variability in naturalness scores assigned by individual raters was evident in the original data presented by Martin et al. (1984), and it has become increasingly more evident (Finn & Ingham, 1994; Martin & Harold-son, 1992; Onslow, Adams, & Ingham, 1992). Indeed, Martin and Haroldson (1992) cautioned against the use of naturalness ratings assigned by a single judge in some situations. Mackey, Finn, and Ingham (in review) also found that monolingual English-speaking judges made bipolar ratings of the naturalness of some speakers whose accents differed from their own; some judged accented speech as natural, while for others it was unnatural. Quite obviously a bipolar distribution of ratings would complicate interpretation of naturalness ratings when speaker and judge had different linguistic backgrounds.

One solution to most of the problems with the naturalness scale would be to develop a series of recorded speech exemplars that judges agree should receive a particular rating. Such exemplars could encompass a variety of speech patterns, to ensure that judges appreciate the multidimensional features of naturalness ratings. Alternatively, scales for individual dimensions of speech quality could be developed, with exemplars derived for each scale (Franken et al., 1995). Another solution, which is more fully developed below, might be to rely on the speaker's own judgments of how natural or acceptable speech sounds or feels (e.g., Finn & Ingham, 1994).

Physiological Stuttering and Subperceptual Stuttering

Contrasting in many ways with the measures described above are the many current physiological measurements of factors claimed to be associated with stuttering. Current perspectives on the nature of stuttering define the problem in terms of internal physiological or neurophysiological processes, rather than in terms of overt behaviors. Many recent studies, therefore, have compared stutterers and nonstutterers on a range of tasks and measures that are claimed to have some direct or indirect relationship to speech production, with the implicit goal being to identify those physiological features that distinguish persons who stutter from those

who do not. Investigated features include oral-motor movements, signal tracking skills, vocal and speech reaction times, coordination of laryngeal and respiratory movements, coordination of laryngeal and articulatory movements, saccadic velocities, and many other physiological parameters (see Armson & Kalinowski, 1994; McClean, 1990; Peters, 1990; Peters, Hulstijn, & Starkweather, 1991, many chapters; Smith, 1990; Starkweather, 1990). They also include such various measures as hemispheric processing of speech (Moore, 1990); relative durations of phonation (Gow & Ingham, 1992; Ingham, Montgomery, & Ulliana, 1983) and pauses (Hillis, 1993); and some differences that might have been introduced by therapies that employ unnatural speech patterns to achieve fluency (see Ingham, 1990b). Significantly, these studies are rarely designed to determine whether there is any relationship between these features and the production of normally fluent speech; this perspective has been primarily focussed on physiological features that may or may not be associated with speech features.

Most of these studies compare a group of persons who are described as displaying normal speech and language skills with a group who are claimed to stutter. Results tend to describe differences between the two groups that may be statistically significant but that are rarely nonoverlapping; that is, most subjects in the stuttering group are often indistinguishable from most subjects in the nonstuttering group, with some subgroup of persons who stutter displaying extreme values, or extremely variable scores, on the dimension of interest. Most, if not all, of the resulting group differences tend to be interpreted as reflecting fundamental deficiencies in the speech-motor system of stutterers (see, for example, Peters, 1990; van Lieshout, Peters, Starkweather, & Hulstijn, 1993). Less often is it acknowledged that these deficiencies may not be causal or even fundamental, but may be consequences of the disorder (see Armson & Kalinowski, 1994; Ingham, 1990b). In either case, these group differences have been repeatedly construed as deficits that limit the ability to produce normally fluent speech—yet there exist no published data confirming that such deficits are incompatible with normally fluent speech production.[2]

The assumptions of neurophysiological differences between all persons who stutter as compared with all persons who do not have yet to be accompanied by convincing explanations for several known features of stuttering. Among these, at the very least, is that environmental variables such as chorus reading can change the speech produced by the same neurophysiological organism from severely stuttered to entirely nonstuttered and back again within just a few seconds. Nor has any plausible neurophysiological explanation been offered for the powerful ameliorative effects of response contingent stimulation on stuttering (Ingham, 1984b; Prins & Hubbard, 1988). These problems are magnified within the most extreme forms of the neurophysiological perspectives, those that claim that neurophysiological deficits in stuttering are so pervasive, or so diagnostic, or both, that the disorder may actually exist "subperceptually," or in the absence of perceived stuttering (see Alfonso, 1990; Armson & Kalinowski, 1994; Starkweather, 1990). Adams, Freeman, and Conture (1984), for example, argued that the stutterings that listeners identify as disfluencies are "only a sampling of the pathophysiological behaviors underlying the disorder" (p. 111). Alfonso argued, similarly, that some dysfluent utterances may not be identified perceptually; "that is, while a segment of a stutterer's speech may be judged 'fluent' by a group of listeners, the acoustic, and/or movement, and/or electromyographic signals underlying the perceptual segment may appear inappropriate or 'dysfluent' " (Alfonso, 1990, p. 18).

Such claims that stuttering can exist at a subperceptual level appear to have emerged from interpretation of physiological measures of stutterers' laryngeal and respiratory behavior during speech and nonspeech tasks. Post hoc interpretation of unpublished data obtained by Freeman (1977), for example, identified brief periods of silence before seven utterances in which activity was recorded for both laryngeal abduction and adduction muscles. These pauses were described by Adams et al. (1984) as "physiological blocks," even though they were "too brief in duration to trigger listener perception of stuttering" (Adams et al., 1984, p. 110). Armson and Kalinowski (1994) provided a similar example, explaining that the reiterative respiratory and laryngeal gestures observed in one example from a study by Story (1990) may be "easily recognized as subperceptual stuttering" because they "closely correspond to . . . repeated articulatory gestures during part-word repetitions" (Armson & Kalinowski, 1994, p. 72). Freeman and Ushijima (1978) and Shapiro (1980) also claimed to have found unusual laryngeal activity during fluent periods of stutterers' speech, and Alfonso, Watson, and Baer (1984; see Alfonso, 1990) reported group differences between stutterers and nonstutterers for photoglottographic, laryngeal EMG, and plethysmograph measures obtained prior to and during the phonation of a vowel /a/.

Closer examination of all of these studies shows that their methods are so questionable that it is difficult to interpret their findings, let alone claim that they have identified subperceptual stuttering. For instance, Freeman and Ushijima (1978) and Shapiro (1980) provided data from a total of only eight stutterers and only one normal control. Neither study provided any data about the reliability of their stuttering and nonstuttering judgments, much less any data to support claims that the stutterers' "abnormal" levels of laryngeal activity were incompatible with the production of normally fluent speech. Alfonso et al. (1984) did

---

[2]The point is illustrated by considering two studies by Prosek and Runyan (1982, 1983) that are often cited in support of the suggestion that there are fundamental neurophysiological differences between speakers who stutter and those who do not. Prosek and Runyan manipulated recorded stutter-free speech samples from treated stutterers, to alter the samples' speech rate and their number of short pauses. Listeners could not distinguish between the altered samples and samples from nonstutterers, a finding that has been interpreted as showing that a slow speaking rate and a high frequency of pause intervals in the stutter-free speech of stutterers is non-normal speech. However, it does not also follow that the speakers themselves would consider the same relatively slow and pause-ridden speech to be problematic or not normally fluent.

not measure stuttering or nonstuttering at all, so their neuromuscular results cannot be related to the presence or absence of occasions of stuttering. At best, their data may show that stutterers are slower than nonstutterers in initiating /a/, but there was no evidence that the measured neuromuscular activity was either experienced as a problem by the speakers or was functionally related to the stuttering perceived by observers.

Many of these issues are exemplified by Story's (1990) much-referenced study of only three speakers who stuttered and two who did not (see Alfonso et al., 1984; Armson & Kalinowski, 1994). The data relevant to inspiratory patterns were provided in terms of the "number of attempts the subject made at inhalation prior to the production of a single [4-word] phrase" (Story, 1990, p. 150). The "typical inhalation pattern observed for nonstutterers" was "a single inhalation prior to inspiration [sic]" (p. 150), but no data from nonstutterers were provided to support this claim. Data were provided for the three stutterers, and they show clearly that the typical pattern for these speakers was also to inhale once and then produce the phrase: Subject KH began 411 of 414 phrases with one inspiration attempt; Subject PC began 370 of 404 phrases with one inspiration attempt (with all multiple attempts recorded in pretreatment tokens); and Subject AB began 372 of 427 phrases with one inspiration attempt. These data simply do not support a conclusion of generalized respiratory-pattern differences between speakers who stutter and those who do not, much less a conclusion that those differences that might occur are related to the presence or absence of stuttering (all phrases analyzed by Story were judged by the speaker and by the experimenter to be fluent productions).

Indeed, a little consideration shows how logically suspect it is to interpret a repetitive pattern in a respiratory trace as necessarily signaling a subperceptual stuttered repetition. This reasoning would suggest that if, for example, the repetitive head movements that sometimes co-occur with overt stuttering happen to be produced during perceptually fluent speech then those head movements should be classified as subperceptual

stutterings. In fact, a strong form of this argument suggests that subperceptual stuttering could occur in speakers who do not believe they stutter, simply because they show repetitive or prolonged respiratory or laryngeal traces. The implications of this strong position are quite intriguing; it would mean that any repetitive or prolonging pattern in physiological data could be diagnostic of a fluency problem, even if the speaker does not experience a fluency problem and observers do not hear or see a fluency problem.[3]

In general, the questions raised by the notion of subperceptual stuttering are whether and how a stuttering problem can exist if it does not manifest itself perceptually. It has long been accepted clinically that some persons may stutter so infrequently that some listeners would never encounter their stuttering; it is also accepted that some persons who stutter may complain of stuttering even when their speech sounds nonstuttered to a listener. As these two possibilities suggest, however, the existence of stuttering is clinically relevant only if the behavior is somehow distinctive, either to the speaker or to the listener, or both. Defining stuttering as an event that is experienced neither by the speaker nor by the listener ruptures the necessary link between a theoretic construct and the disorder it is supposed to describe. Folkins's (1991) conclusions, from his commentary on a major collection of physiologically based papers on stuttering, deserve to be reprinted in their entirety:

> *I believe that it is best to reserve the concept of disfluency (or breakdown, failure, and error) for the level of behavioral output. Of course, there can be unusual processes at any level of the system, [but] atypical physiological processes are not necessarily a problem until they reach the level of transmitted behavior. . . . Unusual processes at any part or level of the system may produce both flexible and*

---

[3]A weaker version of the subperceptual argument might state that the subperceptual stutterings are not perceived by others but are still perceived by the speaker (see Alfonso, 1990; Starkweather, 1990). This notion of subperceptual stuttering seems to be a trivial one, because a speaker-perceived judgment of stuttering is still a judgment of perceptual stuttering.

plastic compensations at other parts or levels. . . .
We cannot label atypical physiology as pathologi-
cal [much less as stuttering] unless we have exam-
ined the [entire system's] limits of flexibility and
plasticity to understand how the physiological lev-
els interact to produce undesired behavioral out-
put. Movements and muscles are not disfluent,
behaviors are. (p. 564)

Demands and Capacities

Dissatisfaction with the behavioral measures described above, and attempts to develop more comprehensive models of stuttering that can incorporate
the neurophysiological perspectives, have led to the
growing influence of multifaceted models of stuttering. Watson et al. (1994), for example, began
with the dubious assertion that "reliable methods
exist for the quantification of moments of disfluency, dysfluency, or nonfluency" (p. 1226), and then
continued with the more supportable claim that
"these measures do not reflect the global phenomenon of fluency" (p. 1226). Working from the assumption that fluency is the successful integration
not only of speech and language components but of
cognitive, linguistic, and motoric processes as a
whole, Watson et al. suggested that fluency failure
occurs when there is disruption to any one of these
processing components, anywhere within the
known parameters of speech-language production,
and that stuttering cannot be understood without
understanding the "substrates of fluency" (p. 1226).
Watson et al. suggested testing models of fluency
such as those proposed by Levelt (1989) and
Perkins, Kent, and Curlee (1991) (see also Kelso,
Tuller, & Harris, 1983; Laver, 1980; Shattuck-Hufnagel, 1983), presumably to determine the level at
which some error or disintegration occurs that leads
to stuttering.

The most influential of these multifaceted
models of stuttering is probably Starkweather's
(1987) demands and capacities model (DCM). The
DCM extends previous behavioral and physiological models of stuttering to consider the influence
on fluency of four domains: speech-motor, linguistic, cognitive, and social-emotional. Starkweath-

er's (1987) description of the DCM traces the development of abnormal fluency in children by stating simply that "when the child lacks the capacity
to meet demands for fluency, stuttering, or something like it, will occur" (p. 75). If demands for fluency continue to exceed a child's capacity for
fluent speech, according to Starkweather, the child
is likely to struggle or try harder to speak; when
that "struggle, tension, and emotional reaction
have become habitual and semiautomatic, stuttering has developed" (Starkweather, 1987, p. 76).
Stuttering may continue even after the child is physiologically capable of producing fluent speech if
"the habits of struggle, forcing, and avoidance . . .
become automatized" (Starkweather, Gottwald, &
Halfond, 1990, p. 14) and resistant to change; alternatively, stuttering may continue because the
child never develops the physiological capacity to
produce fluent speech (see also Adams, 1990).

These descriptions rather obviously lay out a
proposed sequence, based on demands for fluency
and the capacity to produce fluency, for the development and occurrence of fluent and stuttered
speech. However, Starkweather et al. have also
claimed that the DCM is "not an explanation of
the origin of stuttering, but rather an organized description of the relevant facts about the development of stuttering" (Starkweather et al., 1990, p.
22). It is difficult to determine exactly what is
meant by such statements, because the DCM as
presented by Starkweather (1987) and by Starkweather et al. (1990) seems quite clearly to be an
explanation of the beginning of stuttering and, to
a lesser extent, an explanation of the precipitating
factors for individual occurrences of stuttering.

It is equally difficult, in fact, to determine
what exactly the proponents of the DCM believe
this model explains or how it contributes to attempts to measure those features that differentiate
stuttered from nonstuttered speech. In its simplest
form, the DCM states nothing more than that an
organism that lacks the capacity to produce a certain behavior will be unable to produce that behavior, a statement that is essentially vacuous. In
a more complex form, the DCM might be expressed as a purportedly logical argument:

1. Stuttering occurs when capacities are exceeded.
2. Capacities are exceeded in persons who stutter.
3. Therefore, stuttering occurs in persons who stutter.

Or, more problematic yet:

1. If demands exceed capacities, then stuttering will occur.
2. Stuttering occurs.
3. Therefore, demands exceeded capacities.

The DCM reduces, in the first of these arguments, to the simple statement that stuttering occurs in speakers who stutter. The second, which is stated in a traditional logical form, is a clear example of the fallacy of affirming the consequent, or the logical fallacy of asserting that a cause has been identified simply because a result has been obtained. Neither is a particularly useful description of stuttering.

Despite the logical weaknesses of the DCM, this model has undoubtedly provided the structure for much current research on stuttering. Differences obtained between groups who stutter and groups who do not stutter are frequently interpreted as signs that stutterers suffer from deficits in their capacity to cope with demands on their speech fluency, with many of the deficient capacities supposed to be primarily neurophysiological (see Adams, 1990; Andrews, Craig, Feyer, Hoddinott, Howie, & Neilson, 1983; Starkweather, 1987; for reviews).[4] Studies within the linguistic, cognitive, and social-emotional "domains" of the DCM are also common. The DCM, in summary,

has provided a framework for much current work on stuttering, although none of that work has identified features of speech or speech production that are necessarily associated with stuttering or normal fluency, much less identified features that would be sufficient to establish stuttering or fluency.

DEFINITIONS OF FLUENCY: THE "OUTCOME" OF STUTTERING TREATMENT OUTCOME EVALUATION

The major difficulty facing stuttering treatment outcome evaluation is that none of the five features discussed in the preceding section has been shown to define the difference between stuttered speech and normally fluent speech. In general, it remains an open question as to whether a speaker who displays "abnormal" values on these many physiological, neurophysiological, and speech-production measures will stutter. More importantly, it remains an open question as to whether a speaker who displays "normal" values on these measures has satisfied the goals of successful treatment or has achieved normal fluency.

Complicating these questions is the issue of how to define stuttering and fluency for the purposes of measuring stuttering and evaluating treatment. The available definitions of stuttering range from discussions of specific speech behaviors, to descriptions of specific physiological patterns, to references to an overall speech or communication deficit (see Conture, 1990; Cordes, 1994a; Cordes & Ingham, 1994a,b; Prins, 1991). The opposite of stuttered speech, and the implicit or explicit goal of stuttering treatment, is usually labeled fluent speech, or normally fluent speech (see Finn & Ingham, 1989). In common parlance, fluency refers to "having words at one's command and uttering them with facility and smoothness" (*Webster's Dictionary*, 1975, p. 376). This definition encompasses aspects of both speech and language, as reflected in Perkins's suggestion that when observers judge the fluency of a speaker they are probably judging the "adequacy of performance of the semantic, syntactic, morphemic, and prosodic dimensions of speech" (Perkins, 1971, p. 92). This is also the

---

[4]It is not clear whether the DCM claims that persons who stutter will necessarily show lower than normal capacities in some dimensions. Starkweather et al. (1990, p. 14) stated that in some stutterers "the physiological capacities for fluency may never develop sufficiently." However, Adams (1990, p. 137), in an attempt to clarify the DCM, stated that "there is nothing inherent within the DC model that requires that deficits and/or abnormalities be present. . . . All that is necessary is that demands exceed capacities." We suggest that the point is moot, because even in the latter case stutterers could be said to show an abnormally low capacity to respond to demands for speech fluency.

sense in which fluency (i.e., word-finding skill, or the ability to produce multiword utterances) has been defined and measured for adults with acquired language disorders, including the aphasias.

The search for an acceptable measure of normal fluency within stuttering research, however, has generally been restricted to speech fluency, rather than cognitive, linguistic, or word-finding fluency (see Finn & Ingham, 1989). Starkweather, for example, defined speech fluency as "the ability to talk with normal levels of continuity, rate and effort" (1987, p. 12).[5] Implicit in this definition, as in others, is that the speech of persons who have completed some stuttering treatment program should include "normal levels of continuity, rate, and effort." This description would appear to disallow the occurrence of any discontinuity or struggle, or stuttering, in post-treatment speech, and it is consistent with the goal of stutter-free speech that drives many treatment programs (e.g., Costello, 1983).

Some stuttering treatment programs, however, define acceptable post-treatment speech as including disfluencies, or even stutterings, as long as they are acceptably infrequent. Caron and Ladouceur (1989), for example, defined clinical success as clinician ratings of less than 3 percent syllables stuttered; Onslow and his colleagues have defined 1 percent syllables stuttered as an adequate treatment result (e.g., Onslow, Andrews, & Lincoln, 1994). Yet another goal of stuttering treatment is based more on the accessory or secondary characteristics of stuttering than on the primary speech-production features. Thus, the goal of some treatment programs is simply to reduce the secondary avoidance or fear of stuttering, rather than to make any direct change to the speech behavior. In addition, many traditional stuttering treatments, such as those described by Van Riper (1973), focus on modifying moments of stuttering, rather than eliminating them. Acceptable treatment results within such frameworks do not require the absence of stuttering, or even some absolute maximum percentage of stuttering, as long as the stuttering that

occurs happens "fluently" or is sufficiently controllable so as not to cause distress.

This definition of an acceptable treatment outcome differs in fundamental ways from definitions that prescribe normal values of certain speech-production and/or neurophysiological features. It is essentially a complaint-driven definition of stuttering (Baer, 1988, 1990) guided by the subject's sense of handicap (see Prins, 1991) rather than by external prescriptive features. Baer has argued that the client's source of complaint should guide therapy, and that therapy evaluation carries only marginal validity if it fails to establish the extent to which the client's complaint has been resolved. In one sense, this is a self-evident aspect of any treatment; therapy is usually considered unsatisfactory if the patient continues to complain about that disorder that prompted treatment. Within a complaint-driven model of therapy, however, not only is a continuing complaint to be treated as a disorder, but the elimination of complaint, as defined by the subject, is to be trusted as an acceptable outcome.

For stuttering in particular, Baer's complaint-driven definitions of acceptable treatment outcome are consistent with the idea that the ultimate decision as to whether an individual (at least an adult) has a problem with speaking, and whether that problem has ceased, must belong to the speaker. This is similar to the claim made by Perkins (e.g., 1983, 1990) that only the person who stutters is in a position to identify valid occasions of stuttering—although from Baer's perspective complaints can still be considered observable behaviors that are available to external manipulation. Perkins's claim that the definitive feature of stuttering is the speaker's private sensation of loss of control over the ability to proceed with an utterance provoked tremendous debate (see Bloodstein, 1990; Ingham, 1990a; Siegel, 1991; Smith, 1990). The most overlooked and lasting contribution of Perkins's definition, however, might be that it has served to restore attention to the importance of self-measurement in stuttering.

Self-judged acceptability of fluency as an indicator of therapy success does have its own spe-

---

[5]Starkweather also includes rhythm, though he acknowledges its more debatable status.

cial problems. Speakers might simply learn to accept an artificial fluency (Wingate, 1976) or a noticeably abnormal speech pattern in preference to poor fluency. Claims of recovery might also be questionable if subjects report no longer having a problem even though stuttering is obvious to an observer. In the case of children, as well, it is unlikely that their failure to complain about evident stuttering would signify that therapy is unnecessary (Onslow, 1992). But if adults insist that they no longer have a stuttering problem, despite apparently contrary observer-recorded data, then perhaps more serious questions should be raised, not about the validity of their reports, but about the clinical validity of the observer-based data. Ultimately, the self-judged acceptability of fluency may be not only an important part of normal fluency, but perhaps the most critical goal of stuttering treatment. The most critical components of stuttering treatment outcome evaluation, therefore, might be the self-judgments or self-measurements made by the speakers themselves.

INCORPORATING SELF-MEASUREMENT INTO A THREE-FACTOR MODEL FOR STUTTERING TREATMENT OUTCOME EVALUATION

Many diverse methods exist for evaluating the outcome of stuttering treatment for children and adults (see Bloodstein, 1995; Cooper, 1990; Ingham, 1990b, 1990c, 1993a; Ingham & Costello, 1984; *Journal of Fluency Disorders, 18(2)*, 1993), but there seems to be some consensus that thorough treatment outcome evaluation for stuttering should include three elements: (1) establishing that a treatment has produced a clinically significant change in speech production, (2) establishing that the change has generalized across speaking situations, and (3) establishing that the change is maintained over time. The most common method for assessing whether change has occurred uses variations on within-subjects or time-series designs, in which stuttering and related behaviors are measured from repeated speech samples on multiple occasions (see Bellack, Hersen, & Kaz-

din, 1990; Blood, 1993; Conture & Guitar, 1993; Curlee, 1993; Ingham, 1993a; Prins, 1993; Starkweather, 1993). Thus, current methods for stuttering treatment outcome evaluation may be conceived of in terms of a three-factor model that depends on (1) speech performance, (2) speaking situations, and (3) time.

The three-factor model is logically sound, but applying it in treatment research, much less in routine clinical settings, is enormously demanding. Multiple (and nonreactive) recordings of the subject's speech must be obtained across different speaking situations, for months or years after an initial treatment phase has been completed—and that initial phase itself requires multiple recordings. It is no wonder, perhaps, given these complexities, that use of the three-factor model seems to have declined in recent years and that many current treatment methods for stuttering are recommended to clinicians without treatment outcome data at all.[6]

One problem, however, with criticizing recent treatment research for failing to provide adequate speech performance data, is that the currently available measurement procedures are unlikely to provide valid, reliable, objective treatment outcome data about stuttering (see Cordes, 1994b; Cordes & Ingham, 1994a). Some of the many problems with observer-based measurements of stuttering, speech rate, speech quality, and speech physiology were discussed above; this final section suggests that treatment outcome evaluation within the three-factor model might be significantly enhanced and improved, as well as simplified, by the use of self-measurement procedures for stuttering. This final section, therefore, begins with a brief history of self-recording in general, and in stuttering research in particular. The remainder of the chapter then discusses each of the three factors in the current treatment outcome

---

[6]The reader is referred for good examples of recent treatment outcome evaluation to Boberg and Kully (1994) and to Onslow, Andrews and Lincoln (1994). These studies provided some idea of the minimum amount of data necessary to support conclusions about the efficacy of treatment programs for adults and children, respectively.

evaluation model, presenting some of the current problems and suggesting some methods by which inclusion of self-recording procedures might increase the reliability and the validity of measures, thus providing the opportunity for increasing the effectiveness of treatments for stuttering.

Definitions and a Brief History

Self-judgment procedures are neither new to stuttering treatment and research nor new to behavior-based therapies in general. The procedures to be discussed are *self-recording* or *self-monitoring*, two general terms that are used to describe an individual recording occurrences of his or her own behavior (Nelson & Hayes, 1981). This procedure alone often alters the frequency of the target behavior, usually in the desired direction (that is, many behaviors are found to be reactive to self-recording). *Self-evaluation*, another term used in this context, typically means that the subject is required first to self-record then to evaluate the total number of occurrences of the target behavior in relation to some performance criterion, and apply some contingency based on that evaluation. Assessments of *self-efficacy* represent another, more recent, self-measurement procedure. Self-efficacy measures, based on Bandura's (1977) theory of behavior change, require subjects to rate the likelihood of achieving a performance criterion prior to carrying out a certain task (such as speaking in a specified situation).

In general, most of these terms, and the procedures they refer to, have their origins within the framework of applied behavior analysis or operant conditioning. Several studies conducted during the 1960s and 1970s applied self-measurement techniques to stuttering treatment research (e.g., Costello, 1975; Goldiamond, 1965). Results suggested that self-recording of stuttering events while speaking could be a valid measurement methodology and that it often provided self-recorded data trends that differed dramatically from those recorded by observers (Hanson, 1978; Ingham, Adams, & Reynolds, 1978; James, 1981b; La Croix, 1973). Self-delivered contingen-

cies (Flanagan, Goldiamond, & Azrin, 1958; Goldiamond, 1962; Martin & Haroldson, 1982) and self-evaluation of performance criteria in a stuttering therapy schedule (Ingham, 1982) were also shown to reduce stuttering and to contribute to the maintenance of treatment benefits.

These results should have encouraged far more research using self-measurement of stuttering, but publications of research on self-recording of stuttering literally ceased after approximately 1980.[7] Certainly the use of self-judgments was not encouraged by treatment outcome models presented in the early 1980s that emphasized the primacy of observer data (e.g., Ingham & Costello, 1984). Indeed, it is probably understandable from a number of perspectives that most credence would be given to data collected by presumably experienced, objective and disinterested observers, rather than by the subjects themselves. Nonetheless, as was argued above, the methodological problems with the data provided by observers, combined with the theoretical problems with prescribing criteria for fluency that do not recognize the speaker's complaint, may now be combined in the mid-1990s to suggest the need for a renewed emphasis on self-measurement of stuttering.

In general, we suggest that self-recording techniques could be usefully incorporated into all aspects of stuttering measurement, within the three-factor outcome evaluation model and also in other areas. Self-recorded judgments as described below are not meant to replace observer judgments entirely, nor are self-judgments assumed to be necessarily valid, reliable, or useful simply by virtue of being self-recorded. A careful combination of observer and speaker judgments, however, might solve many of the current problems of reliability and validity for stuttering measures, and might contribute significantly to the development of successful treatment programs for this disorder.

---

[7]Some recent therapy evaluation studies have included data from questionnaires that asked subjects whether they are satisfied with their fluency or whether they still consider that they stutter (e.g., Boberg & Kully, 1994). These are useful supplements, but they do not relate directly to speech performance data or to self-judgments of treatment effects.

The Speech Performance Factor

Stuttering. One obvious application of self-recording procedures is as straightforward as asking speakers to count the stuttering events that occur in their own speech. This could be accomplished either during speech or from audiovisual recordings, for spontaneous speech or for oral reading. It could be based on any one of the many potential definitions of stuttering: Subjects could be instructed to count certain types of disfluencies (perhaps those that they themselves had nominated as most problematic), all stuttering events they believe an observer would notice, all stuttering events that bother them, or even all stuttering events that they are aware of producing, whether those are problematic or not.

Several interesting issues arise in trying to determine how such self-recorded data should be used in evaluating treatment outcome. The most important, initially, may be that speakers might consistently identify different behaviors as stuttered, as compared with an experienced clinician or researcher. Debates about who is correct might quickly deteriorate into comparisons of the value of self-judgments versus observer-judgments, or of the value of a subject-driven model versus a professional judgment-driven model of therapy evaluation. A dual stuttering measurement system, incorporating both observer judgments and self-judgments, might solve any such difficulties. In addition, previous research has shown that the most reactive subjects (those who show the greatest reductions in stuttering during self-recording) are often those who count different numbers of stuttering events than observers count (see Ingham, 1984b). From this perspective, therefore, the most clinically important occurrences of stuttering may be those judged by the speaker rather than the observer.

Similar issues will arise in considering the end of treatment programs. Boberg and Kully (1994), for example, reported that some adult and adolescent subjects from their treatment study showed low but consistent stuttering at follow-up, as judged by observers, and yet claimed that they always or almost always felt "like a normal speak-er." There may be no observer-judged behavioral difference between some stutterers who claim to be recovered, or who no longer complain about their stuttering, and others who are seeking treatment. Again, the complaint-driven self-recorded data may prove to be primary, providing the only avenue for clarifying and quantifying the distinction between speakers who are satisfied with their acceptable levels of fluency and speakers who, despite perhaps displaying the same values on observer-judged measures, are dissatisfied enough with their speech to seek treatment.

Speech Rate. In the midst of concerns about the importance of speech rate to normal fluency, there has been relatively little interest in determining whether the speaker can provide a valid source for determining satisfactory speech rate. Perkins's (1973) Breathstream Management program did incorporate procedures designed to achieve a self-determined rate that "should be fast enough to feel satisfying and . . . sound normal to the stutterer on recordings" (p. 299). Recent commentators (e.g., Lees, 1994; Starkweather, 1993) have also suggested incorporating self-based measures of satisfaction with fluency that, presumably, would include rate.

The wide range encompassed by normal speech rates, as discussed above, suggests that satisfactory speaking rates may be highly individualized. Tiffany (1980) reported considerable differences across speakers, but relative within-speaker stability, in syllable production rates under different conditions. In other words, as Tiffany concluded, individual speakers probably have neurophysiologically natural or ideal speech rates. This best rate may emerge for each speaker through judgments of comfortable articulatory rates, as Perkins suggested.

Speech Quality. Ratings of speech naturalness, as discussed above, have been used in preliminary studies of how subjects rate not only how natural their speech sounds, but also how natural it feels (Finn & Ingham, 1994; Ingham, Ingham, Onslow, & Finn, 1989). These investigations were suggested by the frequent complaint that subjects treated by the prolonged speech therapies must use an abnormal or unnatural level of self-monitoring to maintain treatment benefits; that is, their speech may sound normally fluent at the expense of unnatural amounts of attention or self-monitoring. Finn and Ingham (1994) and Ingham et al. (1989) found that subjects listening to recordings of their own speech consistently recognized variations in their own perceived speech naturalness that listeners were unable to recognize. It was also clear that there were marked differences between self-ratings of how natural speech sounds and how natural it feels. Furthermore, in laboratory conditions, subjects showed high replicability for self-judgments of naturalness, making virtually identical ratings of how natural their speech felt when different stimulus conditions were repeated.

In summary, the most promising findings of the speech naturalness studies might be those that show how surprisingly accurate and reliable subjects can be in recording how natural their speech sounds and feels—and this may go a long way towards improving the clinical utility and value of these outcome measures. The important result of the studies on speech naturalness may be a method for quantifying the nonobservable differences between what subjects versus external observers consider to be acceptable fluent speech.

Speaking Situations Factor

The second factor involved in the three-factor evaluation model concerns the speaking situation or speaking environment. Normal speech is assumed to be relatively resilient in different and demanding speaking situations; that is, normal speech is not limited to or limited by certain environmental conditions. Stuttering frequency, however, is known to vary substantially in different speaking situations and in similar situations across time (see Bloodstein, 1995; Ingham, 1984b), and a variety of environmental contingencies on stuttering are known to reduce its frequency of occurrence (Ingham, 1984b; Prins & Hubbard, 1988). In addition, there are ample data demonstrating "clinic-bound fluency": fluency that appears to be controlled by stimuli associated with the therapy setting (see Ingham,

1984a). Thorough treatment outcome evaluation, therefore, requires repeated measurements of speech in multiple situations because measurements made in one situation may not be representative of measurements made in another.

One problem in estimating the resiliency of speech within the three-factor model, however, is that it is extremely difficult to obtain or record observer judgment data in the many speaking situations that constitute a speaker's daily routine. As a substitute, certain selected situations for measurement are generally prescribed for all subjects, but these may not measure the important situations for each speaker. Some stuttering treatment programs include transfer tasks that are designed to provide the necessary links between speaking skills learned in the clinic and speaking skills required in daily life; even the most comprehensive of these, however, prescribe the situations, allowing the speaker to select only the order in which the tasks are to be completed (e.g., Boberg & Kully, 1994).

Self-judgments will obviously be useful in identifying speaking situations that may be functionally associated with variations in stuttering, and in recording speech performance data in those situations. Rather than presupposing the representativeness of, for example, telephone conversations in treatment outcome evaluations, studies could be designed to determine whether speech performance on this task does reflect performance in many other speaking situations. The point is that the clinical relevance of outcome measurement would be better served if subjects were free to identify, and then measure for themselves, their performance in speaking situations that they consider are of most concern.

Time Factor

As mentioned above, subjects who self-record or self-evaluate their stuttering in different speaking situations may not only reduce their stuttering, but also maintain that improvement across time (Ingham, 1982; James, 1981a; Martin & Haroldson, 1982). Craig and Andrews (1985) also reported that subjects who relapsed after treatment and then received a combination of self-recording and self-evaluation training showed improvement on a locus of control of behavior scale, and 5/6 subjects retained their improvement 10 months later. It may also be significant that in these studies the subjects' stuttering frequency counts did tend to match the experimenters' counts.

Despite these few studies, however, there has been relatively little research on the role of self-monitoring in the maintenance of treatment benefits. Two related problems complicate maintenance research, both of which, it would appear, could be ameliorated by the incorporation of self-judgments in the treatment and treatment outcome evaluation processes.

In many treatment research studies, first of all, it is difficult to ascertain the point when active treatment has ceased so that the maintenance of its effects can be monitored. Some years ago Brady (1971) reported the results of stuttering treatment using an earpiece metronome unit called the Pacemaster. Treatment included a schedule for systematically reducing the time that the subject wore the unit, but many of the subjects chose to continue wearing it. Obviously, the evaluation of this treatment would have been confusing if the results of subjects who continued to wear the Pacemaster had been lumped with those who had ceased wearing the unit.

The same principle applies in the evaluation of prolonged speech treatments. Such programs often incorporate rigorous post-treatment practice regimes, including attendance at self-help group meetings for continued practice of fluency-inducing skills. Thus, the point when the treatment process has ceased may not be clear-cut, making it especially difficult to determine if skill practice is ongoing or if a true maintenance phase has been reached. A second and related problem is that it is far from clear in many studies just what is supposed to be maintained. For example, in many prolonged speech therapies stutterers are encouraged to retain certain speech production techniques so as to maintain their therapy gains. Other treatment approaches, however, seem to be based on the assumption that stutter-free speech should become

so automatic that it is no longer controlled by the managed use of specific speech patterns or skills. Hillis (1994), for example, has made some interesting suggestions regarding self-managed strategies that could be used to aid the process of automatizing speech skills.

One solution to both of these problems might be to rely on subjects' judgments of whether their fluency is maintained by the active use, either continuously or intermittently, of specific fluency skills. Such data could provide important reference points for determining how long therapy effects have been maintained under active or passive conditions (see Ingham, 1984a). Another possibility might be some measure of how natural speech feels, perhaps (though not necessarily) along the lines of the speech naturalness scale. Measures of how natural speech feels could even be self-calibrated against different levels of attention required to monitor stutter-free speech production. Differences may certainly be evident at an acoustic level as well, perhaps in terms of the variability in certain dimensions (Packman, Onslow, & van Doorn, 1994; Prins & Hubbard, 1990), a possibility that suggests combining objective acoustic measurements with subjects' judgments about their own speech production.

Self-Measurement in Related Areas

In addition to the factors of speech production, speaking situation, and time, there are several other related aspects of stuttering that lend themselves to self-measurement. Self-rating scales of stutterers' reaction to their problem have a long history of use in stuttering assessment, treatment, and research (see Darley & Spriestersbach, 1978, chapters 9–10). Most of these scales, however, request relatively nonspecific self-judgments of speech and no judgments about the quality of fluency, and they do not lend themselves to repeated measurements. The widely used *Stutterer's Self-Ratings of Reactions to Speech Situations* scale (Williams, 1978) is an example of this type of scale, but it may still have a useful role in treatment. The scale requires the speaker to rate, for forty different speaking situations, levels of avoidance, reaction, and stuttering severity, and the frequency with which each situation is experienced. Some variation on this scale, perhaps limited to self-judged relevant situations and including estimates of stuttering frequency (or fluency), may still prove to be more valid and functional than most current self-rating scales. Other possibilities for self-measurement include anxiety, locus of control of behavior, communication attitudes, self-efficacy, and the effort associated with speaking.

Anxiety.   One stuttering treatment area where self-measurement seemingly has indisputable importance is anxiety, but recent studies in this area appear to have diminished its role. Research on the relationship between anxiety and stuttering, which has waxed and waned over the years (see Bloodstein, 1995; Ingham, 1984b), is currently passing through another period of popularity. An interesting feature of this recent period, which has focused primarily on state or experienced anxiety (rather than trait anxiety, or proneness to anxiety reactions), has been the apparent rejection of self-measurement in favor of physiological measurements of anxiety. Ironically, it seems that the renewed interest in anxiety and stuttering may be traced to Peters and Hulstijn's (1984) claim that state anxiety could not influence stuttering because recorded autonomic arousal levels were similar in stutterers and nonstutterers. Despite the similar physiological measures, however, stutterers reported tenseness during speech to be much higher than did the controls. Subsequent studies by Weber and Smith (1990) and Caruso, Chodzko-Zajko, Bidinger, and Sommers (1994) did not report significantly higher levels of physiologic arousal in stutterers, relative to their controls, during speech tasks, but neither of these studies included self-ratings of state anxiety. Other recent studies (Blood, Blood, Bennett, Simpson, & Susman, 1994; Craig, 1990; Miller & Watson, 1992) have recorded self-ratings of state and trait anxiety when comparing groups of stutterers and nonstutterers, but their findings have been inconsistent. In fact, there is still no compelling evidence of a functional relationship between state anxiety and stuttering. Because it is well established that high autonomic arousal may be related to state anxiety but may also accompany very different emotional states (Schwartz, 1978), this appears to be one area of research where self-measurement should be granted as much credence and importance as physiologic measurement.

Communication Attitudes and Locus of Control. Some other nonbehavioral features, such as attitudes toward communication and the locus of control of behavior, appear to have attracted more recent interest than has anxiety. Craig and Andrews (1985), for example, suggested that when successfully treated stutterers indicate that their lives are not "controlled by outside actions and events," they are more likely to resist relapse (at least as measured from one three-minute telephone task). An even stronger predictor of relapse prevention was reported if subjects' communication attitudes, as measured by the S24 (Andrews & Cutler, 1974), tended towards normalcy.

Many of the issues raised by these features are similar to those raised by the anxiety research, including especially questions about their relationship to stuttering behavior per se. Changes in stuttering, for instance, might cause changes in the perceived locus of control over speech, or changes in perceived locus of control might cause changes in stuttering. It is certainly clear that the sensation of control may be an important predictor variable in the treatment of other disorders (Lefcourt, 1976) and it may be a powerful signature of normal fluency. But it is still not clear that scores on that scale are independent of speech performance in the situations envisaged by the speaker. In the case of communication attitudes, the ratings may reflect a composite of responses to levels of stuttering in certain speaking situations. Ulliana and Ingham (1984) showed that responses on the S24 very accurately reflected the frequency of stuttering in certain speaking situations, and Curlee (1993) recommended including the S24 in outcome measurement, not so much to measure attitudes, but to highlight problematic speaking situations where the subject's speech performance might be measured directly. In short, it may be useful in clinical settings to have clients simply self-record their speech performance in circumstances alluded to in these scales. Such data are then available to guide treatment, a feature that has never characterized locus-of-control-of-behavior or communication-attitude data.

Self-Efficacy.   Further indications that self-assessment might record accurately relevant features of stutterers' speech behavior might appear in self-efficacy measurements. Expectations of success in approaching and producing changed behavior after treatment has been reported to be a powerful predictor of performance in a variety of disorders (see Bandura, Adams, & Beyer, 1977; Kazdin, 1980; Williams, Kinney, & Falbo, 1989). The most common criticism of self-efficacy measurement, however, is the failure to demonstrate its independence from actual behavior (Lee, 1989), an issue that may be relevant to stuttering treatment.

Ornstein and Manning (1985) were the first to develop a scale for adult stutterers for measuring change during treatment. Subjects rated how confident they felt about approaching and maintaining some self-defined "level of fluency" in fifty different speaking situations, using a scale that ranged from 10 ("quite certain") to 100 ("very certain"). Ornstein and Manning obtained relatively poor correlations between self-efficacy scores and communication attitudes, and between self-efficacy scores and stuttering severity ratings, perhaps because they combined the Approach and Performance sections of the scale to calculate these relationships. Hillis (1993) suggested the importance of separating these sections within his report of a single-case treatment study. This interesting study, based on a three-factor model, revealed a close relationship between stuttering frequency (in clinic and home recordings) and repeated self-efficacy scores on Ornstein and Manning's scale. Interestingly, this trend appeared to be more evident for the Performance than Approach part of the scale. For this subject there were strong indications that self-judged expectations of performance closely approximated actual speech performance. Such approximations might be even more pronounced if scale responses were more directly related to speech performance in scale-related speech tasks.

Effort.   Finally, there are also reasons to consider self-measurement of the level of self-perceived effort that is required to produce stuttered or acceptably fluent speech. Starkweather's definition of fluency, discussed above, included the statements that the "facility with which speech is produced is the central idea of fluency. . . . Ease of speaking is a dimension, perhaps the most central dimension, of fluency" (1987, p. 21). Starkweather also found the measurement of effort to be problematic, but a number of recent studies have included psychophysical measures of the "sense of effort" in speech production. Prosek and Montgomery (1969), for example, found that the level of perceived effort involved in speaking loudly was functionally related to the level of subglottic air pressure in normal speakers. Wright and Colton (1972), and Colton and Brown (1972), made similar measurement, with the latter reporting that normal speakers' "sense of effort" may be highly correlated with frequency, intensity, and subglottic pressure during phonation. McCloskey and colleagues (see McCloskey, 1981) have also conducted numerous studies that demonstrate the crucial role that a "sense of effort" can play in the execution of complex motor movements, and Somodi, Robin, and Luschei (in press) found that a "sense of effort," as recorded by hand pressure, can be directly and accurately related to certain levels of tongue pressure. In fact, Somodi et al. (in press) speculated that an accurate sense of effort may be critical for the smooth coordination of temporal relations during speech.

These studies suggest that speakers can accurately quantify perceived changes in the effort levels required for normal speech production, but the relationship between perceived effort and known deficits in speech physiology is, of course, even more relevant to stuttering. This issue has been pursued in studies reviewed recently by Solomon, Robin, Lorell, Rodnitzky, and Luschei (1994) on the level of perceived effort required to maintain tongue pressure in normal and dysarthric speakers. Verdolini-Marston, Hoffman, and McCoy (1992) also reported that magnitude estimations of effort were sensitive to changes in vocal structure and function after adults with voice disorders had received voice therapy. Watterson, McFarlane, and Diamond (1993), similarly, reported that patients with voice disorders, and some normal speaker controls, could recognize differences in the degree of "vocal effort" required for the production of voiceless obstruent consonants when compared with voiced obstruents and, in turn, with sonorants and nasals. A notable feature of Watterson et al.'s study was that a group of experienced listeners did not recognize differences in vocal quality across samples of speech produced with significant differences in speaker-judged vocal effort, a finding that is quite similar to the speech naturalness results reported by Finn and Ingham (1994) and by Ingham et al. (1989).

This growing body of evidence suggests that a "sense of effort" in speech production may be measured validly when referenced against known and controlled impediments to normal speech production. The studies reported by Solomon et al. (1994) are especially interesting because they suggest practical ways to measure the level of effort required while speaking. For instance, subjects squeezed a ball that registered the level of perceived effort involved in sustaining an increasingly fatiguing task. Conceivably, that amount of effort could be calibrated against the effort levels that stutterers report as necessary during certain standardized fluency-inducing conditions, such as chorus reading, to calibrate a level of fluency (i.e., level of effort) that the speaker considers to be acceptable. In fact, defining the goal of stuttering treatment in terms of reducing perceived effort removes many of the differences from treatment methods that are currently seen as disparate because their goals do or do not include the elimination of observer-judged stuttering. The argument could be made that implicit in all stuttering treatments is the goal of reducing the effort of speaking, either through eliminating stuttering or through "stutter fluently" techniques.

Measurement of effort might also help in the identification of sources of impediments to experienced fluency, either within the speech production system or in the environment.

SUMMARY

This chapter has suggested that the evaluation of stuttering treatment might benefit from a renewed focus on self-judged measurement of stuttering. The first section of this chapter reviewed five features that are currently suggested to distinguish stuttering from normal speech, concluding that none of them can establish a necessary and sufficient difference between the two. This problem was considered, in the second section, in terms of suggestions that stuttering can be defined, at least in part, by the speaker's complaint, or by the speaker's sense of handicap. One reasonable goal for stuttering treatment, therefore, might be self-judged acceptability of fluency, a goal that would depend on self-judgments of stuttering and of related behaviors and perceptions. The final section of this chapter then incorporated this possibility into a current three-factor model of treatment outcome evaluation, providing several suggestions for how self-judgments might be used for stuttering treatment and treatment research.

It would be naive to ignore the multitude of problems involved in developing measurement systems that rely on self-judgments. The problem of drift in the accuracy of self-measurement is probably the most serious, and a method for accuracy must be an intrinsic component of any viable self-measurement methodology. One solution might be to make treatment progress contingent on measurement accuracy criteria. Such a solution has been employed in a self-evaluation maintenance schedule within a prolonged speech program devised by the senior author (Ingham, 1987), but its effects have never been carefully established. In this procedure a random selection of the subjects' self-evaluations of their speech was compared with clinician evaluations, with progress in the maintenance phase of the program contingent on clinician-subject agreement. However, as we have suggested, the subject's performance measures may be the more valid reference, whether they agree with the clinician's or not. Perhaps subjects could be intermittently scheduled to remeasure randomly selected samples that they had previously scored under controlled conditions, with progress through a treatment program contingent on some agreement criterion for the two sets of scores.

This complaint-driven concept of normal fluency and of stuttering treatment—one that relies on a sense of effortless speech or acceptable fluency as judged by the speaker—is certainly not a unique suggestion. It is related to a concept of normal health that assumes that individuals recognize the absence of pain or the absence of other complaints as a normal state, and the presence of pain or other self-identified problems as an abnormal state. Obviously, the state of "painlessness" is incompatible with certain externally observable conditions, but neither pain nor the absence of pain can be totally deduced by reference to either biological standards or external observations: Pain is defined by the privately identified sensation of pain. Similarly, fluency might be usefully defined by the speaker's private sensation of acceptable, or acceptably effortless, speech production. Most of this research would probably apply to self-measurement by adult and adolescent stutterers, but the principles are certainly relevant for parents of young stutterers and perhaps some children who stutter.

Finally, we have suggested that research on self-measurement in all phases of treatment might improve the clinical validity of current treatment process and outcome measurement. Clinicians and researchers might find self-judged methods easier to use in evaluating the outcome of stuttering therapy than current methods. Whether this is true or not, self-judgments could provide the much-needed bridge between the current research on the neurophysiology of stuttering and the difficulties faced in developing and evaluating successful treatment programs for this disorder.

REFERENCES

Adams, M.R. (1990). The demands and capacities model I: Theoretical elaborations. *Journal of Fluency Disorders, 15,* 135–141.

Adams, M.R., Freeman, F.J., & Conture, E.G. (1984). Laryngeal dynamics of stutterers. In R.F. Curlee & W.H. Perkins (Eds.), *Nature and treatment of stuttering: New directions* (pp. 89–129). San Diego: College-Hill.

Alfonso, P.J. (1990). Subject definition and selection criteria for stuttering research in adult subjects. *ASHA Reports, 18,* 15–24.

Alfonso, P.J., Watson, B.C., & Baer, T. (1984). Muscle, movement, and acoustic measurements of stutterers' laryngeal reaction times. In M. Edwards (Ed.), *Proceedings of the 19th Congress of the International Association of Logopedics and Phoniatrics, Vol. II,* (pp. 580–585). Perth, Scotland: Danscott Print Limited.

Andrews, G., Craig, A., Feyer, A-M., Hoddinott, S., Howie, P., & Neilson, M. (1983). Stuttering: A review of research findings and theories circa 1982. *Journal of Speech and Hearing Disorders, 48,* 226–246.

Andrews, G., & Cutler, J. (1974). Stuttering therapy: The relation between changes in symptom level and attitudes. *Journal of Speech and Hearing Disorders, 39,* 312–319.

Andrews, J.G., & Ingham, R.J. (1972). An approach to the evaluation of stuttering therapy. *Journal of Speech and Hearing Research, 15,* 296–302.

Armson, J., & Kalinowski, J. (1994). Interpreting results of the fluent speech paradigm in stuttering research: Difficulties in separating cause from effect. *Journal of Speech and Hearing Research, 37,* 69–82.

Baer, D.M. (1988). If you know why you're changing a behavior, you'll know when you've changed it enough. *Behavioral Assessment, 10,* 219–223.

Baer, D.M. (1990). The critical issue in treatment efficacy is knowing why treatment was applied: A student's response to Roger Ingham. In L.B. Olswang, C.K. Thompson, S.F. Warren, & N. Minghetti (Eds.), *Treatment efficacy research in communication disorders* (pp. 31–39). Rockville, Md.: American Speech-Language-Hearing Foundation.

Bakker, K., Brutten, G.J., & McQuain, J. (1995). A preliminary assessment of the validity of three instrument-based measures for speech rate determination. *Journal of Fluency Disorders, 20,* 63–75.

Bandura, A. (1977). Self-efficacy: Toward a unifying theory of behavioral change. *Psychological Review, 84,* 191–215.

Bandura, A., Adams, N.E., & Beyer, J. (1977). Cognitive processes mediating behavior change. *Journal of Personality and Social Psychology, 35,* 125–139.

Bellack, A.S., Hersen, M., & Kazdin, A.E. (Eds.) (1990). *International handbook of behavior modification and therapy.* New York: Plenum Press.

Blood, G.W. (1993). Treatment efficacy in adults who stutter: Review and recommendations. *Journal of Fluency Disorders, 18,* 303–318.

Blood, G.W., Blood, I.M., Bennett, S., Simpson, K.C., & Susman, E.J. (1994). Subjective anxiety measurements and cortisonal responses in adults who stutter. *Journal of Speech and Hearing Research, 37,* 760–768.

Bloodstein, O. (1990). On pluttering, skivering, and floggering: A commentary. *Journal of Speech and Hearing Disorders, 55,* 392–393.

Bloodstein, O. (1995). *A handbook on stuttering* (5th Ed.). San Diego: Singular Publishing Group.

Boberg, E., & Kully, D. (1994). Long-term results of an intensive treatment program for adults and adolescents who stutter. *Journal of Speech and Hearing Research, 37,* 1050–1059.

Brady, J.P. (1971). Metronome-conditioned speech retraining for stuttering. *Behavior Therapy, 2,* 129–150.

Brady, J.P. (1991). The pharmacology of stuttering: A critical review. *American Journal of Psychiatry, 148,* 1309–1316.

Caron, C., & Ladouceur, R. (1989). Multidimensional behavioral treatment for child stutterers. *Behavior Modification, 13,* 206–215.

Caruso, A.J., Chodzko-Zajko, W.J., Bidinger, D.A., & Sommers, R.K. (1994). Adults who stutter: Responses to cognitive stress. *Journal of Speech and Hearing Research, 37,* 746–754.

Colton, R.H., & Brown, W.S. (1972). Some relationships between vocal effort and intra-oral air pressure. Paper presented at the 84th Meeting of the Acoustical Society of America, November.

Conture, E.G. (1990). Childhood stuttering: What is it and who does it? *ASHA Reports, 18,* 2–14.

Conture, E.G., & Guitar, B.E. (1993). Evaluating efficacy of treatment of stuttering: School-age children. *Journal of Fluency Disorders, 18,* 253–287.

Cooper, J.A. (1990). Research directions in stuttering: Consensus and conflict. *Asha Reports, 18,* 98–100.

Cordes, A.K. (1994a). Categorization theory and stuttering: A response to Hamre (1992a, 1992b, 1992c). *Journal of Fluency Disorders, 19,* 65–75.

Cordes, A.K. (1994b). The reliability of observational data: I. Theories and methods for speech-language pathology. *Journal of Speech and Hearing Research, 37,* 264–278.

Cordes, A.K., & Ingham, R.J. (1994a). The reliability of observational data: II. Issues in the identification and measurement of stuttering events. *Journal of Speech and Hearing Research, 37,* 279–294.

Cordes, A.K., & Ingham, R.J. (1994b). Time-interval measurement of stuttering: Effects of interval duration. *Journal of Speech and Hearing Research, 37,* 779–788.

Cordes, A.K., & Ingham, R.J. (1995a). Judgments of stuttered and nonstuttered intervals by recognized authorities in stuttering research. *Journal of Speech and Hearing Research, 38,* 33–41.

Costello, J.M. (1975). The establishment of fluency with time-out procedures: Three case studies. *Journal of Speech and Hearing Disorders, 40,* 216–231.

Costello, J.M. (1983). Current behavioral treatments for children. In D. Prins & R. Ingham (Eds.), *Treatment of stuttering in early childhood: Methods and issues* (p. 69–112). San Diego: College-Hill.

Costello, J.M., & Ingham, R.J. (1984). Assessment strategies for stuttering. In R.F. Curlee & W.H. Perkins (Eds.), *Nature and treatment of stuttering: New directions* (pp. 303–333). San Diego: College-Hill.

Craig, A. (1990). An investigation into the relationship between anxiety and stuttering. *Journal of Speech and Hearing Disorders, 55,* 290–294.

Craig, A., & Andrews, G. (1985). The prediction and prevention of relapse in stuttering. *Behavior Modification, 9,* 427–442

Curlee, R.F. (1993). Evaluating treatment efficacy for adults: Assessment of stuttering disability. *Journal of Fluency Disorders, 18,* 319–331.

Darley, F.L., & Spriestersbach, D.C. (1978). *Diagnostic Methods in Speech Pathology* (2nd Ed.). New York: Harper and Row.

Finn, P., & Ingham, R.J. (1989). The selection of "fluent" samples in research on stuttering: Conceptual and methodological issues. *Journal of Speech and Hearing Research, 32*, 401–418.

Finn, P., & Ingham, R.J. (1994). Stutterers' self-ratings of how natural speech sounds and feels. *Journal of Speech and Hearing Research, 37*, 326–340.

Flanagan, B., Goldiamond, I., & Azrin, N. (1958). Operant stuttering: The control of stuttering behavior through response-contingent consequences. *Journal of the Experimental Analysis of Behavior, 1*, 173–177.

Folkins, J.W. (1991). Stuttering from a speech motor control perspective. In H.F.M. Peters, W. Hulstijn, & C.W. Starkweather (Eds.), *Speech motor control and stuttering* (pp. 561–569). Amsterdam: Excerpta Medica.

Fowler, S.C., & Ingham, R.J. (1986). *Stuttering treatment rating recorder.* Santa Barbara: University of California, Santa Barbara.

Franken, M.C., Boves, L., Peters, H.F.M., & Webster, R.L. (1992). Perceptual evaluation of the speech before and after fluency shaping stuttering therapy. *Journal of Fluency Disorders, 17*, 223–241.

Franken, M.C, Boves, L., Peters, H.F.M., & Webster, R.L. (1995). Perceptual rating instrument for speech evaluation of stuttering treatment. *Journal of Speech and Hearing Research, 38*, 280–288.

Freeman, F.J. (1977). *The stuttering larynx: An electromyographic study of laryngeal muscle activity accompanying stuttering.* Doctoral dissertation. City University of New York.

Freeman, F., & Ushijima, T. (1978). Laryngeal muscle activity during stuttering. *Journal of Speech and Hearing Research, 21*, 358–362.

Goldiamond, I. (1962). The maintenance of ongoing fluent behavior and stuttering. *Journal of Mathetics, 1*, 57–95.

Goldiamond, I. (1965). Stuttering and fluency as manipulatable response classes. In L. Krasner & L.P. Ullman (Eds.), *Research in behavior modification* (pp. 106–156). New York: Holt, Rinehart, & Winston.

Gow, M.L., & Ingham, R.J. (1992). Modifying electroglottograph-identified intervals of phonation: The effect on stuttering. *Journal of Speech and Hearing Research, 35*, 495–511.

Ham, R. (1989). What are we measuring? *Journal of Fluency Disorders, 14*, 231–243.

Hanson, B.R. (1978). The effects of contingent light-flash on stuttering and attention to stuttering. *Journal of Communication Disorders, 11*, 451–458.

Hillis, J.W. (1993). Ongoing assessment in the management of stuttering: A clinical perspective. *American Journal of Speech-Language Pathology, 2*, 24–37.

Hillis, J.W. (1994). Perceptual management of "speech-flow obstructions": A treatment approach for stuttering. Microcomputer Instructional Laboratory, American Speech-Language-Hearing Association annual convention, New Orleans, Louisiana, November 18.

Ingham, R.J. (1982). The effects of self-evaluation training on maintenance and generalization during stuttering treatment. *Journal of Speech and Hearing Disorders, 47*, 271–280.

Ingham, R.J. (1984a). Generalization and maintenance of treatment. In R. Curlee & W.H. Perkins (Eds.), *Nature and treatment of stuttering: New directions* (pp. 447–471). San Diego: College-Hill Press.

Ingham, R.J. (1984b). *Stuttering and behavior therapy: Current status and experimental foundations.* San Diego: College-Hill Press.

Ingham, R.J. (1987). *Residential prolonged speech stuttering therapy manual for clients.* Santa Barbara: University of California, Santa Barbara.

Ingham, R.J. (1990a). Commentary on Perkins (1990) and Moore and Perkins (1990): On the valid role of reliability in identifying "What is stuttering?" *Journal of Speech and Hearing Disorders, 55*, 394–397.

Ingham, R.J. (1990b). Stuttering. In A.S. Bellack, M. Hersen, and A.E. Kazdin (Eds.), *International handbook of behavior modification and therapy* (pp. 599–631). New York: Plenum Press.

Ingham, R.J. (1990c). Theoretical, methodological, and ethical issues in treatment efficacy research: Stuttering as a case study. In L.B. Olswang, C.K. Thompson, S.F. Warren, & N. Minghetti (Eds.), *Treatment efficacy research in communication disorders* (pp. 15–29). Rockville, Md.: American Speech-Language-Hearing Foundation.

Ingham, R.J. (1993a). Current status of stuttering and behavior modification - II: Principal issues and practices in stuttering therapy. *Journal of Fluency Disorders, 18*, 57–79.

Ingham, R.J. (1993b). Stuttering treatment efficacy: Paradigm dependent or independent? *Journal of Fluency Disorders, 18*, 133–145.

Ingham, R.J., Adams, A., & Reynolds, G. (1978). The

effects on stuttering of self-recording the frequency of stuttering on the word "the". *Journal of Speech and Hearing Research, 21*, 459–460.

Ingham, R.J., & Cordes, A.K. (1992). Interclinic differences in stuttering event counts. *Journal of Fluency Disorders, 17,* 171–176.

Ingham, R.J., & Costello, J.M. (1984). Stuttering treatment outcome evaluation. In J.M. Costello (Ed.), *Speech disorders in children: Recent advances* (pp. 313–346). San Diego: College-Hill Press.

Ingham, R.J., Ingham, J.M., Onslow, M., & Finn, P. (1989). Stutterers' self ratings of speech naturalness: Assessing effects and reliability. *Journal of Speech and Hearing Research, 32*, 419–431.

Ingham, R.J., Martin, R.R., & Kuhl, P.K. (1974). Modification and control of rate of speaking by stutterers. *Journal of Speech and Hearing Research, 17*, 489–496.

Ingham, R.J., Montgomery, J., & Ulliana, L. (1983). The effect of manipulating phonation duration on stuttering. *Journal of Speech and Hearing Research, 26*, 579–587.

Ingham, R.J., & Onslow, M. (1985). Measurement and modification of speech naturalness during stuttering therapy. *Journal of Speech and Hearing Disorders, 50*, 261–281.

Jaffe, J., Anderson, S.W., & Rieber, R.W. (1973). Research and clinical approaches to disorders of speech rate. *Journal of Communication Disorders, 6*, 225–246.

James, J.E. (1981a). Behavioral self-control of stuttering using time-out from speaking. *Journal of Applied Behavior Analysis, 14*, 25–37.

James, J.E. (1981b). Self-monitoring of stuttering: Reactivity and accuracy. *Behaviour Research and Therapy, 19*, 291–296.

Johnson, W., & Knott, J.R. (1936). The moment of stuttering. *Journal of Genetic Psychology, 48*, 475–479.

Kazdin, A.E. (1980). Covert and overt rehearsal and elaboration during treatment in the development of assertive behaviour. *Behaviour Research and Therapy, 18*, 191–201.

Kelso, J.A.S., Tuller, B., & Harris, K.S. (1983). A "dynamic pattern" perspective on the control and coordination of movement. In P.F. MacNeilage (Ed.), *The production of speech* (pp. 137–173). New York: Springer-Verlag.

Kent, R.D. (1994). *Reference manual for communication sciences and disorders.* Austin, Tex.: Pro-Ed.

Kully, D., & Boberg, E. (1988). An investigation of interclinic agreement in the identification of fluent and stuttered syllables. *Journal of Fluency Disorders, 13*, 309–318.

La Croix, Z.E. (1973) Management of disfluent speech through self-recording procedures. *Journal of Speech and Hearing Disorders, 38*, 272–274.

Laver, J. (1980). Monitoring systems in the neurolinguistic control of speech production. In V.A. Fromkin (Ed.), *Errors in linguistic performance* (pp. 287–305). New York: Academic Press.

Lee, C. (1989). Theoretical weaknesses lead to practical problems: The example of self-efficacy theory. *Journal of Behaviour Therapy and Experimental Psychiatry, 20*, 115–123.

Lees, R.M. (1994). Of what value is a measure of the stutterer's fluency? *Folia Phoniatrica Logopedia, 46*, 223–231.

Lefcourt, H.M. (1976). *Locus of control current trends: Theory and research.* New York: John Wiley.

Levelt, W.J.M. (1989). *Speaking: From intention to articulation.* Cambridge, Mass.: MIT Press.

Lutz, K.C., & Mallard, A.R. (1986). Disfluencies and rate of speech in young adult nonstutterers. *Journal of Fluency Disorders, 11*, 307–316.

Mackey, L.S., Finn, P., & Ingham, R.J. (in review). Speech dialect and speech naturalness ratings: Effects and reliability in rating stutterers' and nonstutterers' speech. *Journal of Fluency Disorders.*

Martin, R.R., & Haroldson, S.K. (1969). The effects of two treatment procedures on stuttering. *Journal of Communication Disorders, 2*, 115–125.

Martin, R.R., & Haroldson, S.K. (1979). Effects of five experimental treatments on stuttering. *Journal of Speech and Hearing Research, 22*, 132–146.

Martin, R.R., & Haroldson, S.K. (1982). Contingent self-stimulation for stuttering. *Journal of Speech and Hearing Disorders, 47*, 407–413.

Martin, R.R., & Haroldson, S.K. (1992). Stuttering and speech naturalness: Audio and audiovisual judgments. *Journal of Speech and Hearing Research, 35*, 521–528.

Martin, R.R., Haroldson, S.K., & Triden, K.A. (1984). Stuttering and speech naturalness. *Journal of Speech and Hearing Disorders, 49*, 53–58.

McClean, M.D. (1990). Neuromotor aspects of stuttering: Levels of impairment and disability. *Asha Reports, 18*, 64–71.

McCloskey, D.I. (1981). Corollary discharges: Motor commands and perception. In V.B. Brookes (Ed.),

Handbook of physiology: A critical comprehensive presentation of physiological knowledge and concepts. Section I: The nervous system (pp. 1415–1448). Bethesda, Md.: American Physiological Society.

Miller, S., & Watson, B.C. (1992). The relationship between communication attitude, anxiety and depression in stutterers and nonstutterers. *Journal of Speech and Hearing Research, 35,* 789–798.

Moore, W.H., Jr. (1990). Pathophysiology of stuttering: Cerebral activation differences in stutterers vs nonstutterers. *Asha Reports, 18,* 72–80.

Nelson, R.O., & Hayes, S.C. (1981). Theoretical explanations for reactivity in self-monitoring. *Behavior Modification, 5,* 3–14.

Onslow, M. (1992). Identification of early stuttering: Issues and suggested strategies. *American Journal of Speech Language Pathology, 1,* 21–27.

Onslow, M., Adams, R., & Ingham, R.J. (1992). Reliability of speech naturalness ratings of stuttered speech during treatment. *Journal of Speech and Hearing Research, 35,* 994–1001.

Onslow, M., Andrews, C., & Lincoln, M. (1994). A control/experimental trial of an operant treatment for early stuttering. *Journal of Speech and Hearing Research, 37,* 1244–1259.

Ornstein, A.F., & Manning, W.H. (1985). Self-efficacy scaling by adult stutterers. *Journal of Communication Disorders, 18,* 313–320.

Packman, A., Onslow, M., & van Doorn, J. (1994). Prolonged speech and modification of stuttering: Perceptual, acoustic, and electroglottographic data. *Journal of Speech and Hearing Research, 37,* 724–737.

Perkins, W.H. (1971). *Speech pathology: An applied behavioral science.* St. Louis: C.V. Mosby.

Perkins, W.H. (1973). Replacement of stuttering with normal speech: II. Clinical procedures. *Journal of Speech and Hearing Disorders, 38,* 295–303.

Perkins, W.H. (1975). Articulation rate in the evaluation of stuttering treatments. *Journal of Speech and Hearing Disorders, 40,* 277–278.

Perkins, W.H. (1983). Onset of stuttering: The case of the missing block. In D. Prins & R.J. Ingham (Eds.), *Treatment of stuttering in early childhood: Methods and issues* (pp. 1–20). San Diego: College-Hill Press.

Perkins, W.H. (1990). What is stuttering? *Journal of Speech and Hearing Disorders, 55,* 370–382.

Perkins, W.H., Kent, R.D., & Curlee, R.F. (1991) A theory of neuropsycholinguistic function in stuttering. *Journal of Speech and Hearing Research, 34,* 734–752.

Peters, H.F.M. (1990). Clinical application of speech measurement techniques in the assessment of stuttering. In J. Cooper (Ed.), *Assessment of speech and voice production: Research and clinical applications* (pp. 172–182). NIDCD conference proceedings. Bethesda, Md.: U.S. Department of Health and Human Services.

Peters, H.F.M., & Hulstijn, W. (1984). Stuttering and anxiety: The difference between stutterers and nonstutterers in verbal apprehension and physiologic arousal during the anticipation of speech and non-speech tasks. *Journal of Fluency Disorders, 9,* 67–84.

Peters, H.F.M., Hulstijn, W., &. Starkweather, C.W. (Eds.) (1991). *Speech motor control and stuttering.* Amsterdam: Excerpta Medica.

Prins, D. (1991). Theories of stuttering as event and disorder: Implications for speech production processes. In H.F.M. Peters, W. Hulstijn, & C.W. Starkweather (Eds.), *Speech motor control and stuttering* (pp. 571–580). Amsterdam: Excerpta Medica.

Prins, D. (1993). Models for treatment efficacy studies of adult stutterers. *Journal of Fluency Disorders, 18,* 333–349.

Prins, D., & Hubbard, C.P. (1988). Response contingent stimuli and stuttering: Issues and implications. *Journal of Speech and Hearing Disorders, 31,* 696–709.

Prins, D., & Hubbard, C.P. (1990). Acoustical durations of speech segments during stuttering adaptation. *Journal of Speech and Hearing Research, 33,* 494–504.

Prosek, R.A., & Montgomery, A.A. (1969). Some physical correlates of vocal effort and loudness. Paper read to the Annual Convention of the American Speech and Hearing Association, Chicago, Illinois, November 15.

Prosek, R.A, & Runyan, G.M. (1982). Temporal characteristics related to the discrimination of stutterers' and nonstutterers' speech samples. *Journal of Speech and Hearing Research, 25,* 29–33.

Prosek, R.A, & Runyan, G.M. (1983). Effects of segment and pause manipulations on the identification of treated stutterers. *Journal of Speech and Hearing Research, 26,* 510–516.

Ryan, B.P. (1974). *Programmed therapy for stuttering*

in children and adults. Springfield, Ill.: Charles C. Thomas.

Schwartz, G.E. (1978). Psychobiological foundations of psychotherapy and behavior change. In S.L. Garfield & A.E. Bergin (Eds.), *Handbook of psychotherapy and behavior change: An empirical analysis* (pp. 63–99). New York: John Wiley.

Shapiro, A.I. (1980). An electromyographic analysis of the fluent and dysfluent utterances of several types of stutterers. *Journal of Fluency Disorders, 5,* 203–231.

Shattuck-Hufnagel, S. (1983). Sublexical units and suprasegmental structure in speech production planning. In P.F. MacNeilage (Ed.), *The production of speech* (pp. 109–139) New York: Springer-Verlag.

Siegel, G.M. (1990). Conference on treatment efficacy: Concluding remarks. In L.B. Olswang, C.K. Thompson, S.F. Warren, & N. Minghetti (Eds.), *Treatment efficacy research in communication disorders* (pp. 233–237). Rockville, Md.: American Speech-Language-Hearing Foundation.

Siegel, G.M. (1991). Response to Perkins: "What is stuttering?" *Journal of Speech and Hearing Research, 34,* 1081–1083.

Smith, A. (1990). Toward a comprehensive theory of stuttering: A commentary. *Journal of Speech and Hearing Disorders, 55,* 398–401.

Solomon, N.P., Robin, D.A., Lorell, D.M., Rodnitzky, R.L., & Luschei, E.S. (1994). Tongue fatigue testing in Parkinson disease: Indications of fatigue. In J. Till, K. Yorkston, & D. Beukelman (Eds.), *Dysarthria and apraxia of speech* (pp. 147–160). Baltimore, Md.: Paul H. Brookes Publishing Co.

Somodi, L.B., Robin, D.A., & Luschei, E.S. (in press). A model of "sense of effort" during maximal and submaximal contractions of the tongue. *Brain and Language.*

Starkweather, C.W. (1987). *Fluency and stuttering.* Englewood Cliffs, N.J.: Prentice Hall.

Starkweather, C.W. (1990). The assessment of fluency. In J. Cooper (Ed.), *Assessment of speech and voice production: Research and clinical applications* (pp. 30–41) NIDCD conference proceedings. Bethesda, Md.: U.S. Department of Health and Human Services.

Starkweather, C.W. (1993). Issues in the efficacy of treatment for fluency disorders. *Journal of Fluency Disorders, 18,* 151–168.

Starkweather, C.W., Gottwald, S.R., & Halfond, M.M. (1990). *Stuttering prevention: A clinical method.* Englewood Cliffs, N.J.: Prentice Hall.

Story, R.S. (1990). *Articulatory, laryngeal, and respiratory movements in stutterers' fluent speech before and after therapy.* Unpublished doctoral dissertation, University of Connecticut.

Tiffany, W.R. (1980). The effects of syllable structure on diadochokinetic and reading rates. *Journal of Speech and Hearing Research, 23,* 894–908.

Ulliana, L., & Ingham, R.J. (1984). Behavioral and non-behavioral variables in the measurement of stutterers' communication attitudes. *Journal of Speech and Hearing Disorders, 49,* 83–93.

van Lieshout, P., Peters, H.F.M., Starkweather, C.W., & Hulstijn, W. (1993). Physiological differences between stutterers and nonstutterers in perceptually fluent speech: EMG amplitude and duration. *Journal of Speech and Hearing Research, 36,* 55–63.

Van Riper, C. (1973). *Treatment of stuttering.* Englewood Cliffs, N.J.: Prentice-Hall.

Verdolini-Marston, K., Hoffman, H., & McCoy, S. (1992). Non-specific laryngeal granuloma: A literature review and case study involving a professional singer. *National Center for Voice and Speech Status and Progress Report, 3,* 157–174.

Walker, V.G. (1988). Durational characteristics of young adults during speaking and reading tasks. *Folia Phoniatrica, 40,* 12–20.

Watson, B.C., Freeman, F.J., Devous, M.D., Chapman, S.B., Finitzo, T., & Pool, K.D. (1994). Linguistic performance and regional cerebral blood flow in persons who stutter. *Journal of Speech and Hearing Research, 37,* 1221–1228.

Watterson, T., McFarlane, S.C., & Diamond, K.L. (1993). Phoneme effects on vocal effort and vocal quality. *American Journal of Speech-Language Pathology, 2 (2),* 74–78

Weber, C.M., & Smith, A. (1990). Autonomic correlates of stuttering and speech assessed in a range of experimental tasks. *Journal of Speech and Hearing Research, 33,* 690–706.

Williams, D.E. (1978). The problem of stuttering. In F.L. Darley, & D.C. Spriestersbach. *Diagnostic Methods in Speech Pathology* (2nd Ed.) (pp. 284–321). New York: Harper and Row.

Williams, S.L., Kinney, P.J., & Falbo, J. (1989). Generalization of therapeutic changes in agoraphobia: The role of perceived self-efficacy. *Journal of Consulting and Clinical Psychology, 57,* 436–442.

Wingate, M.E. (1964). A standard definition of stuttering. *Journal of Speech and Hearing Disorders, 29,* 484–489.

Wingate, M.E. (1976). *Stuttering: Theory and treatment.* New York: Irvington.

Wright, H.N., & Colton, R.H. (1972). Some parameters of autophonic level. Paper read to the Annual Convention of the American Speech and Hearing Association, San Francisco.

Yorkston, K.M., & Beukelman, D.R. (1980). An analysis of connected speech samples of aphasic and normal speakers. *Journal of Speech and Hearing Disorders, 45,* 27–36.

SUGGESTED READINGS

Baer, D.M. (1990). The critical issue in treatment efficacy is knowing why treatment was applied: A student's response to Roger Ingham. In L.B. Olswang, C.K. Thompson, S.F. Warren, & N. Minghetti (Eds.), *Treatment efficacy research in communication disorders* (pp. 31–39). Rockville, Md.: American Speech-Language-Hearing Foundation.

Cordes, A.K., & Ingham, R.J. (1994a). The reliability of observational data: II. Issues in the identification and measurement of stuttering events. *Journal of Speech and Hearing Research, 37,* 279–294.

Ingham, R.J. (1982). The effects of self-evaluation training on maintenance and generalization during stuttering treatment. *Journal of Speech and Hearing Disorders, 47,* 271–280.

Ingham, R.J. (1993c). Stuttering treatment efficacy: Paradigm dependent or independent? *Journal of Fluency Disorders, 18,* 133–145.

Ingham, R.J., & Costello, J.M. (1984). Stuttering treatment outcome evaluation. In J.M. Costello (Ed.), *Speech disorders in children: Recent advances* (pp. 313–346). San Diego: College-Hill Press.

Prins, D. (1993). Models for treatment efficacy studies of adult stutterers. *Journal of Fluency Disorders, 18,* 333–349.

AFTERWORD

If Wendell Johnson had been even partly right, and there did, in fact, exist a community in the world whose citizens had no knowledge of stuttering, and if we were to ask one of its citizen scientists to ponder what stuttering is like based on just the contents of this book or any similar compendium, the poor chap would have a terrible time, indeed. The scientist might conclude that whatever stuttering is, if it is anything at all, even expert listeners can't agree on when it has occurred, unless the expert is one of the stutterers, and then only during or just after stuttering, although an independent observer might have no clue whether stuttering was or was not occurring at that same moment. Upon reading this book, our bedazzled scientist might alternately conclude that stuttering was in the mind of the speaker, or in the attitude of the listener, or in the circuitry of an acoustic analysis device, or in the interplay of various vocal muscle systems, or in the speaker's phonological system, or perhaps in a particular locus of the brain, or the speech production apparatus it controls.

Our naive scientist might conclude that the authorities agree that stuttering is best treated during early childhood, but couldn't be certain whether that meant as soon as stuttering has been diagnosed or somewhat later, when it seems likely that the disorder will not remit spontaneously.

It would be apparent that systematic therapy is not likely to result in fluent and natural speech in adults who have been stuttering for a long time, although a conversion experience might, quite mysteriously, result in such natural fluency. This inquisitive scientist would learn that some experts advocate treatments designed to make stuttered speech seem less abnormal; others advocate methods to remove it entirely; while still others opt for a combination. But no one can be sure which is likely to have the best results with any particular stutterer in the absence of a body of well-designed research to justify the choice of any treatment method.

Such a scientist would probably come away with a sense that this is an area that is on the verge of enormous breakthroughs in terms of the availability of precise and powerful analytic tools, but that there is still no manual of instructions as to how these tools should be applied—there is no guiding theory, and not even agreement about what form such a theory should take.

On confronting the problem of stuttering in its multiple manifestations as revealed in this book, our scientist might beat a hasty retreat back to the mother country, back to simpler and more amenable problems, like cold fusion or how to achieve lasting world peace. Or, infected by the enthusiasm and the optimism that permeates these chapters, despite the lack of consensus about major issues in stuttering, our visiting scientist might find the challenge of exploring this most fundamental and elusive of human problems to be irresistible, with the promise that every new insight into the origins and the nature of stuttering constitutes an insight into the essence of human behavior so that, while progress may be slow and difficult, it must be pursued simply because we cannot resist probing our own fundamental nature.

Students reading this book, like our hypothetical alien scientist, may understandably be frustrated that the questions concerning stuttering loom so large and current answers are so fragmented and equivocal. And yet, the best among them will find the challenge of working with stuttering—and with persons who stutter—irresistible and the rewards inestimable. It is their energy and enthusiasm that we hoped to recruit as we explored the complexities of stuttering in this volume.

Gerald M. Siegel
University of Minnesota

439

INDEX